General Medicine
For UKMLA and Medical Exams

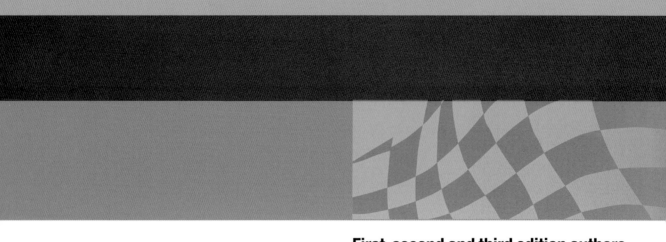

First, second and third edition authors

Rachael Hough

Iftikhar Ul Haq

Robert Parker

Asheesh Sharma

Fourth edition authors

Oliver A. Leach

Gils I. van Boxel

Fifth edition authors

Inez Eiben

Paola Eiben

Kathryn Watson

6th Edition
CRASH COURSE

SERIES EDITOR

Philip Xiu
MA (Cantab), MB BChir, MRCP, MRCGP, MScClinEd, FHEA, MAcadMEd, RCPathME
Honorary Senior Lecturer
Leeds University School of Medicine
PCN Educational Lead
Medical Examiner
Leeds Teaching Hospital Trust
Leeds, UK

FACULTY ADVISOR

Kathryn Watson
MBBS, BSc, MRCP, PGcert, FHEA
Consultant in Nephrology and General Medicine
Portsmouth Hospitals University NHS Trust
Portsmouth, UK

General Medicine
For UKMLA and Medical Exams

Paola Eiben
MBBS, BSc, FRCA
Anaesthetic Registrar
The Royal London Hospital
Barts Health NHS Trust
London, UK

Inez Eiben
MBBS, BSc, MRCS
Plastic Surgery Registrar
St George's University Hospital NHS Foundation Trust
London, UK

Pennylouise Hever
MBBS, BS (Hons), MRCS
Speciality Plastic Surgery Registrar
Royal Free Hospital
London, UK

Megan Giles
MBBS, MRCP (UK), PGCert (MedEd)
ST4 Medical Oncology
University Hospital Southampton
Southampton, UK

ELSEVIER

First edition 1999

Second edition 2005

Third edition 2008

Fourth edition 2013

Updated Fourth edition 2015

Fifth edition 2019

Sixth edition 2025

Notices

Practitioners and researchers must always rely on their own experience and knowledge in evaluating and using any information, methods, compounds or experiments described herein. Because of rapid advances in the medical sciences, in particular, independent verification of diagnoses and drug dosages should be made. To the fullest extent of the law, no responsibility is assumed by Elsevier, authors, editors or contributors for any injury and/or damage to persons or property as a matter of products liability, negligence or otherwise, or from any use or operation of any methods, products, instructions, or ideas contained in the material herein.

ISBN: 978-0-443-11538-7

Content Strategist: Trinity Hutton
Content Project Manager: Taranpreet Kaur
Design: Miles Hitchen
Marketing Manager: Deborah Watkins

Printed in India

Last digit is the print number: 9 8 7 6 5 4 3 2 1

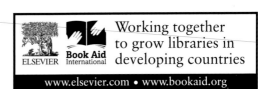

Series editor's foreword

With great honour and pride, we present the latest edition of the *Crash Course* series. This series has traversed a journey of nearly a quarter-century, stemming from the vision of Dr. Dan Horton-Szar, and his legacy continues to walk with us on this pathway of knowledge.

The series has been popular with students worldwide, selling over **1 million copies** and being translated into more than **8 languages**, reinforcing our commitment to global learning.

We remain extremely grateful for your unwavering trust. The series has once again been refreshed and fully upgraded in accordance with the rapidly changing medical guidelines, ensuring the content is comprehensive, accurate and fully up-to-date.

This latest series continues our tradition of integrating clinical practice with basic medical sciences, tailored meticulously for today's medical undergraduate curriculum. A central highlight of this instalment is our emphasis on high-yield exam content designed specifically for the UKMLA curriculum.

The addition of the **Rapid UKMLA Index** at the beginning of the book enhances this offering, serving as a valuable aid to students to track their exam preparation efficiently. We have also revised all self-assessment questions to align with the single best answer format in line with the latest UKMLA examination style. We have also added ***High-Yield Association Tables***. These are essential tools designed to aid students in recognizing clinical patterns and acing vignette-style exam questions. By condensing complex medical scenarios into digestible, manageable insights, these tables ensure efficient learning. They connect symptoms, diagnosis and treatment, bolstering understanding and confidence in tackling the rigorous UKMLA exams. This comprehensive approach makes these tables an indispensable asset in your exam preparations.

Utilizing student feedback, we have strived to maintain the core principles of this series: delivering precise and readable text that brings together depth and clarity. The authors are experienced junior doctors who successfully navigated these exams recently, ensuring practical and tested guidance. A team of expert faculty advisors from across the United Kingdom ensures the content's accuracy, making it resilient and reliable.

As we turn a new chapter with the latest edition, we honour the past, cherish the present, and embrace the promise of the future. We wish you every success in your journey of learning and growth and hope that this series adds value to your life, both as students and as future medical professionals.

Philip Xiu

Prefaces

Authors

We present this textbook as a trusted companion as you embark on your journey as aspiring healthcare professionals. Though as doctors, we are facing the increasing challenge of treating ever complex patients in an overstretched and under-resourced healthcare system, the heart of medical practice; good patient care, remains the same.

Our primary goal in crafting this comprehensive revision aid, is to equip you with the knowledge and skills necessary to excel in your medical education and future practice. Within these pages you will find a wealth of information, including the most up-to-date clinical guidance, as well as red flags, hints and tips, common pitfalls, and key ethical considerations carefully curated through years of experience. Additionally, self-assessment questions, carefully written for each chapter, will help you test your knowledge and better prepare you for medical exams and UKMLA.

Paola Eiben, Inez Eiben, Pennylouise Hever and Megan Giles

Faculty advisor

This latest edition of *Crash Course General Medicine* strikes the balance of being concise, colorful and easy to read whilst comprehensively covering core knowledge and up-to-date evidence and guidance. The images, online resources and detailed self-assessment questions make it a very useful resource for medical students and a platform to start preparing for postgraduate examinations.

I hope this book helps to inspire future generations prepare for a lifetime of clinical practice and learning.

Kathryn Watson

Acknowledgements

To Hannah - our fighter, who despite all the challenges she has had to face continues to amaze us every single day with her positivity, perseverance, grace and strength. You are our superhero!

A huge thank you to our faculty adviser, Katy, series editor, Phil, and everyone on the publishing team for the continuous support and guidance they have given to the authors of this edition. We are extremely grateful and could not have done it without them!

Paola Eiben, Inez Eiben, Pennylouise Hever and Megan Giles

I would like to thank the *Crash Course* editor team for involving me in this exciting project and to the Authors who have kept to deadlines whilst working full-time in clinical practice producing high-quality work, making my task as faculty advisor a stimulating and enjoyable one.

Finally, I would like to thank my husband and children Josie and Xander who have been very patient whilst Mummy escapes to do her "homework".

Kathryn Watson

Series editor's acknowledgement

We would like to express our sincere gratitude to those who have provided their support and expertise in preparing this sixth edition of the *Crash Course* series. Our junior doctor contributors' participation in crafting the manuscript has been indispensable. Their first-hand experience and current medical knowledge have infused realism and practicality into our content.

Our faculty editors deserve a special note of thanks. They have extensively validated the correctness of the information, ensuring that the content is not just accurate but also contemporaneous, credible, and aligns with the latest medical standards.

We extend our heartfelt thanks to our publisher, Elsevier. Their staff have demonstrated an unwavering commitment to quality, maintaining the high standards set since the first edition. Their insights have routinely enriched the content and process alike.

Our Commissioning Editor, Jeremy Bowes, deserves a special mention for his consistent support and guiding hand throughout the development process. His directions and advice have bettered this edition and spurred us on our quest for excellence.

We are greatly indebted to Alex Mortimer for her wisdom, practical insights and valuable guidance. A big thank you to our Content Strategists, Trinity Hutton and Cloe Holland-Borosh, who need special acknowledgement for meticulously outlining the direction and scope of the content. They've managed to mix details with a strategic plan, keeping our readers in mind.

Lastly, much gratitude is owed to our Content Product Managers, Taranpreet Kaur, Ayan Dhar, Shivani Pal and Tapajyoti Chaudhuri, who have juggled the numerous day-to-day tasks with utmost dedication and perseverance. Despite the ever-approaching deadlines, they have shown remarkable patience and steadfast determination, ensuring that each step of the book's development was accomplished seamlessly.

In conclusion, we sincerely thank each of these wonderful people for their outstanding contributions and support, without which this work wouldn't have been achieved. Their passion, commitment and collaborative effort have helped us bring this edition together.

Philip Xiu

Rapid UKMLA Index

The UKMLA Curriculum Conditions Priority levels have been based on the below:

Level 1: Conditions that a newly qualified doctor should have a good knowledge of and be able to recognise and manage.
Level 2: Conditions requiring knowledge for recognising and confirming diagnosis and planning first-line management in straightforward cases.
Level 3: Conditions where recognition of clinical presentation and describing principles of management are important.

UKMLA Conditions and Where to Find Them

continued

UKMLA Conditions and Where to Find Them—cont'd

continued

continued

Contents

Contents

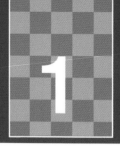

GENERAL PRINCIPLES

Overview

Medical students are often told that '90% of the diagnosis is in the history'. Although this statement has a large amount of truth, this is only the case if your history-taking skills are focused, accurate and relevant. This, in turn, is mainly dependent on your bedside manner and your ability to build up a good rapport with your patient.

There is no easy recipe for developing a suitable bedside manner, but courtesy, patience and letting patients express their ideas, concerns and expectations are essential ingredients. Whenever you meet a patient, introduce yourself politely and do not forget relatives or friends who may also be present. Try to put the patient at ease, as visiting the doctor is very stressful for most people, particularly if they think they have a serious illness. If you cannot speak the same language, get an interpreter. Language Line, a telephone-based translation service, is a useful resource; avoid using family members as interpreters. If a patient has communication difficulties, ask patients themselves or their carers what the best and easiest way to communicate with them is.

The aims of history-taking are:

- to establish rapport with the patient;
- to obtain an accurate, sequential account of the patient's symptoms through open questions and make a differential diagnosis;
- to ask specific questions to focus on the most likely diagnoses;
- to determine risk factors for these possible diagnoses;
- to put this problem or problems into the context of the patient's life.

This chapter provides a framework for taking a comprehensive history. However, the important thing is that you develop an approach with which you are comfortable and then practise it. In this way, you will not miss something, and you will be able to concentrate more on what the patient is telling you rather than what comes next. With experience, you will recognize patterns and explore different avenues in the history.

Make sure not to miss nonverbal clues, as facial expression and body posture can sometimes tell you more than the words themselves. If you are looking up, patients will also feel that you are genuinely listening to what they are saying. It is important to strike a good balance between recording the history accurately and maintaining eye contact. However, when you are learning, it may be easier to make notes as you go along; you can also have prompts on your paper to enable you to fill in all sub-sections of this history detailed below. As you gain experience, you will find it easier to memorize the patient's history and write it down later.

As a general principle, start the consultation by asking very open-ended questions, such as 'How are you?' or 'What has brought you to the clinic today?' This gives patients the opportunity to say what they want. Then ask more specific questions to clarify important aspects.

THE HISTORY

At the start of every history you should always:

- Document the date, time and place of the consultation. This should be done on both sides and each subsequent sheet of paper (remember that the clinical record is a legal document).
- Document your name, grade and role.
- Document who referred the patient and if the patient was seen as an emergency.

CLINICAL NOTES

With the move to electronic notes, some of these steps will be done for you. Only use your own computer log-in details, and if you move away from your computer lock the screen so no patient information is on display.

A comprehensive medical history is detailed later. The separate headings help ensure a good flow and that information is not missed. Depending on the situation, the importance of each part of the history will differ; for instance, family history is crucial with genetic conditions, and a detailed social history is particularly relevant in the elderly. The history needs to be adapted to the situation; it is obviously unsafe and inappropriate to take a detailed history from an acutely unwell patient in the resuscitation unit of the emergency department.

Presenting complaint (PC)

This is a sentence or short list explaining why the patient has seen you today. Resist the temptation to write the entire history in this section, particularly when there are multiple symptoms; however, mentioning an obvious background condition can be helpful (e.g., 'One-week increasing shortness of breath and productive cough. Background: 10-year history of COPD').

History of the presenting complaint (HPC)

This is where the presenting complaint is explored in detail. It is impossible to describe a system that will work for all complaints in every situation. You will need to develop your own techniques, likes and dislikes. Inadequate relevant detail in this section is the most typical problem in medical student histories:

- Aim to obtain a coherent, sequential chronological description of the events leading to the consultation.
- Ask the questions relevant to the symptoms (e.g., for pain, 'Where is it?', 'What is its character?').
- Keep the differential diagnoses for a symptom in your mind and seek evidence to confirm or refute them.
- Use the review of symptoms questions for the system you suspect to fill in extra detail (e.g., if the complaint is a cough, ask about dyspnoea, pain, sputum, etc.).
- Ask about the relevant risk factors (e.g., if pulmonary embolus is suspected, ask about immobility, travel, etc.).
- Recapitulate the history to the patient, as this helps cement the story in your mind and reassures the patient that you are listening.
- If the history is long or vague, the opening question, 'So when did you last feel well?' gives a platform to begin from.
- Seek collateral history from witnesses, friends or family where necessary (e.g., after a seizure). It is always worth asking patients whether they mind you speaking to family or friends first.
- With chronic complaints, ask about how the symptoms affect the patient's life.
- Document relevant negative findings (e.g., headache but no photophobia or neck stiffness).

Finally, ask if the patient has any thoughts or worries about the diagnosis; this can be very enlightening and will help you build a good working relationship as you will be addressing the patient's concerns. What the doctor is interested in and what the patient is interested in can be diametrically different.

HINTS AND TIPS

If the patient presents with pain, the **SOCRATES** principle is a useful framework for remembering to ask all the relevant questions: **S**ite, **O**nset, **C**haracter, **R**adiation, **A**ssociated features, **T**iming, **E**xacerbating/relieving factors and **S**everity.

Past medical history (PMH)

Ask the patient if they suffer from any medical problems or have had any operations. You may have to probe a little about each illness and how the diagnosis was made. Previous histories are sometimes incorrect and can be carried forward from one hospital visit to the next. Record the history in chronological order and, where possible, record the year, hospital and consultant involved for each episode (this is particularly important for rare or long-term diseases). Many patients may forget past illnesses, mainly if they are anxious, and it is worth developing a routine to ask them specifically about the most common conditions.

HINTS AND TIPS

MJTHREADS is a helpful mnemonic for remembering to ask about specific medical conditions: **M**yocardial infarction, **J**aundice, **T**uberculosis, **H**ypertension, **R**heumatic fever, **E**pilepsy, **A**sthma, **D**iabetes and **S**troke.

Medications and allergies (DHX)

Record which medications the patient is currently taking, how often and at what dose. If the prescribed medications are not being taken, ask why. Ask if there have been any recent changes in medication. Always ask what drugs the patient has taken in the past. For example, a patient with pulmonary fibrosis caused by amiodarone may have stopped taking it years before! Ask about any nonprescription medications or herbal remedies the patient may take. Ask about illicit drug use and whether the patient smokes or injects the substance.

Does the patient have any allergies to medications or anything else, no matter how trivial? If yes, what was the exact nature of the reaction? Was it anaphylaxis, or did the patient experience a rash? It is worth asking about penicillin directly as many patients state they have a penicillin allergy. Still, on being questioned more closely, they may describe a nonspecific symptom, and a β-lactam antibiotic can be given safely if the need is there.

If the patient says they have no allergies, it is traditional to write 'No known drug allergies' (NKDA).

> **HINTS AND TIPS**
>
> Some of the prescription abbreviations useful for documentation purposes are:
>
> OD (QD) – once a day
> BD (BID) – twice a day
> TDS (TID) – three times a day
> QDS (QID) – four times a day
> PRN – as needed
> OM – in the morning
> ON (nocte) – at night
> AC – before food
> PC – after food
> PO – oral
> PR – rectal
> SL – sublingual
> IM – intramuscular
> IV – intravenously
> NG – nasogastric
> SC – subcutaneous
> STAT – immediately

Family history (FHX)

Do any diseases run in the patient's family – heart disease, cancer, diabetes and autoimmune disorders? Record illnesses in close relatives, including age of death, where relevant. Generally speaking, family members affected before the age of 60 years are deemed to be appropriate. Drawing a family tree can be helpful for some patients.

Social history (SHX)

This helps to establish how the illness affects the patient's life and whether the patient is coping at home. It also allows determination of the patient's baseline functional status. This is helpful when considering both Treatment Escalation Plan (TEP) and discharge planning.

Ask:

- Who is at home? Are they fit and well?
- What is home like? Are there stairs? Can you manage these? How often do you leave the house? If the patient is in a home, clarify if this is a warden-controlled flat (supported living), a residential home or a nursing home, as these offer different levels of support.
- Do you need help with daily tasks, such as washing, dressing, feeding, cleaning or shopping? Do you have carers or a nearby relative who helps? How often do they come, and what do they help with?
- Have you been more forgetful? Have any of your family or friends commented that you have forgotten things?
- Do you manage your finances? If not, who looks after that for you?
- Do you have dependent children? Who is looking after them now?
- Do you have other responsibilities, such as caring for an infirm parent or pets?
- What is your occupation? Details of the patient's past and present occupation can be important (e.g., industrial lung disease).
- Are you still able to work despite the current problem? Some diagnoses can be critical in relation to work, such as heavy goods vehicle drivers and epilepsy.
- Do you, or did you, smoke? Smoking is a significant cause of many diseases. Record smoking in pack-years.
- How much alcohol do you drink (past and present)? Record the number of units per week (Fig. 1.1).
- Have you recently been abroad, and if so, where? Was this urban or rural? Were you vaccinated?
- Do you have pets (particularly budgerigars, pigeons and parrots)?

Sexual history is not appropriate in every history but may be important (e.g., for hepatitis or human immunodeficiency virus infection).

Systems review (SR)

Patients occasionally focus on one minor symptom while omitting to tell you of another more significant symptom. This can be a deliberate act, asking the doctor to deal with a simple problem (e.g., sore throat) while deciding whether to ask for help with the real worry, such as impotence or rectal bleeding. Performing a quick systems review will ensure you get all the important diseases.

Some of these you will have covered in the history of the presenting complaint, and you do not need to ask about them again.

General symptoms

Fatigue

This is a nonspecific symptom that can accompany many organic and psychiatric diseases. Look particularly for evidence of anaemia or hypothyroidism.

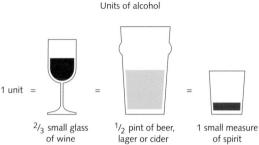

Units of alcohol

1 unit = = =

| $^2/_3$ small glass of wine | $^1/_2$ pint of beer, lager or cider | 1 small measure of spirit |

Fig. 1.1 Units of alcohol. These refer to standard pub measure of wine (12% alcohol by volume), a small pub measure of spirits (40% alcohol by volume) and standard strength beer (3%–4% alcohol by volume). Unit of alcohol is the quantity of pure alcohol in a drink. 1 unit equals 10 mL or 8 g of pure alcohol. An easy way to work out the units for a drink is to remember that the alcohol percentage is equivalent to the number of units in 1 L of the drink (e.g., 1 L of 40% whisky contains 40 units, and a 330-mL bottle of 6% lager contains 2 units).

Table 1.1	Causes of pruritus
Cause	**Examples**
Skin disease	Scabies, eczema, lichen planus, urticaria, dry skin (elderly, hypothyroidism)
Systemic disease	Hepatic (biliary obstruction, pregnancy) Malignancy (particularly lymphoma) Haematological (polycythaemia, iron deficiency) Chronic renal failure Drugs (sensitivity, opiates) Endocrine (diabetes mellitus, hyperthyroidism/hypothyroidism, carcinoid syndrome) Parasitic (trichinosis) Neurological (multiple sclerosis) Psychogenic

Appetite

Anorexia is a feature of many diseases, again organic and psychiatric; increased appetite despite weight loss is seen in hyperthyroidism. Distinguish between reduced appetite, nausea and dysphagia. Unintentional weight loss is seen in malignancy.

Weight change

Weight loss can be deliberate (dieting) or due to chronic disease. The causes are discussed in detail in Chapter 13.

Weight gain is seen in pregnancy, hypothyroidism, Cushing syndrome, polycystic ovary syndrome and 'comfort eating' due to anxiety or depression.

Sweats

Drenching sweats occurring at night are seen in lymphoma, chronic leukaemia and tuberculosis. These are commonly referred to as *B symptoms* (including weight loss and fever).

Pruritus (itching)

Pruritus can be due to local skin disease or systemic disease, as shown in Table 1.1.

Sleep pattern

If there is difficulty sleeping, ask if the problem is in going to sleep or waking early. Difficulty in getting off to sleep is often due to worry or anxiety, whereas early morning wakening is a feature of depression. Sleep apnoea is common, and can be debilitating as excessive sleepiness limits daytime function. The commonest medical condition affecting sleep is obstructive sleep apnoea (see Chapter 29). Ask about snoring, whether sleep is refreshing, morning headaches and restless leg movements. The patient's partner is often the best source of information.

Cardiovascular symptoms

Chest pain

Establish the site, radiation, character, exacerbating and relieving factors and severity; this is discussed in detail in Chapter 4.

Shortness of breath (dyspnoea) and exercise tolerance

Exertional dyspnoea can be due to anaemia, poor left ventricular function, pulmonary oedema, arrhythmia or valvular disease (see Chapter 28).

Orthopnoea is breathlessness on lying flat, usually from increased pulmonary venous congestion. This symptom can be present in heart failure, diaphragmatic weakness and chronic obstructive pulmonary disease, as feedback diaphragmatic input to ventilation is less efficient when lying flat. Ask the patient how many pillows they need to sleep on at night and if they feel breathless without them.

Paroxysmal nocturnal dyspnoea is waking during the night because of severe breathlessness (pulmonary oedema).

Sudden onset of breathlessness, irrespective of body position or exercise, is often due to arrhythmia, pneumothorax or pulmonary embolism (see Chapter 5).

Taking a relevant exercise tolerance history is important. Ask the patient whether they can walk up two flights of stairs (without stopping or being out of breath once upstairs) and how far they can walk on flat. Remember that joint problems rather than cardiorespiratory reserve may be the limiting factor.

Loss of consciousness (syncope)

Syncope is the transient loss of consciousness and motor tone, which may be due to arrhythmia, valvular heart disease, postural hypotension or vertebrobasilar insufficiency (see Chapter 18).

Palpitations

Palpitations mean different things to different people, and they should be explored carefully as they may both be insignificant or life threatening. Most commonly they refer to awareness of one's heart beating (see Chapter 7).

Ankle and calf swelling

This can be due to right ventricular failure, low plasma oncotic pressure (e.g., decreased albumin levels), drugs (e.g., calcium channel blockers) or venous or lymphatic drainage obstruction (e.g., pelvic malignancy), or it can be gravitational.

Calf swelling (especially unilateral) can be due to:
- deep vein thrombosis: consider underlying risk factors such as – recent travel, immobility or surgery, pregnancy, combined oral contraceptive pill use, family history, malignancy;
- ruptured Baker cyst: more common in the elderly and can be secondary to osteoarthritis of the knee;
- muscle trauma;
- cellulitis.

Calf, thigh or buttock pain on exertion (claudication)

Intermittent claudication due to peripheral vascular disease causes calf, thigh or buttock pain on exercise. The amount of exercise required to cause pain tends to be consistent, although it often deteriorates slowly. Pain is relieved within a predictable period of rest.

Spinal claudication due to spinal stenosis also causes calf, thigh or buttock pain on exertion, possibly by causing occlusion of the spinal arteries. However, the claudication distance tends to be variable.

Respiratory symptoms

Dyspnoea

Clarify the degree of dyspnoea and its consequences for everyday tasks; try to separate respiratory dyspnoea from cardiac causes, although there is much overlap (see Chapter 5).

Cough

The causes of cough are multiple. Associated features help develop a sensible differential diagnosis (see Chapter 6).

Sputum

How much sputum is produced? Ask about its colour, texture and time course:
- Yellow/green: usually infection, acute asthma (due to eosinophils).

- Frothy, pink: pulmonary oedema.
- Rusty: lobar pneumonia (pneumococcal).
- Blood: pulmonary embolism, lung cancer, pneumonia (see Chapter 6).
- Taste: foul in bronchiectasis and abscess.
- Smell: foul in bronchiectasis.

Chest pain

This needs a careful assessment of character, position, timing, precipitating factors, etc. Chest pain is usually pleuritic in respiratory disease (see Chapter 4), potentially due to pneumonia, pneumothorax or pulmonary embolus. It can also be of muscular origin when it is worse on inspiration and more localized.

Wheeze

Patients with airway obstruction sometimes notice an audible expiratory wheeze. Stridor is a high-pitched sound.

Hoarse voice

This has multiple origins, but some of the differentials include laryngitis or vocal cord paralysis, as seen in recurrent laryngeal nerve palsy in bronchial carcinoma.

Gastrointestinal disease

Abdominal pain

Establish the site, radiation, character, exacerbating and relieving factors and severity. This is discussed in detail in Chapter 9.

Dysphagia

Dysphagia means difficulty in swallowing. Ask about:
- The onset and progression of symptoms.
- Where things get stuck. This may give a clue as to the site of the lesion.
- If there is difficulty with solids, fluids or both. Neuromuscular disorders present with dysphagia for fluids at onset, whereas mechanical obstruction results in dysphagia for solids at onset.

The causes of dysphagia are outlined in Table 1.2.

Nausea and vomiting

What does the vomitus look like?
- Yellow-green: upper gastrointestinal (GI) tract contents plus bile.
- Brown (feculent): lower small bowel contents.
- Bright-red blood: active upper GI tract bleeding (see Chapter 11).
- 'Coffee grounds': 'old' upper GI tract bleeding.

Table 1.2 Causes of dysphagia

Disorder	Examples
Oropharyngeal lesions	Pharyngitis, quinsy, lymphoma
Intrinsic oesophageal and gastric lesions	Peptic stricture Carcinoma of oesophagus or gastric fundus Foreign body Oesophageal web (Paterson–Brown–Kelly syndrome or Plummer–Vinson syndrome) Infection (*Candida albicans*) Pharyngeal pouch Schatzki ring (lower oesophageal narrowing) Leiomyoma of oesophageal muscle
Extrinsic oesophageal compression	Goitre with retrosternal extension Intrathoracic tumours (lymphoma, bronchial carcinoma) Enlarged left atrium
Neuromuscular disorders	Achalasia Scleroderma Diffuse oesophageal spasm Diabetes mellitus Myasthenia gravis Myotonia dystrophica Bulbar or pseudobulbar palsy, e.g., motor neurone disease or stroke Diphtheria
Psychological	Globus pharyngeus

How 'violent' was the vomiting? Projectile vomiting indicates pyloric stenosis, most commonly seen in infants, but may arise because of duodenal ulceration in adults.

Indigestion

Heartburn or dyspepsia is due to the reflux of gastric contents into the oesophagus. Be aware that heartburn can easily be confused with cardiac chest pain.

Change in bowel habits or stools

Has there been a change? Ask about diarrhoea and constipation or the presence of one alternating with the other (see Chapter 12).

Is there any rectal bleeding? Is the bleeding with or without mucus? The causes of rectal bleeding are summarized in Box 1.1. Anal and rectal lesions result in fresh blood on the outside of the stool, on the paper on wiping or in the pan. Higher lesions result in blood intermixed with the stool. Melaena implies upper GI tract bleeding and the passage of altered blood originating proximal to the hepatic flexure.

Inquire about tenesmus. Tenesmus is the painful desire to defecate when there is no stool in the rectum. This is due to a lesion in the lumen or wall of the rectum mimicking faeces.

BOX 1.1 CAUSES OF RECTAL BLEEDING

Haemorrhoids
Anal fissure
Carcinoma (anus, rectum or colon)
Polyps
Diverticulitis (including Meckel diverticulum) but not diverticulosis
Colitis (infective, ulcerative, Crohn disease, ischaemic)
Angiodysplasia

Jaundice and itch

Jaundice can be insidious or acute, and the patient may therefore not have noticed it. Itching is caused by a build-up of bile salts in the skin and is a feature of obstructive jaundice (see Chapter 14). It may be evident on clinical examination through scratch marks. Jaundice may indicate liver function impairment.

Abdominal swelling

Ask whether the patient has noticed a change in the size of the abdomen. Remember the seven *F*'s: *f*oetus, *f*latus, *f*at, *f*luid, *f*lipping great mass, *f*aeces and a *f*ull bladder.

Genitourinary symptoms

Dysuria

This is discomfort during or after micturition due to urinary tract infection or recent urethral instrumentation (e.g., catheter or cystoscope).

Change in urine appearance

What does the urine look like?
- Cloudy: infection, precipitated urates or phosphates.
- Frothy: proteinuria.
- Orange: very concentrated urine, bilirubin, rifampicin.
- Red/smoky: haematuria, haemoglobinuria, myoglobinuria, rifampicin, blackwater fever due to haemolysis in *Plasmodium falciparum* malaria, eating beetroot.
- Dark on standing or exposure to light: porphyria.
- Green: drugs such as metoclopramide, amitriptyline or propofol.

See Chapter 15 for the causes of haematuria and proteinuria.

Frequency and nocturia

Increased frequency of micturition can be due to the following:
- Bladder irritation: infection, stones, tumour.

- Outflow obstruction: prostatic hypertrophy, urethral stricture.
- Neurological causes: multiple sclerosis, cauda equina syndrome.

In polyuria, there is an increased volume of urine and increased frequency of micturition.

Nocturia can be due to any of the causes of polyuria (see Chapter 15).

Hesitancy
Hesitancy followed by a poor stream with terminal dribbling is a feature of prostatic enlargement. These symptoms are often associated with benign prostatic hypertrophy but could indicate prostate carcinoma.

Loin pain
This can be associated with renal calculus or pyelonephritis (see Chapter 15).

Incontinence
This can be either urge incontinence (e.g., detrusor instability) or stress incontinence (e.g., weak pelvic musculature following childbirth). It can be functional, as people with mobility problems may not be able to get to the toilet quickly enough.

Menstruation
Determine the pattern of the normal cycle. Then ask about flow (heavy or light), intermenstrual bleeding, postcoital bleeding and dysmenorrhoea.

Discharge
Vaginal or penile discharge can indicate infection.

Neurological symptoms

Headache
This is a difficult symptom for the doctor, with the diagnosis ranging from trivial to the fatal. Ask about red flag symptoms (see Chapter 16).

Dizziness and vertigo
Ask about any perceived movement of the room. Establish when it occurs, in bed (classically benign positional vertigo) or with a change in posture (e.g., from sitting to standing as in orthostatic hypotension). Is there any associated tinnitus or recent coryzal symptoms suggesting a vestibular cause? Be aware that the patient may refer to unsteadiness as a sensation of feeling dizzy; consider peripheral neuropathy and visual/hearing impairment (see Chapter 22).

Loss of consciousness
When did it occur (at rest, on sitting to standing or on exertion)? Any warning symptoms, any seizure activity, any postictal period (see Chapter 18).

Visual disturbance
Vision can be affected by lesions of the optic pathway, including the eye itself, and lesions of the nerves controlling eye movements (III, IV and VI cranial nerves).

Altered hearing
Ask about deafness, tinnitus and vertigo (see Chapter 22).

Altered smell
Anosmia can result from head injury, nasal polyps, following viral upper respiratory tract infections (e.g., COVID-19) or frontal lobe tumours and can be a feature of Parkinson disease.

Speech disturbance
There are three types of disordered speech:
- Dysarthria: difficulty in articulating speech, but language content is normal.
- Dysphonia: difficulty in voice production.
- Dysphasia: difficulty understanding or expressing language caused by lesions affecting the dominant cerebral hemisphere (usually the left).

Table 1.3 shows the characteristic speech abnormalities that result from lesions at specific anatomical sites.

Limb weakness, paraesthesiae and sensory loss
This may result from a stroke leading to weakness or sensory loss symptoms. Paraesthesiae or pins and needles can be seen in nerve injury, migrainous conditions or seizures (see Chapter 34).

Metabolic and endocrine symptoms
Symptoms associated with metabolic and endocrine problems are varied and multiple and are described in detail in Chapter 33. The two commonest endocrine conditions to consider and ask about are thyroid disorders (Table 1.4) and diabetes (Table 1.5).

Musculoskeletal symptoms

Pain
Pain can arise in the muscles, joints (see Chapter 23) or bones (see Table 1.6).

Weakness
This can be either secondary to a neurological condition or from nutritional deficiency, medications (e.g., long-term steroid

Table 1.3 Causes and features of abnormalities of speech arising from lesions at specific anatomical sites

Site of lesion	Causes	Features of speech
Dysarthria		
Mouth	Ulcers, macroglossia	Slurred
Lower cranial nerve lesions (IXth to XIIth)	Bulbar palsy (stroke, poliomyelitis, motor neurone disease, syringobulbia, malignancy)	Nasal quality, slurred Associated features such as dysphagia
Upper cranial nerve lesions (IXth to XIIth)	Pseudobulbar palsy (stroke, motor neurone disease, multiple sclerosis)	Spastic speech, like 'Donald Duck' Associated features such as dysphagia and emotional lability
Cerebellum	Multiple sclerosis, stroke, tumour, hereditary ataxias, alcohol, hypothyroidism	Scanning (staccato) speech Flow is broken Syllables explosive
Extrapyramidal	Parkinsonism	Difficulty initiating speech Monotonous and slightly slurred
Toxic	Acute alcohol intoxication	Slurred
Dysphonia		
Neuromuscular junction	Myasthenia gravis	Weak, nasal speech Deteriorates on repetition
Vocal cord disease	Tumour, viral laryngitis, tuberculosis, syphilis	Weak volume, husky quality
Vocal cord paralysis	Recurrent laryngeal nerve palsy (mediastinal carcinoma, intrathoracic surgery or trauma, aortic aneurysm)	Weak volume, husky quality
Dysphasia		
Broca area (inferior frontal gyrus)	Infarction, bleeding, space-occupying lesion	Expressive dysphasia Comprehension intact Difficulty in finding appropriate words and so speech nonfluent
Wernicke area (superior temporal gyrus)	Infarction, bleeding, space-occupying lesion	Receptive dysphasia Fluent speech but words are disorganized or unintelligible Comprehension impaired
Frontotemporoparietal lesion Posterior part of superior temporal/inferior parietal lobe	Infarction (left middle cerebral artery), bleeding, space-occupying lesion and raised intracranial pressure, dementia	Global dysphasia Marked receptive and expressive dysphasia Nominal aphasia Unable to name specific objects Other aspects of speech preserved

use) or underlying arthritis or myositis leading to muscle wasting and atrophy; this is covered in detail in Chapter 35.

Stiffness
Stiffness, particularly after inactivity (e.g., early morning stiffness), is a feature of inflammation.

Joint swelling
This can be caused by infection, inflammation, blood (haemarthrosis) or crystal deposition.

Disability
How do the symptoms affect lifestyle? Consider if the disability is affecting the patient's work.

Skin symptoms

Rash
The distribution and character help determine the diagnosis (see Chapter 24).

Table 1.4 Differences in the history between hyperthyroidism and hypothyroidism

Symptom	Hyperthyroidism	Hypothyroidism
Temperature intolerance	Heat	Cold
Weight	Decreased	Increased
Appetite	Increased	Decreased
Bowel habit	Diarrhoea	Constipation
Psychiatric	Anxiety, irritability	Poor memory, depression
Menstruation	Oligomenorrhoea	Menorrhagia
Other symptoms	Palpitations, sweating, eye changes, pretibial myxoedema, acropachy	Dry skin, brittle hair, arthralgia, myalgia

Table 1.5 Symptoms of diabetes mellitus

Mechanism	Symptoms
Due to hyperglycaemia	Polyuria Polydipsia Fatigue Blurred vision Recurrent infections, e.g., *Candida* Weight loss (type 1)
Due to complications	Peripheral neuropathy Retinopathy Vascular disease Nephropathy

Table 1.6 Causes of bone pain

Cause	Example
Tumour	Primary tumour (benign or malignant), metastases
Infection	Osteomyelitis (*Staphylococcus*, *Haemophilus influenzae*, *Salmonella*, tuberculosis)
Fracture	Traumatic, pathological
Metabolic	Paget disease, osteomalacia

Precipitants

Has there been any recent change in detergents, soap, shampoo, etc., used?

Haematological symptoms

Excessive bleeding or bruising

Has the patient been aware of easy bruising, prolonged bleeding with minor injuries, such as bleeding gums, or menorrhagia (see Chapter 26)?.

Recurrent infections

Has the patient been getting more frequent infections which are harder to recover from, suggesting an underlying immunosuppressive state?

Glandular swelling

Ask how long the swelling has been there. Is it enlarging? Is there any tenderness or B symptoms such as weight loss or night sweats? Has the patient had a recent systemic illness? The differentials here are between normal reactive lymph nodes following infection and lymphoma (see Chapter 25).

CONCLUSION OF HISTORY TAKING

The way to become skilled in history taking for both clinical practice and examinations is to record as many patients as possible with the range of listed presentations. It is important to write these up with a list of diagnoses and plans, and then practise presenting them to others. Then ask yourself how you could do it better next time.

COMMUNICATION

Use 'ICE'; this stands for *ideas*, *concerns and expectations*. Has the patient got any ideas as to what the problem is? What is the patient concerned about it being? What would they like to get out of the consultation/Has the consultation met the patient's expectations? Use of these questions helps ensure a patient-centred approach.

COMMON PITFALLS

Be careful not to label a patient's symptoms as 'functional'. All organic causes must be ruled out before making this diagnosis – it is a diagnosis of exclusion.

● Chapter Summary

- A good history is the key to getting the correct diagnosis.
- To achieve this, try to put the patient at ease and establish a good rapport.
- Good history taking is a skill doctors develop and improve on throughout their careers.
- There is a structure to taking the history, which helps ensure all details are covered; this needs to be adapted to the situation and the patient.
- A thorough history is more likely to lead to the correct diagnosis, but it is inappropriate in a time-critical emergency.

Clinical examination

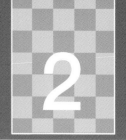

When it comes to examining patients, practice really does make perfect. Examiners will be able to tell whether you have examined many patients or not within the first few seconds of seeing you in action! Therefore take every opportunity you have to rehearse your technique.

In this chapter we describe the technique for each system and how to interpret the clinical signs you will find. However, there are situations where a full examination is not appropriate, such as when you are assessing the acutely unwell patient. In these cases, an ABCDE approach should be used to rapidly assess and treat the patient.

ABCDE APPROACH

This systematic approach ensures that the clinician prioritizes the most life-threatening problem first. Using this systematic approach, the patient is simultaneously examined, basic investigations are performed and treatment is commenced.

A: Airway. This needs to be addressed first as hypoxia kills quickest. Can the patient speak? If so you can be reassured the airway is maintained and move on to B. If not, is the patient cyanosed? Can you see an obvious airway obstruction? Can you hear gurgling or snoring suggesting a compromised airway? If you can, perform basic airway manoeuvres such as a head tilt, chin lift (if there are no concerns of a neck injury) or jaw thrust. Simple airway adjuncts can be used, such as a nasopharyngeal or oropharyngeal (Guedel) airway. If the latter is being tolerated, this suggests a very low Glasgow Coma Scale (GCS) score, and a more secure airway, such as a supraglottic airway device (e.g., laryngeal mask airway or I-gel), should be considered or even endotracheal intubation. Ensure high-flow oxygen is given; oxygen should also be administered before intubation. If the airway is compromised, call for help and anaesthetic support early.

B: Breathing. Can you see the chest wall moving, is it moving symmetrically? Is the trachea central? Listen to the chest, can you hear air entry? A trachea deviated away from a hyper-resonant chest with no breath sounds is consistent with a tension pneumothorax. Measure the oxygen saturation (this can be unreliable in the hypothermic or shocked patient with poor peripheral perfusion; take an arterial blood gas measurement to provide more accurate information). Treat the patient with oxygen. High-flow oxygen at 15 L through an oxygen mask with an inflated reservoir bag should be the initial choice in most emergency scenarios. In the case of a tension pneumothorax, emergency decompression is needed (see Chapter 29).

C: Circulation. Is the patient cyanosed or pale? Feel the temperature of the peripheries. Are they cold and clammy, suggesting hypovolemic shock, or warm and vasodilated, suggesting septic shock? Measure capillary refill (normal is < 2 s). This should be performed by pressing on the sternum for 5 s, noting the time needed for the colour to return once the pressure is released. Measure the heart rate and note the character of the pulse. Is it weak and thready, such as in hypovolemic shock, or bounding, such as in septic shock? Measure the blood pressure. Attach the patient to a cardiac monitor and, where possible, perform an ECG. Consider whether intravenous (IV) fluids are needed, and what the most appropriate resuscitation fluid is.

D: Disability. Measure the patient's neurological status using the GCS. It is divided into eyes, verbal and motor domains, with the patient's best response taken in each (see Chapter 18). The best score is 15, and the worst score is 3. Patients whose GCS score is 8 or less are at risk of not being able to maintain their own airway with this degree of neurological compromise. Examine the pupils, and see whether they are dilated (mydriasis) or constricted (miosis). Are the pupils equal? Do they react to light?

Do not forget to measure the blood glucose level. Hypoglycaemia is defined as a blood glucose level below 4 mmol/L and needs urgent treatment.

E: Exposure. Expose the patient. Look for evidence of haemorrhage, injury such as fractured limbs, rashes or hot swollen limbs. Do not forget to check the back – roll the patient safely with adequate assistance and appropriate protection of the vertebral spine, airway and the rest of the body.

Following the A to E assessment, it is important to go back and reassess the patient, particularly if there are any interventions, or any change in the patient's condition. If the situation changes during the A to E assessment, go back to A and recheck the patient.

> ### RED FLAG
>
> Hypoxia can kill within minutes. Never move on from the airway unless you are happy. Call for help and particularly for anaesthetic support early. There will be an anaesthetist in the cardiac arrest team, and putting out a cardiac arrest call in patients with severe airway compromise is appropriate.

Massive blood loss protocol

In the bleeding patient who is haemodynamically unstable or deteriorating, blood needs to be given quickly. Hospitals have a major haemorrhage protocol, sometimes called a 'code red'. Variations exist between hospitals, so it is important to know your local National Health Service Trust policy on how to activate this emergency response. Activating the major haemorrhage protocol will usually bring a porter, O-negative blood and fresh frozen plasma. It is important to state the emergency (e.g., whether it is obstetric or trauma) and the location of the patient. Whilst you are waiting for the blood, quick access or 'flying squad' O-negative blood will be available and can usually be found in the fridge of the emergency department, in the operating theatre or in the maternity unit. It is important to perform a crossmatch with blood from your patient as soon as possible so that group-specific blood can be given. The blood bank will continue to issue blood until called to stand down. If platelets or cryoprecipitate are needed, these need to be requested in addition to the code red.

GENERAL PRINCIPLES

Outside the situation of a time-critical medical emergency, performing a clinical examination is a lengthy process, and it is extremely important to ensure the patient is comfortable, appropriately exposed and in the best position to allow you to conduct a thorough examination.

There are four essential things you must do whenever you see a patient:

- Introduce yourself, wash your hands and explain to the patient what you would like to do and why, thereby obtaining the patient's consent for the examination.
- Ask the patient to move into the position required for the system you are looking at, expose the area concerned and then make sure that the patient is comfortable and that the patient's privacy is respected and modesty maintained. It is usual practice that all clinical examinations are performed from the right-hand side of the patient.
- Ask the patient if he or she has any pain. A good phrase to use is 'Are you in any pain currently? If I cause you any discomfort during my examination, please let me know and I will stop immediately'.
- From the moment you first see the patient, try to decide whether the patient looks well or ill.

You will probably find that all clinical teachers will show you a slightly different routine for the examination technique. The important thing is to develop an approach that you are comfortable with and then keep practising it until it becomes second nature.

In your medical school or professional examinations, you will almost always be asked to examine a particular system: 'Examine this gentleman's chest', 'What do you notice about this lady's face?' This chapter describes the technique for each system and how to interpret the clinical signs you will find. However, in clinical practice you will generally be performing a full examination of your patient.

VISUAL SURVEY

The most important thing is to decide how well or ill the patient is, as described earlier. Other specific abnormalities should then be looked for.

Patient position, general behaviour and around the bed

Is the patient comfortable? Is the patient anxious? Is the patient breathless? Is the patient in pain? Can the patient walk? Are there any handy clues around the bed (e.g., a wheelchair, stick or hearing aids, a nebulizer, catheter, oxygen or visible drains)? Taking time to assess these factors has several advantages: it will help you with the diagnosis, to support your clinical reasoning, to prioritize your approach and it will calm your nerves in clinical examinations.

Pallor

This is a pale colour of the skin and mucous membranes, and is the result of a reduced amount of oxyhaemoglobin or decreased peripheral perfusion. Look for evidence of pallor in the lower palpebral conjunctiva, soft palate, nail beds, palmar creases and general body skin. Pallor can be a result of anaemia, shock or respiratory distress or can be physiological in a fair-skinned patient.

Cyanosis

This is a bluish discolouration which is seen when the absolute concentration of reduced (deoxygenated) haemoglobin in the blood is greater than 50 g/L. Central cyanosis is seen best in the tongue. It is caused by underlying respiratory or cardiovascular disease. Peripheral cyanosis can be due to either central cyanosis or reduced peripheral circulation, as poorly perfused peripheral tissue will take up oxygen more readily. Remember that a patient with central cyanosis is always peripherally cyanosed, yet peripheral cyanosis can occur in the absence of central cyanosis. Reduced peripheral circulation is seen in shock, cold weather and vascular abnormalities. Cyanosis is seen rarely in anaemia but occurs more readily in polycythaemia.

Jaundice

Jaundice is a yellow discolouration of the skin, sclera and mucous membranes due to serum bilirubin concentrations greater than 30 µmol/L. Jaundice can be due to increased bilirubin production (prehepatic), abnormal bilirubin metabolism in the liver (hepatic) or reduced bilirubin excretion (posthepatic) (see Chapter 14). It is much easier to see in natural as opposed to artificial lighting.

Yellow skin (particularly palms and soles) with normal sclera can be due to excessive consumption of carrots (carotenaemia), hypothyroidism or uraemia.

Fluid status

Signs of dehydration include dry mucous membranes, tachycardia, postural hypotension and reduced skin turgor. If the patient is in hospital, hydration status should be monitored more accurately with use of urine output, fluid balance charts and daily weights.

Overhydration can sometimes result from the overenthusiastic administration of IV fluids, particularly in the elderly or in the context of renal or heart failure. Clinical signs include a raised jugular venous pressure (JVP), pulmonary oedema, a third heart sound and peripheral oedema.

Fluid status can be hard to assess, and a central line may be inserted to allow central venous pressure monitoring. This is generally limited to the high-dependency or critical care units.

Pigmentation

Generalized pigmentation is usually of racial origin but may also arise in haemochromatosis (greyish-bronze), in occupational exposure (e.g., a slate-grey appearance with argyria in silver workers) and with some drugs (e.g., slate-grey with amiodarone).

Pigmentation may also be raised with increased ACTH levels, such as in Addison disease or Cushing disease (ACTH-secreting pituitary tumour). Chronic illness may be associated with pigmentation, common examples being chronic liver disease, chronic uraemia and chronic haemolysis.

Local areas of pigmentation may be seen in Addison disease (palmar creases), Peutz–Jeghers syndrome (brown lesions around the lips) and neurofibromatosis (café au lait patches).

Localized areas of depigmentation, particularly affecting the back of the hand and neck, are seen in vitiligo. This is often associated with other autoimmune diseases.

THE FACE AND BODY HABITUS

Examiners will often take you to a patient and simply ask, 'What is the diagnosis in this patient?' or 'What do you notice about

Table 2.1 Common 'spot diagnoses'

Disease	Examples
Endocrine	Hypothyroidism, hyperthyroidism, acromegaly, Cushing syndrome, Addison disease
Metabolic	Paget disease, chronic liver disease, uraemia/stigmata of dialysis
Neuromuscular	Parkinson's disease, myotonia dystrophica, facial nerve palsy, Horner syndrome, ptosis, choreoathetosis
Connective tissue	Systemic lupus erythematosus, scleroderma, Marfan syndrome, ankylosing spondylitis
Hereditary	Turner syndrome, Down syndrome, Klinefelter syndrome, achondroplasia
Cardiovascular	Mitral facies, cyanotic congenital heart disease
Physiological	Chloasma of pregnancy
Haematological	Thalassaemia
Infection	Congenital syphilis
Dermatology	Pigmentation, purpura, psoriasis, neurofibromatosis, hereditary haemorrhagic telangiectasia, herpes zoster, pemphigoid/pemphigus, necrobiosis lipoidica diabeticorum

All these 'spot diagnoses' have characteristic physical signs.

this patient's face?'. The conditions in Table 2.1 are often known as 'spot diagnoses' – they have characteristic physical features and often come up in examinations.

THE HANDS

The hands can provide a wealth of information for the alert clinician. They should be part of examining each system (e.g., cardiac, respiratory and abdominal) but you may be asked to examine the hands in isolation. The hand examination will be discussed later in this chapter. In general, when you are looking at the hands, nails and skin, note:

Hands

- Blue: peripheral cyanosis, Raynaud phenomenon.
- Pallor: anaemia (skin creases).
- Pigmentation: Addison disease (skin creases).
- Depigmentation: vitiligo.
- Palmar erythema (Table 2.2).

Nails

- Koilonychia: spoon-shaped nails seen in iron deficiency.
- Leuconychia: white nails due to hypoalbuminaemia (Table 2.3).
- Clubbing: loss of the nail bed angle. The causes are shown in Table 2.4.
- Splinter haemorrhages: terminal lesions are usually due to trauma; proximal lesions are found in infective endocarditis and vasculitis.

Table 2.2 Causes of palmar erythema

Causes	Examples
Physiological	Pregnancy Puberty Familial
Pathological	Chronic liver disease Rheumatoid arthritis Thyrotoxicosis Oral contraceptive pill use Polycythaemia

Table 2.3 Causes of hypoalbuminaemia

Causes	Examples
Reduced intake	Malnutrition
Reduced synthesis	Liver disease
Increased utilization	Chronic illness
Increased loss	Nephrotic syndrome (kidneys) Protein-losing enteropathy (gut) Severe burns (skin)

Table 2.4 Causes of clubbing

Causes	Examples
Respiratory	Tumour: bronchial carcinoma, mesothelioma Chronic suppuration: abscess, bronchiectasis, empyema Fibrosis: from any cause Vascular: arteriovenous malformation
Cardiovascular	Congenital cyanotic heart disease Infective bacterial endocarditis Atrial myxoma
Gastrointestinal	Inflammatory bowel disease Lymphoma Cirrhosis
Endocrine	Thyrotoxicosis (acropachy)
Familial	Autosomal dominant

- Quincke sign: capillary pulsation in the nail bed due to aortic regurgitation.
- Beau lines: horizontal grooves in the nails caused by temporary arrest of nail growth as a result of acute severe illness.
- Onycholysis: separation of the nail from the nail bed as a result of psoriasis, trauma, fungal infection and hyperthyroidism.
- Yellow nails: yellow nail syndrome with lymphatic hypoplasia (peripheral oedema and pleural effusions).

Tendons

- Xanthomata: hypercholesterolaemia.
- Dupuytren contractures (thickening of the palmar fascia): associated with alcoholic liver disease, people with epilepsy treated with phenytoin, vibrating tools and familial and idiopathic causes.

Joints

- Destructive arthropathy: e.g., rheumatoid arthritis.
- Heberden nodes: osteophytes of the distal interphalangeal joints.
- Bouchard nodes: osteophytes of the proximal interphalangeal joints.
- Gouty tophi: deposits of urate crystals.

Neuromuscular

- Localized wasting of the hypothenar eminence with an ulnar nerve lesion or thenar eminence with a median nerve lesion.
- Generalized wasting: e.g., with C8/T1 anterior horn cell, nerve root or brachial plexus damage, combined median and ulnar nerve damage, disuse atrophy in severe arthritis, profound cachexia.
- Myotonia: failure to relax after voluntary contraction. It is seen in myotonic dystrophy, for instance, after shaking the patient's hand.

Miscellaneous

- Sclerodactyly (tightening of the skin causing tapering of the fingers), which along with calcinosis and Raynaud phenomenon, is a feature of systemic sclerosis.
- Large hands with doughy swelling seen in acromegaly (often called 'spade-like hands').
- Asterixis: a coarse flapping tremor is seen when the hand is outstretched with the wrist extended and fingers apart. It is caused by metabolic encephalopathy (e.g., liver failure, carbon dioxide retention, uraemia).
- Action tremor: this is rapid and fine in amplitude. It is worsened by holding the hands in a particular posture (e.g.,

hands outstretched) or by movement. It is characteristic of benign essential tremor, thyrotoxicosis and excessive caffeine intake and is an exaggeration of physiological tremor.

- Resting tremor: the thumb moves across the tips of the fingers. This 'pill-rolling' tremor is worst at rest and is characteristic of Parkinson's disease.
- Intention tremor: this is absent at rest, present on maintaining a posture and exaggerated by movement. It is characteristic of disorders of the cerebellum and its connections. See Table 2.22 for causes of tremor.

THE CARDIOVASCULAR SYSTEM

Visual survey

- Does the patient look well or ill? Is the patient comfortable? Is the patient breathless or in pain? Is the patient lying flat? Is the patient pale or cyanosed?
- Is there evidence of a congenital syndrome associated with cardiac abnormalities such as Marfan syndrome or Down syndrome?

Position

Help the patient to adopt a comfortable position at 45 degrees with the chest exposed. In women, cover the chest until you are ready to examine the precordium.

Hands

Specifically look for:

- Clubbing: seen with infective bacterial endocarditis (IBE) and congenital cyanotic heart disease.
- Cyanosis: present with peripheral vasoconstriction pulmonary oedema, right-to-left cardiac shunt.
- Splinter haemorrhages: IBE.
- Janeway lesions: nontender macules in the palms due to IBE.
- Osler nodes: painful nodules on the pulps of the fingers due to IBE.
- Quincke sign: aortic regurgitation.
- Xanthomata: hypercholesterolaemia (vascular disease).

Radial pulse

- Rate: normally between 60 and 100 bpm (see Chapter 7).
- Rhythm: regular or irregular (see Chapter 7).
- Radioradial delay: dissecting thoracic aortic aneurysm.
- Radiofemoral delay: coarctation of the aorta.

- Character: best determined by palpation of a larger artery (e.g., brachial or carotid arteries).

Blood pressure

- This is an important component of the cardiac examination. Blood pressure can be measured at rest in the hospital setting, referred to as 'office blood pressure', but patients may measure their blood pressure at home or occasionally 24-hour ambulatory blood pressure monitoring is performed when white coat syndrome or postural blood pressure drops are a concern.
- Lying and standing: postural hypotension. Should be measured when the patient is lying, and then at 1 and 3 minutes after standing. A 30-mmHg drop is deemed a significant drop. However, if a patient experiences symptoms such as dizziness on standing, this is deemed to be significant regardless of actual blood pressure measurements.
- Right and left arm: the pressure in the left arm may be lower than in the right arm in aortic dissection.
- Pulse pressure (the difference between systolic and diastolic pressure): a wide pulse pressure is more common in the elderly and is a feature of aortic regurgitation.
- Narrow pulse pressure: aortic stenosis.
- Pulsus paradoxus: exaggerated fall in pulse pressure during inspiration resulting in a faint or absent pulse in inspiration; caused by severe asthma or cardiac tamponade.

Brachial and carotid artery

- Character: collapsing (Table 2.5), slow rising (aortic stenosis), alternans (severe left ventricular failure), jerky (hypertrophic obstructive cardiomyopathy).
- Corrigan sign: prominent carotid pulsation due to aortic regurgitation.

Jugular Venous Pressure

When you are assessing JVP, the patient should be at 45 degrees with their head resting on a pillow (this relaxes the sternocleidomastoid muscles). Pulsation should be up to 3 cm above the sternal angle (8 cm above the right atrium). Differences between JVP and carotid pulsation in normal individuals are shown in Table 2.6. The JVP acts as a manometer for right atrial pressure, and is raised when right atrial pressure is raised (Box 2.1). Abnormalities in the waveform result from specific underlying diseases (Fig. 2.1).

Restrictive cardiomyopathy, constrictive pericarditis and pericardial tamponade are all associated with Kussmaul sign (JVP that rises during inspiration).

Table 2.5 Causes of a collapsing pulse

Causes	Examples
Physiological	Elderly
	Pregnancy
	Exercise
Pathological	Aortic regurgitation
	Patent ductus arteriosus
	Fever
	Thyrotoxicosis
	Anaemia
	Arteriovenous shunts

Table 2.6 Differences between jugular venous pressure and carotid pulsation

Feature	Carotid pulsation	JVP
Palpable	Yes	No
Number of visible peaks	One	Two
Occlusion by gentle pressure	No	Yes (fills from above)
Sitting upright	No change	Height falls
Lying flat	No change	Height rises
Gentle pressure on liver	No change	Height rises (hepatojugular reflux)
Deep inspiration	No change	Height rises

JVP, Jugular venous pressure.

BOX 2.1 CAUSES OF A RAISED JUGULAR VENOUS PRESSURE

Right ventricular failure

Volume overload (e.g., overenthusiastic administration of intravenous fluids)

Superior vena cava obstruction (jugular venous pressure is nonpulsatile)

Tricuspid valve disease (stenosis and regurgitation)

Pericardial effusion causing tamponade

Constrictive pericarditis

HINTS AND TIPS

If the jugular venous pressure is not visible at 45 degrees, try sitting the patient upright or laying the patient flat and eliciting the hepatojugular reflux, as it may be either too high or too low to be seen.

Face

- Central cyanosis: right-to-left shunt.
- Anaemia: possible high-output cardiac failure.
- Malar flush: mitral valve disease.
- Jaundice: haemolysis due to mechanical valves.
- Xanthelasmata: hypercholesterolaemia (vascular disease).
- Mouth: high-arched palate in Marfan syndrome.
- De Musset sign: head nodding because of aortic regurgitation.
- Roth spots in the retina: IBE.

Praecordium

Look for scars and deformities, including:

- Sternotomy scar: arterial bypass grafts and valve replacements.
- Mitral valvotomy scar under the left breast: always look for it, as it indicates a previously closed mitral valvotomy.
- Skeletal deformities: can cause an ejection systolic flow murmur.

Apex beat

The apex beat should be at the midclavicular line in the fifth left intercostal space.

- Lateral displacement: left or severe right ventricular dilatation. Lung pathology may also cause displacement.
- Impalpable: obesity, pleural effusion, pericardial effusion, chronic obstructive airway disease and dextrocardia (palpable on the right!).
- Tapping: mitral stenosis (palpable first heart sound).
- Heaving: 'pressure overload' in aortic stenosis or hypertension.
- Thrusting: 'volume overload' in aortic regurgitation, mitral regurgitation (ventricle usually markedly displaced).

Palpation

Parasternal heave is caused by the enlargement or hypertrophy of the right ventricle.

A thrill is a palpable murmur and indicates significant valve disease; it can be systolic or diastolic, and therefore its position in the cardiac cycle should be assessed by timing its relation to a central pulse. Palpate in all valve areas (Fig. 2.2).

Auscultation

- Listen in all four areas with the bell and diaphragm (see Fig. 2.2).
- Roll the patient to the left-hand side to listen with the bell at the axilla for mitral stenosis.

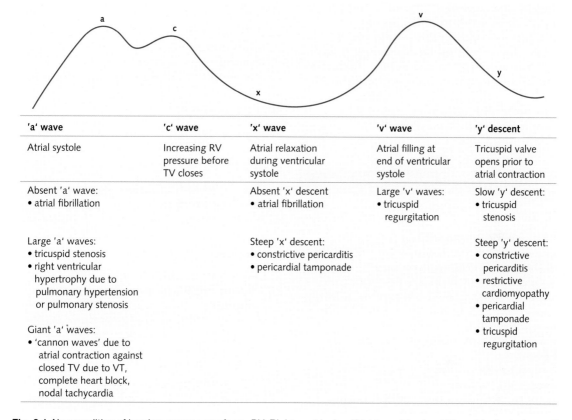

'a' wave	'c' wave	'x' wave	'v' wave	'y' descent
Atrial systole	Increasing RV pressure before TV closes	Atrial relaxation during ventricular systole	Atrial filling at end of ventricular systole	Tricuspid valve opens prior to atrial contraction
Absent 'a' wave: • atrial fibrillation		Absent 'x' descent • atrial fibrillation	Large 'v' waves: • tricuspid regurgitation	Slow 'y' descent: • tricuspid stenosis
Large 'a' waves: • tricuspid stenosis • right ventricular hypertrophy due to pulmonary hypertension or pulmonary stenosis Giant 'a' waves: • 'cannon waves' due to atrial contraction against closed TV due to VT, complete heart block, nodal tachycardia		Steep 'x' descent: • constrictive pericarditis • pericardial tamponade		Steep 'y' descent: • constrictive pericarditis • restrictive cardiomyopathy • pericardial tamponade • tricuspid regurgitation

Fig. 2.1 Abnormalities of jugular venous waveform. *RV*, Right ventricular; *TV*, tricuspid valve; *VT*, ventricular tachycardia.

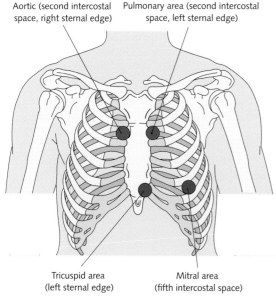

Aortic (second intercostal space, right sternal edge)　Pulmonary area (second intercostal space, left sternal edge)

Tricuspid area (left sternal edge)　Mitral area (fifth intercostal space)

Fig. 2.2 Positions of auscultation of the cardiac valves.

- Sit the patient forward to listen with the diaphragm at the left sternal edge in expiration (with breath held) for aortic regurgitation.
- Listen to the first and second sounds, then to third and fourth sounds.
- Are there any murmurs? (See Chapter 28.)
- Listen for additional sounds, including opening snap, ejection click, pericardial knock or rub and mechanical valves.
- Time any abnormalities against the carotid pulsation.
- Listen to the carotid arteries for bruits (atheroma) or radiation of aortic stenotic murmur.

Summary

Following auscultation of the heart, finish the cardiovascular examination by:

- Examining the lung bases, checking for pulmonary oedema.
- Palpating for hepatomegaly, which occurs in right ventricular failure.

- Looking for pitting oedema and note the level (e.g., to knees) and for sacral oedema.
- Palpating peripheral pulses: pulses in the legs may be diminished in peripheral vascular disease. Systolic and diastolic murmurs may be heard in the femoral arteries that are due to aortic regurgitation (pistol shots and Duroziez sign).
- Performing the full set of observations and an ECG.
- Dipping the urine for blood and protein (IBE).

THE RESPIRATORY SYSTEM

Visual survey

- Does the patient look well or ill? Is the patient alert?
- Respiratory rate: is the patient breathless at rest? A normal respiratory rate is 12 to 16 breaths per minute.
- Is the patient on oxygen? If so, how is this being administered (i.e., venturi mask or by nasal speculum), and how much (i.e., what is the FiO_2)?
- Is the patient cyanosed?
- Look for cachexia: suggesting COPD or an underlying malignancy.
- Sputum pot: note the contents.
- Nebulizer and medications.
- Pursed lip breathing and accessory muscle use: chronic small airway obstruction.
- Voice: hoarse in bronchial carcinoma (recurrent laryngeal nerve palsy).
- Note if a chest drain is present and look at the contents.

Position

Help the patient to adopt a comfortable position at 45 degrees with the chest exposed. In women, cover the chest until you are ready to examine it.

Hands

- Clubbing: see Table 2.4.
- Cyanosis: respiratory failure.
- Wasting of small muscles: infiltration of T1 by bronchial neoplasm (Pancoast tumour).
- Tar-stained fingers: increased likelihood of malignancy and obstructive airway disease.
- Asterixis (flap): carbon dioxide retention.
- Fine tremor: recent salbutamol use.
- Evidence of conditions which may involve the lungs (e.g., systemic sclerosis, rheumatoid arthritis) (see Chapter 29).

Pulse

- Tachycardia: severe respiratory disease (e.g., pulmonary embolism, acute asthma or pneumonia).
- Bounding: carbon dioxide retention.
- Atrial fibrillation: e.g., sepsis secondary to pneumonia.

Blood pressure

Pulsus paradoxus is seen in severe acute asthma.

Jugular venous pressure

- Right ventricular failure: chronic respiratory disease with pulmonary hypertension.
- Superior vena caval obstruction: bronchial carcinoma.

Face and mouth

- Central cyanosis: respiratory failure.
- Anaemia: chronic respiratory disease, particularly malignancy.
- Horner syndrome: apical carcinoma (Pancoast tumour) involving cervical sympathetic nerves (see Chapter 29).
- Fine tremor: β-agonists.
- Plethoric facies: secondary polycythaemia.

Trachea

Warn the patient before you palpate the trachea! Note the following:

- Tracheal deviation reflects disease in the upper mediastinum (Table 2.7).
- Feel for tracheal tug in acute respiratory distress.
- The distance from the cricoid cartilage to the suprasternal notch should be 2 to 3 cm – this distance reduces in hyperinflation.

COMMUNICATION

Always take care to explain what you are doing to the patient when you are examining the trachea. If done badly, it may be uncomfortable, and if you hurt the patient, you are likely to fail.

Thorax

Perform inspection, palpation, percussion and auscultation on the front of the chest first. Then sit the patient forward, palpate the front of chest for lymphadenopathy and then repeat the

Table 2.7 Causes of tracheal deviation

Towards lesion	Away from lesion
Collapse	Tension pneumothorax
Apical fibrosis	Massive pleural effusion
Pneumonectomy	Large mass (e.g., thyroid)

examination on the back of the chest. Typical patterns of respiratory abnormalities are shown in Table 2.8.

Inspection

On inspecting the chest, assess:

- Respiration: use of accessory muscles (respiratory distress).
- Recession: intercostal and subcostal (respiratory distress).
- Scars: including previous surgery and chest drains.
- Deformity: barrel chest (seen in long-standing airways obstruction as a result of hyperinflation), pectus excavatum, pectus carinatum.
- Radiotherapy: tattoos or skin changes indicate previous treatment for malignancy.

Expansion

- Ask the patient to take a deep breath in and note symmetry and comfort.
- The chest circumference should expand by at least 5 cm on deep inspiration.
- Any significant pulmonary disease will reduce expansion.
- In unilateral disease, the affected side will move less than the other.
- Note any chest wall tenderness, which is usually caused by musculoskeletal abnormalities.

Tactile fremitus and vocal fremitus

Ask the patient to say '99' and palpate with the ulnar border of the hand. Increased vocal fremitus indicates consolidation; decreased vocal fremitus indicates pleural effusion or collapse.

Percussion

Compare one side with the other and remember the axillae. The following signs are important:

- Hyperresonance: pneumothorax.
- Dull: solid organ (liver or heart), consolidation, collapse, pleural thickening, peripheral tumours, severe fibrosis, previous old pneumonectomy.
- Stony dull: pleural effusion.

Auscultation

- Normal breath sounds are termed 'vesicular'.

- Bronchial breathing, whispering pectoriloquy, increased vocal resonance: consolidation (sometimes fibrosis and above pleural effusion).
- Wheeze: small airway obstruction (polyphonic), large airway obstruction (e.g., bronchial carcinoma (monophonic or localized)) and cardiac failure.
- Fine crackles: pulmonary fibrosis, pulmonary oedema.
- Coarse crackles: infection.
- Absent breath sounds: pleural effusion.
- Pleural rub: pleural irritation due to pneumonia or pulmonary embolus.

HINTS AND TIPS

The upper border of the liver is normally at the sixth intercostal space in the right midclavicular line. If the percussion note remains resonant below this, the lungs are hyperinflated.

Summary

To conclude the examination, look for:

- Pitting oedema indicating right ventricular failure, or low albumin level from chronic disease.
- Sputum inspection, peak flow, oxygen saturation, temperature and chest X-ray: these can be remembered by the mnemonic SPOT-X.

THE ABDOMEN

Visual survey

- Appearance: does the patient look well or ill?
- Is the patient in pain?
- Patient's position: think of peritonism if the patient is very still, appendicitis (psoas irritation) if the knees are flexed and renal colic if the patient is rolling around in agony.
- Cachexia: chronic disease, particularly malignancy.
- Drowsy: encephalopathy (hepatic or uraemia).
- Hydration status, you can assess this more carefully with attention to mucous membranes, height of the JVP, capillary refill time, patient weight, urine output and postural blood pressure.

Position

The patient can initially be assessed sitting at 45 degrees. For examination of the abdomen itself, the patient should be as flat as can be tolerated comfortably (this relaxes the abdominal

Table 2.8 Findings on clinical examination of common respiratory diseases

Pathology	General signs	Tracheal deviation	Palpation	Percussion note	Breath sounds	Causes
Pneumothorax	Tachycardia and hypotension in tension pneumothorax	Away from affected side if tension	Reduced expansion, reduced TVF	Normal or hyperresonant	Reduced or absent	Spontaneous (particularly tall healthy males and Marfan syndrome), trauma, airway obstruction, cystic fibrosis, pulmonary abscess
Consolidation	Pyrexia, tachycardia	None	Reduced expansion, increased TVF	Dull	Increased vocal resonance, whispering pectoriloquy, bronchial breath sounds	Pneumococcus, *Haemophilus influenzae*, *Staphylococcus aureus*, *Klebsiella*, *Pseudomonas*, *Mycoplasma*, *Legionella*, influenza type A, *Aspergillus*
Pleural effusion		Away from affected side if large	Reduced expansion, reduced TVF	Stony dull	Absent	Transudate (protein < 30 g/L): cardiac failure, liver failure, nephrotic syndrome, Meigs syndrome, myxoedema
Exudate (protein > 30 g/L): malignancy, pneumonia, pulmonary embolus, rheumatoid arthritis, SLE, subphrenic abscess, pancreatitis, trauma, Dressler syndrome
Collapse		Towards affected side	Reduced expansion, reduced TVF	Dull	Reduced or absent	Foreign body or mucous plugs (asthma, aspergillosis) within the bronchial lumen, bronchial carcinoma arising from the bronchus itself, extrinsic compression by enlarged lymph nodes (malignancy, tuberculosis)
Fibrosis	Clubbing	Towards affected side if apical disease	Reduced expansion, increased TVF	Normal or dull	Fine inspiratory crepitations	Cryptogenic fibrosing alveolitis, sarcoidosis, drugs (amiodarone, bleomycin), radiation, inhalation of dust (asbestos, coal), extrinsic allergic alveolitis, ankylosing spondylitis, rheumatoid arthritis, systemic sclerosis, tuberculosis
Bronchiectasis	Clubbing, purulent sputum	Normal	Normal or reduced expansion, normal or increased TVF	Normal or dull	Coarse inspiratory crepitations, occasional polyphonic wheeze	Congenital (cystic fibrosis, Kartagener syndrome, hypogammaglobulinaemia), idiopathic, bronchial obstruction (foreign body, carcinoma, lymphadenopathy), infection (childhood measles or whooping cough, tuberculosis, aspergillosis, postpneumonia)
Bronchospasm	Hyperexpanded chest, tremor (if taking a β-agonist), Harrison sulci, pectus carinatum	Normal	Reduced expansion, normal TVF	Normal, hyper-resonant over bullae, reduced liver dullness	Polyphonic wheeze, crepitations in chronic obstructive airways disease	Anaphylaxis

SLE, *Systemic lupus erythematosus*; TVF, *tactile vocal fremitus*.

muscles). Exposure should be from 'nipples to knees', but bear in mind the patient's dignity.

Hands

- Clubbing: cirrhosis, inflammatory bowel disease.
- Leukonychia: clinical sign of hypoalbuminaemia. Consider liver disease, nephrotic syndrome, protein-losing enteropathy.
- Koilonychia: chronic iron deficiency. Consider occult neoplasm, particularly in the stomach and caecum.
- Palmar erythema: cirrhosis.
- Hyperpigmented palmar creases: Addison disease.
- Asterixis: hepatic encephalopathy and uraemia.
- Dupuytren's contracture: alcoholic liver disease.

Arms

- Scratch marks: obstructive jaundice (particularly primary biliary cirrhosis), uraemia and lymphoma.
- Needle track marks, tattoos: viral hepatitis.
- Muscle wasting: proximal myopathy due to alcohol, steroid excess or underlying malignancy (paraneoplastic).
- Bruising: hepatic impairment.

Face and mouth

- Jaundice: prehepatic, hepatic or posthepatic (see Chapter 14).
- Pallor suggesting anaemia from any cause.
- Xanthelasmata: hypercholesterolaemia (primary biliary cirrhosis or nephrotic syndrome).
- Kayser–Fleischer rings: Wilson disease (best seen by slit-lamp examination).
- Glossitis and stomatitis: iron deficiency and megaloblastic anaemia.
- Telangiectasia: associated with limited systemic sclerosis (CREST syndrome), cirrhosis and hereditary haemorrhagic telangiectasia (Osler–Weber–Rendu disease).
- Crohn disease: mucosal ulceration.

Neck

Look for left supraclavicular lymphadenopathy – caused by metastasis from underlying gastrointestinal carcinoma (Virchow node or Troisier sign).

> **HINTS AND TIPS**
>
> Always palpate the neck from behind the patient with the neck slightly flexed to relax the sternocleidomastoid muscles.

Trunk and back

Spider naevi arise in the distribution of the superior vena cava – five or more suggest underlying chronic liver disease, pregnancy or hyperthyroidism. Look for gynaecomastia (increased breast tissue) in men. This is most commonly associated with chronic liver disease or drugs (e.g., spironolactone).

Abdomen

Inspection

Observe closely, looking for:

- Scars: previous surgery or trauma.
- Distension (Table 2.9).
- Obvious mass: including movement with respiration.
- Bruising: Cullen (paraumbilical) and Grey Turner (flanks) signs in acute pancreatitis (these are rare).
- Dilated veins and caput medusae: portal hypertension or inferior vena cava obstruction (venous flow is upwards).
- Striae: pregnancy or Cushing syndrome.
- Node: umbilical nodule (Sister Mary Joseph nodule) is a metastasis from intraabdominal malignancy.
- Peristalsis: if visible, this indicates an obstruction, although it may be normal in a thin or elderly patient.

Palpation

Before you touch the patient, ask if the patient is tender anywhere and start palpation away from that area. Feel gently in each of the nine abdominal regions, noting tenderness or masses. Then feel more deeply in each region to determine the characteristics of any mass found (Box 2.2).

> **HINTS AND TIPS**
>
> Always look at the patient's face when palpating the abdomen to ensure that you know immediately if you are causing discomfort. You should palpate the abdomen with your arm level to the patient.

Table 2.9 Causes of generalized abdominal swelling

Cause	Example
Fluid	Ascites
Faeces	Constipation
Foetus	Pregnancy
Flatus	Bowel obstruction
Fat	Obesity
Fibroids	And any other tumour or organomegaly

BOX 2.2 FEATURES TO DETERMINE FOR ANY MASS

Site
Shape
Size, including upper, lower and lateral limits
Consistency
Tenderness
Fluctuance
Fixation to underlying or overlying structures
Transillumination (where appropriate)
Local lymph node involvement
Bruit

Table 2.10 Causes of hepatomegaly

Cause	Examples
Infection	Viral hepatitis,[a] abscess, syphilis, Weil disease,[a] hydatid disease, brucellosis
Tumour	Benign, malignant, primary (hepatocellular carcinoma) and metastases
Venous congestion	Right ventricular failure, Budd–Chiari syndrome, tricuspid disease
Autoimmune	Autoimmune liver disease, primary biliary cirrhosis and primary sclerosing cholangitis
Cysts	Polycystic disease
Haematological	Lymphoproliferative disease,[a] myeloproliferative disease[a]
Metabolic	Nonalcoholic fatty liver, storage diseases,[a] amyloidosis,[a] haemochromatosis, Wilson disease
Toxic/drug	Alcoholic liver disease,[a] drug-induced hepatitis, e.g., statins

The liver may appear large in the absence of true hepatomegaly when it is pushed down by a hyperinflated lung (as in acute asthma or chronic obstructive airway disease) and when a Riedel lobe is present (normal anatomical variation of the right hepatic lobe).
[a]*Cause of hepatosplenomegaly.*

If a mass is present, consider what structures normally lie at that site and what disease processes might affect that structure (see Chapter 9). Next, palpate for hepatomegaly and splenomegaly, starting in the right iliac fossa. Examine the patient for renal masses by bimanual palpation. If hepatomegaly or splenomegaly is present, comment on consistency (smooth or irregular), whether tender and size in centimetres (not finger breadths) beneath the costal margin (the causes of hepatomegaly are shown in Table 2.10; the causes of splenomegaly are

Table 2.11 Causes of unilateral and bilateral palpable kidneys

Type	Cause
Unilateral	Tumour (hypernephroma, nephroblastoma) Hydronephrosis, pyonephrosis Hypertrophy of single-functioning kidney Perinephric abscess or haematoma Polycystic disease (only one kidney palpable)
Bilateral	Polycystic kidneys (autosomal dominant in adults, autosomal recessive in children) Amyloidosis Bilateral hydronephrosis

Table 2.12 Causes of ascites

Type	Cause
High SAAG, >1.1 g/dL	Cardiac failure Liver failure Hypoproteinaemia Meigs syndrome Myxoedema Budd–Chiari syndrome Constrictive pericarditis (rare) Cirrhosis with portal hypertension
Low SAAG, <1.1 g/dL	Intraabdominal malignancy Infection (tuberculosis, perforation, spontaneous) Pancreatitis Lymphatic obstruction (chylous)

SAAG is a better discriminant than older measures of transudate (high SAAG) and exudate (low SAAG).
SAAG, Serum ascites albumin gradient.

discussed in detail in Chapter 25). The causes of renal mass are summarized in Table 2.11.

Finally, palpate for abdominal aortic aneurysm and examine the groins for lymphadenopathy and hernias.

Percussion

Always percuss from resonance to dullness. Use percussion to determine the size of the liver and spleen, starting at the chest, moving inferiorly. Percuss over any masses to determine their consistency. Always assess for ascites by looking for a fluid thrill and shifting dullness. Table 2.12 summarizes the causes of ascites. Look for tenderness on percussion; this is a useful clinical sign that may indicate peritoneal irritation.

Auscultation

- Bowel sounds may be normal, increased or decreased. Increased bowel obstruction (high-pitched and tinkling) and absent with an ileus (functional motor paralysis of the bowel) of any cause (Box 2.3).

BOX 2.3 CAUSES OF ILEUS

Following intraabdominal surgery
Peritonitis
Pancreatitis
Hypokalaemia
Diabetic ketoacidosis
Intraabdominal haemorrhage
Retroperitoneal haematoma
Retroperitoneal trauma, e.g., surgery for aortic
    aneurysm
Anticholinergic drugs

Table 2.13 Causes of lower limb oedema

Cause	Examples
Pitting	Unilateral: • deep vein thrombosis • unilateral compression of veins (tumour or lymph nodes) • following hip/knee replacement • local infection or trauma Bilateral: • right ventricular failure • constrictive pericarditis • hepatic failure • nephrotic syndrome • protein-losing enteropathy • immobility • pregnancy • kwashiorkor
Lymphatic (nonpitting)	Blocked lymph channels: surgical damage, radiation, malignant infiltration, infection (filariasis) or congenital (Milroy disease)

- Arterial bruits: may be heard over stenosed vessels such as renal arteries.
- Succussion splash: any cause of gastric outlet obstruction.

Concluding your examination

- If the patient has symptoms or signs of rectal bleeding, has iron deficiency or reports a change in bowel habit, you should perform a digital rectal examination.
- You may have to examine the patient's genitals in some circumstances.
- For both of these, in your clinical examinations you should say that you would like to go on to examine the genitalia and perform a rectal examination, but generally you will not be asked to perform this.
- If there is hepatosplenomegaly, go on to examine all lymph node sites, bearing in mind the multitude of potential causes (see Chapter 25).
- Examine the legs for pitting oedema (Table 2.13).
- Do not forget to examine hernial orifices.

THE NERVOUS SYSTEM

Although it is true that neuroanatomy is complicated and many different diseases can affect each part, the end result is a limited repertoire of patterns of signs. The best approach is to identify which signs are present using a well-rehearsed technique and consider where the lesion is likely to be. You can then think of which diseases affect that part of the nervous system and look for additional evidence to support the diagnosis.

The clinical signs and common diseases associated with different parts of the nervous system are discussed in detail in Chapter 21. This section covers a practical approach to the examination technique itself. It is particularly important to practice this routine repeatedly.

Visual survey

- Appearance: does the patient look well or ill?
- Level of consciousness: is the patient alert, drowsy or unresponsive?
- Age: for instance, a young patient is more likely to have multiple sclerosis, motor neurone disease or an inherited disease; an elderly patient is more likely to have had a stroke.
- General clues: does the patient need a wheelchair or walking stick?
- Posture: how is the patient sitting? Is the patient leaning towards one side (hemiparesis)? Is there a tremor at rest (parkinsonism)?
- Speech: when the patient speaks, does the speech sound normal? (See Table 1.3.)

Cranial nerves

Features and examinations of the cranial nerves include the following.

Cranial nerve I (olfactory nerve)
- This is a sensory nerve only.
- Ask the patient if he or she has noticed anything abnormal about the sense of smell.
- Sense of smell can be tested with bottles containing essences, although this test is rarely performed. (Note that ammonia should not be used as it also stimulates the trigeminal nerve.)
- Anosmia can result from head injury (fracture of the cribriform plate), upper respiratory tract infection or tumour (olfactory groove meningioma or glioma), or can be

Table 2.14 Visual field defects

Defect	Site of lesion	Causes
Tunnel vision	Retina	Glaucoma, retinitis pigmentosa, laser therapy for diabetic retinopathy
Enlarged blind spot	Optic nerve	Papilloedema (from any cause)
Central scotoma	Macula, optic nerve	Optic atrophy, optic neuritis, retinal disease affecting macula
Monocular visual loss	Eye, optic nerve	Extrinsic compression, toxic optic neuropathy
Bitemporal hemianopia	Optic chiasm	Pituitary tumour, craniopharyngioma, sella meningioma
Quadrantic hemianopia	Temporal lobe (superior), parietal lobe (inferior)	Stroke, tumour
Homonymous hemianopia	Occipital cortex, optic tract	Stroke, tumour

a feature of Parkinson's disease or Kallmann syndrome (anosmia with hypogonadotrophic hypogonadism).

Cranial nerve II (optic nerve)

- This is a sensory nerve only.
- Visual acuity: test each eye separately. Ask the patient to read some print or a Snellen chart (with spectacles if worn normally). Any lesion from the cornea, lens, retina, optic nerve, optic chiasm, optic radiation or occipital cortex can result in reduced acuity.
- Visual fields: test each eye individually. Make sure your eyes are on the same level as the patient's. Move your fingers from beyond your visual field inwards and ask the patient to tell you when he or she can see them. Check each quadrant. Use a red hatpin to determine the blind spot. Typical field defects are shown in Table 2.14. Vision can be formally assessed by perimetry. If the visual fields are intact, look for inattention by simultaneously stimulating both the left and the right.
- Pupillary reflexes: the pupillary reactions to light and accommodation should be tested. Remember sympathetic innervation causes mydriasis (dilated pupil), and parasympathetic innervation causes miosis (constricted pupil). Pupillary abnormalities in patients who are in a coma are described in Chapter 18. Other clinical abnormalities include:
  - Physiological anisocoria: slight difference in size.
  - Senile miosis: small, irregular pupils in old age.
  - Total afferent pupillary defect (complete lesion of optic nerve): if, for instance, the left eye is affected, shining a light in it fails to cause pupillary constriction in either eye – absent direct and consensual reflexes. However, if a light is shone in the right eye, the left pupil constricts (i.e., the right eye consensual reflex is intact).
  - Relative afferent pupillary defect (RAPD), which occurs if there is incomplete damage to the afferent pathway (e.g., previous retrobulbar neuritis due to multiple sclerosis). The swinging light test is performed (i.e., the light is moved from one eye to the other alternately). If

the left eye has an RAPD, there will be reduced conduction along its afferent pathway. Therefore if the light is initially shone in the left eye, both pupils will constrict; when the light is moved to the right eye, bilateral constriction occurs again; when the light returns to the left eye, the pupil dilates because of its reduced afferent conduction. This is diagnostic of an RAPD.

- Horner syndrome: a triad of a constricted pupil (miosis), an eyelid droop (ptosis) and decreased sweating (anhidrosis) caused by interruption of the sympathetic chain at any level from the brainstem to the ciliary ganglion (see Chapter 34).
- Argyll Robertson pupil: a small, irregular pupil that 'accommodates but does not react' (i.e., fixed to light but constricts on convergence). Almost diagnostic of neurosyphilis (occasionally occurs in diabetes mellitus).
- Myotonic pupil (Holmes–Adie pupil): a dilated pupil that reacts very slowly to light and constricts incompletely to convergence. Most common in young females, and if combined with absent tendon reflexes, this is Holmes–Adie syndrome.
- Ophthalmoscopy: common abnormalities on ophthalmoscopy are papilloedema (Table 2.15), optic atrophy (Table 2.16), diabetic retinopathy (Table 2.17) and hypertensive retinopathy and in examinations, retinitis pigmentosa. Pigmentary retinal degeneration may also occur in other conditions, such as Refsum disease and Laurence–Moon–Biedl syndrome.

COMMUNICATION

Prolonged gazing with an ophthalmoscope can be uncomfortable for the patient. Be aware of this, and consider giving the patient a short break every so often.

Table 2.15 Causes of papilloedema

Cause	Examples
Raised intracranial pressure	Tumour, abscess, hydrocephalus, haematoma, idiopathic intracranial hypertension, cerebral oedema (trauma)
Venous occlusion	Central retinal vein thrombosis, cavernous sinus thrombosis
Malignant hypertension	Grade IV hypertensive retinopathy
Acute optic neuritis	Multiple sclerosis, sarcoidosis
Metabolic	Hypercapnia, hypoparathyroidism
Haematological (rare)	Severe anaemia, acute leukaemia

Table 2.16 Causes of optic atrophy

Cause	Examples
Pressure on optic nerve	Tumour, glaucoma, aneurysm, Paget disease
Demyelination	Multiple sclerosis
Vascular	Central retinal artery occlusion
Metabolic	Diabetes mellitus, vitamin B_{12} deficiency
Toxins	Methyl alcohol, tobacco, lead, quinine
Trauma	Including surgery
Consecutive	Extensive retinal disease such as chorioretinitis
Hereditary prolonged papilloedema	Friedreich ataxia, Leber optic atrophy

Table 2.17 Stages of diabetic retinopathy

Stage	Features
Background nonproliferative	At least one microaneurysm
Moderate nonproliferative	Microaneurysms or intraretinal haemorrhages with or without cotton wool spots, venous beading and intraretinal microvascular abnormality
Severe nonproliferative or preproliferative	Findings as for moderate nonproliferative, but needs to be present in a minimum number of retinal quadrants
Proliferative	All of the above, plus new vessel formation on the disc, retina or iris (rubeosis iridis). Also, retinal detachment and vitreous haemorrhage
Diabetic maculopathy	Focal or diffuse macular oedema Ischaemic maculopathy Thickening of the retina and hard exudates

The classification of diabetic retinopathy is based on which part of the retina is affected and the degree of pathology, and does not necessarily correlate with the patient's degree of vision. Note that cataracts are also more common in diabetes, and that retinopathy may have been treated by laser photocoagulation (burns around the periphery of the retina, destroying ischaemic tissue and thus reducing the drive for new vessel formation).

IV and VI are responsible. Cranial nerve IV innervates the superior oblique muscle to cause downward movement of the eye in the midline, and cranial nerve VI innervates the lateral rectus muscle for abduction of the eye.

- Ask the patient to follow your finger with his or her eyes while you slowly draw out the shape of two large letter H's joined in the middle. You should ensure that the vertical movements are at extremes of lateral gaze as well as in the midline.
- Ask the patient if he or she sees double (i.e., does the patient have diplopia). Note when it occurs, and in which direction. Diplopia in all directions of gaze may result from myasthenia gravis, ocular myopathy or disease in the surrounding tissue of the eye, such as Graves disease, tumour or orbital cellulitis.
- Look for inability of the patient to move the eye (i.e., ophthalmoplegia). If this is present, carefully note the exact movement the patient was not able to make, and whether it was at extreme gaze or in the midline.
- Look for nystagmus. This is involuntary rhythmic eye oscillation. It occurs physiologically at the extremes of lateral gaze, and more than two beats are required for it to be significant.

HINTS AND TIPS

A mnemonic to help you remember all the parts of the second cranial nerve (optic nerve) examination is AFRO; which stands for visual *a*cuity, visual *f*ields, pupillary *r*eflexes and *o*phthalmoscopy.

Cranial nerves III, IV and VI and eye movements

- It is best to assess the function of these cranial nerves together as they are all involved in the movement of the eye. Cranial nerve III (the oculomotor nerve) is responsible for all eye movements except for those for which cranial nerves

Then assess conjugate gaze by asking the patient to look at your hand and then at a finger on your other hand, and then from one to the other as quickly as possible. If there is an internuclear ophthalmoplegia (a lesion in the medial longitudinal fasciculus), there will be slow movement in the adducting eye and nystagmus in the abducting eye. If one eye is covered, or if convergence is attempted, adduction is normal, as this is a disorder of conjugate gaze. Internuclear ophthalmoplegia is usually caused by multiple sclerosis but may occasionally result from vascular lesions.

Cranial nerve III (oculomotor nerve)

You have already partly tested cranial nerve III (oculomotor nerve); however, you also need to test its innervation of the levator palpebrae superioris (allowing elevation of the upper eyelid), and its parasympathetic component, which causes a miosis (constricted pupil).

Cranial nerve IV (trochlear nerve)

This supplies motor innervation to the superior oblique muscle, allowing downward eye movement in the midline. The patient is likely to report diplopia on downward gaze and have difficulty with vision when walking downstairs or reading a book.

Cranial nerve VI (abducens nerve)

This motor nerve innervates the lateral rectus. A cranial nerve VI palsy results in an inability to abduct the orbit. The patient will report diplopia (double vision) on abduction of the affected eye.

Cranial nerve V (trigeminal nerve)

This has both sensory and motor functions, providing sensation to the face with ophthalmic, maxillary and mandibular branches and motor supply to the muscles of mastication (temporalis, masseter and pterygoid muscles).

When you are testing this nerve, test sensation in the distribution of each division and compare one side with the other. Remember the corneal reflex; this tests the sensory function of the trigeminal nerve but also motor function of cranial nerve VII, allowing them to blink in response to the stimulus.

When you are testing the motor function:

- Ask the patient to clench the teeth.
- Ask the patient to keep the mouth open and resist you trying to shut the jaw.
- Then test jaw jerk, which is increased in pseudobulbar palsy (an upper motor neurone lesion) and reduced or absent in bulbar palsy (a lower motor neurone lesion).

The causes of cranial nerve V lesions are shown in Table 2.18.

Cranial nerve VII (facial nerve)

This nerve has sensory and motor functions: supplying the sensation of taste from the floor of the mouth, the soft palate and anterior two-thirds of the tongue and motor supply to the muscles of

Table 2.18 Causes of a trigeminal nerve lesion

Anatomical site	Examples
Brainstem	Tumour, infarction, demyelination, syringobulbia
Cerebellopontine angle	Acoustic neuroma, meningioma
Petrous temporal bone	Trauma, tumour, middle ear disease, herpes zoster
Cavernous sinus	Tumour, thrombosis, aneurysm of internal carotid artery
Peripheral	Meningeal tuberculosis, syphilis, lymphoma, carcinoma, sarcoid

Table 2.19 Causes of facial nerve palsies

Anatomical site	Examples
Upper motor neurone central	Stroke, tumour
Lower motor neurone pons angle	Stroke, tumour, demyelination, motor neurone disease
Cerebellopontine angle	Acoustic neuroma, meningioma
Petrous temporal bone	Bell palsy, herpes zoster (Ramsay Hunt syndrome)
Middle ear disease	Infection, tumour
Peripheral	Trauma, parotid disease, mononeuritis multiplex, sarcoid, Guillain–Barré syndrome

facial expression and the stapedius muscle. It also carries parasympathetic nerve fibres to the salivary and lacrimal glands.

The sensory part of this nerve is not usually examined formally, but ask the patient if he or she has noticed any change in taste, or increased sensitivity to high-pitched or loud sounds from impaired function of the stapedius muscle.

To test the main motor functions of this nerve, ask the patient to wrinkle the forehead, screw the eyes tightly shut, show the teeth and blow the cheeks out. Table 2.19 summarizes the causes of facial nerve palsies.

HINTS AND TIPS

When you are assessing power for both cranial nerves and with neurological examination of the limbs, it is often best to test resistance. For example, get the patient to screw the eyes shut and say, 'screw your eyes tight shut and stop me from opening them' or 'blow out your cheeks and stop me from squashing them' (you can demonstrate the blowing out of cheeks). This is a good way of assessing power and facilitating communication of these actions, which the patient may find hard to understand.

CLINICAL NOTES

In lower motor neurone lesions affecting cranial nerve VII, all the muscles are affected. In upper motor neurone lesions, the forehead is spared (e.g., there is normal eye closure and wrinkling of the forehead).

HINTS AND TIPS

Crossed signs – cranial nerve abnormalities contralateral to limb abnormalities – should alert you to the possibility of a brainstem lesion.

Cranial nerve VIII (vestibulocochlear nerve)

This nerve provides sensation to the utricle, saccule and semicircular canals (vestibular) and to the organ of Corti (cochlea).

To assess the function, ask the patient if he or she has noticed any difficulty with hearing. Assess the ability of the patient to hear whispered numbers with the other ear covered.

CLINICAL NOTES

There are two important tests you should perform: a Rinne test and a Weber test. To perform a Rinne test, place a vibrating tuning fork on the mastoid process and then at the external auditory meatus. The test result is positive if the sound is louder when the fork is held at the external auditory meatus (i.e., air conduction) than when placed on the mastoid process (i.e., bone conduction). This is normal. An abnormal test result (Rinne negative) indicates conductive deafness.

If there are concerns about ability to hear, perform the Weber test to differentiate between a sensorineural and conductive deafness. This is done by placing a vibrating tuning fork at the centre of the forehead. The sound will be heard towards the normal ear in sensorineural deafness or towards the affected ear in conductive deafness.

Vestibular disease is discussed further in Chapter 22. The causes of conductive and sensorineural deafness are described in Table 2.20.

Cranial nerve IX (glossopharyngeal nerve)

This supplies sensation to the pharynx and carotid sinus and taste to the posterior third of the tongue. It has motor functions,

Table 2.20 Causes of deafness

Type	Examples
Conductive	Wax, foreign body, otitis externa, injury to tympanic membrane, otitis media, otosclerosis (e.g., Paget disease), middle ear tumour (e.g., cholesteatoma)
Sensorineural	Presbycusis (due to old age), noise-induced, drugs (aminoglycosides, aspirin overdose), infection (meningitis, syphilis, measles), congenital (maternal rubella, cytomegalovirus, toxoplasmosis), Ménière disease, acoustic neuroma, trauma, Paget disease

Table 2.21 Causes of glossopharyngeal, vagus and accessory nerve palsies

Anatomical site	Examples
Central (brainstem)	Tumour, infarction, syringobulbia, motor neurone disease
Peripheral	Tumour or aneurysm near the jugular foramen, trauma of skull base, Guillain–Barré syndrome, poliomyelitis

supplying the stylopharyngeus muscle. It also carries parasympathetic nerve fibres to the parotid gland.

This nerve is tested simultaneously with the vagus nerve (cranial nerve X).

Cranial nerve X (vagus nerve)

This has sensory and motor functions; it provides sensation to the larynx, and motor innervation to the cricothyroid and the muscles of the pharynx and larynx. It carries parasympathetic nerve fibres to the bronchi, heart and gastrointestinal tract.

The glossopharyngeal nerve (cranial nerve IX) and vagus nerve (cranial nerve X) are tested simultaneously by assessment of palatal movement (ask the patient to say 'Aah'). Lesions cause reduced palatal elevation on the affected side, with the uvula pulled towards the normal side.

Check for a gag reflex; this tests the sensory function of the glossopharyngeal nerve and motor innervation of the vagus nerve.

Cranial nerve XI (accessory nerve)

This provides motor innervation to some muscles of the soft palate and larynx and the trapezius and sternocleidomastoid muscles. Test the function of this nerve by asking the patient to shrug the shoulders, and resist as you attempt to press them down. Then ask the patient to turn his or her head against your resisting hand, and test the sternocleidomastoid muscle bulk.

Causes of glossopharyngeal, vagus and accessory nerve palsies are summarized in Table 2.21.

Cranial nerve XII (hypoglossal nerve)

This provides the motor supply to the styloglossus, hyoglossus and all intrinsic muscles of the tongue. Test this nerve by asking the patient to open the mouth. Look for wasting and fasciculation. This indicates a lower motor neurone lesion of the tongue. Then ask the patient to protrude the tongue. If the tongue

deviates to one side, this suggests a hypoglossal nerve lesion. If it is a lower motor neurone lesion, the tongue will deviate towards the side of the lesion; with an upper motor neurone lesion it will deviate away from the side of the lesion.

> **CLINICAL NOTES**
>
> Upper motor neurone lesions are due to stroke, tumour or motor neurone disease.
>
> Lower motor neurone lesions affecting the hypoglossal nerve are due to diseases in the posterior fossa, skull base and neck, including tumour, motor neurone disease, syringobulbia, trauma and poliomyelitis.

Upper limb

Visual survey

When you are performing a neurological examination, good inspection is key. Look carefully for:

- Muscle wasting: seen with lower motor neurone lesions, muscle disease and disuse.
- Fasciculation: a feature of a lower motor neurone lesion;
- Scars, particularly from surgery.
- Deformity, which may cause mononeuropathy by entrapment and contractures may be the result of neurological disease.
- Tremor (Table 2.22).

Tone

Reduced tone is a feature of a lower motor neurone lesion or cerebellar lesion. Increased tone, hypertonia, is a feature of an upper motor neurone lesion. Hypertonia may manifest itself as either spasticity or rigidity. 'Spasticity' describes the sudden build-up of increased tone during the first few degrees of passive movement. The resistance lessens as the movement is continued, and this is characteristic of upper motor neurone

Table 2.22 Causes of tremor

Type	Features	Causes
Resting	Seen when patient relaxed with hands at rest	Parkinsonism
Postural	Seen when hands held outstretched	Benign essential tremor Anxiety Thyrotoxicosis β_2-agonists
Intention	Seen when patients try to touch examiner's finger with their own finger	Cerebellar disease

Table 2.23 Medical Research Council grading system for muscle power

Grade	Features
0	No muscle contraction and no movement at all
1	Muscle contraction visible, but no joint movement
2	Movement only when gravity excluded
3	Movement can overcome gravity but not resistance from the examiner
4	Movement can overcome gravity and move against some resistance from the examiner
5	Normal power against resistance

lesions. This is often described as the 'clasp-knife' phenomenon. 'Rigidity' describes the sustained resistance to passive movement seen in extrapyramidal conditions (e.g., parkinsonism). This may be described as 'lead pipe' rigidity, and when associated with a tremor gives rise to 'cogwheel' rigidity.

Power

All muscle groups should be tested and scored (Table 2.23). You will need to learn the root value for each movement (Fig. 2.3). Remember to compare muscle power of one side with muscle power of the other side for each group.

Look for pronator drift by asking the patient to hold the arms outstretched, hold the palms upward and close the eyes. Marked weakness will be easily apparent. If an upper motor neurone lesion affecting the parietal lobe is present, the arm will drift downwards and the hand will pronate.

Coordination

Ask the patient to alternately touch his or her nose and your finger. In cerebellar disease, there will be an intention

tremor and past pointing (i.e., the patient overshoots the examining clinician's finger consistently towards the side of the lesion). Ask the patient to tap one palm with alternating sides of the other hand as quickly as possible (demonstrate to the patient what you would like the patient to do). In cerebellar disease, this will be slow and poorly coordinated and the action of the moving hand has a high amplitude – this is dysdiadochokinesis.

Reflexes

Practice as often as you can. Test the biceps, triceps and supinator reflex, and learn the root value for the reflex (Fig. 2.4). Reflexes can be reduced, normal or increased. They will be reduced or absent in lower motor neurone lesions, sensory neuropathy and severe muscle disease (disruption of reflex arc), and will be exaggerated in upper motor neurone lesions.

Sensation

Test each dermatome (Fig. 2.5) for the sensation of light touch, pinprick and temperature. Then, starting distally, check vibration and joint position sense. Remember the different pathways these senses take (Fig. 2.6). The tests for the various sensory modalities are shown in Table 2.24.

Lower limb

Visual survey

Like the upper limbs, look for wasting, fasciculation and scars. Specific to the lower limb, take time to look at the feet. Look for ulceration (may suggest a lack of pain reception). Look at the soles, for pes cavus, high arched sole, a feature of hereditary motor and sensory neuropathy type 1 (formerly known as Charcot–Marie–Tooth disease) and Friedreich ataxia.

Tone

This is best assessed with the patient relaxed on the bed, and rolling patient's leg from side to side. Then pick up the patient's knee to a flexed position and note how easy it is to flex the relaxed leg. Test for clonus, present with upper motor neurone lesion. This is best elicited at the ankle through quick dorsiflexing of the foot of the patient. The patient's foot will beat up and down if clonus is present; more than five beats is significant.

Power

In the lower limbs, as for the upper limbs, test all muscle groups and score them using the Medical Research Council grading system for power (see Table 2.23), and consider the nerve roots (see Fig. 2.3).

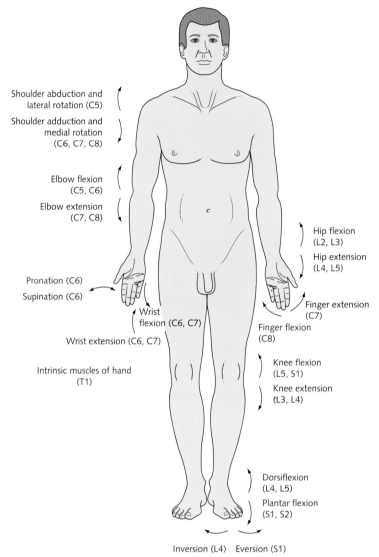

Shoulder abduction and lateral rotation (C5)

Shoulder adduction and medial rotation (C6, C7, C8)

Elbow flexion (C5, C6)

Elbow extension (C7, C8)

Pronation (C6)

Supination (C6)

Wrist flexion (C6, C7)

Wrist extension (C6, C7)

Intrinsic muscles of hand (T1)

Hip flexion (L2, L3)

Hip extension (L4, L5)

Finger extension (C7)

Finger flexion (C8)

Knee flexion (L5, S1)

Knee extension (L3, L4)

Dorsiflexion (L4, L5)

Plantar flexion (S1, S2)

Inversion (L4)   Eversion (S1)

Fig. 2.3 Nerve roots for each muscle group movement.

Coordination

To check coordination in the lower limbs, ask the patient to lift the leg, place the heel on the knee of the opposite leg and gently run it down the shin and repeat this motion. In cerebellar disease, this will be slow and clumsy.

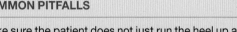

COMMON PITFALLS

Make sure the patient does not just run the heel up and down the shin. The movement should be down the shin and then up in an arc back to the knee, otherwise coordination is not being appropriately assessed.

Reflexes

Test reflexes at the knee and ankle and check plantar responses. This is normally downgoing but will be upgoing in upper motor neurone lesions, giving a Babinski response (see Fig. 2.7).

HINTS AND TIPS

Reflexes can be hard to elicit, in particular the ankle reflex. Ensure the patient is at ease and the muscle is relaxed. Use of reinforcement techniques such as asking the patient to clench the teeth or pull on clasped hands when you are trying to elicit the reflex can help.

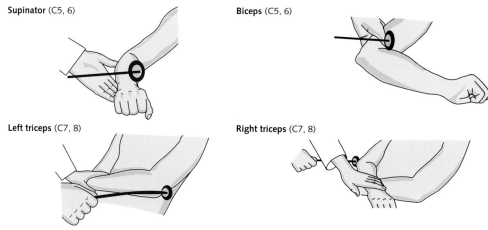

Supinator (C5, 6)

Biceps (C5, 6)

Left triceps (C7, 8)

Right triceps (C7, 8)

Fig. 2.4 Eliciting reflexes. Upper limb tendon reflexes.

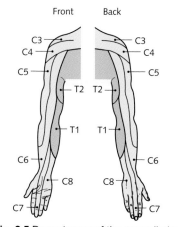

Front   Back

C3 — C3
C4 — C4
C5 — C5
T2 T2
T1 T1
C6 — C6
C8 C8
C7 — C7

Fig. 2.5 Dermatomes of the upper limbs.

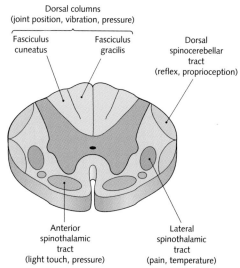

Dorsal columns
(joint position, vibration, pressure)

Fasciculus
cuneatus

Fasciculus
gracilis

Dorsal
spinocerebellar
tract
(reflex, proprioception)

Anterior
spinothalamic
tract
(light touch, pressure)

Lateral
spinothalamic
tract
(pain, temperature)

Fig. 2.6 Anatomy of sensory pathways within the spinal cord.

Table 2.24 Tests for different sensory modalities

Sensation	Tested using	Pathway	Level of decussation
Pain	Neurotip	Lateral spinothalamic tract	At level of sensory root within one spinal segment
Temperature	Tuning fork for cold	Lateral spinothalamic tract	At level of sensory root within one spinal segment
Light touch	Cotton wool	Anterior spinothalamic tract	At level of sensory root within several spinal segments
Vibration	Tuning fork	Posterior columns (fasciculus gracilis and fasciculus cuneatus)	Medulla oblongata
Joint position sense	Move fixed joints	Posterior columns (fasciculus gracilis and fasciculus cuneatus)	Medulla oblongata
Two-point discrimination	Orange stick	Posterior columns (fasciculus gracilis and fasciculus cuneatus)	Medulla oblongata

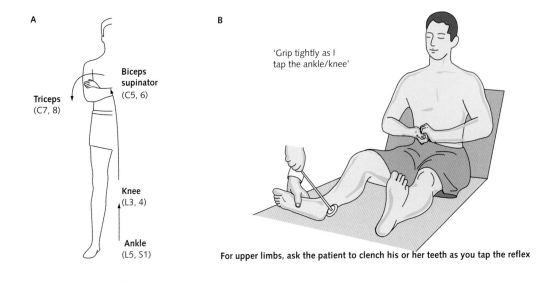

A

Triceps
(C7, 8)

Biceps
supinator
(C5, 6)

Knee
(L3, 4)

Ankle
(L5, S1)

B

'Grip tightly as I
tap the ankle/knee'

For upper limbs, ask the patient to clench his or her teeth as you tap the reflex

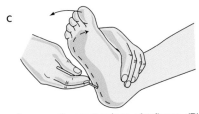

C

Fig. 2.7 Eliciting reflexes. (A) A simple way to remember root values of reflexes. (B) Testing ankle jerk with reinforcement. (C) The normal response is a downgoing hallux. In an upper motor neurone lesion, the hallux dorsiflexes and other toes fan out (the Babinski response).

Sensation

Test different modalities of sensation, as per the upper limb. See Table 2.24. Look for patterns. Is there the glove and stocking distribution sensation loss (a feature of diabetic neuropathy), or is the sensation dermatomal (Fig. 2.8)?

CLINICAL NOTES

A glove and stocking distribution does not follow a dermatomal distribution but affects peripheral nerves. When you are assessing the patient for this, test sensation distally and work your way proximally, noting a sensory level. Test the different modalities of sensation, touch, pain, temperature and proprioception in this way on both feet and arms. Lower limbs are more commonly affected than hands.

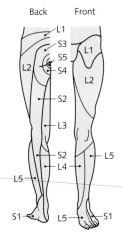

Back   Front

L1
S3
S5
L2   S4
L1
L2
S2
L3
S2   L5
L4
L5
S1   L5   S1

Fig. 2.8 Dermatomes of the lower limbs.

When you are assessing proprioception (joint position sense), it is best to start with the big toe. Get the patient to close their eyes. Hold either side of the interphalangeal joint and move the toe up and down, telling the patient which is which to orient the patient. Then move the toe and ask the patient which way has it moved (up or down?) If the patient lacks proprioception in the toe, move on to the ankle. Loss of proprioception is commonly seen in diabetes, and is a feature of dorsal column disease.

Sensory testing is difficult and subjective. A thorough inspection and examination of tone, power, coordination and reflexes may help to predict which sensory abnormality should be expected.

Gait

An immense amount of information can be gained by careful study of a patient's gait; for this reason you may wish to start your neurological examination by getting the patient to walk. In clinical practice, pay careful attention to how your patient walks into your clinic room. Observe the symmetry of the gait, the smoothness, how comfortably the patient turns and how many steps this takes, the height of the step and whether there is any evidence of pain. To test gait, ask your patient to walk for 2 to 3 m, turn and walk back, then walk heel to toe (cerebellar ataxia) and finally stand on toes and on heels (any muscle weakness will now manifest itself).

Whilst the patient is standing, perform a Romberg test. Do this by asking the patient to stand with the eyes closed. This assesses posterior column function (proprioception).

PATIENT SAFETY

Make sure you are ready to catch the patient should the patient become unsteady with the Romberg test, and when asking the patient to walk.

MUSCULOSKELETAL EXAMINATION

When you are examining a joint, use a systematic look, feel and move approach. Look around the bed and at the patient as a whole, not just the joint in question. Diseases affecting the musculoskeletal system are discussed in detail in Chapter 35.

Visual survey

Look at the patient. Does the patient look well or ill?

Look for any evidence of systemic connective tissue disorders, such as features of systemic sclerosis (microstoma, telangiectasia, sclerodactyly), or systemic lupus erythematosus (butterfly rash), or evidence of long-term steroid use (cushingoid facies, buffalo hump, thin skin and bruising); see Chapter 33. Note the patient's posture (e.g., any kyphoscoliosis suggestive of ankylosing spondylitis or osteoporosis) and any rashes (e.g., psoriatic rash).

Look

- Deformity.
- Scars: previous surgery.
- Erythema: acute inflammation or infection.
- Swelling: osteophytes, gouty tophi, synovial hypertrophy and acute inflammation.
- Muscle wasting: disuse, nerve entrapment, mononeuritis multiplex or long-term steroid therapy.

Feel

- Increased temperature: acute inflammation or infection.
- Tenderness.
- Effusions.
- Crepitus on movement.

Move

- Assess both active (patient moves his or her own limb) and passive movement (you move the patient's limb).
- Is pain associated with movement?
- Is the joint stable? Are there intact ligaments and supporting musculature?

Assessment of disability

It is very important to get an impression of how limiting the joint problem is. For example, in a patient with rheumatoid arthritis, ask the patient to undo some buttons or write their name with a pen.

Hands

Examining the hands makes up an important part of the general musculoskeletal examination and can be very informative when you are looking for evidence of underlying arthritic diseases. It is common for you to be asked to examine the hands. This should be performed in the same way as examination of a joint, using the look, feel, move and assessment of disability approach.

First get the patient to put his or her hands on a white sheet or pillow. Take time to inspect the hands, nails and elbows. Note any erythema, rashes, swelling, bony deformity, muscle wasting, scars and rheumatoid nodules (seen at the back of the elbow). Feel across each joint in turn, examining them for warmth and swelling. If they are swollen ask yourself if it is a spongy/boggy swelling or if it is hard and bony. Assess power of movement of fingers and wrist, in particular abduction of the thumb in the palmar position, testing the median nerve, and abduction of the fingers against resistance, testing the ulnar nerve, and interphalangeal extension of the thumb against resistance, testing the radial nerve. Go on to examine the functional use of the hand (e.g., ask the patient to undo a button or pick up a pen). This is particularly important in neurological abnormalities and destructive arthritides (e.g., rheumatoid arthritis).

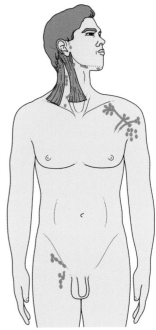

Fig. 2.9 Examination of lymph node sites.

HINTS AND TIPS

When you are examining the hands, always look at the elbows for a psoriatic rash, rheumatoid nodules or gouty tophi. Most information can be gained from inspection; do not rush this part of the examination. Always ensure you do not cause the patient pain. Ask them if their hands are painful before you start.

SKIN AND LYMPHADENOPATHY

The clinical approach to rashes will be discussed in detail in Chapter 24. When you are asked to look at a rash, you will be awarded marks for giving a good description, even if you are unable to make a diagnosis. Remember to describe:

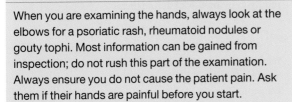

- Distribution: this can be diagnostic in itself.
- Shape.
- Size.
- Colour.
- Consistency.
- Temperature.
- Tenderness.

- Margins.
- Relation to the surface: raised, flat or ulcerated.
- Fixation to underlying structures.

When you are examining a patient for lymphadenopathy, it is important to examine all lymph node sites (Fig. 2.9). Always examine the cervical lymph nodes standing behind the patient. The causes of generalized and localized lymphadenopathy are discussed in Chapter 25. If lymphadenopathy is present, pay special attention to examination of the spleen and liver.

BREAST EXAMINATION

Breast examination should be performed in women who have symptoms of breast disease or when an underlying malignancy is suspected. Occasionally it is also necessary in men. Follow the systematic approach of inspection, palpation and movement. Pay close attention to the nipple. Is it inverted? Look for overlying skin changes or dimpling. Palpate the breast moving clockwise around the nipple, and feel for any masses. If any masses are found, note the size, texture, regularity, tenderness and whether they are fixed to the muscle (see Box 2.2). Do not forget that breast tissue extends into the axillae. Palpate the breast for lymph nodes. Ask the patient to move his or her hands behind the head; this can help assess whether the mass is fixed to muscle. A breast examination must be approached sensitively with a full explanation. Ask for a female chaperone; this is important and helps put the patient at ease and protects you against accusations of inappropriate behaviour.

NECK EXAMINATION

In clinical examinations, when you are asked to examine the neck, there will usually be a thyroid mass or lymphadenopathy. However, do not forget the salivary glands, branchial cyst, pharyngeal pouch, cervical rib, carotid body tumour and cystic hygroma. Causes of lymphadenopathy are described in Chapter 25. Table 2.25 lists the causes of thyroid enlargement.

First, look very carefully at the neck. Look for obvious masses, scars, skin changes or deformity. If there is a mass in the region of the thyroid gland, ask the patient to take a sip of water into the mouth and then swallow – a goitre will move upwards on swallowing. In addition, ask the patient to open the mouth and then watch as the tongue protrudes – a thyroglossal cyst will move upwards. Stand behind the patient to palpate the neck for a mass. If a mass is present, assess its properties as described in Box 2.2. Percussion is useful to determine retrosternal extension of a goitre. Bruits may be audible in the thyroid gland (thyrotoxicosis) or carotid artery (atheroma). If you find a thyroid mass, you should go on to assess thyroid status as shown in Table 2.26.

HINTS AND TIPS

If the neck is normal, examine the jugular venous pressure, listen to the carotid artery for bruits and reexamine the patient for a cervical rib.

Table 2.25 Causes of thyroid gland enlargement

Form of enlargement	Causes
Diffuse enlargement (goitre)	Idiopathic Physiological: puberty, pregnancy Autoimmune: Hashimoto and Graves diseases Iodine deficiency: endemic, e.g., Derbyshire neck Thyroiditis: de Quervain thyroiditis (viral), Riedel thyroiditis (autoimmune) Drugs: carbimazole, lithium, sulphonylureas Genetic: dyshormonogenesis (Pendred syndrome)
Solitary nodule	Thyroglossal cyst Prominent nodule in multinodular goitre Adenoma Cyst Carcinoma (papillary, follicular, anaplastic, medullary) Lymphoma

Table 2.26 Examination of thyroid status

	Hyperthyroidism	Hypothyroidism
Mood	Irritability, anxiety	Depression, slowness
Weight	Underweight	Overweight
Hands	Fine tremor, palmar erythema, sweaty palms, acropachy[a]	Puffiness, anaemia, Tinel sign (carpal tunnel syndrome)
Pulse	Tachycardia, atrial fibrillation	Bradycardia
Face	Lid lag, lid retraction, exophthalmos,[a] ophthalmoplegia,[a] chemosis[a]	Loss of outer third of eyebrow, puffy eyes and face causing characteristic appearance, xanthelasmata
Skin	Pretibial myxoedema (shins)[a]	Dry, thin hair
Neuromuscular	Proximal myopathy	Slow-relaxing ankle jerks, cerebellar signs

[a]Feature that is specific to Graves disease.

Chapter Summary

- Communicate effectively with patient to explain process, get consent, address concerns to make comfortable.
- Carefully position and expose areas needed while maintaining privacy as much as possible.
- Conduct visual assessment by looking over patient and surroundings, note observations.
- Tailor examination based on clinical situation - full exam may not be advisable for unstable patient.

Writing in the medical notes

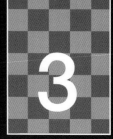

3

GENERAL PRINCIPLES

Writing in the medical notes includes any form of clinical documentation that you undertake. It includes 'clerking' (a written summary of the patient's history and examination), recording the ward round, documenting discussions with the patient, the patient's friends and family or other healthcare professionals or any other communication relating to patient care. Any documentation you make is a legal record, and should be precise, complete and legible. You will see many abbreviations in most medical notes you read, and you will need to be familiar with the most common ones (Table 3.1). If you choose to use abbreviations, you should consider if the meaning will be the same to other healthcare professionals, if they could be interpreted differently by professionals in a different specialty or in a different hospital or if a non-medically trained person were to read them. Best practice is to avoid the use of abbreviations for these reasons.

When you are documenting your clerking, the 'history of presenting complaint' section is a useful place to document the most relevant positive and negative historical points. Less relevant details can be recorded in their appropriate subsection. For example, in the case presented here, the relevant negative historical points have been included in the 'history of presenting complaint' rather than elsewhere in the clerking.

At the end of the clerking, the salient points should be emphasized in a summary statement. You should then compile a 'problem list'. This is often forgotten by students and junior doctors alike, but is invaluable in planning appropriate investigations and management. In some patients, it will not be appropriate, or even possible, to take a full history and perform a full clinical examination (e.g., in an emergency situation). We have outlined a clinical example.

As a student, it is good practice to be very thorough as it helps you to learn the relevant questions and to avoid missing anything important. However, with practice, you will learn to tailor carefully the clinical approach to each patient based on individual, and often very different, needs.

Table 3.1 Common abbreviations used in medical documentation

Abbreviation	Meaning
Titles	
• OT	• Occupational therapy/therapist
• PT	• Physiotherapy/physiotherapist
• SALT	• Speech and language therapy/therapist
Dosing	
• OD	• Once daily
• OM	• Every morning
• ON	• Every night
• BD	• Twice daily
• TDS	• Three times daily
• QDS	• Four times daily
• PRN	• Pro re nata (as required)
History	
• ATSP	• Asked to see patient
• PC	• Presenting complaint
• HPC	• History of presenting complaint
• DHx	• Drug history
• NKDA	• No known drug allergies
• FHx (FamHx)	• Family history
• SHx (SocHx)	• Social history
Examination	
• AE	• Air entry
• BS	• Bowel sounds
• CN	• Cranial nerve
• CP	• Chest pain
• CR	• Capillary refill
• HS	• Heart sounds
• MSK	• Musculoskeletal
• PEARLA	• Pupils equal and reactive to light and accommodation
• SNT	• Soft nontender
• SOB	• Shortness of breath
• WOB	• Work of breathing
Other	
• CA	• Cancer
• CAMHS	• Child and Adolescent Mental Health Services
• DNA	• Did not attend
• FU	• Follow up
• GA	• General anaesthetic
• RTA	• Road traffic accident

SAMPLE CLERKING

Hospital No. X349282   BLOGGS, Joe   DOB 29/4/54
                                                                     63 year old man

01/01/2018 07.20   Referred by General practitioner

PC   shortness of breath

> 1. Presenting complaint should be brief, but it is helpful to mention relevant background information.

HPC   4-day history of worsening dyspnoea. Gradual onset over hours.
            Initially noted while climbing stairs at home. Over the last 12 hours
            has become short of breath at rest. No periods of relief since onset.
            Relieving/exacerbating factors:
            Relieved by rest. Exacerbated by exertion.
            Associated symptoms:
            Cough productive of green sputum for 3 days.
            Sharp left sided posterior chest pain worsened by coughing and inspiration.
            Feels 'feverish'.
            Relevant direct questions:
            Usually unlimited exercise tolerance
            Lifelong non-smoker
            No asthma, tuberculosis exposure, occupational exposure to
            chemicals or asbestos.
            No pets or travel abroad
            No haemoptysis, worsening of chest pain on exertion, ankle swelling, calf pain
            palpitations, trauma to chest wall, orthopnoea or paroxysmal nocturnal dyspnoea.

> 2. Mention only the relevant negatives.

> 3. A useful way of recording important negatives on one line.

PMH   1971   appendectomy
            1980   duodenal ulcer (no symptoms since)

            No diabetes, hypertension, rheumatic heart disease, epilepsy, jaundice, cerebrovascular disease

S/E   General - fatigue lately, appetite unchanged, weight stable, no sweats or pruritus
            CVS - as above
            RS - As above
            GIT - No current indigestion. No symptoms like previous duodenal ulcer.
                        No vomiting/dyspnoea/abdominal pain
            GUS - No urinary symptoms
            NS - No headache/syncope. No dizziness/limb weakness/sensory loss. No disturbed vision/
                        hearing/smell/speech
            MS - No joint pain/stiffness/swelling. No disability
            Skin - No rash/pruritus/bruising

DH   No regular or over the counter medication.
            Penicillin allergy - facial swelling and
            rash as young child

> 4. Always record the dose and frequency of any drugs – remember you'll be writing the drug chart later! Always document that you have asked about drug allergies.

Fam Hx   Father died of 'heart attack' aged 60
            Mother died of 'old age' at 96

Social Hx   Lives with wife who is fit and well
            Own house. stairs
            Completely independent
            Never smoked
            Alcohol: 24 units per week
            Sexual history: not appropriate
            No recent overseas travel
            No pets
            Occupation: hotel porter

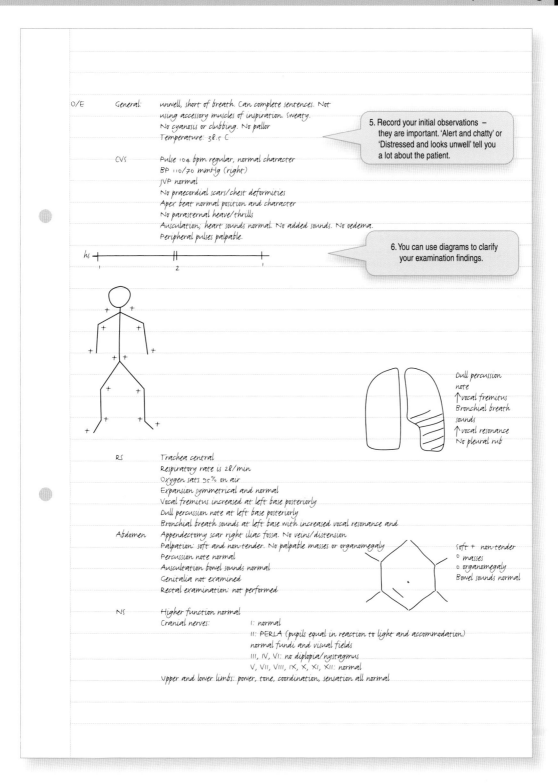

O/E General: unwell, short of breath. Can complete sentences. Not
using accessory muscles of inspiration. sweaty.
No cyanosis or clubbing. No pallor
Temperature: 38.5 C

5. Record your initial observations –
they are important. 'Alert and chatty' or
'Distressed and looks unwell' tell you
a lot about the patient.

CVS Pulse 104 bpm regular, normal character
BP 110/70 mmHg (right)
JVP normal
No praecordial scars/chest deformities
Apex beat normal position and character
No parasternal heave/thrills
Ausculation; heart sounds normal. No added sounds. No oedema.
Peripheral pulses palpable.

6. You can use diagrams to clarify
your examination findings.

Dull percussion
note
↑vocal fremitus
Bronchial breath
sounds
↑vocal resonance
No pleural rub

RS Trachea central
Respiratory rate is 28/min
Oxygen sats 95% on air
Expansion symmetrical and normal
Vocal fremitus increased at left base posteriorly
Dull percussion note at left base posteriorly
Bronchial breath sounds at left base with increased vocal resonance and

Abdomen Appendectomy scar right iliac fossa. No veins/distension
Palpation: soft and non-tender. No palpable masses or organomegaly
Percussion note normal
Auscultation bowel sounds normal
Genitalia not examined
Rectal examination: not performed

soft + non-tender
° masses
° organomegaly
Bowel sounds normal

NS Higher function normal
Cranial nerves: I: normal
II: PERLA (pupils equal in reaction to light and accommodation)
normal fundi and visual fields
III, IV, VI: no diplopia/nystagmus
V, VII, VIII, IX, X, XI, XII: normal
Upper and lower limbs: power, tone, coordination, sensation all normal

Reflexes		Right	Left
	Biceps	++	++
	Supinator	++	++
	Triceps	++	++
	Knee	++	++
	Ankle	+	+
	Plantar	↓	↓

Joints and skin	Normal
Summary	63 year old male non-smoker presents with a 4 day history of worsening exertional dyspnoea associated with a productive cough, pleuritic left sided chest pain and symptoms of fever.
	On examination he is short of breath and tachypnoeic. He has a pyrexia and signs of consolidation at the left base. The most likely diagnosis is left-sided community acquired pneumonia.
Problem list	Dyspnoea? Left basal pneumonia.
	Penicillin allergy.
Plan	Full blood count, Urea and Electrolytes, C-Reactive protein
	Blood and sputum for microscopy and culture
	Chest X-ray
	CURB-65 score when blood results available
	Antibiotics as per local protocol
	Arterial Blood Gas
	Urine for pneumococcus/legionella antigens
	Intravenous access and fluid
	Senior Review

> 7. Sign your notes, including printed surname and bleep number.

Oliver Leach,
ST2 medicine
Bleep 1234

Clinical Presentations

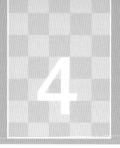

Chest pain | 4

INTRODUCTION

Chest pain is one of the commonest reasons for hospital attendance. The causes can range from a simple musculoskeletal strain to a life-threatening myocardial infarction (MI) (Table 4.1). A thorough clear assessment is essential in making the correct diagnosis and identifying or excluding a serious cause needing immediate hospital treatment.

CLINICAL NOTES

DIFFERENT TYPES OF PAIN AND THEIR DIFFERENTIAL DIAGNOSIS

Central chest pain

The differential diagnosis of pain in the centre of the chest includes:

- Angina: crushing/tightness.
- Acute coronary syndromes (ACS): angina-like but commonly long-lasting and with associated symptoms (see Chapter 28).
- Dissecting aortic aneurysm: tearing interscapular pain.
- Oesophagitis: burning.
- Oesophageal spasm.

Pleuritic chest pain

This is sharp pain caused by irritation of the pleura that is worse on deep inspiration, coughing or movement. The differential diagnosis includes:

- Pneumothorax.
- Pneumonia.
- Pulmonary embolism.
- Pericarditis: retrosternal (see Chapter 28).

Chest wall tenderness

The differential diagnosis of chest wall tenderness includes:

- Rib fracture.
- Shingles (herpes zoster): pain precedes rash; dermatomal distribution.
- Costochondritis (Tietze syndrome).

CLINICAL NOTES

DEFINITION OF ANGINA-TYPE PAIN

The National Institute for Health and Care Excellence (NICE) describes angina pain as:

- Constricting discomfort in the anterior chest, neck, shoulders, jaw or arms.
- Precipitated by physical exertion.
- Relieved by rest or glyceryl trinitrate within 5 minutes.

HISTORY AND EXAMINATION FINDINGS

History

A carefully taken history will lead to the most likely underlying diagnosis and determine whether the chest pain is of cardiac origin. Once this has been established, enquire about the presence of cardiovascular risk factors, previous investigations for chest pain and history of coronary heart disease and any previous treatment.

Table 4.1 Differential diagnosis in chest pain

Cardio-vascular	Respiratory	Gastrointes-tinal	Musculoskel-etal
Angina	Pneumonia	Gastritis	Rib fracture
ACS/myocardial infarction	Pulmonary embolism	Pancreatitis	Varicella zoster
Pericarditis	Pneumothorax	Gastro-oesophageal reflux disease and spasm	Costochondritis
Dissecting aortic aneurysm		Biliary colic/cholecystitis	Vertebral

ACS, *Acute coronary syndromes.*

Type of chest pain

Onset and progression

Cardiac ischaemic pain typically builds up over a few minutes and may be brought on by exercise, emotion or cold weather. In angina, the pain resolves on resting or with the use of glyceryl trinitrate. It is often reproducible with consistent effort. Spontaneous pneumothorax and pulmonary embolism (PE) usually cause sudden onset of pleuritic pain and breathlessness.

CLINICAL NOTES

NICE advises that the following symptoms may indicate ACS:

- Pain in the chest and/or other areas (the arms, back or jaw) that lasts more than 15 minutes.
- Chest pain associated with nausea and vomiting, marked sweating, breathlessness or a combination of these.
- Chest pain associated with haemodynamic instability.
- New-onset chest pain, or abrupt deterioration in previously stable angina, with frequent recurrent episodes that last more than 15 minutes and are brought on by little or no exertion.

Site and radiation

Cardiac ischaemia and pericarditis cause retrosternal pain. With ischaemia, the pain is tight and crushing, band-like, etc., often radiating to the neck, jaw or arms. Pericarditis produces pleuritic chest pain; it is classically worse on lying flat and relieved by sitting up and leaning forward. A dissecting aortic aneurysm causes tearing pain radiating through to the back. Pulmonary disease may cause unilateral pain, which the patient can often localize specifically. Oesophageal disease can also cause retrosternal pain mimicking cardiac pain. Referred pain from vertebral collapse or shingles will follow a dermatomal pattern.

Nature of pain

The precise nature of the pain gives important clues as to the underlying diagnosis. Most commonly the pain is dull/tight or sharp/stabbing.

Associated symptoms

Important associated symptoms include:

- Breathlessness: PE, pneumonia, pneumothorax, pulmonary oedema, hyperventilation in anxiety (these patients will often report dizziness and tingling in their lips and extremities which is due to respiratory alkalosis).
- Cough: purulent sputum in pneumonia, haemoptysis in PE, frothy pink sputum in pulmonary oedema.
- Rigors: pneumonia (particularly lobar pneumococcal pneumonia).
- Palpitations: arrhythmia (e.g., new-onset atrial fibrillation) can cause angina or result from cardiac ischaemia, PE or pneumonia.
- Clamminess, nausea, vomiting and sweating are features of MI or massive PE.

CLINICAL NOTES

RISK FACTORS

Important risk factors include:

- Coronary heart disease: smoking, family history, hypercholesterolaemia, hypertension, diabetes, chronic kidney disease.
- Pulmonary embolism: recent travel, immobility, surgery, family history, pregnancy, malignancy, nephrotic syndrome, oral contraceptive pill use.
- Pneumothorax: spontaneous (young, thin men, more commonly smokers), trauma, emphysema, asthma, malignancy, Marfan syndrome.

RED FLAG

In patients with altered pain perception (e.g., diabetes) MI can present without the classical symptoms such as chest pain. This can also be the case in the elderly where pain can be a minor feature.

Examination

The examination should focus on determining the cause of the pain, and then looking for risk factors and consequences of the underlying problem. A schematic guide to examining the patient with chest pain is given in Fig. 4.1. Remember to assess the patient for the presence of complications of ACS (e.g., pulmonary oedema, cardiogenic shock). Patients with aortic dissection will have a discrepancy in blood pressure between the left and right arms and possibly a murmur of aortic regurgitation. Patients with tension pneumothorax, massive PE or MI will be shocked.

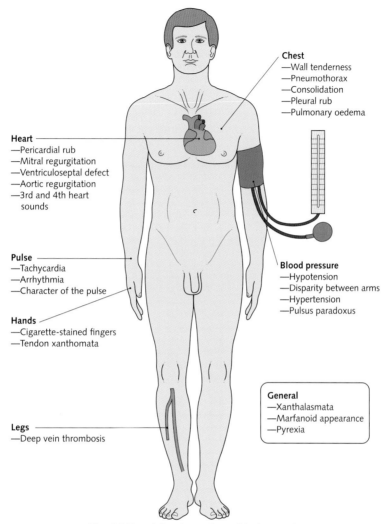

Fig. 4.1 Examining the patient with chest pain.

Chest
—Wall tenderness
—Pneumothorax
—Consolidation
—Pleural rub
—Pulmonary oedema

Heart
—Pericardial rub
—Mitral regurgitation
—Ventriculoseptal defect
—Aortic regurgitation
—3rd and 4th heart
  sounds

Blood pressure
—Hypotension
—Disparity between arms
—Hypertension
—Pulsus paradoxus

Pulse
—Tachycardia
—Arrhythmia
—Character of the pulse

Hands
—Cigarette-stained fingers
—Tendon xanthomata

General
—Xanthalasmata
—Marfanoid appearance
—Pyrexia

Legs
—Deep vein thrombosis

HINTS AND TIPS

Patients who have a median sternotomy scar are common in final examinations. This most commonly represents previous heart surgery (e.g., coronary artery bypass graft, valve replacement). Always check the legs for vein harvesting scars and listen for a metallic valve sound.

INVESTIGATIONS

Consider the following investigations in a patient presenting with chest pain:

- Resting 12-lead ECG: regional ST-segment elevation or presumed new left bundle branch block (LBBB) should be treated as ACS until proven otherwise (Table 4.2). Regional ST-segment depression or deep T-wave inversion suggests a non-ST-segment elevation MI or unstable angina. A normal ECG does not exclude ACS, and serial ECGs are often helpful. Changes suggestive of PE are listed in the Clinical Notes box later. Look for signs of ventricular hypertrophy (Fig. 4.2) and arrhythmias.
- Chest X-ray: look for signs of heart failure, pneumothorax, consolidation (pneumonia), widened mediastinum (aortic dissection), pulmonary oedema, wedge infarct (PE) and fractured ribs.
- Full blood count, urea and electrolytes, glucose, C-reactive protein (CRP), liver function tests: look for anaemia,

Table 4.2 Causes of ST-segment elevation on ECG

Cause	Distribution of ST-segment elevation
Myocardial infarction	Inferior aVF, II, III Anteroseptal V_{1-4} Lateral I, aVL, V_{4-6} Posterior V_7, V_8, V_9 (posteriorly placed leads)
Pericarditis	Across all leads (saddle-shaped ST change)
Prinzmetal angina	Leads of affected coronary artery (spasm)
Aortic dissection	Only if coronary artery involved
Left ventricular aneurysm	Persistent elevation for 6 months following infarct

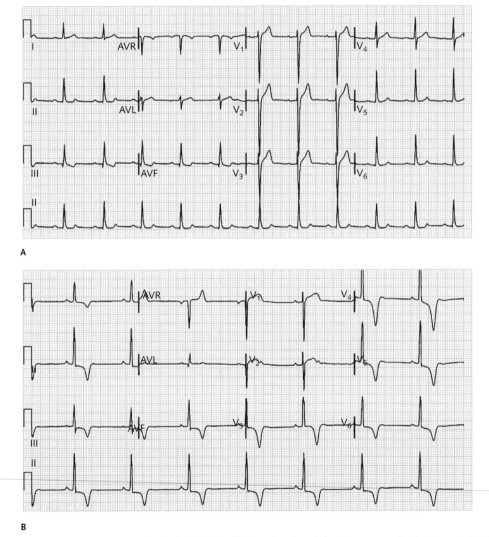

Fig. 4.2 Left ventricular hypertrophy, shown in 12-lead ECGs. (A) Note the size of the S wave seen in V_1 (26 mm); S in V_1 + R in V_6 = >35 mm. (B) Left ventricular hypertrophy in a patient with hypertrophic cardiomyopathy, with additional repolarization changes of deep T-wave inversion in leads V_3–V_6 and leads I, II, III and AVF. (From Feather A, Randall D, Waterhouse M. *Kumar and Clark's Clinical Medicine.* 10th ed. Elsevier; 2021.)

leucocytosis, electrolyte disturbances, hyperglycaemia, signs of inflammation, cholecystitis or pancreatitis.

- Cardiac markers: troponin I and troponin T are biological markers of cardiac muscle death, and measurement of their levels can be used to signify the occurrence of myocardial ischaemia. Troponin levels are classically measured at 4 hours and 10 to 12 hours after the onset of pain. Serial measurements are useful.
- Echocardiography: can be used acutely to demonstrate cardiac dysfunction, valvular pathology, pericardial effusion and aortic dissection (particularly transoesophageal echocardiography, see Chapter 28).
- Percutaneous coronary intervention: angioplasty and coronary artery stenting can be used to reopen occluded arteries in acute MI. Coronary angiography allows direct visualization of the coronary arterial anatomy (see Chapter 28).
- Other tests to exclude alternative diagnoses including PE (see Chapter 5) and gastro-oesophageal reflux disease (see Chapter 10).

CLINICAL NOTES

ECG changes associated with pulmonary embolism
- Sinus tachycardia
- Atrial arrhythmia (e.g., atrial fibrillation)
- Right-sided heart strain
- Right axis deviation
- Right bundle branch block
- $S_1Q_3T_3$ (i.e., deep S wave in lead I, Q wave in lead III, T-wave inversion in lead III)

HINTS AND TIPS

Although troponin is a useful enzyme to investigate potential myocardial ischaemia, its level may also be raised in renal impairment, heart failure, sepsis, PE, acute pericarditis, myocarditis and aortic dissection. Serial measurements are useful to assess trends and point towards the diagnosis.

HINTS AND TIPS

Although not always possible, it is very useful to compare the ECG done in the acute setting with an old ECG. Changes such as left bundle branch block and T-wave inversion may indeed be long-standing, which would alter your management.

● Chapter Summary

- Numerous underlying diseases can present as chest pain.
- In patients presenting with a history of chest pain suggestive of a cardiac origin, acute coronary syndromes (ACS) should be excluded.
- ACS is a medical emergency and needs immediate treatment.
- Troponin is a cardiac biomarker usually measured at 4 hours and 10 to 12 hours from the onset of pain.
- Patients presenting with ACS should be urgently assessed for reperfusion therapy. See Chapter 28 for detailed recommendation.
- A new left bundle branch block should be treated as ACS until proven otherwise.

UKMLA Conditions
Acute coronary syndromes
Aortic aneurysm
Aortic dissection
Arrhythmias
Pulmonary embolism
Deep vein thrombosis

UKMLA Presentations
Chest pain
Breathlessness

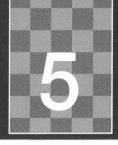

Shortness of breath 5

INTRODUCTION

Shortness of breath (dyspnoea) is the subjective sensation of breathlessness, which is excessive for a given level of activity. Dyspnoea may be due to any of the following:

- Pulmonary disease: disorders of the airways, lung parenchyma, pleura, pulmonary vasculature, respiratory muscles or chest wall.
- Cardiac disease: right or left ventricular dysfunction, arrhythmias, ischaemic heart disease, valvular disease;
- Systemic diseases (e.g., anaemia, thyrotoxicosis or ketoacidosis).
- Nonorganic causes (e.g., anxiety or chronic hyperventilation syndrome).

HISTORY AND EXAMINATION FINDINGS

History

Onset
The onset of breathlessness and rate of progression helps indicate its cause. It can be thought of in terms of acute or chronic onset – see Table 5.1).

Severity
Exercise tolerance is a good measure of how severe the dyspnoea is (e.g., distance walked on the flat or on hills, while dressing or climbing stairs). Has this changed recently? Does it affect daily activities?

Precipitating and aggravating factors
- Precipitating factors: exercise increases the demand for oxygen and as such, many pulmonary and cardiac causes of dyspnoea are aggravated by exercise. Cold and airborne material (e.g., pollen) can irritate the airways and can cause dyspnoea in the context of bronchoconstriction. Dyspnoea that improves at weekends or on holiday may imply an environmental or occupational cause.
- Aggravating factors: position can affect dyspnoea; 'orthopnoea' is the term used for shortness of breath on lying flat. Paroxysmal nocturnal dyspnoea is breathlessness that wakes the patient from sleep. Both generally indicate underlying cardiac dysfunction.

COMMUNICATION

When you are clarifying the duration of symptoms, asking your patient 'When were you last well?' and then 'Take me through what has happened since' often opens the consultation better than the more direct 'How long has this been going on?'

COMMUNICATION

Asking the patient how many pillows they sleep on is a good way of quantifying the level of orthopnoea, and if this has changed, it helps to assess the severity.

Associated features
- Cough: a chronic persistent cough has many causes; for example, underlying lung disease, malignancy, asthma, gastro-oesophageal reflux, postnasal drip or drugs (especially angiotensin-converting enzyme inhibitors, where patients may have a dry cough). How long has the cough been present? Is the cough worse at any particular time of day?
- Sputum: how much does the patient produce? What does it look like?
- Haemoptysis: coughing up blood, either frank blood or blood-tinged sputum. It needs to be distinguished from haematemesis and nasopharyngeal bleeding (see Chapter 6).
- Stridor: a harsh sound caused by turbulent airflow through a narrowed airway. Inspiratory stridor suggests upper airway obstruction, and may indicate impending airway compromise, which requires urgent evaluation by someone with appropriate expertise. Inspiratory and expiratory stridor can indicate fixed obstruction.
- Wheeze: a whistling noise, most commonly in expiration caused by turbulent airflow through narrowed intrathoracic airways. Present in conditions such as asthma, chronic obstructive pulmonary disease (COPD) and pulmonary oedema.
- Pain: is the dyspnoea associated with pain? Acute onset of both symptoms may be cardiac acute coronary syndrome (ACS) or trauma (rib fracture). Is the pain pleuritic in nature indicating a pulmonary embolism or pneumothorax?

Table. 5.1 Differential diagnosis of dyspnoea

	Respiratory	Cardiac	Systemic	Other
Acute	Asthma exacerbation COPD exacerbation PE Pneumonia Pneumothorax	Pulmonary oedema Arrhythmia Tamponade	Anaphylaxis Metabolic acidosis	Anxiety Foreign body
Chronic	Bronchiectasis COPD Pleural effusion Pulmonary fibrosis	Heart failure Valvular disease	Anaemia Malignancy	Chronic hyperventilation syndrome

---

HINTS AND TIPS

Asthma typically has a nocturnal cough. Chronic bronchitis-associated cough is often worse in the morning.

Other factors

- Occupational history, including exposure to asbestos and dusts: changing the working environment may relieve symptoms.
- Known lung disease: current, such as asthma, or previous, such as tuberculosis.
- History of atopy: asthma, seasonal allergic rhinitis (hay fever) or eczema.
- Pets: can exacerbate asthma or cause chronic lung diseases (extrinsic allergic alveolitis, e.g., 'pigeon fanciers' lung').
- Current medications: noncardioselective β-blockers may exacerbate wheeze.
- Previous medications: can cause interstitial lung disease (amiodarone, bleomycin).
- Angina or previous myocardial infarction: symptoms of cardiac dyspnoea.
- General health: e.g., weight loss, appetite.
- Recent foreign travel.
- Smoking tobacco, marijuana and other inhaled compounds.
- Contacts: friends, family or colleagues unwell.

Examination

The examination of the respiratory system is covered in Chapter 2. Findings of common respiratory conditions are listed in Table. 5.2, and the approach to examining a patient with breathlessness is summarized in Fig. 5.1. For more detailed description of examination findings in respiratory disease, see Chapter 29. In those with shortness of breath, the following are important to consider.

Inspection/palpation

- Shape of the chest and chest movements. A barrel-shaped chest is common in COPD. Kyphoscoliosis may affect chest expansion and therefore effectiveness of respiration. Paradoxical abdominal movement may indicate diaphragmatic weakness.
- Assess the pattern of breathing (clinical note: patterns of respiration).
- Central cyanosis (bluish discolouration of the buccal mucosa due to excess deoxygenated haemoglobin).
- Tar staining of the fingers.
- Clubbing: respiratory causes include carcinoma, suppurative lung disease (e.g., empyema, lung abscess, bronchiectasis, cystic fibrosis), interstitial lung disease, tuberculosis and mesothelioma.
- Cervical lymphadenopathy: malignant disease (lung cancer or metastatic disease) or infection (upper or lower respiratory tract infections, pneumonia).
- Trachea: deviation may indicate underlying chest or cardiac disease.

Auscultation

- Expiration: may be prolonged in COPD.
- Breath sounds: diminished over an effusion, pneumothorax and in an obese person.
- Bronchial breathing: consolidation, cavitation or at the top of an effusion.
- Rhonchi or wheeze: partially obstructed bronchi; found in asthma, COPD and occasionally left ventricular failure. If polyphonic, this usually suggests multiple small-airway narrowing. If monophonic and fixed, it can indicate a fixed single obstruction (e.g., a central malignant lesion).
- Crepitations or crackles (sudden opening of small closed airways): pulmonary congestion (fine crepitations in early inspiration); fibrosing alveolitis (fine crepitations in late inspiration); bronchial secretions (coarse crepitations).

Table. 5.2 Findings on examination of common respiratory conditions

Condition	Movement on side of lesion	Position of trachea	Percussion	Tactile vocal fremitus	Breath sounds
Pleural effusion	↓	Central or deviated away from effusion if massive	↓ ('stony dull')	↓	↓ with bronchial breathing at top of effusion
Pneumothorax	↓	Central or deviated away	↑	↓	↓
Pneumonia	↓	Central or deviated towards the affected side if associated with collapse	↓	↑	Increased vocal resonance Bronchial breathing (absent if obstruction of bronchus) Coarse crepitations
Pulmonary fibrosis	↓	Central or deviated towards the affected side if upper lobe involvement	↓	↑	Fine crepitations

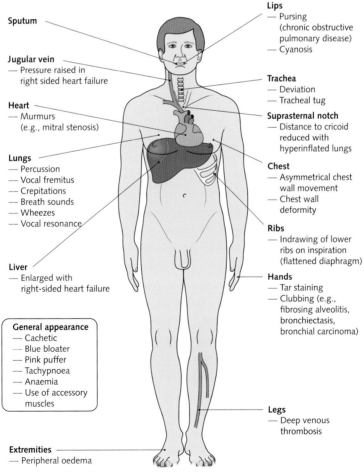

Lips
— Pursing (chronic obstructive pulmonary disease)
— Cyanosis

Trachea
— Deviation
— Tracheal tug

Suprasternal notch
— Distance to cricoid reduced with hyperinflated lungs

Chest
— Asymmetrical chest wall movement
— Chest wall deformity

Ribs
— Indrawing of lower ribs on inspiration (flattened diaphragm)

Hands
— Tar staining
— Clubbing (e.g., fibrosing alveolitis, bronchiectasis, bronchial carcinoma)

Legs
— Deep venous thrombosis

Sputum

Jugular vein
— Pressure raised in right sided heart failure

Heart
— Murmurs (e.g., mitral stenosis)

Lungs
— Percussion
— Vocal fremitus
— Crepitations
— Breath sounds
— Wheezes
— Vocal resonance

Liver
— Enlarged with right-sided heart failure

General appearance
— Cachetic
— Blue bloater
— Pink puffer
— Tachypnoea
— Anaemia
— Use of accessory muscles

Extremities
— Peripheral oedema

Fig. 5.1 Examining the patient with breathlessness.

Central cyanosis is visible when there is more than 5 g of deoxygenated haemoglobin per 100 mL of blood. Despite this, it is an unreliable guide to the severity of hypoxaemia, it is difficult to appreciate in anaemic patients and it is common in patients who have polycythaemia associated with chronic respiratory and cardiac disease. Peripheral cyanosis can be due to poor peripheral circulation (e.g., cardiac failure, peripheral vascular disease, cold environment).

CLINICAL NOTES

Lip pursing is common in patients with COPD and alveolar air trapping. Pursing the lips allows the creation of positive end-expiratory pressure, which eases the work of breathing.

CLINICAL NOTES

PATTERNS OF RESPIRATION

- Cheyne–Stokes respiration: cyclical variation in the depth of breathing with periods of rapid and deep inspiration and apnoea. Causes include neurological disease (brainstem lesions, raised intracranial pressure), left ventricular failure and altitude sickness.
- Kussmaul respiration: deep and laboured breathing. It is most often associated with metabolic acidosis.
- Biot respiration: periodic breathing characterized by quick shallow inspirations followed by apnoea. Causes include pontine damage and opioid use.

HINTS AND TIPS

Always look in the sputum pot:
- Purulent, moderate quantity – bronchitis or pneumonia.
- Purulent, copious quantity – bronchiectasis or pneumonia.
- Pink and frothy – pulmonary oedema.
- Blood stained – causes of haemoptysis.
- Rust coloured – pneumococcal lobar pneumonia.

INVESTIGATIONS

Acute presentation

- Full blood count: anaemia; leucocytosis in pneumonia.
- Urea and electrolytes: renal failure.
- Blood glucose: diabetic ketoacidosis.
- Chest X-ray: hyperexpanded lungs in COPD; consolidation in pneumonia; lack of lung markings in pneumothorax; blunting of the costodiaphragmatic angle(s) in pulmonary effusion or empyema; ground glass opacifications in infections or malignancy. Cardiomegaly in heart failure; fluid in the horizontal fissure, upper lobe pulmonary venous diversion, air space opacifications classically in a batwing distribution in pulmonary oedema.
- Electrocardiogram: to look for evidence of
  - acute or chronic cardiac disease (acute myocardial infarction, arrhythmias);
  - respiratory disease (right axis deviation, P pulmonale, low voltage QRS).
- Arterial oxygen saturation: easy to perform and may obviate the need for blood gas analysis.
- Arterial blood gases: pH, Po_2 and Pco_2, base excess, bicarbonate concentration and lactate level (see Chapter 29).
- Computed tomography (CT) scanning: used to assess causes of both acute and chronic dyspnoea.

HINTS AND TIPS

Nail varnish, in particular red nail varnish, will interfere with pulse oximetry measurements and should be removed.

Chronic presentation

- Spirometry: distinguish between obstructive and restrictive lung pathology. This is best done for diagnosis when the patient is not acutely unwell. Lying and standing vital capacity will screen the patient for diaphragm weakness.
- Peak expiratory flow rate: useful for assessing acute decline, especially in asthmatic patients who often know their best results.
- Full pulmonary function tests: transfer factor, flow–volume loop and lung volumes.
- Bronchoscopy: if an endobronchial lesion is suspected.
- Echocardiogram: assess cardiac structure and function, including pulmonary hypertension.
- CT scanning: to diagnose and quantify interstitial lung disease, bronchiectasis and malignancies.

HINTS AND TIPS

The upper lobes of the lungs are best heard on the anterior chest wall, middle lobe in the axilla and lower lobes on the posterior chest wall.

● Chapter Summary

- Shortness of breath can be a manifestation of disease of different systems, including respiratory, cardiovascular, metabolic and neurological.
- Careful history taking and examination will guide you towards the cause. Suspected disease will guide investigations.

UKMLA Conditions
Acute coronary syndrome
Arrhythmias
Asbestos-related lung disease
Asthma
Bronchiectasis
Cardiac failure
Chronic obstructive pulmonary disease
Cystic fibrosis
Fibrotic lung disease
Influenza
Lower respiratory tract infections
Lung cancer
Metastatic disease
Occupational lung disease
Pneumonia
Pneumothorax
Pulmonary embolism
Pulmonary hypertension
Upper respiratory tract infection

UKMLA Presentations
Breathlessness
Chest pain
Cough
Cyanosis
Pain on inspiration
Pleural effusion
Stridor
Wheeze

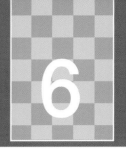

Cough and haemoptysis

INTRODUCTION

Cough is a reflex reaction to irritation anywhere in the respiratory tract from the pharynx to the alveoli. A chronic cough lasts more than 8 weeks and a cough lasting more than 3 weeks should be investigated (see Chapter 29). Haemoptysis is the coughing of blood from the respiratory tract. This chapter covers the approach to a patient presenting with a cough and/or haemoptysis, followed by potential differential diagnoses.

HISTORY AND EXAMINATION FINDINGS

History

The nature of the cough may help in diagnosis (Table 6.1). Assess the following in patients with cough or haemoptysis:

- Onset: acute or chronic?
- Character: dry or productive cough? Fresh or old blood? Are there clots?
- Severity.
- Associated factors: is the cough worse at night? Is there postnasal drip?
- Weight loss or other systemic symptoms? Think of carcinoma or lung abscess.
- Has the patient been in contact with any person with any infections? Think of COVID-19 and tuberculosis, especially in at-risk patient groups.
- History of recent foreign travel?
- History of chest trauma?
- Any gastro-oesophageal reflux disease? The lack of overt indigestion or waterbrash does not exclude reflux as a cause of chronic cough.
- Drug history – particularly angiotensin-converting enzyme (ACE) inhibitors. 10% to 20% of people taking ACE inhibitors report having a dry, tickly cough (related to increased levels of bradykinin). Angiotensin receptor blockers are better tolerated as they do not interact with the bradykinin activation pathway.
- Do they smoke? Cigarette smoke can cause a cough by acting as an irritant but is also strongly associated with bronchial malignancy.

- Occupational agents or exposure to dusts that might account for the cough.

Examination

A full respiratory examination should be undertaken, of which the approach to the examination is summarized in Fig. 6.1. See also Chapters 2, 5 and 29. If available, inspection of sputum (in sputum pot or tissues) is useful to review colour and consistency as well as amount of haemoptysis.

INVESTIGATIONS

Bedside

- Vital signs: heart rate, respiratory rate, oxygen saturations, temperature.
- Sputum: microscopy, culture and cytology, acid-fast bacillus test for tuberculosis.
- Nasal/throat swabs: influenza, COVID-19.
- Peak expiratory flow rate.

Table 6.1 Conditions with characteristic cough

Pressure on trachea	'Brassy' cough—hard and metallic
Tracheitis	'Hot poker' cough—often associated with retrosternal pain
Laryngeal nerve paralysis (e.g., secondary to tumour)	'Bovine' cough – often associated with hoarse voice
Laryngitis (e.g., croup)	'Seal' cough – barking, hoarse cough
Pharyngitis	'Hacking' cough – frequent, irritating
Small airways (e.g., asthma)	'Wheezy' cough – often associated with shortness of breath

Blood tests

- Full blood count: anaemia is associated with malignancies, a raised white cell count is associated with infection and pulmonary eosinophilia is associated with several intrinsic and extrinsic conditions (see clinical notes: conditions associated with eosinophilia).

- Urea and electrolytes: vasculitis can affect renal function; electrolytes may be deranged in malignancy (e.g., small cell carcinoma releasing antidiuretic hormone (ADH)); urea level may be raised if bleeding is not haemoptysis but haematemesis and used as a marker of severity in pneumonia (CURB-65 score – see Chapter 29).
- Arterial blood gas.

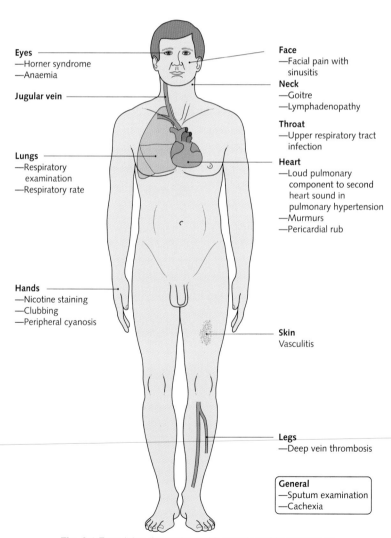

Eyes
—Horner syndrome
—Anaemia

Jugular vein

Lungs
—Respiratory examination
—Respiratory rate

Hands
—Nicotine staining
—Clubbing
—Peripheral cyanosis

Face
—Facial pain with sinusitis

Neck
—Goitre
—Lymphadenopathy

Throat
—Upper respiratory tract infection

Heart
—Loud pulmonary component to second heart sound in pulmonary hypertension
—Murmurs
—Pericardial rub

Skin
Vasculitis

Legs
—Deep vein thrombosis

General
—Sputum examination
—Cachexia

Fig. 6.1 Examining the patient with cough and haemoptysis.

CONDITIONS ASSOCIATED WITH EOSINOPHILIA

Intrinsic eosinophilic syndromes are most commonly autoimmune or idiopathic. These include:

- Chronic eosinophilic pneumonia.
- Eosinophilic granulomatosis with polyangiitis (previously known as Churg–Strauss syndrome): small and medium vessel vasculitis.
- Eosinophilic granuloma: the benign form of Langerhans cell histiocytosis; an interstitial lung disease.
- Asthma.
- Eosinophilic bronchitis without asthma.

Extrinsic eosinophilic syndromes are caused by inhaled or ingested extrinsic factors (e.g., pathogens, medications); these include:

- Loeffler syndrome: eosinophilic pneumonia in response to infection (most commonly parasitic).
- Drug rash with eosinophilia and systemic symptoms (DRESS) syndrome; a hypersensitivity reaction to a medication.
- Parasitic and fungal infections, schistosomiasis or infections with other pathogens.

Imaging

- Chest X-ray is the first-line investigation. It may reveal a pulmonary cause for presentation (e.g., pneumonia, carcinoma, bronchiectasis, bilateral hilar lymphadenopathy).
- Computed tomography (CT): to assess malignancy, interstitial lung disease and bronchiectasis.
- CT pulmonary angiogram: if pulmonary embolism is suspected. A V/Q (ventilation/perfusion) scan is an alternative imaging modality which reduces need for ionizing radiation.

Further investigations

Other investigations may be required as directed by initial tests and symptoms:

- Pharyngoscopy: if an upper respiratory tract cause is suspected.
- Bronchoscopy: with or without washings, brushings or biopsies (infection, malignancy).
- Endobronchial ultrasonography (EUS): with or without fine-needle aspiration (malignancy).
- Spirometry: if airway disease is suspected.
- Gastroscopy, barium swallow or 24-hour oesophageal pH recording: to investigate possible gastro-oesophageal reflux disease.

DIFFERENTIAL DIAGNOSIS

Cough

- Postnasal drip: rhinitis, sinusitis.
- Upper respiratory tract infections: viral or bacterial, causing laryngitis, tracheobronchitis, etc.
- Pressure on the trachea: e.g., from a goitre; this may be associated with stridor.
- Lower respiratory tract causes: acute infection – pneumonia, COVID-19, infective/noninfective exacerbation of chronic lung disease. Chronic – almost any lung disease may be associated with cough. Particularly asthma (classically a nocturnal cough), chronic obstructive pulmonary disease, bronchiectasis, interstitial lung disease or carcinoma.
- Left ventricular failure.
- Drugs: especially ACE inhibitors and irritants (e.g., occupational agents).
- Gastro-oesophageal reflux disease: reflux is a common cause of a chronic cough and may not be obvious from symptoms.
- Psychogenic/habitual cough.

Haemoptysis

- Acute infections: e.g., pneumonia, exacerbations of chronic obstructive pulmonary disease.
- Bronchiectasis: can be responsible for massive haemoptysis.
- Malignancy: bronchial carcinoma. Secondary malignancies and benign tumours can also lead to haemoptysis but are less common.
- Pulmonary tuberculosis.
- Other chronic infection: e.g., lung abscess, pulmonary aspergillosis.
- Pulmonary embolus: due to lung infarction.
- Left ventricular failure: typically, pink, frothy sputum.
- Alveolar haemorrhage: usually due to a systemic vasculitis (e.g., anti-glomerular basement membrane disease (Goodpasture syndrome) and granulomatosis with polyangiitis (previously known as Wegener granulomatosis)).
- Trauma: e.g., contusions to the chest, inhalation of foreign bodies or after intubation. In up to 15% of cases, no cause for haemoptysis is found.

CLINICAL NOTES

Rare causes of haemoptysis:

- Bleeding diatheses.
- Interstitial lung disease.
- Mitral stenosis.
- Idiopathic pulmonary haemosiderosis.

- Arteriovenous malformations: hereditary haemorrhagic telangiectasia (previously known as Osler–Weber–Rendu disease), a favourite in examinations but rare in practice.
- Eisenmenger syndrome.
- Pulmonary hypertension.
- Cystic fibrosis.

● Chapter Summary

- Cough can be of acute or chronic nature. Cough lasting more than 3 weeks in high-risk patients warrants further investigations.
- Haemoptysis without a known cause should always be investigated.
- Cough and haemoptysis are mainly caused by the dysfunction of the respiratory system but cardiac or gastrointestinal causes should also be considered.

UKMLA Conditions
Acute bronchitis
Adverse drug effects
Asthma
Bronchiectasis
Cardiac failure
Chronic obstructive pulmonary disease
Cough
COVID-19
Fibrotic lung disease
Gastro-oesophageal reflux disease
Influenza
Lower respiratory tract infection
Lung cancer
Metastatic disease
Occupational lung disease
Pneumonia
Pulmonary embolism
Tuberculosis
Upper respiratory tract infection

UKMLA Presentations
Breathlessness
Cough
Gastro-oesophageal reflux disease
Haemoptysis
Lower respiratory tract infection
Weight loss

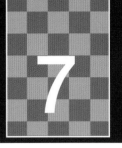

Palpitations 7

INTRODUCTION

Palpitations are a symptom where the patient is uncomfortably aware of and abnormally perceiving their heartbeat. The most common cause is an arrhythmia or dysrhythmia; other causes include conditions causing an increase in stroke volume (e.g., regurgitant valvular disease) or cardiac output (e.g., exercise, thyrotoxicosis, anaemia or anxiety). If an arrhythmia is suspected, determine whether there is an underlying cause. The differential diagnosis of palpitations is illustrated in Fig. 7.1.

HISTORY

A carefully taken history will often lead to the correct diagnosis and is especially important as, between episodes, examination and investigation findings may be unremarkable. Are the palpitations continuous or intermittent? Are they regular or irregular? When did the palpitations start? This can range from a few minutes to decades ago. If the onset dates back years and there have been no serious complications (e.g., syncope), the palpitations are usually benign (but you should enquire if there is any reason why your patient has chosen to seek help now).

How often do the palpitations occur and how long do they last? They may last for days or seconds, with intervals between episodes of a few hours to years. Are there any associated features? These may be related to the underlying cause (e.g., angina, features of hyperthyroidism) or may be a consequence of the palpitations (e.g., dizziness or syncope).

RED FLAG

Palpitations associated with exercise can indicate serious underlying pathology.

COMMUNICATION

Asking the patient to tap out the rhythm they have been experiencing may be a good way of characterizing an intermittent arrhythmia.

CAUSES AND CONTRIBUTING FACTORS

Ask about smoking, alcohol, work, stress, caffeine (tea, coffee, cola) intake and illicit drug use. These may contribute to extrasystolic beats.

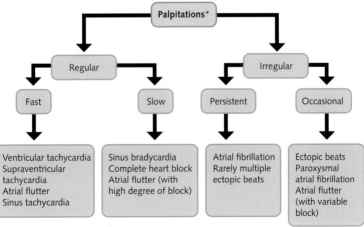

* Bradycardia is rarely referred to as palpitations.

Fig. 7.1 Differential diagnosis of palpitations.

A history of ischaemic and valvular heart disease (including rheumatic fever) should be sought. Structural heart problems are a predisposing factor for pathological arrhythmias.

A family history of palpitations or sudden cardiac death may be important (e.g., hypertrophic obstructive cardiomyopathy or long-QT syndromes).

Symptoms that point towards a sinister cause include breathlessness, chest pain and syncope or near syncope.

A full drug history of both prescribed and over-the-counter medications should be taken. Many drugs, both cardiac and noncardiac, can promote palpitations. Most antiarrhythmic drugs are also potentially pro-arrhythmic. Drug causes of palpitations include cardiac stimulants (dopamine, dobutamine), antimuscarinics (atropine), vasodilators (isosorbide mononitrate, losartan), antiarrhythmics (digoxin, flecainide, quinidine) and calcium channel blocker withdrawal (verapamil, diltiazem) or β-blocker withdrawal (bisoprolol, atenolol).

Noncardiac causes of palpitations include:

- Thyrotoxicosis: may cause sinus tachycardia, paroxysmal atrial tachycardia and atrial flutter/atrial fibrillation (AF).
- Anxiety: a very common cause of palpitations.
- Noncardiac causes of sinus tachycardia and causes of sinus bradycardia are outlined below.

CLINICAL NOTES

NONCARDIAC CAUSES OF SINUS TACHYCARDIA

- Exercise.
- Fever.
- Anaemia.
- Thyrotoxicosis.
- Pregnancy.
- Arteriovenous fistulae.
- Anxiety/emotional stress.
- Lack of sleep.
- Pain.
- Cigarettes, alcohol, caffeine.
- Sympathomimetic drugs (e.g., cocaine).

CLINICAL NOTES

CAUSES OF SINUS BRADYCARDIA

- Physiological (e.g., athletes)
- Hypothyroidism.
- Obstructive jaundice.

- Raised intracranial pressure.
- Hypopituitarism.
- Hypothermia.
- Cardiac causes: including ischaemia, drugs (e.g., digoxin, β-blockers), inflammation and degeneration/fibrosis.

CLINICAL NOTES

CONSEQUENCES OF PALPITATIONS

Palpitations can cause a range of problems, from minor anxiety to syncope or sudden death. If a benign arrhythmia is present, reassurance that the condition is not serious is often all that is required. Rate changes may be more serious, compromising coronary blood supply and leading to symptoms of myocardial ischaemia or cardiac failure.

Tachycardia or bradycardia may lead to a reduction in cardiac output and cause dizziness or collapse (e.g., Stokes–Adams attacks). Ventricular tachycardia (VT) is potentially life-threatening. Any broad complex tachycardia is VT unless proven otherwise.

CLINICAL NOTES

STOKE–ADAMS ATTACKS

Arrhythmia-mediated periodic syncope is most commonly associated with bradycardias in sick sinus syndrome, second-degree heart block or complete heart block. The syncope is a consequence of a brief period of loss of output with resultant hypoperfusion of the brain.

EXAMINATION

A guide to examining the patient with palpitations is given in Fig. 7.2. Look for signs of systemic diseases. Feel the pulse. Note:

- Rate: beats per minute. The pulse rate felt at the radial artery may be slower than the apical rate in AF (pulse deficit).

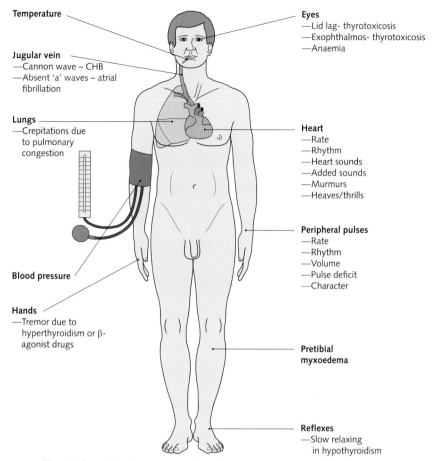

Temperature

Jugular vein
—Cannon wave – CHB
—Absent 'a' waves – atrial fibrillation

Lungs
—Crepitations due to pulmonary congestion

Blood pressure

Hands
—Tremor due to hyperthyroidism or β-agonist drugs

Eyes
—Lid lag- thyrotoxicosis
—Exophthalmos- thyrotoxicosis
—Anaemia

Heart
—Rate
—Rhythm
—Heart sounds
—Added sounds
—Murmurs
—Heaves/thrills

Peripheral pulses
—Rate
—Rhythm
—Volume
—Pulse deficit
—Character

Pretibial myxoedema

Reflexes
—Slow relaxing in hypothyroidism

Fig. 7.2 Examining the patient with palpitations. *CHB*, Complete heart block.

- Rhythm: regular, regularly irregular (e.g., Wenckebach second-degree heart block), irregularly irregular (e.g., multiple ectopic beats or AF).
- Volume/character: e.g., a collapsing pulse of hyperdynamic circulation or aortic regurgitation or a low-volume pulse of shock or aortic stenosis. Remember, this may be positional, so raising the arm above the heart may exaggerate a collapsing pulse.

The jugular venous pressure may be elevated if cardiac failure is present. A displaced apex beat may indicate cardiomyopathy. Feel for heaves and thrills with associated right ventricular enlargement and valvular heart disease.

HINTS AND TIPS

An irregularly irregular pulse is irregular in *both* rhythm and volume.

INVESTIGATIONS

The following tests should be considered.

- Bedside observations: pulse, blood pressure, respiratory rate, saturations, temperature.
- Full blood count: anaemia.
- Urea and electrolytes: disturbances of potassium or, less commonly, magnesium and calcium may contribute to refractory arrhythmias.
- Thyroid function tests: hypothyroidism/hyperthyroidism.
- Drug concentration if appropriate (e.g., digoxin levels in suspected toxicity).
- ECG: although this is mandatory for everyone with palpitations, paroxysmal events may not be caught on a resting 12-lead ECG. Wolff–Parkinson–White syndrome will be seen at rest, as will persistent AF. Ectopic beats may be seen. Look for signs of ischaemia. For infrequent

symptoms, a 24/48/72-hour ECG (Holter monitoring) may record the rhythm disturbance.

- It should be performed with a diary of symptoms to see if they correlate with any rhythm disturbances found. It can also help detect paroxysmal AF. Occasionally an implantable loop recorder is used (fitted subcutaneously, allows continuous recording and review of the heart rhythm for up to 3 years). See Table 7.1 for some common ECG features of some arrhythmias.
- Echocardiogram: to exclude any underlying structural heart disease.
- Exercise test: the induction of symptoms under controlled conditions with ECG monitoring may be appropriate.
- Electrophysiological studies: more rarely, patients may be referred for specialized studies. These can be used to induce arrhythmias, locate the origin of any arrhythmic foci, assess the response to drug treatment or destroy any aberrant pathway via radiofrequency ablation.

Table 7.1 ECG features of some arrhythmias

Arrhythmia	ECG features
AF	No distinct P-waves Irregularly irregular rhythm
Atrial flutter	Saw-tooth appearance Irregular rhythm Rate ~300 bpm Patterns include: 2:1, 3:1 and 4:1 (QRS complex rate of 150 bpm, 100 bpm and 75 bpm, respectively)
SVT	P-waves present but not identifiable due to the fast rate (150–300 bpm) QRS is regular and narrow (<120 ms)
VT	No P-waves Broad QRD complex (>120 ms) Rate ~160 bpm
Ventricular ectopics	Early wide abnormally shaped QRS complex No P-waves Abnormal T-wave

AF, *Atrial fibrillation;* SVT, *supraventricular tachycardia;* VT, *ventricular tachycardia.*

Chapter Summary

- Ensure that both you and the patient have the same understanding of the word palpitations.
- Palpitations can be of cardiac or noncardiac origin. They can be a manifestation of a sinister disease, and therefore need to be investigated.
- Worrying symptoms include dizziness, syncope, chest pain and breathlessness.
- Palpitations can be of regular or irregular character. The most common cause of regular palpitations is sinus tachycardia. The most common cause of irregular palpitations is atrial fibrillation.

UKMLA Conditions

Arrhythmias
Acute coronary syndromes
Aortic valve disease

UKMLA Presentations

Breathlessness
Chest pain
Dizziness
Palpitations

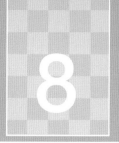
INTRODUCTION

Fever is a common symptom and often a cause is obvious (e.g., respiratory or urinary tract infection). Pyrexia of unknown origin (PUO) is defined as a temperature above 38.3°C measured on multiple occasions, present with an illness lasting at least 3 weeks and where a diagnosis has not been reached despite investigations. PUO is a challenging presentation for medical professionals. There may be a variety of causes, including infection, malignancy and autoimmune disease. Thorough clinical history taking and examination are essential for prompt diagnosis and management.

HISTORY AND EXAMINATION FINDINGS

The history and examination is vital and must be thorough in PUO. Systematic enquiry should be rigorous, with any symptoms explored in detail.

It is important to pay attention to:

- Symptoms such as sweats, weight loss, itch, lumps and rash.
- Past medical history, particularly recurrent infection and immunosuppression.
- Surgical history, including complications and trauma.
- Travel and contact with animals. Has there been exposure to endemic diseases or disease-carrying vectors (e.g., malaria, toxoplasmosis, borreliosis)?
- Sexual history.
- Drug history, including prescribed, over-the-counter, recreational and immunizations.
- Family history (may point to inherited disorders such as familial Mediterranean fever).

COMMUNICATION

A thorough sexual history is important and becomes easier to elicit with practice.

Examination of a patient with PUO should include all systems (Fig. 8.1). Consider the need for appropriate personal protective equipment (PPE). Ensure the following are reviewed:

- Teeth and throat signs (e.g., periodontal disease/dental abscess)
- Joint signs (including spinal tenderness) and temporal artery tenderness
- Eye signs (e.g., conjunctival petechiae)
- Skin lesions (e.g., rashes, petechiae, vasculitic infarction)
- Lymphadenopathy and organomegaly
- Heart murmurs and stigmata of endocarditis
- Rectal and vaginal examination findings (abscesses, masses, retained items)

INVESTIGATIONS

Investigations are best directed by the history and examination. Frequently there will be few clues, and general nonspecific screening tests may direct more specific investigations.

Bedside investigations

Blood tests

The full blood count may yield useful information, and although it is often nonspecific, it may show:

- Neutrophilia: bacterial infections, myeloproliferative disease, malignancy or connective tissue disease.
- Lymphocytosis: acute viral infection, chronic bacterial infection (e.g., tuberculosis (TB) and brucellosis) or protozoal infection. Atypical lymphocytosis can suggest infectious mononucleosis (Epstein–Barr virus (EBV)) or cytomegalovirus infection (CMV).
- Monocytosis: subacute bacterial endocarditis, inflammatory disease such as Crohn disease, connective tissue disease, Hodgkin lymphoma or TB.
- Eosinophilia: helminth infection (e.g., schistosomiasis, filariasis), malignancy (especially Hodgkin disease) or drug reaction.
- Leucopoenia: viral infections, lymphoma, systemic lupus erythematosus, TB or drugs.

Inflammatory markers such as C-reactive protein level (CRP) and erythrocyte sedimentation rate (ESR) are raised in many conditions and can be unspecific. CRP can be particularly high in viral infections. A significant rise in ESR can suggest:

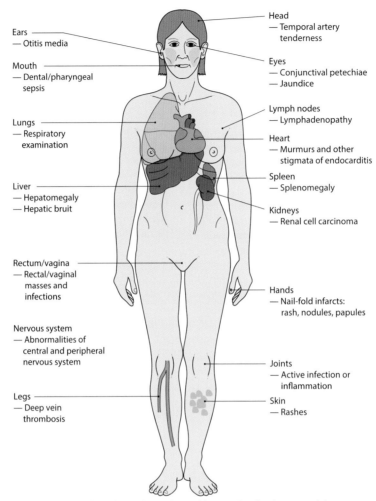

Fig. 8.1 Examining the patient with pyrexia of unknown origin.

- multiple myeloma;
- connective tissue disease (e.g., systemic lupus erythematosus, giant cell arteritis, polymyalgia rheumatica);
- Still disease;
- rheumatic fever;
- lymphoma.

Procalcitonin (PCT) testing is now often used as it is raised in proinflammatory states, particularly bacterial infection.

Renal and liver function tests are useful in narrowing down the cause of fever. Liver function tests showing raised alkaline phosphatase (ALP) level can point to biliary origin, bone disease, myeloproliferative disorder or connective tissue disease.

Many specific serological blood tests are available. They should be directed by clinical assessment. You should always ask for an HIV test, with the patient's consent.

Urinalysis

Urine dipstick may demonstrate presence of infection (leucocytes, nitrites, blood) and can be sent for microbiology testing (as discussed in the following section). Consider possible malignancy if nonvisible haematuria is persistent (see Chapter 15) or if presence of protein and blood, this may indicate glomerulonephritis (see Chapter 31).

Microbiology tests

Samples for microbiology testing can be taken from multiple sites, depending on indication, including:

- Urine: for infections, TB, sexually transmitted disease or haematuria.
- Blood cultures: for septicaemia.

- Culture of any indwelling lines (central venous catheters, Hickman lines).
- Faeces: for infections and inflammatory bowel conditions.
- Genital swabs: for sexually transmitted disease.
- Throat and nose swabs.
- Sputum samples.
- Wound swabs.
- Joint aspiration: for septic arthritis.
- Bone marrow.
- Cerebrospinal fluid.

Further investigations

Simple investigations including chest X-ray and ultrasound scan are first-line investigations. Further imaging including CT/MRI/positron emission tomography (PET) scans or echocardiogram can help.

When you are considering PUO, sometimes further investigations need to proceed 'blindly' rather than be directed by the clinical picture, simply because of lack of an apparent diagnosis. Noninvasive tests should be performed first, and can involve autoimmune antibody screening, immunoglobulins, protein electrophoresis and tumour markers.

DIFFERENTIAL DIAGNOSIS

The differential diagnosis associated with PUO is very wide ranging (Table 8.1). Infections including undiagnosed abscesses, TB, endocarditis, hepatobiliary infections (cholangitis) and osteomyelitis are common. Viral causes include herpes viruses and HIV. The most likely neoplasm which causes fever is lymphoma, although PUO can also be attributed to solid tumours, particularly renal cell and gastrointestinal carcinoma. Drug fever can be caused by antibiotics and is usually associated with rash. Rarer causes include hyperthyroidism, peripheral pulmonary emboli and familial Mediterranean fever.

> **HINTS AND TIPS**
>
> Remember to go over the history and examination findings repeatedly, even when investigations are in progress.

Table 8.1 Differential diagnosis of pyrexia of unknown origin

Causes	Percentage of cases
Infections	25–40
Autoimmune disorders	10–20
Malignancy	10–30
Miscellaneous (e.g., drugs, thyroid disorders)	5–14
Undiagnosed	15–20

Chapter Summary

- Persistent fever can prove problematic for medical professionals to diagnose when no cause can be found.
- When assessing PUO, ensure you conduct a thorough, systematic history and examination and that appropriate investigations are conducted to aid in diagnosis.
- The most common causes of PUO include infectious disease and malignancy, and therefore their prompt diagnosis will improve disease management and patient survival.

UKMLA Conditions
Fever
Human immunodeficiency virus
Lymphadenopathy
Malaria
Notifiable disease
Tuberculosis

UKMLA Presentations
Fever
Lymphadenopathy
Lymphoma
Night sweats
Organomegaly

Abdominal pain

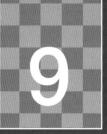

9

INTRODUCTION

Abdominal pain is a common presentation to the emergency department. The differential diagnosis is multiple, ranging from benign disease, such as mesenteric adenitis, to life-threatening causes, such as a ruptured abdominal aortic aneurysm. Consideration of the anatomical structures at the site of the pain will often provide clues to its cause. Table. 9.1 summarizes the common causes of abdominal pain in reference to the site.

HISTORY AND EXAMINATION FINDINGS

History

An 'acute abdomen' describes sudden-onset, severe abdominal pain that may signify a life-threatening condition. It presents as an emergency with no history of trauma, and requires urgent assessment. As with all pains, a certain number of key features should be elicited in the history.

The SOCRATES approach is an easy-to-remember, commonly used approach to taking a history of pain (see Hints and Tips).

It is also helpful to consider the underlying aetiology when classifying the type of abdominal pain. In broad terms, an acute abdomen is most often caused by one of the following:

1. Pain due to perforation or rupture of a viscus (e.g., ruptured aortic aneurysm or perforated colon). Described as sudden onset and severe.
2. Pain due to inflammation (i.e., peritonitis, hepatitis, cholecystitis). Described as gradual onset and consistent.
3. Pain due to obstruction of a hollow viscus (colicky type pain, e.g., gallstones, ureteric stones). Described as pain that 'comes and goes'.
4. Referred pain due to nerve root compression (e.g., pancreatic and aortic pain may radiate to the back as these are retroperitoneal structures, ureteric pain often radiates from 'loin to groin' and diaphragmatic irritation caused by subphrenic disease (e.g., an abscess) may cause pain which is referred to the shoulder tip.)

Associated symptoms may also direct to a particular cause of pain (see Hints and Tips).

Table 9.1 Differential diagnosis of abdominal pain

Site of pain	Causes
Epigastric	**Lower oesophagus**: oesophagitis, malignancy, perforation **Stomach**: peptic ulcer, gastritis **Pancreas**: pancreatitis, malignancy See Chapter 30
Right hypochondrium	**Biliary tree**: biliary colic, cholecystitis, cholangitis **Liver**: hepatitis, malignancy, abscess, right ventricular failure **Subphrenic space**: abscess See Chapters 29 and 30
Left hypochondrium	**Spleen**: traumatic rupture, infarction (sickle cell disease) **Pancreas**: pancreatitis, malignancy **Subphrenic space**: abscess See Chapter 30
Central abdomen	**Abdominal aorta**: ruptured aortic aneurysm **Pancreas**: pancreatitis, malignancy **Small/large bowel**: obstruction, perforation, intussusception, ischaemia, Crohn disease, lymphoma, IBS, adhesions, early appendicitis **Lymph nodes**: mesenteric adenitis, lymphoma See Chapter 30
Right iliac fossa	**Terminal ileum**: Crohn disease, infection (e.g., tuberculosis), Meckel diverticulum **Appendix**: appendicitis, tumour (including carcinoid) **Caecum/ascending colon**: diverticulitis, paracolic abscess, ulcerative colitis, malignancy **Ovary/fallopian tubes**: malignancy, ectopic pregnancy, pelvic inflammatory disease, cyst (bleeding or torsion) See Chapter 30
Left iliac fossa	**Sigmoid/descending colon**: diverticulitis, paracolic abscess, ulcerative colitis, malignancy **Ovary/fallopian tubes**: malignancy, ectopic pregnancy, pelvic inflammatory disease, cyst (bleeding or torsion) See *Crash Course: Obstetrics and Gynaecology*
Loin	**Kidneys**: malignancy, pyelonephritis, polycystic disease **Ureters**: colic due to stone or clot See Chapter 31
Suprapubic	**Bladder**: UTI, acute urinary retention **Uterus**: pregnancy (see *Crash Course: Obstetrics and Gynaecology*)
Other causes of abdominal pain	**Gynaecological**: pelvic inflammatory disease, endometriosis, pregnancy (see *Crash Course: Obstetrics and Gynaecology*) **Anxiety** (see *Crash Course: Psychiatry*) **Myocardial infarction** (especially inferior causing epigastric discomfort) (see Chapter 28) **Lower lobe pneumonia** (causing hypochondrial or loin pain) (see Chapter 29) **Vasculitis** (especially HSP and PAN) (see Chapter 35) **Diabetic ketoacidosis** (see Chapter 33) **Addison disease** (see Chapter 33) **Sickle cell crisis** (see Chapter 37) *Very rarely*: lead poisoning, porphyria, familial Mediterranean fever

HSP, Henoch–Schönlein purpura; IBS, irritable bowel syndrome; PAN, polyarteritis nodosa; UTI, urinary tract infection.

COMMUNICATION

It may be challenging to elicit a history from a patient who is in pain. Offer analgesia and antiemetics early. This will not only help build rapport between you and the patient but will also facilitate communication.

Examination

The first question that must be asked is, 'Is the patient acutely ill?' Signs of shock and peritonism should be looked for. The examination should then focus on specific signs. Fig. 9.1 summarizes the examination approach.

The typical patient with peritonism looks pale and sweaty. They often lie still, as movement exacerbates the pain. Look for

Table 9.2 Causes of peritonism	
Cause	**Examples**
Infection	Spread from paracolic/ subphrenic abscess following surgery or paracentesis
Chemical irritation (from solid organ perforation)	Bile Faeces Gastric acid Pancreatic enzymes
Transmural inflammation	Crohn disease Salpingitis

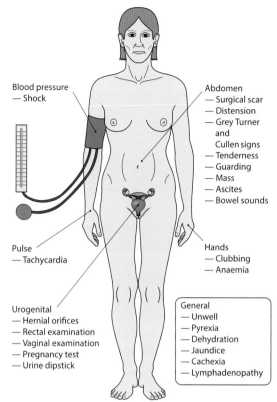

Blood pressure
— Shock

Pulse
— Tachycardia

Urogenital
— Hernial orifices
— Rectal examination
— Vaginal examination
— Pregnancy test
— Urine dipstick

Abdomen
— Surgical scar
— Distension
— Grey Turner and Cullen signs
— Tenderness
— Guarding
— Mass
— Ascites
— Bowel sounds

Hands
— Clubbing
— Anaemia

General
— Unwell
— Pyrexia
— Dehydration
— Jaundice
— Cachexia
— Lymphadenopathy

Fig. 9.1 Examining the patient with abdominal pain.

rebound tenderness (pain that becomes more severe when the examining hand is removed) and guarding (involuntary spasm of the abdominal wall on palpation). When peritonism becomes generalized, the abdomen will be rigid and bowel sounds may be scanty and high pitched or absent because of paralysis of peristalsis. Causes of peritonism are summarized in Table 9.2.

HINTS AND TIPS

SIGNS OF SHOCK

These include tachypnoea, tachycardia and hypotension, delayed capillary refill (beware that in early sepsis, the peripheries may be warm because of vasodilation) and reduced urine output. Consider sepsis (particularly gram-negative), severe bleeding (ruptured abdominal aortic aneurysm, splenic rupture), significant fluid loss (vomiting, diarrhoea, third spacing in bowel obstruction and pancreatitis) and, rarely, acute Addisonian crisis.

Clinical signs

- General
  - Pyrexia – high temperature (infection), low-grade pyrexia (malignancy, bowel infarction, inflammatory bowel disease or pancreatitis).
  - Rigors – visible shaking accompanied by fever (sepsis, particularly common with gram-negative infection).
  - Cachexia – suggests a chronic disease (malignancy, cirrhosis, pancreatitis).
- Head and neck
  - Eyes – sclera for jaundice (hepatitis, gallstones or pancreatitis), conjunctival pallor (anaemia), xanthelasma (hyperlipidaemia in cholestasis).
  - Mouth/tongue – glossitis/stomatitis (iron/vitamin B_{12} deficiency), aphthous ulcers (inflammatory bowel disease).
  - Neck – supraclavicular lymphadenopathy (lymphoma, Virchow's node associated with abdominal malignancy).
- Chest
  - Spider naevi, gynecomastia, loss of axillary hair (indicate raised oestrogen levels with malignancy).
- Hands
  - Asterixis (hepatic encephalopathy/ severe uraemia in advanced renal disease).
  - Nails – clubbing (cirrhosis, inflammatory bowel disease, coeliacs), leukonychia (hypoalbuminaemia in cirrhosis), koilonychia (iron deficiency anaemia).
  - Pulse – tachycardia and low volume indicate shock.
- Abdomen
  - Scars – recent surgical scar may indicate a source of peritoneal sepsis (anastomotic leak); older surgical scar may indicate the presence of adhesions.
  - Cullen sign (periumbilical or central bruising) and Grey Turner sign (bruising in the flanks) are signs of retroperitoneal bleeding (seen in haemorrhagic

pancreatitis, rarely leaking abdominal aortic aneurysm).
- Abdominal distension – bowel obstruction (accompanied by resonant percussion, quiet or absent bowel sounds and, occasionally, visible peristalsis).
- Tenderness – consider which anatomical structures lie at the site of tenderness (see Table 9.1). Assess for rebound and percussion tenderness (peritonitis).
- Mass – this can be neoplastic or inflammatory (as Crohn disease).
- Ascites – dullness to percussion, fluid thrill (malignancy, peritoneal sepsis, pancreatitis, portal hypertension).
- Bowel sounds – high-pitched (tinkling) suggest obstruction; absence indicates an ileus (the paralysis of bowel).
- Hernial orifices (inguinal and femoral) – these must be examined, particularly if obstruction is suspected.
- Pelvic and rectal examination – pelvic inflammation, cervical excitation, ectopic pregnancy, rectal mass or bleeding, stool consistency. Vaginal discharge will often be present in pelvic inflammatory disease.
- Cardiorespiratory examination – consider myocardial infarction and pneumonia.

HINTS AND TIPS

Murphy sign: classically associated with cholecystitis; place two fingers just inferior to the liver border and ask the patient to take a deep breath in. The patient reports pain, and inspiration is limited as the inflamed gallbladder descends onto your fingers. A similar examination in the left upper quadrant does not halt inspiration or cause pain.
Rovsing sign: a sudden release of pressure in the left iliac fossa causes pain in the right iliac fossa in appendicitis. Both are common examination questions.

INVESTIGATIONS

Investigations will depend on a focused differential diagnosis. The diagnostic pathway is outlined in Fig. 9.2.

Bedside investigations

- Blood glucose: hypoglycaemia in advanced liver failure or Addison disease; hyperglycaemia in ketoacidosis and may complicate acute pancreatitis.

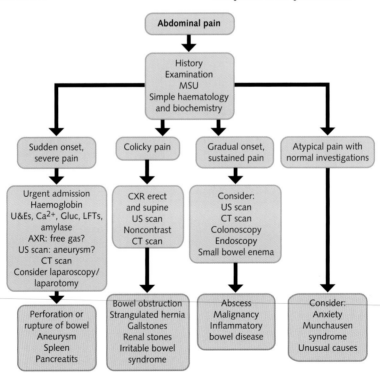

Fig. 9.2 Diagnosis in the patient with abdominal pain. *AXR*, Abdominal X-ray; *CT*, computed tomography; *CXR*, chest X-ray; *Gluc*, glucose; *LFTs*, liver function tests; *MSU*, midstream urine; *U&Es*, urea and electrolytes; *US*, ultrasound.

- Urine dipstick test: positive for nitrites and leucocytes indicates urinary tract infection; ketone positive may indicate dehydration, anorexia or diabetic ketoacidosis.
- Pregnancy test: any female of childbearing age with abdominal pain must have a pregnancy test.

Blood tests

- Full blood count: leucocytosis is seen in infection and occasionally inflammation and malignancy. Anaemia may be due to acute blood loss or chronic disease such as malignancy.
- Serum amylase: hallmark of acute pancreatitis, but its level may also be raised in perforated peptic ulcer, diabetic ketoacidosis, cholecystitis, ectopic pregnancy, abdominal trauma and myocardial infarction. Note that in chronic pancreatitis, serum amylase level may not be raised.
- Urea and electrolytes: dehydration, acute kidney injury, deranged electrolytes (e.g., low potassium level in diarrhoea), high urea level in an upper gastrointestinal tract bleed.
- Serum calcium: hypercalcaemia may cause renal stones and pancreatitis; it may also indicate malignancy; hypocalcaemia may be a consequence of pancreatitis.
- Liver function tests: abnormal with liver disease and biliary disease.
- Arterial blood gas: high lactate level in dehydration or ischaemic bowel.

Imaging

- Abdominal X-ray: obstruction (dilated loops of bowel); pancreatitis (sentinel loop due to ileus in the overlying loop of the small bowel); volvulus (sigmoid and caecal); infarction ('thumb printing' representing mucosal oedema); renal stone (90% are radio-opaque).
- Erect chest X-ray: check for free gas under the diaphragm – a sign of perforated viscus.
- Abdominal ultrasound scan: dilatation of biliary tree; intraabdominal mass; ascites; abscess; hydronephrosis.
- Computed tomography (CT): useful in the diagnosis of abdominal aortic aneurysm, perforation of a viscus, and abdominal malignancy. Noncontrast CT scans are used where renal stone disease is suspected.

Further investigations

- Urine sample: microscopy, culture and sensitivity of midstream urine.
- ECG to rule out myocardial infarction.
- Stool sample: microscopy, culture and sensitivity. Toxin testing for *Clostridium difficile*.
- Endoscopic tests: upper gastrointestinal tract endoscopy, flexible sigmoidoscopy and colonoscopy.
- Diagnostic laparoscopy: occasionally, the investigations mentioned above do not yield a diagnosis, and the abdominal pain persists. Diagnostic laparoscopic surgery can help make a diagnosis, but is more commonly useful in ruling out a specific disease.

● Chapter Summary

- Acute abdomen can signify a medical emergency, such as septic shock or ruptured abdominal aortic aneurysm, and requires urgent assessment and management.
- Careful history taking and examination will point towards the diagnosis and guide investigations and management.
- Cardiorespiratory conditions such as myocardial infarction or chest infection can present as abdominal pain and mimic abdominal diseases.

UKMLA Conditions
Acute pancreatitis
Ascites
Cholecystitis
Diverticular disease
Ectopic pregnancy
Gastric cancer
Gastro-oesophageal reflux disease
Gastrointestinal perforation
Hepatitis
Inflammatory bowel disease
Irritable bowel syndrome
Mesenteric adenitis
Pancreatic cancer
Peptic ulcer disease and gastritis

UKMLA Presentations
Acute abdominal pain
Abdominal distension
Ascites
Chronic abdominal pain
Organomegaly
Peritonitis

Heartburn and indigestion 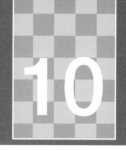 10

INTRODUCTION

'Heartburn' and 'indigestion', also known as 'dyspepsia', describe a group of symptoms that relate to the upper gastrointestinal tract. These include upper abdominal discomfort, retrosternal chest pain, anorexia, nausea, vomiting, bloating and early satiety with fullness after meals. Causes range from benign, e.g., gastro-oesophageal reflux disease (GORD), or *Helicobacter pylori* infection, to malignant (oesophageal or gastric cancer). A full list of potential causes is listed in the Clinical Notes section.

The presence of 'alarm' symptoms warrants urgent investigation, with referral for endoscopy. In those <55 years of age with no alarm symptoms, a 'test and treat' approach (test for *H. pylori*) can be safely adopted, and is more successful than acid suppression alone.

CLINICAL NOTES

ALARM SYMPTOMS

Anaemia

Loss of weight

Anorexia

Recent onset of progressive symptoms/**R**esistant to treatment

Melaena

CAUSES OF DYSPEPSIA (SEE CHAPTER 30)

Duodenal ulcer[a,b]

Gastric ulcer[a,b]

Oesophageal/gastric cancer[a]

Oesophagitis/GORD

Gastritis/duodenitis[a,b]

Nonulcer dyspepsia[a,b]

Hiatus hernia

Oesophageal motility disorders

Biliary disease

[a] Condition associated with *H. pylori* infection. It is unclear whether this infection is causative in all the conditions.
[b] Responds favourably to eradication of *H. pylori*.
GORD, Gastro-oesophageal reflux disease.

HISTORY AND EXAMINATION FINDINGS

Ask about the following, although correlation between symptoms and the underlying cause is poor:

- Dyspepsia: usually retrosternal discomfort, often worse with leaning forward or lying flat. May be associated with waterbrash (excessive sour or tasteless saliva in the back of the mouth, either in response to acid in the lower oesophagus or due to reflux of fluid into the upper pharynx).
- Chest pain: burning retrosternal pain, not related to exertion (unlike angina), which may radiate between the shoulder blades. This can relate to acid-provoked oesophageal spasm, which, like angina, is relieved by nitrates.
- Nocturnal cough/asthma: occasionally due to acid reflux.
- Epigastric pain: feature of peptic ulcer disease (PUD). Classically, a gastric ulcer is aggravated by food, and a duodenal ulcer is aggravated by fasting, but these are unreliable symptoms.

Aggravating factors for reflux include:

- Increased intraabdominal pressure (stooping/bending/ obesity/pregnancy).
- Spicy or fatty foods.
- Alcohol ingestion (also causes gastritis).
- Cigarettes, caffeine, theophylline, calcium channel blockers, β-blockers, anticholinergic drugs; all of which reduce lower oesophageal sphincter tone.
- Nonsteroidal antiinflammatory drugs, which interfere with prostaglandin cytoprotection of the gastric mucosa.
- Hiatus hernia.

Identifying patients who require endoscopy is key Fig. 10.1. This depends on the presence of the 'alarm' features listed in Clinical Notes. An urgent endoscopy (i.e., within 2 weeks) is indicated for any patient over the age of 55, with dyspepsia and one of the alarming symptoms, as they are at high risk for an upper gastrointestinal cancer.

INVESTIGATIONS

An approach to the dyspeptic patient is outlined in Fig. 10.1. The management of specific conditions is further explained in Chapter 30.

The investigations used are explained later. Specialized investigations are used predominantly in cases such as persistent symptoms not responding to the approach in Fig. 10.1 or atypical symptoms (e.g., laryngeal discomfort or atypical chest pain that may result from acid reflux or oesophageal dysmotility). It is important to remember that most patients with dyspepsia can be managed safely without extensive investigations.

HINTS AND TIPS

Although dyspepsia or heartburn is usually a gastrointestinal complaint, some older patients with 'dyspepsia' actually have angina pectoris. Make sure you take an adequate history to ensure that the problem is gastrointestinal in origin, and not cardiac.

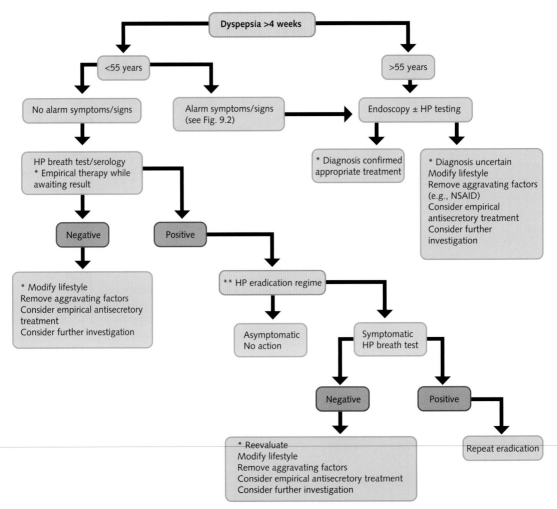

Fig. 10.1 Algorithm for the investigation and management of patients with dyspepsia. See Chapter 30. Seek local microbiological advice. Further information on the management of dyspepsia can be obtained from https://www.nice.org.uk/guidance/cg184. *HP, Helicobacter pylori; NSAID,* nonsteroidal antiinflammatory drug.

Common investigations

- Full blood count: iron-deficiency anaemia and/or thrombocytosis may suggest gastrointestinal blood loss and needs further investigation.
- Electrocardiography: to rule out cardiac ischaemia causing atypical chest pain.
- *Helicobacter pylori* testing: H. pylori is commonly diagnosed with the Carbon-13 urea breath test or with the Stool Helicobacter Antigen test. These are the most accurate of the tests available and can also confirm eradication post treatment. However, these tests should not be performed within 2 weeks of proton pump inhibitor use or within 4 weeks of antibacterial treatment, as this can lead to false negative results.
- Endoscopy (oesophagogastroduodenoscopy): a relatively safe investigation. It allows visualization of the upper gastrointestinal tract to the second part of the duodenum. It allows biopsy and therapeutic manoeuvres (see Chapter 30).

- Barium meal: an alternative for patients in whom endoscopy is not possible (e.g., elderly frail patients in whom sedation is dangerous). It is useful in diagnosing strictures and dysmotility, but does not allow intervention at the time of the procedure.

Specialized investigations

- Oesophageal motility studies – demonstrates motility disorders (e.g., achalasia, systemic sclerosis, diffuse oesophageal spasm).
- Twenty-four-hour intraluminal pH monitoring (confirms acid reflux in difficult cases).
- Abdominal ultrasound scan (if a mass or biliary disease is suspected) (see Chapter 30).

● Chapter Summary

- Symptom management is an approach appropriate for most patients presenting with dyspepsia.
- Identifying patients at increased risk of a sinister cause for symptoms is key.

UKMLA Conditions
Gastro-oesophageal reflux disease
Hiatus hernia
Peptic ulcer disease and gastritis
Swallowing problems

UKMLA Presentation
Chest pain

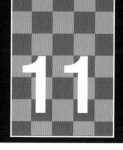

INTRODUCTION

Haematemesis is the vomiting of blood; it can be fresh bright red blood or altered ('coffee ground' vomit). Melaena is black, tarry, offensive smelling stool; it is usually due to bleeding in the gastrointestinal (GI) tract above the hepatic flexure. Both are typical signs of an upper GI tract bleed. Occasionally, very brisk bleeding may present as haematochezia (fresh blood per rectum). GI bleeding is an emergency, and treatment is usually initiated before a diagnosis can be made (see Chapter 30).

Table 11.1 gives the differential diagnosis of haematemesis and melaena. It is important to note that melaena which occurs in the absence of haematemesis may be caused by disease in the small bowel or ascending colon.

HISTORY AND EXAMINATION FINDINGS

The management of patients with GI bleeding includes resuscitation followed by a full history and examination to identify stigmata of liver disease.

History

In a patient presenting with haematemesis, it is important to clarify whether the blood has been vomited or coughed up (haemoptysis). Food mixed with the blood or an acid pH suggests haematemesis. Haematemesis may also be due to blood swallowed from the nasopharynx or mouth.

You must ask about:

- Nonspecific symptoms of hypovolaemia: faintness, weakness, dizziness, sweating, palpitations, dyspnoea, pallor, collapse. These symptoms may precede the actual haematemesis/melaena.
- Pain:
  - Intermittent epigastric pain relieved with antacids: *peptic ulceration.*
  - Sudden severe abdominal pain: *possible bowel perforation.*
  - Heartburn: *oesophagitis.*
  - Odynophagia (pain on swallowing): oesophageal carcinoma or oesophagitis.
- Retching, especially after an alcohol binge: *Mallory–Weiss tear.*

- Symptoms of the blood loss being chronic, associated with weight loss and anorexia: *carcinoma.*
- History of chronic excessive alcohol intake and other causes of liver disease (see Chapter 14): *oesophageal varices.*
- A history of GI bleeds and their cause.
- Family history: inherited bleeding disorders.
- Current drugs: antiplatelet agents, nonsteroidal antiinflammatory drugs, steroids or excessive alcohol consumption are suggestive of gastric erosions; anticoagulation will exacerbate bleeding.

HINTS AND TIPS

Iron therapy causes black stools but this is not melaena!

Table 11.1 The differential diagnosis of haematemesis and melaena

Cause	Notes
PUD	Causes 50% of major upper GI tract bleeds. Mortality 10%
Gastritis/gastric erosions	Causes 20% of upper GI tract bleeds, rarely severe
Mallory–Weiss tear	Laceration in GOJ mucosa, often following retching (e.g., after alcohol binge) Causes 10% of upper GI tract bleeds
Oesophagitis	Due to GORD
Ruptured oesophageal varices	Due to portal hypertension, most commonly in cirrhosis Causes 10%–20% of upper GI tract bleeds High mortality
Drugs	NSAIDs, aspirin, steroids, anticoagulants
Gastric neoplasm	Causes 5% of upper GI tract bleeds
Rare causes	Oesophageal ulcers or tumours, aorto-enteric fistula, angiodysplasia, bleeding disorders, pancreatic tumour, biliary bleeding

GI, Gastrointestinal; GOJ, gastro-oesophageal junction; GORD, gastro-oesophageal reflux disease; PUD, peptic ulcer disease.

Examination

The approach to examining the patient with haematemesis and melaena is given in Fig. 11.1.

Step back from the patient for a few seconds. Does the patient look well, or pale and clammy? If the patient is clearly unwell, follow the ABCDE approach (see Chapter 2). Volume replacement in actively bleeding patients should be started quickly, and the source of bleeding should be identified and the 'blood tap' turned off. Once it is recognized that the patient needs transfusion, resuscitation with O-negative blood should be commenced until group-specific crossed-matched blood is available. Consider the need for further blood products, platelets, clotting factors and cryoprecipitate and whether a major transfusion protocol needs to be initiated.

Examination and findings include:

- Signs of shock: peripherally shut down, cool and clammy, reduced capillary refill time, oliguria.
- Pulse and blood pressure: tachycardia is a reflex response to hypovolaemia (due to bleeding) and usually precedes a blood pressure fall. A young and healthy patient may lose more than 500 mL of blood before a rise in heart rate or fall in blood pressure occurs. If these signs are present give early resuscitation with intravenous fluids and/or blood products.
- Stigmata of chronic liver disease (see Chapter 14): look for signs of chronic liver disease and portal hypertension such as jaundice, clubbing, spider naevi, and bruising – these could indicate variceal bleeding as a source.
- Anaemia: assess mucous membranes. If the patient is clinically anaemic, this may indicate chronic blood loss.
- Cachexia.
- Mouth: pharyngeal lesions; pigmented macules (Peutz–Jeghers syndrome).
- Lymphadenopathy (especially Virchow node – left supraclavicular lymph node): associated with gastric carcinoma (Troisier sign).
- A rigid abdomen: bowel perforation.

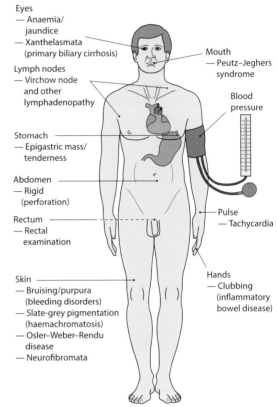

Fig. 11.1 Examining the patient with haematemesis and melaena.

- Epigastric tenderness: peptic ulcer disease, oesophagitis or gastric carcinoma.
- Epigastric mass: gastric carcinoma.
- Lymphadenopathy: especially Virchow node (left supraclavicular lymph node) associated with gastric carcinoma (Troisier sign).
- Rectum: A rectal examination should be preformed (with a chaperone present), to look for malaena, or rectal source of bleed e.g., haemorrhoids, rectal tumour.

INVESTIGATIONS

An algorithm for investigating the patient with a GI bleed is given in Fig. 11.2. Investigations will aid in diagnosis and contribute to estimating mortality and morbidity (see Further Investigations and Tables 11.2 and 11.3). The Glasgow-Blatchford bleeding score can be applied for adult patients being considered for hospital admission due to upper GI bleeding to stratify patients who are 'low-risk' and appropriate for outpatient investigation and management (see Table 11.4).

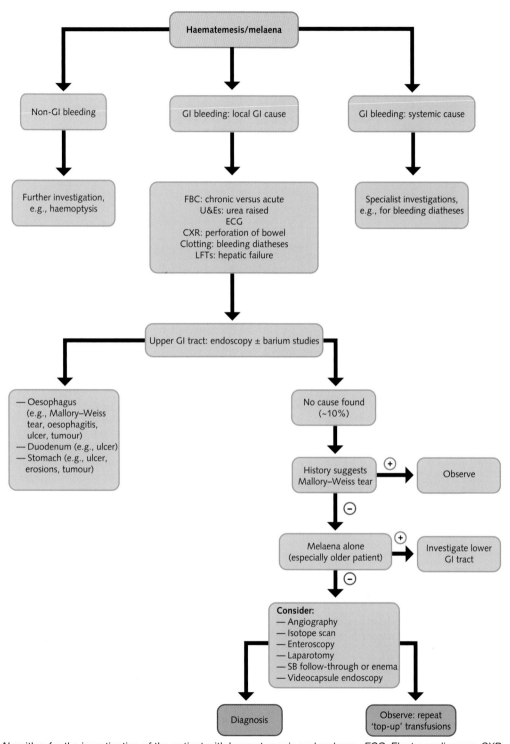

Fig. 11.2 Algorithm for the investigation of the patient with haematemesis and melaena. *ECG*, Electrocardiogram; *CXR*, chest X-ray; *FBC*, full blood count; *GI*, gastrointestinal; *LFTs*, liver function tests; *SB*, small bowel; *U&Es*, urea and electrolytes.

Table 11.2 Rockall score*

	Variable	Score			
		0	1	2	3
Pre-endoscopy	*Preendoscopy Age (years)*	<60	60–79	>80	
	Shock	No shock (HR <100/min, SBP >100 mmHg)	HR >100/min, SBP >100 mmHg	SBP <100 mmHg	
	Comorbidity	Nil major		Any major comorbidity except renal or liver failure and/or metastases	Renal failure, liver failure and/or metastases
Post-endoscopy	*Postendoscopy Diagnosis*	Mallory–Weiss tear; no sign of recent bleeding	All other diagnoses	Upper GI malignancy	
	Evidence of recent bleeding	None		Blood, adherent clot, spurting vessel	

CHF, *Congestive heart failure;* GI, *gastrointestinal;* HR, *heart rate;* SBP, *systolic blood pressure.*
Rockall score: A scoring system that helps to identify high-risk patients presenting with an upper GI tract bleed. It is used to predict the risk of rebleeding and mortality (before and after endoscopy) (Tables 11.2 and 11.3). A score of less than 3 carries good prognosis (Table 11.3).

Table 11.3 Prediction of rebleeding and mortality from the Rockall score

Score	Pre-endoscopy initial score (%)	Final score after endoscopy (%)
0	0.2	0
1	2	0
2	6	0.2
3	11	2.9
4	25	5.3
5	40	10.8
6	50	17.3
7	50	27
8 +	—	41.1

for haemodilution to occur. Low haemoglobin level on initial presentation and/or mean corpuscular volume (MCV) suggests chronic blood loss. White cell count may be raised after a GI bleed. Platelet count may be reduced (acute bleed) or increased (chronic blood loss). A very low platelet count should raise suspicion of a bleeding diathesis.
- Clotting screen: prothrombin time is raised in liver disease. More specific investigations may be indicated (e.g., in patients with haemophilia or von Willebrand disease).
- Urea levels: intestinal absorption of blood will lead to an elevated urea level. Intravascular volume depletion causing prerenal impairment also contributes.
- Liver function tests: deranged in chronic liver disease.

HINTS AND TIPS

Elevated blood urea level with normal serum creatinine level suggests gastrointestinal blood loss.

Bedside investigations

Closely monitor vital signs including heart rate, blood pressure, respiratory rate, oxygen saturations, temperature, urine output (once catheterized).

Blood tests

All patients presenting with signs of shock should have two large-bore cannulas sited for fluid resuscitation, and bloods sent for urgent group and save and cross match in addition to:

- Full blood count: haemoglobin level may be normal in the acute phase, despite a large GI bleed, as it takes some hours

Further investigations

- An erect chest X-ray may be considered to look for pneumoperitoneum; suggestive of bowel perforation.
- Endoscopy: endoscopy is the mainstay of diagnosis and treatment, and should be performed urgently in unstable patients or those with significant comorbidity. It allows direct visualization of the disease and provides a diagnosis in around 90% of cases. This will determine the most appropriate form of medical therapy. The risk of rebleeding (the major cause of

death) may be estimated through use of the Rockall risk score (Table 11.2). Endoscopic intervention may take the form of banding or sclerosing a bleeding varix, or adrenaline injection into a bleeding vessel.

- If endoscopy findings are negative, **colonoscopy** should be performed to rule out a proximal colonic bleed (see Fig. 11.2).

Most patients do not require further tests, but occasionally these are performed under the guidance of a specialist when the diagnosis remains uncertain (see Fig. 11.2):

- Mesenteric angiography requires significant, active bleeding to localize the source. It can also be used to visualize the portal venous system.
- Computed tomography (CT)/magnetic resonance imaging (MRI) with or without capsule endoscopy to investigate disease of the small intestine.
- Diagnostic laparoscopy before laparotomy and surgically assisted enteroscopy are occasionally performed.

Despite extensive investigation, a small minority of patients will remain undiagnosed. If bleeding is severe, laparotomy may be required, but if it is mild, the patient may attend hospital for 'top-up' transfusions or iron infusions as required while investigations continue.

Table 11.4 Glasgow-Blatchford bleeding score (GBS)

Admission risk marker		Score
Blood urea (mmol/L)	≥6.5–<8	2
	≥8–<10	3
	≥10–<25	4
	≥25	6
Haemoglobin for men (g/L)	≥120–<130	1
	≥100–<120	3
	<100	6
Haemoglobin for women (g/L)	≥100–<120	1
	<100	6
Systolic blood pressure (mmHg)	≥100–<109	1
	≥90–<100	2
	<90	3
Other measures	Pulse ≥100	1
	Melaena	1
	Syncope	2
	Hepatic disease	2
	Cardiac failure	2

Low risk = score of 0. Any score higher than 0 is high risk for needing intervention: transfusion, endoscopy, or surgery.

● Chapter Summary

- Haematemesis and melaena are signs of gastrointestinal bleeding.
- Melaena suggests a bleed originating above the hepatic flexure.
- Endoscopy is the main diagnostic and therapeutic investigation in this presentation and should not be delayed.

UKMLA Conditions
Haemorrhoids
Peptic ulcer disease and gastritis

UKMLA Presentations
Bleeding from upper GI tract
Change in stool colour
Melaena

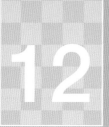

Change in bowel habit | 12

INTRODUCTION

Change in bowel habit is an important symptom and may suggest an underlying disease. Always ask about the patient's normal bowel habit because there are considerable differences between people.

Constipation is defined as <2 bowel movements/week, or less than the patient's normal habit, with passage of dry hardened stool with difficulty and/or pain. Diarrhoea is defined as abnormally frequent intestinal evacuations with stools which are mostly fluid. Tables 12.1 and 12.2 summarize the causes of diarrhoea and constipation, respectively.

COMMUNICATION

Make sure that by 'constipation' and 'diarrhoea' you and the patient mean the same thing.

RED FLAG

Note the features of acute gastrointestinal obstruction: absolute constipation (no passage of either faeces or gas), vomiting, pain and abdominal distension – this is a surgical emergency.

HISTORY AND EXAMINATION FINDINGS

History

Ask about:

- Normal bowel habit and diet.
- Onset: if acute suspect gastroenteritis, i.e., infective diarrhoea – any risk factors?
- Has the patient been in contact with anyone with diarrhoea? Any recent poorly cooked food? Or other household contacts also affected? Recent foreign travel? Diet change? New medication changes (e.g., antibiotics)?
- Frequency of defecation.
- Stool appearance: Formed, loose or watery; colour – normal, bloody (*Campylobacter, Shigella/Salmonella, Escherichia*

coli, ulcerative colitis, Crohn disease, colonic polyps, ischaemic colitis), black (melaena), yellow (high fat content, or mucus and slime), 'redcurrant jelly' (intussusception), putty coloured (obstructive jaundice); volume; do the stools float? (high fat content—malabsorption).
- Associated features (e.g., pain, fever, vomiting, weight loss, extraintestinal manifestations of inflammatory bowel disease) (see Chapter 30).
- Nocturnal symptoms: these go against a functional disorder.
- Tenesmus (a sense of incomplete evacuation).
- Smell: offensively malodorous in malabsorption; melaena has a particularly offensive characteristic smell.
- Symptoms of thyrotoxicosis.
- Relationship to food.
- Stress.
- Drugs: antacids, laxatives, proton pump inhibitors, digoxin, antibiotics, alcohol.
- Surgical history (e.g., multiple bowel resections for Crohn disease can result in malabsorption).

RED FLAG

All patients >50 presenting with a change in bowel habit associated with rectal bleeding should be considered for urgent investigation on a 2-week-wait suspected cancer pathway referral. For patients >60, this pathway should be followed for change in bowel habit even without symptoms of rectal bleeding. In patients with a change in bowel habit without rectal bleeding who do not meet criteria for a 2-week-wait referral, a quantitative faecal immunochemical test (FIT) should be performed (see Investigations section).

Examination

The examination approach in the patient with a change in bowel habit is given in Fig. 12.1.

Look for:

- Dehydration: dry mucous membranes, decreased skin turgor, signs of shock.
- Cachexia, anaemia.
- Fever.

Table 12.1 Differential diagnosis of diarrhoea (see Chapter 30)

Causes	Examples
Infective	Bacterial: *Campylobacter* (poultry), *Salmonella* (meat, poultry and dairy), *Shigella* (faecal–oral transmission) Viral: rotavirus, Norwalk virus, cytomegalovirus Protozoa: *Giardia lamblia*, *Cryptosporidium*, *Entamoeba histolytica*
Inflammatory	Inflammatory bowel disease (Crohn disease and UC) Malignancy Radiation enteritis
Ischaemic	Emboli or mesenteric atheromatous disease
Functional	Irritable bowel syndrome
Secretory	Infection (e.g., cholera) VIPoma/Zollinger–Ellison/carcinoid Villous adenoma Factitious diarrhoea (e.g., laxative abuse) Bile salt malabsorption (disruption of enterohepatic circulation)
Osmotic	Medications (e.g., antacids and lactulose) Disaccharidase deficiency Factitious diarrhoea
Malabsorption	See Chapter 30 for causes
Systemic illness	Hyperthyroidism, diabetes mellitus, Addison disease (see Chapter 33)
Overflow diarrhoea	Faecal impaction in elderly patients
Drugs	Alcohol, digoxin, metformin, proton pump inhibitors, GLP-1 receptor agonists, bisphosphonates

UC, *Ulcerative colitis.*

Table 12.2 Differential diagnosis of constipation (see Chapter 30)

Causes	Examples
Congenital	Hirschsprung disease
Mechanical obstruction	Inflammatory stricture (e.g., Crohn disease, diverticulitis) Neoplasm Extraluminal mass (e.g., pelvic) Rectocele
Lifestyle	Diet Dehydration Immobility Lack of privacy (e.g., hospital ward)
Pain	Fissure-in-ano Thrombosed haemorrhoids Postoperative
Metabolic/endocrine (see Chapter 33)	Hypothyroidism Hypercalcaemia Diabetic neuropathy
Drugs	Opiates, anticholinergics, diuretics
Neurological (see Chapter 34)	Paraplegia Multiple sclerosis
Functional	Irritable bowel syndrome Idiopathic megacolon/rectum

- Clubbing, rashes, extraintestinal signs of inflammatory bowel disease.
- Any goitre/hyperthyroid signs?
- Abdominal masses or scars.
- Rectal examination: masses or impacted faeces.

INVESTIGATIONS

The wide range of possible diagnoses in patients with altered bowel habit is reflected by the large number of tests that may be performed. Some of these are used commonly, whereas others are used much less frequently and only under the guidance of specialists.

Bedside investigations

- Observations – to detect signs of shock
- Stool chart (see reference 'Bristol stool chart' – a diagnostic scale which classifies stools into seven groups, ranging from hardest to softest)

Blood/laboratory tests

- Full blood count: anaemia of chronic disease (e.g., coeliac or colon cancer), raised white cell count in infections, raised

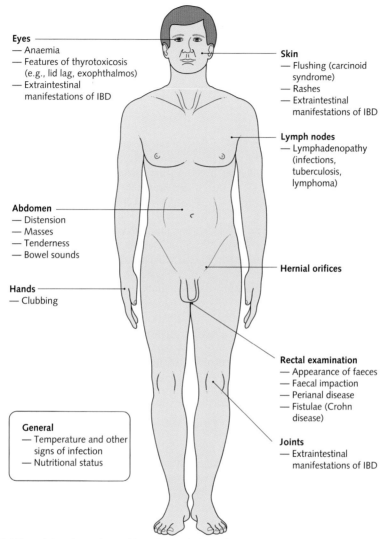

Eyes
— Anaemia
— Features of thyrotoxicosis
   (e.g., lid lag, exophthalmos)
— Extraintestinal
   manifestations of IBD

Skin
— Flushing (carcinoid
   syndrome)
— Rashes
— Extraintestinal
   manifestations of IBD

Lymph nodes
— Lymphadenopathy
   (infections,
   tuberculosis,
   lymphoma)

Abdomen
— Distension
— Masses
— Tenderness
— Bowel sounds

Hernial orifices

Hands
— Clubbing

Rectal examination
— Appearance of faeces
— Faecal impaction
— Perianal disease
— Fistulae (Crohn
   disease)

General
— Temperature and other
   signs of infection
— Nutritional status

Joints
— Extraintestinal
   manifestations of IBD

Fig. 12.1 Examining the patient with a change in bowel habit. *IBD*, Inflammatory bowel disease.

mean corpuscular volume (MCV) if history of alcohol abuse; may also indicate vitamin B_{12} deficiency in malabsorption (request folate, iron and other fat-soluble vitamin tests if malabsorption is suspected).

- Urea and electrolytes, including calcium: acute kidney injury secondary to dehydration, hyponatraemia/hypokalaemia/hypomagnesaemia in profound secretory diarrhoea.
- Thyroid function tests: constipation in hypothyroidism and diarrhoea in hyperthyroidism.
- Blood glucose: diabetes.
- Liver function tests: pale stools in obstructive or posthepatic jaundice.

- Albumin: level decreased in malabsorption, protein-losing enteropathies, inflammatory diseases.
- Inflammatory markers (erythrocyte sedimentation rate and C-reactive protein): levels raised in infection/inflammation.
- Antitissue transglutaminase antibodies if coeliac disease is suspected.
- Stool microscopy, culture and detection of *Clostridium difficile* toxin if infection is suspected.
- Quantitative faecal immunochemical test ('FIT' test) to look for evidence of blood in the stool not visible to the eye (recommended for adoption in primary care to guide referral for suspected colorectal cancer in people without rectal bleeding who have unexplained symptoms but do not

meet the criteria for a suspected cancer pathway referral outlined in *NICE's guideline on suspected cancer*)

Imaging

Noninvasive
- Abdominal X-ray: distended intestinal loops and fluid levels suggest obstruction, pancreatic calcification suggests chronic pancreatitis and gross dilatation of the colon suggests Hirschsprung disease (rare). Featureless colon, with loss of haustral markings, may indicate colitis.
- Abdominal ultrasound scan and/or computed tomography (CT) for suspected masses and pancreatitis.
- Occasionally MRI enterography is used for detailed visualization of the small bowel.
- Videocapsule endoscopy for small bowel disease.

Invasive
- Rigid sigmoidoscopy – performed without sedation (e.g., in an outpatient setting); allows inspection and/or biopsy of rectal mucosa.
- Flexible sigmoidoscopy/colonoscopy – examination of the large bowel; allows biopsies (even if the large bowel is macroscopically normal to exclude microscopic colitis). Flexible sigmoidoscopy examines the colon up to the sigmoid, whereas colonoscopy examines the whole large bowel.

- Oesophagastroduodendoscopy (OGD) and duodenal (D2) biopsy for malabsorption.
- Magnetic resonance cholangiopancreatography, endoscopic retrograde cholangiopancreatography or endoscopic ultrasonography for suspected biliary and pancreatic pathology.

Further investigations

- Faecal calprotectin as a means of differentiating inflammatory from noninflammatory diarrhoea.
- Faecal elastase test for pancreatic exocrine function.
- Assessment of bile salt absorption using radioisotope-labelled bile acids (SeHCAT scan).
- Faecal clearance of α_1-antitrypsin to investigate protein-losing enteropathy.
- Laxative screen.
- Colonic transit study: to confirm constipation and measure the transit time.
- Studies of pelvic floor function: defecating proctography and anal manometry.
- Fasting gut hormones: serum vasoactive intestinal polypeptide (VIPoma); serum gastrin (Zollinger–Ellison syndrome); chromogranin calcitonin (medullary thyroid carcinoma); cortisol (Addison disease); 24-hour urinary 5-hydroxyindoleacetic acid (carcinoid syndrome).

● Chapter Summary

- Change in bowel habit can indicate serious disease; if indicated, patients presenting with this symptom should undergo full assessment to exclude a sinister cause.
- Local or systemic causes can be the reason for the presentation. In most cases, careful history taking and examination will lead to the correct diagnosis. Occasionally specialized testing is necessary.

UKMLA Conditions	UKMLA Presentations
Constipation	Change in bowel habit
Colorectal tumours	Constipation
Diverticular disease	Diarrhoea
Hyperthyroidism	
Hypothyroidism	
Infectious colitis	
Inflammatory bowel disease	
Irritable bowel syndrome	
Malabsorption	

INTRODUCTION

Weight loss is due to either decreased energy intake or increased energy output, or both. Distinguish deliberate weight loss from involuntary weight loss. Involuntary weight loss is a common manifestation of physical or psychological illness and always warrants further investigation. It can be a manifestation of disease in any system. Table 13.1 summarizes the differential diagnosis of weight loss.

Table 13.1 The differential diagnosis of weight loss

Causes	Examples
Psychiatric/psychological	Anorexia nervosa Depression or agitation Catatonia Schizophrenia Laxative or diuretic abuse Neglect (e.g., 'tea and toast' diet)
Drugs	Alcohol, tobacco, laxatives or diuretics, opiates, amphetamines and some antihyperglycaemic drugs (e.g., dulaglutide, dapagliflozin)
Infections	Tuberculosis HIV infection Other chronic infections and infestations See Chapter 38
Chronic inflammation	Inflammatory bowel disease Connective tissue disease See Chapters 30 and 35
Malignancy	Almost every type of malignancy is associated with weight loss
Chronic illness	Cardiac failure ('cardiac cachexia') Chronic obstructive pulmonary disease Chronic renal failure See Chapters 28–30
Endocrine	Uncontrolled diabetes mellitus Hyperthyroidism and rarely hypothyroidism Adrenal insufficiency Phaeochromocytoma Hypopituitarism Severe diabetes insipidus See Chapter 33
Gastrointestinal	Peptic ulcer disease Dysphagia Malabsorption liver disease See Chapter 30
Neurological	Motor neurone disease Myopathies Poliomyelitis See Chapter 34

HIV, *Human immunodeficiency virus.*

HISTORY AND EXAMINATION FINDINGS

History

Try to confirm weight loss objectively with records of previous weights.
Ask about:

- The amount of weight lost, over what period the weight was lost and if the weight loss was intentional.
- Diet: detailed intake and any recent changes in diet history. Assess alcohol intake and illicit drug use.
- Physical activity: any changes in level.

Systems review:

- Symptoms of chronic infection, inflammation or malignancy: fever and night sweats, rashes, general malaise, lethargy, anorexia, easy bruising.
- Cardiorespiratory: shortness of breath, cough, haemoptysis.
- Gastrointestinal: dysphagia, change in bowel habit, melaena, rectal bleeding, change in stool consistency, haematemesis.
- Genitourinary: polyuria and polydipsia (diabetes), haematuria, obstructive urinary symptoms (prostate), menstrual history.
- Oral health: assess for poor dentition and gum disease – tooth loss can increase the risk of swallowing difficulty leading to change in food preference, avoidance of foods, and a decreased energy intake. Poor nutrition can also cause periodontal disease, with vitamin deficiencies (particularly C and D) linked to gingivitis.
- Neurological: vitamin and mineral deficiencies can result in neurological symptoms such as paraesthesia.
- Endocrine: assess the patient for thyrotoxicosis (tremor, heat intolerance, palpitations); adrenal insufficiency (skin pigmentation, weakness); phaeochromocytoma (headache, sweating and tachycardia is the classic triad); panhypopituitarism (pallor, dizziness, loss of body hair, loss of libido, visual field defects, symptoms of hypothyroidism).
- Psychiatric: depression screen and assessment for anorexia nervosa.

Examination

The examination approach in the patient with weight loss is given in Fig. 13.1. Does the patient look as if he or she has lost weight (loose skin, loose clothes)? Does the patient look well or ill? Is the patient pyrexial? The patient's weight, height and body mass index should be documented.
Check for:

- Clubbing: malignancy, cirrhosis, inflammatory bowel disease and infections (chronic suppurative lung disease, infective endocarditis, chronic obstructive pulmonary disease (COPD)).
- Leuconychia and palmar erythema: liver disease (leuconychia reflects hypoalbuminaemia).
- Koilonychia: iron deficiency anaemia.
- Pigmentation: increased in Addison disease (particularly in palmar creases) but decreased in anaemia.
- Joint swelling and decreased range of movement: connective tissue diseases.
- Tremor, goitre and eye signs: hyperthyroidism (see Chapters 17 and 33).
- Jaundice and other signs of liver failure (e.g., spider naevi) (see Chapter 14).
- Muscle wasting.
- Rashes.
- Raised blood pressure: phaeochromocytoma.
- Mouth changes: dentition, periodontitis, malignancies.
- Lymphadenopathy.

The following individual systems should be examined:

- Cardiorespiratory.
- Gastrointestinal: including careful palpation for abdominal masses, rectal examination and organomegaly (e.g., liver metastases). Always do a digital rectal examination.
- Neurological system: motor neurone disease, myopathy, paraneoplastic or metastatic manifestations of malignancy.
- Breast lumps.

INVESTIGATIONS

As the potential causes of weight loss are multiple, investigations need to be tailored to the history and clinical examination findings. Nonetheless, the following investigations should be performed.

Blood tests

- Full blood count: anaemia with malignancy, iron deficiency, vitamin B_{12} deficiency or folate deficiency, with inadequate dietary intake.
- Urea and electrolytes for uraemia and chronic kidney disease; calcium, phosphate, magnesium and potassium.
- C-reactive protein: level raised in infection and inflammation but also in myeloma and other malignancies.
- Blood cultures if indicated (e.g., in sepsis or endocarditis).

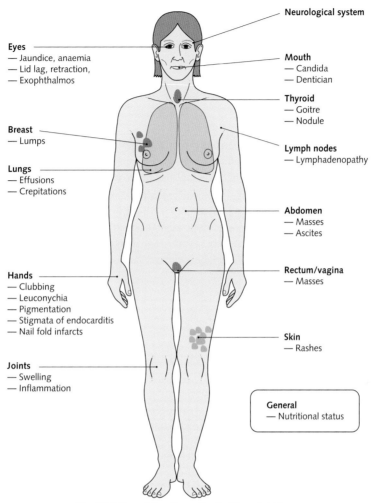

Eyes
— Jaundice, anaemia
— Lid lag, retraction,
— Exophthalmos

Breast
— Lumps

Lungs
— Effusions
— Crepitations

Hands
— Clubbing
— Leuconychia
— Pigmentation
— Stigmata of endocarditis
— Nail fold infarcts

Joints
— Swelling
— Inflammation

Neurological system

Mouth
— Candida
— Dentician

Thyroid
— Goitre
— Nodule

Lymph nodes
— Lymphadenopathy

Abdomen
— Masses
— Ascites

Rectum/vagina
— Masses

Skin
— Rashes

General
— Nutritional status

Fig. 13.1 Examining the patient with weight loss.

- Liver function tests (importantly albumin!) and clotting: liver failure.
- Blood glucose: diabetes, low glucose level in liver failure, Addison disease.
- Thyroid function tests.

Imaging

- Chest X-ray: infection or tuberculosis, and malignancy.
- CT/MRI/ultrasound scan (dependent on differential diagnosis).

CLINICAL NOTES

Malnutrition in the elderly is frequently undetected and untreated causing a wide range of adverse consequences, which include:

- Impaired immune response
- Impaired wound healing
- Reduced muscle strength and fatigue
- Impaired psychosocial function

In the community, elderly patients identified as malnourished are more likely to be admitted to hospital and to visit their GP more frequently. In hospital, patients identified as being at risk of malnutrition stay in hospital significantly longer, and are more likely to be discharged to healthcare facilities other than home.

Risk of weight loss is particularly high for inpatients who are repeatedly being kept nil by mouth for surgery, and those who are assessed as having an unsafe swallow, e.g., post stroke and severe dementia. For this reason, the 'Malnutrition Universal Screening Tool' ('MUST') has been designed to help identify adults who are underweight and at risk of malnutrition, as well as those who are obese. It is the most widely used nutrition screening tool in the UK. Patients identified as being malnourished using this tool are managed with careful input from dieticians, speech and language therapy (SALT).

Note: See Crash Course Endocrine/Nutrition volumes for further detail.

● Chapter Summary

- It is very important to distinguish between intentional and unintentional weight loss. Intentional weight loss may be a sign of a mental health disorder, and this should be screened for.
- Unintentional weight loss is a nonspecific symptom that may be a manifestation of sinister pathology such as malignancy.
- It occurs with inadequate energy intake, increased energy expenditure, malabsorption and/or increased metabolic rate.
- The history and examination and good clinical reasoning should guide the choice of investigations.
- The MUST score has been designed to help identify adults who are underweight and at risk of malnutrition. This should be monitored annually by the GP in patients identified as being high risk.

UKMLA Conditions
Eating disorders
Malabsorption
Malignancy
Malnutrition

UKMLA Presentations
Abnormal eating or exercising behaviour
End-of-life care/symptoms of terminal illness
Food intolerance
Nausea
Weight loss

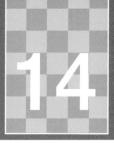

Jaundice 14

INTRODUCTION

Jaundice (icterus) is the yellow discoloration of the skin, sclera and mucosae that is detectable when serum bilirubin concentrations exceed approximately 35 µmol/L. Normal bilirubin metabolism is summarized in Fig. 14.1. Jaundice can arise because of increased red blood cell breakdown, disordered bilirubin metabolism or reduced bilirubin excretion.

The causes of jaundice are outlined in Table 14.1. **Prehepatic** jaundice (unconjugated hyperbilirubinaemia) usually results from the excessive production of bilirubin by haemolysis (see Fig. 14.1), in haemolytic anaemia for instance, but it can also result from inherited metabolic defects – the commonest of which is Gilbert syndrome, or due to impaired hepatic uptake with certain drugs (contrast agents, rifampicin). **Hepatic** jaundice results from hepatocyte dysfunction causing disordered bilirubin metabolism. Hepatocellular dysfunction usually causes some cholestasis and may cause 'pale stools/dark urine'. **Posthepatic** jaundice (cholestasis) is caused by reduced bilirubin excretion due to intrahepatic or extrahepatic biliary obstruction. Both cause a conjugated hyperbilirubinaemia.

HISTORY AND EXAMINATION FINDINGS

History

Ask about:

- Abdominal pain: the episodic, colicky, right hypochondrial pain of biliary colic will commonly be due to gallstones. A dull, persistent epigastric or central pain radiating to the back may suggest a pancreatic origin.
- Fevers or rigors: cholangitis.
- Weight loss: underlying malignancy, particularly pancreatic cancer.
- Duration of illness: a short history of malaise, anorexia and myalgia is suggestive of viral hepatitis.
- Drug history: particularly paracetamol, oral contraceptive pill.
- Alcohol consumption: acute alcoholic hepatitis, cirrhosis.
- Infectious contacts: hepatitis A.
- Recent foreign travel to areas of high hepatitis risk.
- Recent surgery: surgery for known malignancy, biliary stricture due to previous endoscopic retrograde cholangiopancreatography (if the patient had a sphincterotomy).
- Intravenous drug abuse, tattoos, unprotected sex, blood transfusions: increased risk of hepatitis B and hepatitis C.

- Occupation: sewage workers and people who participate in open water sports and activities are at increased risk of leptospirosis.
- Pregnancy.

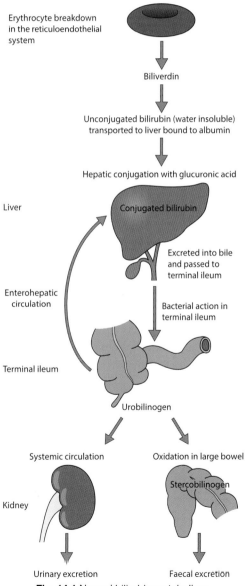

Fig. 14.1 Normal bilirubin metabolism.

Table 14.1 The differential diagnosis of jaundice

Prehepatic (see Chapter 37)	Hepatic (see Chapter 30)			Posthepatic (see Chapter 30)	
	Acute hepatocellular damage	Chronic hepatocellular damage		Extrahepatic obstruction	Intrahepatic obstruction
Haemolysis	Viral infection (e.g., hepatitis A, B, C, E; EBV; CMV) Alcohol	Inherited defects (e.g., primary haemochromatosis, Wilson disease, α_1-antitrypsin deficiency, autoimmune hepatitis)		Gallstones	Primary biliary cirrhosis

CMV, *Cytomegalovirus*; EBV, *Epstein–Barr virus*.

- Personal history of other autoimmune conditions such as ulcerative colitis (associated with primary sclerosing cholangitis). Important to ask about duration of jaundice, presence of joint ache, rash and other systemic features of autoimmune disease as part of the screening process.
- Family history of recurrent jaundice: inherited haemolytic anaemias and Gilbert syndrome.

Examination

The causes of jaundice are multiple and may therefore indicate underlying disease in one of many organ systems. There are three important groups of abnormalities that should specifically be looked for in the jaundiced patient:

- How severe is the jaundice? Is there any evidence of encephalopathy?
- Is this an acute or a chronic problem? Are there any signs of chronic liver disease?
- Are there any signs of specific disorders?

This approach is summarized in Fig. 14.2.

HINTS AND TIPS

Important to take a thorough drug history, including herbal medications which can be hepatotoxic.

CLINICAL NOTES

ENCEPHALOPATHY

Encephalopathy is defined as disordered brain function. The following suggest encephalopathy:

- Drowsiness: this will eventually progress through stupor to coma.
- Slurred speech.
- Asterixis: flapping tremor of outstretched hands.
- Seizures.
- Constructional apraxia: test for this by asking the patient to copy a five-pointed star.

- Hepatic fetor: mercaptans pass directly into the lungs because of portal hypertension, causing a characteristic odour of the patient's exhaled breath.

Hepatic encephalopathy can arise because of fulminating acute liver failure or when chronic disease decompensates. Precipitating factors, grading and management are described in Chapter 30.

CLINICAL NOTES

SIGNS OF CHRONIC LIVER DISEASE

- Palmar erythema.
- Leuconychia and oedema: hypoalbuminaemia.
- Clubbing.
- Dupuytren contractures: particularly in alcoholic cirrhosis.
- Spider naevi: more than five in the distribution of the superior vena cava.
- Scratch marks: cholestasis.
- Gynaecomastia, loss of body hair and testicular atrophy: elevated oestrogen level.
- Bruising: disordered coagulation.
- Hepatomegaly: not in well-established cirrhosis.
- Splenomegaly, ascites and caput medusae: portal hypertension.

SIGNS OF SPECIFIC DISEASES

- Xanthelasmata: primary biliary cirrhosis.
- Kayser–Fleischer rings: Wilson disease.
- Slate-grey pigmentation: haemochromatosis.
- Hard, irregular hepatomegaly: malignant metastases.
- Nontender, palpable gallbladder: jaundice is unlikely to be caused by gallstones (Courvoisier's law).
- Parotid gland enlargement: alcohol.
- Needle marks or tattoos: hepatitis B, hepatitis C.

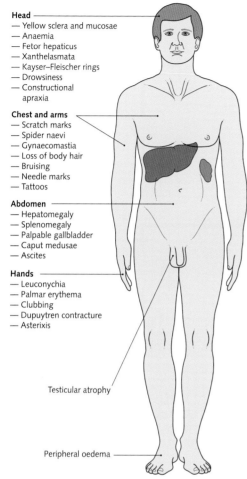

Head
— Yellow sclera and mucosae
— Anaemia
— Fetor hepaticus
— Xanthelasmata
— Kayser–Fleischer rings
— Drowsiness
— Constructional
  apraxia

Chest and arms
— Scratch marks
— Spider naevi
— Gynaecomastia
— Loss of body hair
— Bruising
— Needle marks
— Tattoos

Abdomen
— Hepatomegaly
— Splenomegaly
— Palpable gallbladder
— Caput medusae
— Ascites

Hands
— Leuconychia
— Palmar erythema
— Clubbing
— Dupuytren contracture
— Asterixis

Testicular atrophy

Peripheral oedema

Fig. 14.2 Examining the patient with jaundice.

INVESTIGATIONS

The investigation of jaundiced patients falls into two stages. First the type of jaundice must be determined (prehepatic, hepatic or posthepatic); then more detailed tests should be performed to determine the specific cause. Fig. 14.3 summarizes this approach.

Table 14.2 describes biochemical abnormalities in different types of jaundice.

- Blood tests: conjugated bilirubin, alanine transaminase, aspartate transaminase, alkaline phosphatase, γ-glutamyltransferase will give a reasonable indication as to the type of abnormality present. Alkaline phosphatase level is commonly raised in biliary disorders, but is also elevated in pregnancy and seen with high bone turnover, e.g., puberty and bony metastasis. A raised alkaline phosphatase level due to biliary injury can be differentiated from bone disorder by ordering γ-glutamyltransferase serum profile, where increased levels confirm hepatic origin. Isolated raised γ-glutamyltranspeptidase level occurs in alcohol excess. Raised alanine transaminase and aspartate transaminase levels indicate hepatocellular dysfunction.
- Urinary bilirubin and urobilinogen: urine is normally free of bilirubin. Dark urine indicates the presence of conjugated bilirubin. Low urobilinogen level suggests obstructive jaundice, whereas raised urobilinogen level suggests haemolysis or intrahepatic damage.
- Abdominal ultrasound scan, computerized tomography (CT) scan, magnetic resonance cholangiopancreatography (MRCP), endoscopic retrograde cholangiopancreatography (ERCP): to investigate the cause.

Haemolysis screen

The haemolysis screen is detailed in Chapter 30.

Hepatocellular screen

- Viral serology: hepatitis A, B and C; EBV, CMV.
- Autoantibody screen: antimitochondrial antibodies (levels raised in primary biliary cirrhosis), anti-smooth muscle antibodies, antinuclear antibodies.
- Ferritin: haemochromatosis.
- Serum caeruloplasmin: Wilson disease.
- α_1-Antitrypsin.
- Liver biopsy: definitive diagnostic test for intrinsic liver disease.
- Fasting lipid profile: triglycerides for steatosis.

HINTS AND TIPS

Liver dysfunction affects the synthesis of clotting factors, and therefore the prothrombin time must be checked and corrected before an invasive procedure (e.g., liver biopsy).

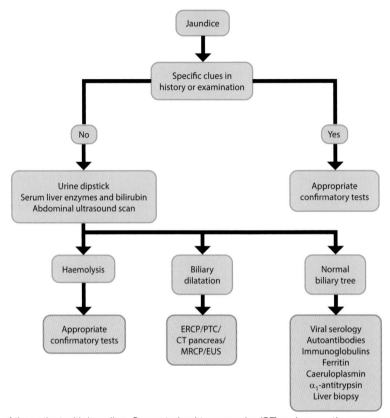

Fig. 14.3 Investigation of the patient with jaundice. Computerized tomography *(CT)* and magnetic resonance cholangiopancreatography *(MRCP)* are usually performed before endoscopic retrograde cholangiopancreatography *(ERCP)* or percutaneous transhepatic cholangiography *(PTC)*. *EUS*, Endoscopic ultrasonography.

Table 14.2 Biochemical abnormalities in different types of jaundice

Specimen	Test	Haemolysis	Hepatocellular	Cholestasis
Urine	Urobilinogen	Raised level	Normal or raised level	Decreased level or absent
	Conjugated bilirubin	Absent	Present	Raised
Faeces	Stercobilinogen	Raised level	Normal or decreased level	Decreased level or absent
Blood	Bilirubin	Unconjugated	Unconjugated and conjugated	Conjugated
	Liver enzymes	Normal levels	AST, ALT raised	Alkaline phosphatase, GGT raised

ALT, *Alanine transaminase;* AST, *aspartate transaminase;* GGT, *γ-glutamyltransferase.*

Chapter Summary

- Bilirubin is the breakdown product of haemoglobin.
- Jaundice becomes apparent if bilirubin level is greater than 35 µmol/L.
- Jaundice can be of prehepatic, hepatic or posthepatic origin.
- The history and examination, together with investigations, will point towards the cause.
- Management depends on the underlying disease.

UKMLA Conditions
Alcoholic hepatitis
Hepatitis
Jaundice
Liver failure

UKMLA Presentations
Ascites
Change in stool colour
Jaundice
Pruritis

Urinary symptoms and haematuria

INTRODUCTION

In this chapter we review the approach to assessing and managing urinary symptoms including polyuria, dysuria and incontinence. We focus on causes and approach to managing haematuria.

The volume of water in the circulation is under constant physiological control. Water is reabsorbed from the loop of Henle as it passes through the hyperosmolar renal medulla, and is also reabsorbed from the collecting ducts under the control of antidiuretic hormone (ADH, also called 'vasopressin') (Fig. 15.1). ADH is synthesized by the hypothalamus and released from the posterior pituitary in response to a rise in serum osmolality or fall in plasma volume.

MICTURITION DISTURBANCES

Urinary symptoms:

- Polyuria: the passage of excessive volumes of urine (>3 L in 24 hours). Urine output depends on fluid intake and loss via other routes (e.g., respiration, sweat, faeces), and typically ranges from 1 to 3 L/day.
- Polydipsia: excessive thirst, often manifested as the ingestion of excessive volumes of fluid. Usually a consequence of polyuria.
- Frequency: the frequent passage of small volumes of urine.
- Dysuria: pain on passing urine.
- Nocturia: passage of urine at night. May be associated with frequency or polyuria.

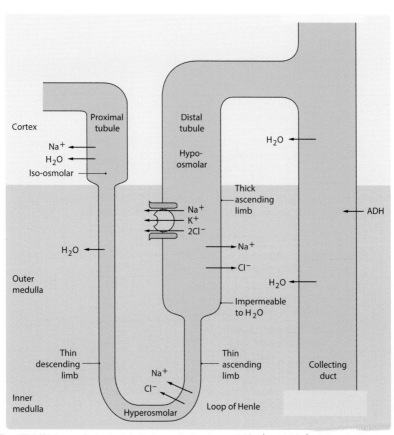

Fig. 15.1 Water and electrolyte balance in the loop of Henle. *ADH,* Antidiuretic hormone.

- Oliguria: the passage of small volumes of urine.
- Anuria: no passage of urine.
  - Oliguria and anuria may be due to renal impairment or urinary tract obstruction (see Chapter 31).

HINTS AND TIPS

There are many causes of polyuria, but those seen most commonly in clinical practice are hyperglycaemia and hypercalcaemia.

The differential diagnosis of polyuria/polydipsia is summarized in Table 15.1.

Frequency is often due to bladder irritation, which is commonly due to infection but can also be caused by chemical irritation, tumours or bladder calculi. Dysuria is most commonly due to infection, but can also be caused by chemical irritation. When accompanied by frequency, it may indicate cystitis, and in men may also be caused by prostatitis.

Symptoms of bladder outflow obstruction, such as those caused by an enlarged prostate gland, include hesitancy (difficulty initiating micturition), terminal dribbling and poor stream.

Urinary incontinence is common, and is broadly divided into stress incontinence and urge incontinence. Stress incontinence is common in women and is often due to weakened pelvic floor muscles resulting from physical changes following pregnancy and childbirth. Urge incontinence is associated with detrusor instability and inappropriate contraction, which may be a consequence of local factors such as infection or inflammation, or may be due to damage to the nerve supply. Innervation is mainly from the autonomic nervous system, although there is voluntary control of the external urinary sphincter, and higher control of urination in the micturition centre of the pons.

CLINICAL NOTES

Symptoms of prostatic hypertrophy include poor stream, hesitancy, postmicturition dribbling and incomplete emptying. Nocturia is a troubling symptom – ask the patient about sleep disturbance.

Table 15.1 Differential diagnosis of polyuria

Causes	Examples/notes
Cranial DI (insufficient ADH secretion)	Idiopathic (often familial and commonest form) Following pituitary surgery/irradiation Following head trauma Malignancy (e.g., craniopharyngioma, pinealoma, glioma, metastases) Infections (e.g., meningitis) Infiltrations (e.g., sarcoid and histiocytosis X) Drugs (e.g., alcohol)
Nephrogenic DI (inability of kidney to respond to ADH)	Congenital (primary renal tubular defect) Electrolyte imbalance (hypokalaemia and hypercalcaemia) Lithium toxicity Long-standing pyelonephritis or hydronephrosis
Chronic kidney disease	Can result in depressed kidney concentrating ability and therefore higher urine volume to excrete a given solute load
Acute renal failure	Diuretic phase of ATN Following relief of obstructive uropathy Early stages of analgesic nephropathy
Osmotic diuresis	Glucose (diabetes mellitus) Calcium (hypercalcaemia)
ANP release	Arrhythmia (e.g., after SVT)
Psychogenic polydipsia	Relatively common psychiatric disturbance characterized by excessive water intake (if prolonged can cause temporary 'renal medullary washout' with reduction of kidney's concentrating ability)

ADH, *Antidiuretic hormone;* ANP, *atrial natriuretic peptide;* ATN, *acute tubular necrosis;* DI, *diabetes insipidus;* SVT, *supraventricular tachycardia.*

HISTORY AND EXAMINATION FINDINGS

History

For many urinary symptoms, there will be a simple explanation, for instance infection or prostatic hypertrophy. The history should focus on the following points:

- Frequency: is there coexistent fever, dysuria or cloudy urine (pyuria) which may indicate infection? If so, is there a history of recurrent infection that might indicate a predisposition (e.g., diabetes, urinary stasis, immunosuppression)? In men, are there associated symptoms of prostatic hypertrophy? Is there urinary stasis from incomplete bladder emptying?
- Does the patient have loin pain, or a history of renal calculi?
- Is there associated haematuria? In the presence of other lower urinary tract symptoms this could be due to infection, calculus or a bladder tumour.
- If incontinence is present, determine the circumstances in which it occurs (i.e., coughing, standing) and the effect it is having on the patient's everyday activities.
- Consider medication causes (e.g., is the patient taking diuretics?).

Polyuria and polydipsia may pose a more difficult diagnostic challenge, after general questions the enquiry should focus on the following:

- Differentiation between polyuria and frequency.
- Weight loss: associated with malignancy which may result in hypercalcaemia.
- Headache: primary or secondary brain tumours can cause diabetes insipidus.
- Family history: this is relevant in diabetes mellitus, both forms of diabetes insipidus (cranial and nephrogenic) and renal stone disease.
- Medical history: particularly consider previous neurosurgery or radiotherapy, head injuries and meningitis.
- Drug history: lithium may cause nephrogenic diabetes insipidus; vitamin D or milk–alkali syndrome may lead to hypercalcaemia.
- Recurrent infections: may be due to diabetes mellitus.
- Features of hypercalcaemia (see Chapter 32).
- Brief psychiatric history: especially if thirst is predominant. These patients may drink surreptitiously, resist investigation, have other symptoms and lack nocturnal symptoms.

Examination

The examination approach in the patient with urinary symptoms is summarized in Fig. 15.2. Consider the following:

General
- Wasting/cachexia (malignancy and initial presentation of type 1 diabetes mellitus)
- Hydration status.
- Skin manifestations: diabetes mellitus and malignancy (see Chapter 36).
- Nails: clubbing – associated with bronchogenic carcinoma, which may produce parathyroid hormone (and result in hypercalcaemia), or may metastasize to the brain.
- Anaemia: malignancy or chronic kidney disease (CKD).
- Lymphadenopathy: malignancy or infiltrative disorder.
- Optic signs: fundal changes of hypertension or diabetes.
- Blood pressure for hypertensive nephropathy.

Abdominal examination
- Palpate the kidneys carefully as they may be enlarged in polycystic kidney disease or with a hydronephrosis.
- A large bladder may indicate urinary tract obstruction.
- The liver and spleen may be enlarged in malignancy and infiltrative disorders.
- An enlarged or craggy prostate can often be palpated on rectal examination.

Neurological examination
- Peripheral neuropathy (caused by diabetes or infiltrative disorders).
- Hypotonia and areflexia with hypokalaemia.
- Visual fields (classically bitemporal hemianopia with pituitary disease) and papilloedema (raised intracranial pressure).
- In idiopathic urge incontinence if there is evidence of any underlying neurological abnormality.

INVESTIGATIONS

The following investigations should be considered:

Urine tests
- Urinalysis (urine dip): pH, protein, blood, glucose and ketones, as well as leucocytes and nitrites, the presence of which may indicate infection.
- Laboratory urine analysis can measure urine osmolality and quantify protein loss (protein/creatinine or albumin/creatinine ratios). Urinary electrolytes, including sodium, potassium, phosphate, calcium and oxalate, can be measured. Urine microscopy may reveal the presence of blood cells, bacteria or casts, and culture may reveal a pathogenic organism.

Blood tests
- Biochemistry: acute kidney injury or CKD (see Chapter 31), hypercalcaemia, hypokalaemia (see Chapter 32) and hyperglycaemia.

- Full blood count: anaemia with CKD or malignancy. Raised white cell count suggests infection.

Imaging

- Chest X-ray: if any suspicion of sarcoidosis, primary or secondary malignancy.
- Renal tract ultrasound scan can detect abnormal kidney size, cysts and masses, congenital defects of the renal tract, hydronephrosis or hydroureter.
- CT of the kidneys/ureters/bladder (CT KUB – noncontrast CT scan) if there is suspicion of renal tract calculi.

- CT or MRI of brain to investigate intracranial disease (e.g., if considering a space-occupying lesion).

Further investigations

- Renal concentration tests in polyuria: if either a hypothalamic or a pituitary cause or renal tubular dysfunction is suspected. It is mandatory to exclude other potential causes of polyuria, as renal concentration tests may be dangerous. The patient is asked to drink nothing from 16:00 the day before attending the outpatient department. If the urine osmolality the next morning is not greater than

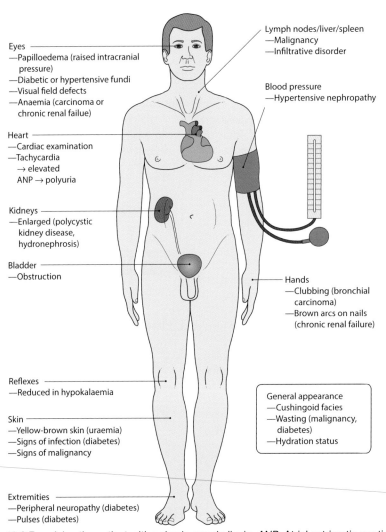

Eyes
—Papilloedema (raised intracranial pressure)
—Diabetic or hypertensive fundi
—Visual field defects
—Anaemia (carcinoma or chronic renal failue)

Heart
—Cardiac examination
—Tachycardia
 → elevated
 ANP → polyuria

Kidneys
—Enlarged (polycystic kidney disease, hydronephrosis)

Bladder
—Obstruction

Reflexes
—Reduced in hypokalaemia

Skin
—Yellow-brown skin (uraemia)
—Signs of infection (diabetes)
—Signs of malignancy

Extremities
—Peripheral neuropathy (diabetes)
—Pulses (diabetes)

Lymph nodes/liver/spleen
—Malignancy
—Infiltrative disorder

Blood pressure
—Hypertensive nephropathy

Hands
—Clubbing (bronchial carcinoma)
—Brown arcs on nails (chronic renal failure)

General appearance
—Cushingoid facies
—Wasting (malignancy, diabetes)
—Hydration status

Fig. 15.2 Examining the patient with polyuria or polydipsia. *ANP*, Atrial natriuretic peptide.

800 mmol/kg, inpatient tests are required (Box 15.1 and Table 15.2).

- Urodynamic tests: these commonly measure the prevoid and postvoid bladder volume and flow rate to assess bladder emptying.
- Nuclear renography: radioisotope uptake scans (e.g., dimercaptosuccinic acid (DMSA) or mercaptoacetyltriglycine (MAG3) scans) can provide detailed information about asymmetric kidney function and can evaluate kidney scarring.

BOX 15.1 PROCEDURE FOR TESTING INPATIENTS WITH POLYURIA AND POLYDIPSIA

- Weigh the patient.
- Deprive the patient of all fluids the night before the tests.
- The next morning, weigh the patient every 2 h (a decrease in weight by >3% indicates dehydration, so stop the test).
- Collect urine and blood for osmolality measurement.
- If the urine osmolality fails to reach 800 mmol/kg, intramuscularly administer desmopressin (which is synthetic vasopressin), which acts in the same way as ADH.
- Collect blood and urine for osmolality measurement.

HAEMATURIA

Haematuria (blood in the urine) is classified as visible or nonvisible, painful or painless and whether it is associated with proteinuria. Haematuria and proteinuria together are suggestive of intrinsic renal damage, and are discussed in Chapter 31. Painful haematuria may suggest renal calculus or urinary tract infection; painless haematuria suggests the possibility of renal tract malignancy. Remember that red urine may also be due to haemoglobinuria, myoglobinuria, porphyria, drugs (e.g., rifampicin) or even the ingestion of beetroot.

Haematuria can come from anywhere in the urogenital tract. It can be classified by the site of disease (see Table 15.3). Systemic conditions (e.g., thrombocytopenia) or anticoagulants can predispose to bleeding.

HISTORY AND EXAMINATION FINDINGS

- Ask about the appearance of the urine. Is there frank blood (malignancy) or clots?
- Ask about associated urinary symptoms (see earlier).
- Is the haematuria worse with exercise?
- Is there loin pain (present with pyelonephritis or renal calculi)?
- Is there colicky pain (ureteric calculus)?
- Is there a history of trauma?
- Does the patient have vaginal or penile discharge?

CLINICAL NOTES

If haematuria is present in a young woman, it is important to ask about the menstrual cycle and whether she was menstruating when the haematuria was noticed.

Table 15.2 Interpretation of patient test results

	Fluid deprivation		After intramuscular administration of desmopressin	
	Plasma osmolality	Urine osmolality	Plasma osmolality	Urine osmolality
Pituitary DI	↑	→	↑	↑
Psychogenic polydipsia	↑	↑a	↑	↑
Nephrogenic DI	↑	→	↑	→

aUrine is concentrated, but less than in normal response.

DI, *Diabetes insipidus*; ↑, *increase in osmolality*; →, *no significant change in osmolality*.

Table 15.3 Differential diagnosis of haematuria

Site	Causes
Kidney	Infections (pyelonephritis, tuberculosis) Tumours (renal cell carcinoma) Trauma (spontaneous or after renal biopsy) Papillary necrosis (associated with diabetes) Glomerulonephritis (e.g., IgA nephropathy)
Ureters	Renal calculi Malignancy Trauma
Bladder	Cystitis; infection, post-radiation cystitis Malignancy Trauma Bladder calculi Infections; tuberculosis and schistosomiasis
Prostate	Prostate carcinoma Benign prostatic hypertrophy Infection; prostatitis
Urethra	Calculi Trauma Malignancy Foreign bodies

CLINICAL NOTES

Ask *when* in the urinary stream the patient notices the blood. Patients may not volunteer this information because they do not think it is important.

- If the urine is bloodstained at the start of micturition and clears later, the site of disease is likely to be the urethra or prostate.
- If the urine is more bloodstained towards the end of micturition, the site of disease is likely to be the bladder.
- If the urine is evenly bloodstained throughout micturition, the site of disease is likely to be the kidney or ureter.

INVESTIGATIONS

Initial tests

- Gross appearance: visible, asymptomatic, haematuria in patients older than 45 years should always make you consider malignancy (Fig. 15.3).
- Urinalysis (urine dip): as earlier.
- Microscopy and culture (midstream urine): infection.
- Early morning urine: acid-fast bacilli if tuberculosis is suspected.
- Cytology: malignancy.

Other investigations

Imaging: as discussed in micturition disturbances, renal ultrasound and CT KUB common investigations. Consider further imaging (CT chest/abdomen/pelvis) in malignancy staging.

- Cystoscopy: bladder lesions.
- Ureteroscopy: ureter lesions.

RED FLAG

Visible asymptomatic haematuria in patients over 45 years and persistent nonvisible haematuria in patients over 60 years need urgent urological investigation to exclude a renal tract malignancy (see Fig. 15.3).

PROTEINURIA

Small amounts of proteinuria can occur in nonrenal diseases such as urinary tract infection and with vaginal mucus; however, significant proteinuria (more than 1 g/day) usually indicates primary renal pathology. Proteinuria is discussed in further detail in Chapter 31.

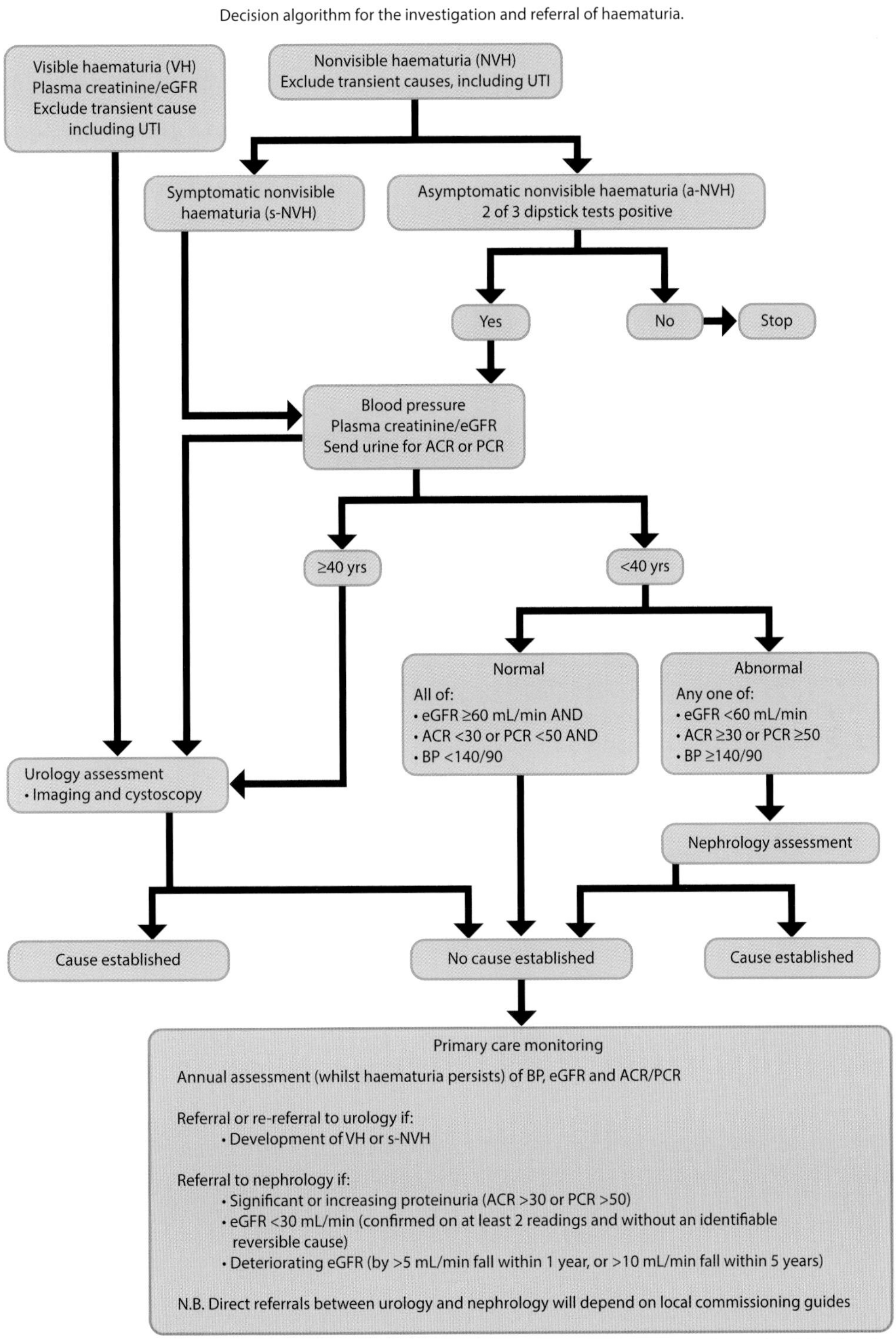

Decision algorithm for the investigation and referral of haematuria.

Fig. 15.3 BAUS/RA Guidelines: Initial assessment of haematuria, July 2008. *ACR*, Albumin/creatine ratio; *BP*, blood pressure; *eGFR*, estimated glomerular filtration rate, *PCR*, protein/creatinine ratio; *UTI*, urinary tract infection.

Chapter Summary

- Urinary symptoms include symptoms of irritation (frequency, dysuria) or obstruction (hesitancy, poor stream, postmicturition dribbling, incomplete voiding).
- Polydipsia and polyuria can be driven by high glucose levels, hypercalcaemia and diabetes insipidus.
- Diabetic insipidus can be cranial or nephrogenic; focus your history taking and examination on potential causes.
- Haematuria can occur from anywhere in the urogenital tract. It can be classified into visible and nonvisible, painful and painless. Painless visible haematuria in patients over 45 years and persistent nonvisible haematuria in patients over 60 years should prompt urological referral to exclude an underlying malignancy.

UKMLA Conditions
Acute kidney injury
Adverse drug effects
Anaemia
Bladder cancer
Brain metastases
Chronic kidney disease
Dehydration
Diabetes insipidus
Diabetes mellitus type 1 and 2
Haematuria
Incidental findings
Lung cancer
Metastatic disease
Pituitary tumours
Polydipsia (thirst)
Prostate cancer
Urinary incontinence
Urinary symptoms
Urinary tract calculi
Urinary tract infection

UKMLA Presentations
Abnormal urinalysis
Acute kidney injury
Chronic kidney disease
Dehydration
Diabetes mellitus type 1 and 2
Electrolyte abnormalities
Haematuria
Oliguria
Polydipsia (thirst)
Urinary incontinence
Urinary symptoms

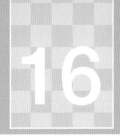
INTRODUCTION

Headache (see Chapter 34) is one of the most common presenting symptoms. There are often few clinical signs, and the history is the main diagnostic tool. Many different pathological processes can result in headaches and facial pain. The International Headache Society classification divides headaches into primary (where the headache is itself the disease; e.g., migraine), secondary (where the headache is due to other conditions; e.g., infection, trauma, vascular disorder) and other headaches, facial pains and cranial neuropathies (e.g., trigeminal neuralgia).

The differential diagnosis of headache and facial pain are summarized in Table 16.1.

HISTORY AND EXAMINATION FINDINGS

History

Characteristics of the headache will point towards the diagnosis.

> **HINTS AND TIPS**
>
> If patients struggle to describe the headache or suffer from multiple episodes, advise them to keep a headache diary where they can record all the information in chronological order.

Solitary acute episode

This pattern is seen in vascular events, infection and trauma. It may also be the first presentation of the other causes of headaches.

Subarachnoid haemorrhage presents with a sudden onset of severe pain 'as if someone had hit them on the head'. Often most severe occipitally, with maximal severity at onset or within seconds. Nausea, vomiting, neck stiffness and photophobia can result from meningeal irritation and raised intracranial pressure (ICP).

Cerebral venous sinus thrombosis can lead to seizures, focal neurological signs and symptoms of raised ICP (see later). Causes include inherited coagulation disorders, pregnancy, oral contraceptive pill use, dehydration, an extension of local infection (e.g., paranasal sinuses or middle ear) and severe intercurrent illness.

Patients with infective meningitis present with a short history of headache, symptoms of infection (malaise, fever, rigors), meningeal irritation (vomiting, photophobia, neck pain and/or stiffness) and possibly a rash or altered mental state. Encephalitis, acute brain inflammation, may present with features similar to meningitis.

Cerebral abscess may cause fevers, rigors, headaches, seizures and symptoms of raised ICP as the lesion enlarges. The infection may have spread from a local or distant primary focus, such as lung (bronchiectasis, abscess), heart (endocarditis), middle ear or sinuses (paranasal sinusitis).

Acute angle-closure glaucoma can cause a severe headache associated with blurred vision, eye pain, cloudiness of the cornea, conjunctival injection and a dilated pupil. There may be nausea and vomiting. It should be considered in hypermetropic patients. It may occur intermittently with repeated acute attacks.

> **HINTS AND TIPS**
>
> Ask the patient when was the last time they were headache free – this can help differentiate between a progressive headache and a migraine.

Progressive headache

A headache that comes on gradually over days or weeks and increases in severity is often a feature of a 'space-occupying lesion' (such as a tumour or abscess), idiopathic intracranial hypertension, chronic subdural haematoma or hydrocephalus. Hydrocephalus can be due to either blockage of cerebrospinal fluid (CSF) flow ('noncommunicating', e.g., haemorrhage, cysts, malformations) or failure of CSF reabsorption ('communicating', e.g., following meningitis or subarachnoid haemorrhage).

In these, the headache results from raised ICP and has the characteristic features outlined below.

> **CLINICAL NOTES**
>
> **SYMPTOMS OF RAISED ICP**
>
> - Headache worse on coughing, sneezing and stooping down.
> - Headache worse in the morning.
> - Visual disturbance due to papilloedema.
> - Nausea and vomiting.
> - Diplopia (false localizing cranial nerve VI palsy).

Table 16.1 Differential diagnosis of headache and facial pain (see Chapter 34)

Pattern	Causes
Solitary acute episode	Infection: meningitis, encephalitis, abscess Vascular event: intracranial haemorrhage (especially subarachnoid), venous sinus thrombosis, occasionally infarction (especially if arterial dissection occurred) Trauma First migraine or benign thunderclap headache
Progressive headache	Raised ICP (including idiopathic intracranial hypertension) Giant cell arteritis
Episodic headache/facial pain	Migraine Cluster headache and other trigeminal autonomic cephalalgias Trigeminal neuralgia Coital cephalalgia
Chronic headache/facial pain	Tension headache/analgesic rebound headache Postherpetic neuralgia Head injury Paget disease of the skull
Other causes of facial pain	Dental problems Temporomandibular joint Ears/nose/sinuses Cervical spine Eye – especially acute or intermittent angle-closure glaucoma

ICP, *Intracranial pressure.*

CLINICAL NOTES

SIGNS OF RAISED ICP

- Papilloedema
- False localizing sign (ipsilateral then bilateral cranial nerve VI palsy)
- Altered level of consciousness
- Bradycardia with hypertension (the Cushing reflex – a late sign); may indicate imminent brain herniation and death

HINTS AND TIPS

Consider temporal arteritis in any patient older than 50 years with a headache (see Chapter 34).

Recurrent episodic headache and facial pain

Migraine and cluster headaches present with episodes of pain (often severe) interspersed with long symptom-free periods. Paroxysms of pain are also a feature of trigeminal neuralgia and other cranial neuralgias.

Although classically, migraine is preceded by an aura, migraine without aura is more common. Premonitory symptoms precede both types, occur hours to days before the migraine and include fatigue, nausea and sensitivity to light and noise. Aura can consist of visual features (positive, e.g., flickering lights, spots or lines, or negative, e.g., visual loss), sensory symptoms (paraesthesia or numbness), speech disturbance and focal neurology. These symptoms can occur with or without a headache and are fully reversible (see Chapter 34).

Cluster headache is a severe unilateral pain centred around one eye. It is more common in men and may be precipitated by alcohol. The pain occurs up to eight times per day for several weeks, often waking the patient from sleep. There may be ipsilateral nasal congestion or rhinorrhoea, and the eye can become watery and red; miosis and ptosis can also develop

Headache associated with temporal arteritis is also of gradual onset; however, the nature of it is different from that described earlier. The condition predominantly affects older people (mean age at onset is over 70 years). Presentation is with superficial headache overlying the temporal arteries; scalp tenderness, which may be exacerbated by brushing or combing the hair, is often present. Jaw claudication, and occasionally tongue claudication, may arise because of inflammation of the branches of the external carotid artery. Visual loss may be temporary (amaurosis fugax) or permanent if the ciliary or central retinal arteries are affected. Weight loss, anorexia, fever and proximal muscle stiffness (but not tenderness) may also occur.

and occasionally become permanent. Symptom-free periods of many months occur between attacks.

Trigeminal neuralgia is characterized by paroxysms of lancinating pain in the distribution of cranial nerve V. It is often stimulated by the touching of 'trigger zones' on the face, such as the lips, or by eating or drinking but can occur spontaneously.

Chronic headache and facial pain

Persistent pain is a feature of postherpetic neuralgia, posttraumatic headache, Paget disease of the skull and tension headache.

Postherpetic neuralgia is persistent burning pain in the nerve distribution that develops following the nerve's infection by varicella zoster virus (commonly known as 'shingles').

Tension-type headache is often described as 'a tight band around the head'. It is most often constant and bilateral and tends to worsen towards the end of the day or at times of stress.

People with headaches that developed or worsened while using analgesic medication for more than 3 months may have a medication-overuse headache. It can occur with practically any medicines commonly used to treat headache, including nonsteroidal antiinflammatory drugs (NSAIDs), paracetamol, aspirin, triptan, opioid and ergot drugs.

HINTS AND TIPS

Opiate-based analgesia is most frequently seen as the cause of medication-overuse headaches.

Examination

On examination, look for evidence of pathological processes, such as raised ICP and meningism. Focal neurological deficits, if present, help to determine the site of the lesion. Fig. 16.1 summarizes the examination approach.

CLINICAL NOTES

SIGNS OF MENINGISM

- Irritability: with a preference for a quiet, darkened room
- Neck stiffness and photophobia
- Positive Kernig sign: spasm and pain in hamstrings on knee extension
- Positive Brudzinski sign: neck flexion causes hip and knee flexion
- Delirium, fever and petechial rash: may be present in infectious meningitis

---

CLINICAL NOTES

SUBARACHNOID HAEMORRHAGE

Look for subhyaloid (retinal) haemorrhage, bruit of an arteriovenous malformation and a cranial nerve III palsy caused by direct pressure from a posterior communicating artery aneurysm.

CLINICAL NOTES

SIGNS OF TEMPORAL ARTERITIS

- Temporal artery tenderness
- Loss of temporal artery pulsation – there may be overlying erythema
- Optic atrophy (seen as optic disc pallor)
- Low-grade pyrexia

INVESTIGATIONS

An algorithm for investigating the patient with headache and facial pain is shown in Fig. 16.2. Investigations include the following.

Blood tests

- Full blood count: normochromic normocytic anaemia suggests chronic disease (e.g., temporal arteritis, tuberculous meningitis); leucocytosis in infection.
- Erythrocyte sedimentation rate and C-reactive protein (CRP): high in temporal arteritis but may also be raised in infection and malignancy.
- Clotting studies may be important in the context of intracerebral bleeding.

Imaging

- CT or MRI scans of the head: presence of blood, space-occupying lesion (tumour, abscess) or hydrocephalus. Contrast enhancement may help determine the nature of a lesion.
- CT angiography, magnetic resonance angiography or digital subtraction angiography: to identify the precise cause (e.g., berry aneurysm or arteriovenous malformation) in subarachnoid haemorrhage.

Further tests (Fig. 16.2)

- Temporal artery biopsy: temporal arteritis. This is a definitive test, but a negative result does not exclude the diagnosis as there is often patchy vascular involvement ('skip lesions').

- Lumbar puncture: this should never be performed when raised ICP is a possibility, as it may cause cerebellar tonsil herniation ('coning'). CSF should be sent to the laboratory to assess glucose, protein, microscopy, culture and cytology (see Chapter 21). CSF sampling may also diagnose subarachnoid haemorrhages not detected on CT (xanthochromia).

- Visual fields: these should be serially measured in patients with idiopathic intracranial hypertension (because of the risk of optic nerve infarction and visual field defects).
- Electroencephalography: herpes simplex encephalitis shows abnormal patterns.
- Intraocular tonometry: pressure will be raised in glaucoma.

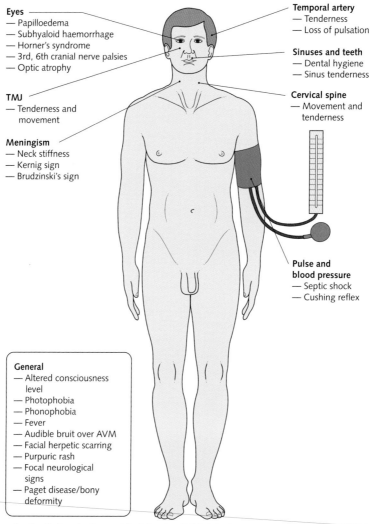

Eyes
— Papilloedema
— Subhyaloid haemorrhage
— Horner's syndrome
— 3rd, 6th cranial nerve palsies
— Optic atrophy

TMJ
— Tenderness and movement

Meningism
— Neck stiffness
— Kernig sign
— Brudzinski's sign

Temporal artery
— Tenderness
— Loss of pulsation

Sinuses and teeth
— Dental hygiene
— Sinus tenderness

Cervical spine
— Movement and tenderness

Pulse and blood pressure
— Septic shock
— Cushing reflex

General
— Altered consciousness level
— Photophobia
— Phonophobia
— Fever
— Audible bruit over AVM
— Facial herpetic scarring
— Purpuric rash
— Focal neurological signs
— Paget disease/bony deformity

Fig. 16.1 Examining the patient with headache and facial pain. *AVM*, Arteriovenous malformation; *TMJ*, temporomandibular joint.

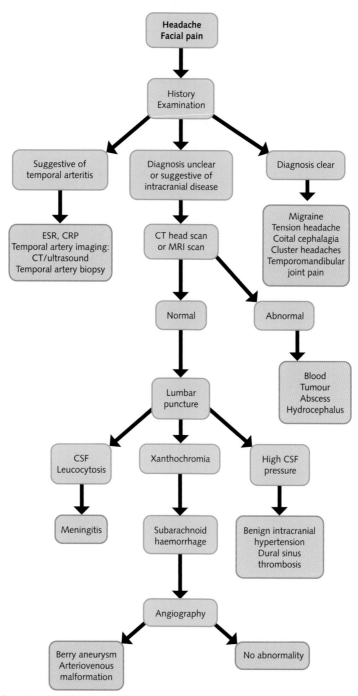

Fig. 16.2 Algorithm for the investigation of the patient with headache and facial pain. *CSF*, Cerebrospinal fluid; *CT*, computed tomography; *ESR*, erythrocyte sedimentation rate; *MRI*, magnetic resonance imaging.

Chapter Summary

- Tension headache is the most common type of headache.
- The history and examination are the most useful diagnostic tools for a patient with a headache.
- Brain imaging is not routinely performed in patients with no worrying features.
- Raised ICP is a contraindication to performing a lumbar puncture.

UKMLA Conditions
Encephalitis
Meningitis
Migraine
Raised intracranial pressure
Tension headache
Visual field defects

UKMLA Presentations
Facial pain
Headache
Neck pain/stiffness

Goitre, thyroid disease and thyroid malignancy 17

INTRODUCTION

The control of thyroid hormone production and release is outlined in Fig. 33.4. Thyroid disease results from either under or over production of these hormones. The spectrum of thyroid disease encompasses conditions including hypo- and hyperthyroidism, and thyroid cysts which may be benign or malignant. Some of these disorders will present with an enlarged thyroid gland (i.e., a goitre). In this chapter we will discuss each in turn.

GOITRE

'Goitre' means an enlarged thyroid gland. It may be a single enlarged gland or composed of a single nodule or multiple nodules. The leading cause of a goitre worldwide is iodine deficiency; in the United Kingdom, however, where iodine is added to foods as a supplement, autoimmune conditions (e.g., Hashimoto thyroiditis and Graves disease) are the most common causes.

Thyroid nodules are common, and are often incidental findings on ultrasonography or at autopsy. In adults, only around 5% of these nodules are malignant. Thyroid nodules are less common in children, but a greater proportion are malignant.

CLINICAL NOTES

The incidence of thyroid cancer peaks between 30 and 50 years and is around three times more common in women.

HISTORY AND EXAMINATION FINDINGS

Goitre may be noticed by someone else or may be seen by the patient in the mirror. The history taking should aim to reveal any features of compression from the goitre, whether the metabolic function of the gland is altered, and to elucidate whether a malignant cause is likely:

- Duration of goitre and rate of change: long-standing goitres suggest benign disease.

- Local symptoms: ask about dysphagia, dyspnoea and hoarseness.
- Tenderness: subacute thyroiditis.
- Symptoms of hypothyroidism or hyperthyroidism.
- Pregnancy/menopause (associated with thyroid enlargement).
- Previous or current use of goitrogenic drugs (e.g., lithium, amiodarone).
- Smoking (the evidence is conflicting but smoking is certainly a risk factor for other malignancies which may cause neck lumps).
- Diet, lack of iodine or conversely very high iodine intake (e.g., seaweed); both can lead to goitre formation.
- Exposure to environmental factors such as previous radiotherapy or environmental radiation such as fallout from the Hiroshima or Chernobyl disasters, or living in an area of high volcanic activity such as Iceland or Hawaii (all are risk factors for benign and malignant thyroid nodules).
- Family history: ask about a history of goitre (suggesting autoimmune disease) or of thyroid cancer (suggesting familial thyroid cancer or multiple endocrine neoplasia).

Physical examination should look for:

- Signs related to the patient's thyroid status (see sections on hypo-/hyperthyroidism).
- Whether the goitre is smooth or nodular.
- Whether there are nodules and whether these are multiple nodules or a single nodule.
- Whether the nodule is hard or soft, regular or irregular and fixed or mobile and whether there is lymphadenopathy.

HINTS AND TIPS

When examining the patient, ask them to drink some water, and note the thyroid moving as the patient swallows. Does the mass move with swallowing? If it does, this suggests it is part of the thyroid. Look for enlargement and asymmetry. Stand behind a seated patient and use your fingers to examine the gland as the patient swallows. Feel for lumps and tenderness. Percuss down below the thyroid onto the anterior chest wall to detect any retrosternal thyroid mass.

INVESTIGATIONS

The following investigations are important in patients with goitre/thyroid nodule:

- Thyroid function tests: screening for hypo- or hyperthyroidism. Thyroid-stimulating hormone (TSH) level is usually checked first; if it is abnormal, free triiodothyronine (T_3) and thyroxine (T_4) levels are measured.
- Calcitonin secretion: increased in medullary thyroid cancer, and should be measured only in patients in whom there is high clinical suspicion of medullary thyroid cancer.

Imaging

- Thyroid size and nature: assessed by ultrasound, CT or magnetic resonance imaging (MRI) scan. Ultrasonography is quick to perform and can differentiate between cystic and solid nodules. It cannot distinguish benign from malignant lesions. CT or MRI is useful in assessing compression or invasion of other structures.
- Radionuclide imaging (thyroid scintigraphy): can distinguish 'hot nodules' (high uptake of radioisotope) from 'cold nodules' (due to lack of concentration of radioisotope). Unfortunately, there are no specific features that indicate the benign or malignant nature of a thyroid nodule. Malignant nodules are more likely to be cold than hot, although most cold nodules are benign. Even so, the presence of a hot nodule does not exclude malignancy.
- Respiratory function tests, including flow–volume loop: if signs of upper airway obstruction are present.

Further investigations

- Fine-needle aspiration cytology: performed on nodules where there are suspicious features in the history or examination findings. It can be performed in outpatients, and is well tolerated; cytology is not completely reliable as false-positive and false-negative results occur.

DIFFERENTIAL DIAGNOSIS

- Diffuse:
  - Graves disease
  - Hashimoto thyroiditis
  - de Quervain thyroiditis
  - Iodine deficiency
- Nodular:
  - Nontoxic multinodular goitre: nonfunctioning nodules with normal thyroid function test results (e.g., pregnancy, puberty and menopause).
  - Thyroid adenoma or cyst.
  - Thyroid carcinoma.
  - Nonthyroid lumps including thyroglossal cyst, brachial cyst and pharyngeal pouch

Hypothyroidism

Hypothyroidism results from deficiency of T_4 or T_3. The prevalence is up to 2% in women; it is around five times less common in men.

Aetiology

Primary thyroid failure may take the following forms:

- Chronic autoimmune (Hashimoto) thyroiditis: this is around five to eight times more common in women than in men, and tends to affect the middle-aged and elderly. Patients may present with a firm, nontender goitre, hypothyroidism or both. It is associated with vitiligo, pernicious anaemia, insulin-dependent diabetes mellitus, Addison disease and premature ovarian failure. Biopsy shows a lymphocytic infiltrate with destruction of follicles and variable fibrosis.
- Primary atrophic hypothyroidism: goitre due to lymphocytic infiltration of the thyroid, leading to atrophy and hence no goitre. The incidence increases with age, and it is more common in women.
- Previous treatment for hyperthyroidism: postthyroidectomy or radioiodine.
- Drug-induced hypothyroidism: can occur with amiodarone and lithium carbonate.
- Secondary thyroid failure is rare and can be caused by hypothalamus or pituitary disease resulting in reduced levels of thyrotropin-releasing hormone or TSH.
- Iodine-deficient hypothyroidism: this is a major cause of hypothyroidism and goitre worldwide, although most iodine-deficient people are euthyroid even though they have a goitre.
- Congenital hypothyroidism: the prevalence in the United Kingdom is 1 in 3500 to 4000 infants, and it is diagnosed in the first week of life by routine screening,

measuring TSH or T_4. It is usually due to thyroid agenesis, which is mostly sporadic, or dyshormonogenesis, which is due to autosomal recessively inherited enzyme defects.

Clinical features

The onset is insidious, and symptoms are often nonspecific, therefore patients may not be aware that anything is wrong. Common presenting symptoms include tiredness, lethargy, weight gain, cold intolerance, constipation, hoarseness and dryness of the skin. However, virtually any organ system can be affected. Very rarely it presents as myxoedema coma (see Chapter 33).

HINTS AND TIPS

Mnemonic for remembering signs:
BRADYCARDIC
Reflexes (slow)
Ataxia (cerebellar)
Dry, thin skin/hair
Yawning/drowsy/coma
Cold hands
Ascites/nonpitting oedema (eyelids, shins, feet)
Round, puffy face
Demeanour (dull, blank, defeated)
Ileus
CCF

Investigations

Blood tests
- Thyroid function tests: these include tests for TSH. If the level of TSH is abnormal, then tests for T_4 and T_3 are performed.
- Antibodies to thyroglobulin or thyroid peroxidase (microsomal antibodies): typically strongly positive in Hashimoto thyroiditis.
- Cholesterol level is often raised.
- Full blood count: anaemia is often present, possibly with a mild macrocytosis.
- Urea and electrolytes; hyponatraemia is a feature of hypothyroidism.

Other
- ECG: sinus bradycardia, low-voltage complexes.

Imaging
- Ultrasonography, CT, MRI or radionuclide imaging (thyroid scintigraphy) may be performed if nodules are present.

CLINICAL NOTES

- In primary disease, the free and total T_4 levels are reduced and serum TSH level is high.
- In subclinical hypothyroidism, T_4 level may be normal, with a high serum TSH level.
- In secondary hypothyroidism, the free and total T_4 levels are reduced and the TSH level is usually also low. This picture is also seen in unwell people without thyroid disease ('sick euthyroid') and in patients taking steroids and anticonvulsants.

Hyperthyroidism

Thyrotoxicosis is the condition resulting from raised levels of circulating free T_4 and free T_3. It affects approximately 10 in 1000 women and 1 in 1000 men. 'Hyperthyroidism' indicates thyroid gland overactivity, which may cause thyrotoxicosis. However, the terms 'thyrotoxicosis' and 'hyperthyroidism' are often used interchangeably.

Aetiology

Primary hyperthyroidism

Graves disease – This accounts for up to 80% of cases of hyperthyroidism. It is caused by the production of autoantibodies that stimulate the TSH receptor. There is a painless diffuse goitre in more than 90% of patients. In addition to the general features of thyrotoxicosis (see later), features specific to Graves disease may occur, including ophthalmopathy, pretibial myxoedema and thyroid acropachy.

- The ophthalmopathy includes periorbital oedema, conjunctival oedema (chemosis), proptosis, diplopia, impaired visual acuity and corneal ulceration due to exposure. It is clinically obvious in up to 50% of patients with Graves disease but subclinical ophthalmopathy can be detected in more than 90% of patients by CT scan or MRI, revealing enlargement of the extraocular muscles caused by lymphocytic infiltration, oedema and later fibrosis.
- Pretibial myxoedema occurs in 1% to 5% of patients with Graves disease, and consists of painless thickening of the skin in nodules or plaques, generally over the shin.
- Thyroid acropachy occurs in less than 1% of patients, and resembles finger clubbing.

Other causes of primary hyperthyroidism
- Toxic multinodular goitre
- Toxic adenoma

Less common:
- Ectopic thyroid tissue (e.g., metastatic follicular cancer or 'struma ovarii', ovarian teratoma with ectopic thyroid tissue).
- Exogenous – high iodine load (e.g., dietary intake, contrast medium or drugs such as lithium, amiodarone and anticancer drugs including interferon alpha, interleukin IL-2 and tyrosine kinase inhibitors (see Clinical Notes)).

CLINICAL NOTES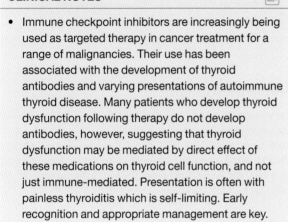

- Immune checkpoint inhibitors are increasingly being used as targeted therapy in cancer treatment for a range of malignancies. Their use has been associated with the development of thyroid antibodies and varying presentations of autoimmune thyroid disease. Many patients who develop thyroid dysfunction following therapy do not develop antibodies, however, suggesting that thyroid dysfunction may be mediated by direct effect of these medications on thyroid cell function, and not just immune-mediated. Presentation is often with painless thyroiditis which is self-limiting. Early recognition and appropriate management are key.

Secondary hyperthyroidism

This is very uncommon. Causes include TSH-secreting pituitary adenoma and trophoblast or germ cell tumours secreting large amounts of human chorionic gonadotrophin, which has mild thyroid-stimulating effects.

Subacute (de Quervain) thyroiditis

Various viruses (e.g., enterovirus or Coxsackie virus) can cause subacute thyroiditis. Patients present with pain, a small, tender goitre and initially thyrotoxicosis caused by release of stored thyroid hormones. There may be a history of preceding 'influenza-like' illness. Some weeks later, there is a period of hypothyroidism followed by the recovery of normal thyroid function 3 to 6 months after onset.

The erythrocyte sedimentation rate is raised, and there is low radioisotope uptake by the thyroid. Liver function test results may be abnormal. Treatment is with NSAIDs for mild symptoms and with high-dose prednisolone for moderate or severe thyroiditis. The dose is gradually tailed off in subsequent weeks.

Thyrotoxicosis without hyperthyroidism

This may occur with destructive thyroiditis such as in postpartum thyroiditis, autoimmune thyroiditis, subacute/de Quervain thyroiditis and amiodarone-induced thyroiditis, or with excessive T_4 administration or self-administered T_4.

Clinical features

The general symptoms of hyperthyroidism include:

- weight loss
- increased appetite
- heat intolerance and sweating
- fatigue and weakness
- hyperactivity, irritability and sleep disruption
- tremor

Less common symptoms include:

- depression
- oligomenorrhoea
- pruritus
- diarrhoea and vomiting
- polyuria

Signs include:

- goitre, possibly with a bruit
- tremor
- tachycardia and atrial fibrillation
- warm, moist skin
- lid retraction and lid lag (indicating Graves disease)
- proximal myopathy
- cardiac failure

Investigations

- Thyroid function tests, including tests for TSH, secretion of which is suppressed, and T_4 and T_3, the levels of which are raised. In Graves disease, the levels of TSH receptor antibodies are elevated.
- Check thyroid autoantibodies.
- ECG; may show tachycardia and atrial flutter/fibrillation.
- If ophthalmopathy, test visual fields, acuity and eye movements.
- Thyroid imaging: if a toxic nodule or thyroiditis is suspected, a radioisotope thyroid scan may be performed. In the case of thyroiditis, a low level of uptake is seen; a toxic nodule appears as a 'hotspot'. In Graves disease, there is diffusely increased uptake.

CLINICAL NOTES

Thyroid function tests: secretion of TSH will be suppressed in thyrotoxicosis because of negative feedback (the exception to this being secondary hyperthyroidism). It may also be suppressed in euthyroid patients with Graves ophthalmopathy, large goitres, recent treatment for thyrotoxicosis or severe nonthyroid illness.

Thyroid malignancy

The incidence of thyroid cancer has risen greatly in the last 50 years. This may be due to improved diagnosis of small tumours. Prognosis is generally good, but worse in older age groups, if metastases are present at presentation, and with anaplastic carcinoma.

Papillary thyroid carcinoma

This accounts for 80% to 85% of thyroid malignancies, and is more common in women; the peak age of onset is 30 to 50 years. It may be locally invasive or multifocal. Treatment is by surgical excision, and the 5-year survival rate is 95%.

> **HINTS AND TIPS**
>
> Papillary carcinoma is the most common thyroid carcinoma, and has a tendency to spread to local lymph nodes.

Follicular thyroid carcinoma

This occurs in older people (peak incidence at 40–60 years) and accounts for around 10% of thyroid cancers. Distant metastases develop in around 15% of patients. Treatment is by thyroidectomy and radioiodine ablation of the thyroid remnant. The 5-year survival rate is 80% in men and almost 100% in women. Fine-needle aspiration biopsy may not be able to distinguish between follicular adenoma and carcinoma, and these patients often undergo surgery, with the diagnosis being confirmed on pathology of the excised specimen.

Anaplastic carcinoma

Anaplastic carcinoma is uncommon. The peak incidence is at 60 to 70 years. The malignant cells are atypical and undifferentiated, and the mean survival is only 6 months from diagnosis.

Medullary thyroid carcinoma

This is rare, accounting for around 4% of thyroid cancer. The cells secrete calcitonin and other hormones. The prognosis is poor. Family members should be screened as it is a feature of multiple endocrine neoplasia.

Primary thyroid lymphoma

Lymphoma arising in the thyroid is almost always non-Hodgkin lymphoma. There is an increased risk in patients with autoimmune thyroiditis. Most are B-cell tumours, which are treated with chemotherapy, often combined with radiotherapy.

● Chapter Summary

- The hypothalamus–pituitary–thyroid axis is a neuroendocrine feedback loop responsible for the production of thyroid hormone.
- The spectrum of thyroid disease encompasses both benign and malignant conditions that manifest with features of either hyper- or hypothyroidism.
- Careful history and examination can easily distinguish between symptoms and signs of hyper- and hypothyroidism.
- Papillary carcinoma is the most common thyroid malignancy.
- Anticancer medications have been linked with self-limiting thyroiditis of both autoimmune and non-immune-mediated causes.

UKMLA Conditions
Hyperthyroidism
Hypothyroidism
Thyroid eye disease
Thyroid nodules
Thyrotoxicosis

UKMLA Presentations
Neck lump
Palpitations
Weight gain
Weight loss

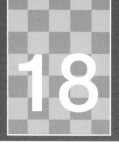
INTRODUCTION

Loss of consciousness may be transient (blackouts) or ongoing (coma). The causes of blackouts are summarized in Table 18.1. In a coma, the patient remains unconscious and is unarousable. The causes of coma are summarized in Table 18.2.

Many patients are admitted to the hospital with 'collapse'. This term is rarely helpful as patients (and doctors) use the word 'collapse' to describe various situations, and it is essential to determine whether or not the patient has actually lost consciousness.

COMMUNICATION

Many people use the terms 'dizziness', 'light-headedness', 'fall', 'faint', 'loss of consciousness' and 'collapse' interchangeably. Careful questioning is needed to establish whether the patient had a true loss of consciousness episode, which is key to making the correct diagnosis.

HISTORY AND EXAMINATION FINDINGS

History

COMMUNICATION

Always try to obtain a collateral history from a witness, even if the patient has regained consciousness.

The history of a patient presenting with loss of consciousness should include the following:

Before the event
- What was the patient doing at the time of the attack?
  - Was there a change in posture or position before the event? Syncope due to postural hypotension often occurs after standing up suddenly.

Table 18.1 Differential diagnosis of blackouts

Causes	Subgroups	Examples and notes
Syncope (see Chapters 28 and 34)	Orthostatic (postural) syncope	Old age, drugs (e.g., antihypertensives), autonomic neuropathy
	Neurocardiogenic (vasovagal) syncope	Characterized by inappropriate vagal outflow in response to stimulus (e.g., prolonged standing, fear, pain)
	Carotid sinus syndrome	Syncope on minor stimulation of the carotid sinus (e.g., head-turning, shaving)
	Situational syncope	Cough, micturition, defecation
	Cardiogenic syncope	Arrhythmia (Stokes–Adams attack) or structural heart disease (e.g., AS, HCM)
	TIA/vertebrobasilar insufficiency	Transient ischaemia in posterior circulation causing LOC (i.e., needs to affect RAS in the brainstem; as this is diffuse, TIAs rarely cause LOC alone – other brainstem structures are affected), subclavian steal
Epilepsy (see Chapter 34)	Focal onset seizure with impaired awareness	Focal epileptic activity with altered consciousness (e.g., temporal lobe epilepsy)
	Generalized onset seizure	Generalized epileptic activity
	Pseudoseizure	Behaviour mimicking a seizure but no epileptic activity in the brain
Hypoglycaemia (see Chapter 33)	Fasting	See the list in Chapter 33
	Postprandial	Dumping syndrome

AS, Aortic stenosis; HCM, hypertrophic cardiomyopathy; LOC, loss of consciousness; RAS, reticular activating system; TIA, transient ischaemic attack.

Table 18.2 Differential diagnosis of coma

Causes	Examples
Neurological (see Chapter 34)	Trauma – especially closed head injury
	Cerebrovascular event – intracranial haemorrhage or infarction
	Epilepsy (postictal or nonconvulsive status epilepticus)
	Meningitis, encephalitis, overwhelming septicaemia
	Space-occupying lesion
Metabolic	Hypoglycaemia or hyperglycaemia
	Myxoedema or Addisonian crisis (see Chapter 33)
	Hypothermia (see Chapter 33)
	Hypoxia or CO_2 narcosis (see Chapter 29)
	Severe electrolyte disturbance (see Chapter 32)
	Uraemic encephalopathy
	Hepatic encephalopathy (see Chapter 30)
	Drugs and toxins (see Chapter 39)

- Exertional syncope is seen in aortic stenosis and hypertrophic cardiomyopathy (HCM).
- Occasionally, syncope can occur following cough, micturition, swallowing or straining during defecation (mediated by the vasovagal reflex).
- Syncope on head-turning may suggest carotid sinus hypersensitivity or rotational vertebrobasilar insufficiency.
- Did any symptoms occur before the event?
  - Was there any aura? Aura often precedes an epileptic seizure.
  - Were there any chest symptoms (e.g., palpitations, chest pain or dyspnoea)? Note that episodes of bradycardia may cause collapse without warning (Stokes–Adams attacks, see Chapter 7).

The event itself
- Try to obtain an eyewitness account of the event if available.
- Duration of loss of consciousness.
- Prolonged seizure activity associated with tongue biting, particularly the side of the tongue, is suggestive of epilepsy. Any cause of cerebral hypoxia may result in brief anoxic seizures, which may be more prolonged if the patient is upright. Urinary incontinence can be a feature of both syncope and epilepsy; faecal incontinence is usually not a feature of syncope.

- In Stokes–Adams attacks, the patient typically becomes very pale, flushing on recovery.
- If available, the pulse rate during the episode can help (e.g., bradycardia or absent pulse in Stokes–Adams attack). If the attack occurs in the hospital, the blood pressure and blood glucose level should be recorded during the episode.

HINTS AND TIPS

It is helpful to get a video recording of any seizure/syncopal event from an eyewitness if it is safe to do so.

After the event
- How quickly did the patient recover? Syncope is generally followed by rapid recovery. In epilepsy, there is typically postictal sleepiness or disorientation.
- Focal neurological impairment after recovery of consciousness may suggest a stroke or Todd paresis following a seizure (see Chapter 34).

Risk factors
- A history of similar episodes, epilepsy, cardiac disease, cerebrovascular disease, obstructive airway disease and diabetes (especially if the patient is taking medication known to cause hypoglycaemia, such as insulin, sulphonylureas and sodium-glucose cotransporter 2 inhibitors).
- Cardiovascular risk factors or relevant family history (e.g., HCM, early cardiac death).
- History of drug abuse or depression.
- Previous head trauma.

Examination

Fig. 18.1 summarizes the examination approach. The emphasis of the examination differs between the sick comatose patient and one with recurrent blackouts. The different approaches are outlined below.

Comatose patient
- Start with the ABCDE approach. Calculating the patient's Glasgow Coma Scale (GCS) score (Table 18.3) is a part of D – disability. Examine the pupils and eye movements (Table 18.4).
- Survey for injuries: especially closed head injury and evidence of skull fractures such as blood or cerebrospinal fluid in ears or Battle sign (bruising over the mastoid process).

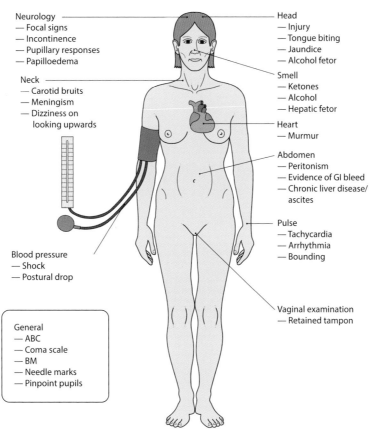

Neurology
— Focal signs
— Incontinence
— Pupillary responses
— Papilloedema

Neck
— Carotid bruits
— Meningism
— Dizziness on
   looking upwards

Blood pressure
— Shock
— Postural drop

General
— ABC
— Coma scale
— BM
— Needle marks
— Pinpoint pupils

Head
— Injury
— Tongue biting
— Jaundice
— Alcohol fetor

Smell
— Ketones
— Alcohol
— Hepatic fetor

Heart
— Murmur

Abdomen
— Peritonism
— Evidence of GI bleed
— Chronic liver disease/
   ascites

Pulse
— Tachycardia
— Arrhythmia
— Bounding

Vaginal examination
— Retained tampon

Fig. 18.1 Examining the patient with loss of consciousness. *ABC*, The airway–breathing–circulation first-aid mnemonic; *BM*, stick test for blood glucose; *GI*, gastrointestinal.

- Systems:
  - Respiratory: consolidation, carbon dioxide retention.
  - Abdomen: Consider hepatic encephalopathy and opiate or another overdose. Check for injection sites and hypo/hyperglycaemia (diabetic coma).
  - Neurological: focal neurology suggests intracranial cause.

HINTS AND TIPS

Remember to look for items hinting at the cause of loss of consciousness (e.g., MedicAlert bracelets, neck tags or wallet cards, insulin in patients' medication).

Patient with blackouts
- Lying and standing blood pressure
- Thorough cardiovascular and neurological examination
- Survey for any possible injuries sustained

INVESTIGATIONS

HINTS AND TIPS

A blood glucose test should be performed urgently in all unconscious patients to exclude hypoglycaemia.

Investigation will be guided by findings in the history and clinical examination.

- Full blood count: anaemia (e.g., severe haemorrhage or haemolysis); leucocytosis (e.g., sepsis).
- Arterial blood gas: hypoxia, hypercapnia, acidosis (e.g., in diabetic ketoacidosis). Raised lactate is often seen following a seizure.
- Urea and electrolytes: electrolyte disturbances, renal failure.
- Calcium: hypocalcaemia.
- Glucose: hypoglycaemia/hyperglycaemia.

Table 18.3 The Glasgow Coma Scale

Category	Response	Score
Eye opening	Spontaneous	4
	In response to voice	3
	In response to pain	2
	No eye opening	1
Best verbal response	Orientated	5
	Confused conversation	4
	Inappropriate speech	3
	Incomprehensible sounds	2
	No response	1
Best motor response (i.e., best response of any limb)	Obeys commands	6
	Localizes to pain	5
	Withdraws to pain	4
	Flexion to pain (decorticate)	3
	Extension to pain (decerebrate)	2
	No movements	1

GCS is used in assessing loss of consciousness in a patient.

Table 18.4 Examination of the eyes in the comatose patient

Test	Findings	Interpretation
Visual fields (by visual threat – normal response is to blink)	Hemianopia	Suggests contralateral hemisphere lesion
Pupil reactions	Normal direct and consensual	Intact midbrain
	Mid position, unreactive to light, irregular	Midbrain lesion
	Unilateral, fixed, dilated	Third nerve compression (e.g., due to tentorial herniation)
	Small, reactive	Pontine lesion, opiate overdose
	Horner syndrome	Ipsilateral lateral medullary or hypothalamic lesion
Doll's head manoeuvre to test vestibuloocular reflex (*perform only if cervical spine intact*)	Normal if pupils fixed on same point in space when head moved quickly	Brainstem from third to seventh nerve nucleus intact
Fundoscopy	Papilloedema	Raised ICP (occasionally CO_2 narcosis)
	Subhyaloid haemorrhage	Subarachnoid haemorrhage
	Hypertensive retinopathy	Hypertensive encephalopathy

ICP, Intracranial pressure.

- Creatine kinase: rhabdomyolysis (if the patient has been lying unconscious for a prolonged period).
- Liver function tests (biochemistry and synthetic function): liver failure, hepatic encephalopathy.
- Thyroid function tests and cortisol level: hypothyroidism (myxoedema coma).
- ECG: arrhythmia, left ventricular hypertrophy in aortic stenosis and HCM.
- Chest X-ray: pulmonary disease, aspiration pneumonia.
- Blood and urine drug screen.
- Brain imaging: head computed tomography (CT) is usually more readily available than magnetic resonance imaging (MRI).

- Lumbar puncture: meningitis, subarachnoid haemorrhage.
- Doppler studies of the carotid arteries: carotid artery stenosis.
- 24/48-hour or 7-day ECG monitoring for arrhythmia.

- Echocardiogram: source of emboli, aortic stenosis, HCM.
- EEG: epilepsy (including nonconvulsive status epilepticus), viral encephalitis.

Chapter Summary

- In all patients presenting with loss of consciousness should investigate the cause of the episode. Circumstances surrounding the episode will often guide the clinician to the cause.
- In an emergency, when a patient presents with loss of consciousness, follow the ABCDE approach. Once the patient has been stabilized and initial interventions have been performed, brain imaging is an important investigation in a patient who remains unconscious despite appropriate treatment.
- The GCS is a useful score that enables the assessment of consciousness. It also allows monitoring of patients for deterioration/improvement.

UKMLA Conditions
Arrhythmias
Decreased/loss of consciousness
Head injury
Vasovagal syncope

UKMLA Presentations
Blackouts and faints
Decreased/loss of consciousness
Dizziness

INTRODUCTION

Dementia and delirium are frequent challenges in the hospital, particularly with our ageing population. Individuals with a background of dementia are more likely to have delirium, but delirium can occur without dementia. Acute confusion may be the first sign of infection, particularly in the elderly. Identifying delirium and dementia early is important for the best patient care and can minimize in-patient complications such as falls. Delirium is a risk factor for prolonged in-patient stay.

HINTS AND TIPS

Advanced care planning and treatment escalation ceilings should be ascertained early in patients with dementia to ensure the most appropriate care. Patient's previously expressed wishes and communication with next of kin are vital.

Confusion can be a manifestation of delirium or dementia. Delirium is a clinical syndrome of acute (or subacute) onset, often fluctuating and presenting as a disturbance of consciousness, perception or cognitive function. Dementia, on the other hand, is a progressive disease of the brain causing impairment of higher cortical function without impairment of consciousness. The most common causes of delirium are summarized in Table 19.1, whereas the causes of dementia are described in Table 19.2. The diagnosis of delirium is clinical.

COMMUNICATION

In confused patients, a good account from relatives, carers or friends is almost always the only way of getting an accurate picture of the disease pattern. It is important to establish the patient's baseline level of cognitive function, whether this presentation is a new problem or part of a long-standing issue.

HINTS AND TIPS

Depression can sometimes mimic dementia ('pseudodementia'). Other psychiatric illnesses, causing psychosis and severe anxiety, can present similarly to acute confusional state.

CLINICAL NOTES

RISK FACTORS FOR DELIRIUM

Previous delirium
Age
Male > female
Dementia
Severe illness
Certain drugs (e.g., benzodiazepines, steroids)
Substance misuse
Sensory impairment
Reduced mobility
Admission to the intensive care

HISTORY AND EXAMINATION FINDINGS

History

Establish whether the patient is newly confused or if there is a history of dementia, and if so, whether the confusion is worse than usual. The history-taking should then focus on possible underlying causes.

Pattern of confusion

Delirium typically develops over 1 to 2 days. It is characterized by clouding of consciousness that fluctuates in severity, often worse at night with lucid periods in the day. It can be accompanied by poor recent memory, disorientation and hallucinations. Abnormalities of the sleep–wake cycle are common. Delirium

Table 19.1 Differential diagnosis of delirium

Causes	Examples
Infection	Any – commonly urinary tract, pneumonia, cellulitis, meningitis, encephalitis
Drug intoxication	Opiates, anxiolytics, steroids, tricyclics, anticonvulsants, drugs of abuse (see Chapter 39)
Drug withdrawal	Alcohol, benzodiazepines
Metabolic	Liver, kidney, cardiorespiratory failure (hypoxia and hypercapnia), hypernatraemia or hyponatraemia, hypoglycaemia, hypercalcaemia
Endocrine	Thyroid disorders, electrolyte and glucose abnormalities, diabetes and parathyroid disorders
Vitamin deficiency	Wernicke–Korsakoff syndrome (thiamine deficiency)
Cerebral disease	Abscess, tumour, haemorrhage, infarction, trauma, epilepsy/postictal, encephalitis (both infectious and autoimmune) (see Chapter 34)
Pain, urinary retention, constipation, dehydration	Any cause
New surroundings	Hospital ward, possibly without hearing (hearing aid?) or vision (spectacles?)

Table 19.2 Differential diagnosis of dementia (see *Crash Course: Psychiatry*)

Categories	Causes
Common causes	Alzheimer disease, vascular dementia, Lewy body dementia, frontotemporal dementias
Rarer causes	Long-term alcohol abuse, Huntington chorea, Creutzfeldt–Jakob disease, Parkinson disease, Pick disease, HIV, subacute sclerosing panencephalitis, progressive multifocal leucoencephalopathy, pellagra (niacin deficiency)
Treatable causes (which *must* therefore be excluded)	Vitamin B_{12}/folate deficiency, hypothyroidism, thiamine deficiency, subdural haematoma, normal pressure hydrocephalus, neurosyphilis, resectable tumour, depression (pseudodementia)

can be hypoactive (patients are withdrawn, quiet and sleepy), hyperactive (patients are restless, agitated and aggressive) or mixed (features of both).

Dementia has a gradual onset over months or years. It is a progressive global deterioration in higher cerebral function without effect on the level of consciousness. The symptoms are often exacerbated if the patient is removed from familiar surroundings.

RED FLAG

Assess the following:
- Symptoms of infection (see Chapter 8).
- Symptoms of raised intracranial pressure (see Chapter 16).
- Alcohol intake: long-term alcohol abuse can cause dementia; it is also associated with thiamine deficiency (Wernicke–Korsakoff syndrome) and folate and B_{12} deficiency.
- Previous head injury or evidence of falls: subdural haematoma.
- Evidence of chronic disease: long-standing renal disease (uraemia), liver disease (encephalopathy), malignancy (cerebral metastases, hypercalcaemia or paraneoplastic syndromes), diabetes (hypoglycaemia), Addison disease, hypo-/hyperthyroidism.
- Drug history: use of sedatives, anticonvulsants and/or steroids. Might the patient have consumed illicit drugs?
- Social history: confused patients often need a referral to the safeguarding team, and understanding their social circumstances may help contextualize the presentation.
- Family history: Wilson disease (autosomal recessive); Huntington chorea (autosomal dominant).
- Brief psychiatric history: notably for features of depression or psychosis.
- Sexual history may provide information regarding possible HIV infection, hepatitis or syphilis.

CLINICAL NOTES

CONFUSION ASSESSMENT METHOD

The Confusion Assessment Method (CAM) is a delirium-screening tool that helps identify patients with the condition. It comprises four questions:

1. Acute onset and fluctuating course?
2. Inattention?
3. Disorganized thinking?
4. Altered level of consciousness?

Delirium is suggested if 1 *and* 2 and either 3 *or* 4 are present. The patient is then said to be 'CAM-positive'.

HINTS AND TIPS

Severe symptoms of delirium tremens due to alcohol withdrawal may occur more than 72 hours after the patient's last drink and long after the patient has been admitted to the hospital.

Examination

The approach to examining a patient presenting with confusion is summarized in Fig. 19.1. Attention should be given to the following:

- Signs of infection: measure temperature, look for neck stiffness, consolidation in the chest, signs of endocarditis, abdominal tenderness, otitis media on otoscopy and check pressure areas and skin for evidence of cellulitis (see Chapter 8).
- Assess for urinary retention or constipation.
- Mental state: the 10-point abbreviated mental test score is useful to assess the level of confusion and may be used serially to monitor progress.
- Signs of chronic liver disease (CLD): hepatic encephalopathy can cause confusion. The presence of CLD may also indicate long-term alcohol abuse or rarer disorders, such as Wilson disease.

CLINICAL NOTES

Abbreviated mental test score

One point is awarded for each correct answer. A score of less than 7/10 strongly suggests confusion.

- Age.
- Date of birth.
- Time (to the nearest hour).
- Current year.
- Address for recall at the end of the test – to be repeated by the patient to ensure it has been heard correctly (e.g., 42 West Street).
- Name of the place where we are.
- Recognition of two people (e.g., nurse and doctor).
- Beginning of the First World War or similar.
- Name of monarch/prime minister/president.
- Count backwards from 20 to 1.

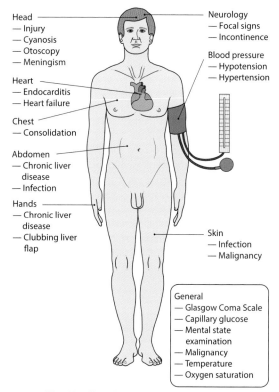

Fig. 19.1 Examining the confused patient.

INVESTIGATIONS

The investigations used in diagnosing delirium and dementia are very similar, although the urgency with which they are required is different. The following tests should be considered.

Bedside investigations

Routine observations, including oxygen saturation, capillary glucose, urinalysis and ECG.

Blood tests

- Full blood count: infection or inflammation; anaemia with raised mean corpuscular volume in vitamin B_{12} or folate deficiency.
- Erythrocyte sedimentation rate: raised in malignancy, infection and inflammation.
- Urea and electrolytes: hyponatraemia or hypernatraemia, renal failure, uraemia.
- Liver function tests: abnormal results in liver disease.
- Thyroid function tests: hypo-hyperthyroidism.
- Serum calcium: hypercalcaemia or hypocalcaemia.
- Glucose: hypoglycaemia or hyperglycaemia; diabetic ketoacidosis or hyperosmolar hyperglycaemic state.
- Arterial blood gas: hypoxia and/or CO_2 retention.
- Blood cultures if indicated.

- Vitamin B_{12} and folate levels: deficiency.
- Syphilis serology: tertiary syphilis may cause dementia.

Further tests

Consider the following:

- Chest X-ray: pneumonia, cardiac failure, malignancy.
- Computed tomography/magnetic resonance imaging (CT/MRI) of the brain: tumour, stroke, age-related changes, subdural haematoma.
- Urine: dipstick and microscopy, toxicology screen.
- Lumbar puncture and cerebrospinal fluid (CSF) examination: cell counts, protein, glucose, microscopy, culture.
- Ammonia – level often raised in liver disease and metabolic disorders (see Chapter 33).
- Serum copper and caeruloplasmin (reduced) and 24-hour urinary copper excretion (increased): Wilson disease.
- *Borrelia* serology for Lyme disease.
- Thick and thin blood films: malaria.
- HIV serology.

CLINICAL NOTES

CONFUSION SCREEN

Patients presenting with new-onset confusion should undergo various tests collectively termed the 'confusion screen'. These include:

- Full blood count, urea and electrolytes, liver function tests, clotting, thyroid function tests, calcium, vitamin B_{12} and folate, and glucose
- CT of the head
- Urine dipstick
- ECG for evidence of myocardial infarction
- Assess for dehydration or pain
- Assess for urinary retention or constipation

MANAGEMENT

Delirium

Treat the underlying cause. Support and reorientate the patient often. Use clear communication techniques. Have a clock available and remind them of the date and location daily. Nurse them in a well-lit, calm environment with familiar objects (including glasses, hearing aids and walking aids) and family involvement. Encourage physiotherapy and mobilization. Ensure adequate nutrition.

Pharmacological management should be avoided unless necessary, as it can worsen delirium. A short-term course of low-dose haloperidol or olanzapine can be considered if needed, with the aim of treatment being to calm the patient but not sedate them. Benzodiazepines are generally avoided unless delirium is due to alcohol withdrawal, where benzodiazepines are preferred (chlordiazepoxide is the drug of choice).

Dementia

Management of dementia is symptomatic. The patient should be encouraged to perform activities that promote well-being, independence and cognition. Pharmacological measures include acetylcholinesterase inhibitors (such as donepezil or rivastigmine) or memantine.

Chapter Summary

- Delirium is very common among hospital patients.
- Delirium is difficult to diagnose and often goes unnoticed for prolonged periods. It is also challenging to treat. Pharmacological interventions should be used only as a last resort.
- As opposed to delirium, dementia is a condition of gradual onset that progresses over time. It is most common in the elderly population.
- There can be many causes of dementia, but the most common one is Alzheimer disease.

UKMLA Conditions
Decreased/loss of consciousness
Delirium
Dementias
Wernicke's encephalopathy

UKMLA Presentations
Confusion
Decreased/loss of consciousness
Memory loss

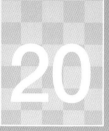
INTRODUCTION

Stroke is a clinical syndrome where acute focal or global signs of cerebral dysfunction develop rapidly and persist for more than 24 hours. Deficits lasting less than 24 hours are termed 'transient ischaemic attacks' (TIAs). Different types of stroke and their causes are described in Table 20.1. Eighty-five percent of strokes are ischaemic, and 15% haemorrhagic.

Around 100,000 people have strokes per year, and the number rises with age; the incidence of TIA is approximately 50 in 100,000. The risk of developing a stroke following a TIA is as high as 17% at 3 months. Stroke patients are at increased risk of experiencing another event. The 90-day recurrence is 5%, and 5-year recurrence is around 20%. The Clinical Notes box shows the main risk factors for stroke; many are common to all vascular diseases (see Chapter 28).

CLINICAL NOTES

RISK FACTORS FOR STROKE AND TIA

- Previous stroke or TIA
- Age
- High blood pressure
- Atrial fibrillation
- Established vascular disease (carotid bruit, coronary artery disease, peripheral vascular disease)
- Diabetes
- Chronic kidney disease
- Hypercholesterolaemia
- Family history
- Smoking
- Oral contraceptive pill use
- Obesity
- Excessive alcohol intake
- Thrombophilia
- Sickle cell disease

CAUSES AND PATHOPHYSIOLOGY

The main causes of ischaemic stroke are thromboembolism from arteries (e.g., atherothromboembolism from carotid arteries) and heart emboli (in atrial fibrillation, left ventricular thrombi such as after myocardial infarction, or infective endocarditis). Uncommon causes include vasculitis, arterial dissection, venous sinus thrombosis (which may also cause haemorrhage) and polycythaemia. Thrombus in situ may also occur in perforating arteries, often due to lipohyalinosis as a complication of hypertension. Around 20% of ischaemic strokes occur in the posterior cerebral circulation. The

Table 20.1 Types of stroke

Type	Causes
Haemorrhagic	Hypertension Aneurysm (particularly Charcot–Bouchard microaneurysms; also berry and mycotic aneurysms) Arteriovenous malformation Tumours Bleeding tendency (thrombocytopenia, coagulopathy, anticoagulants) Drugs (amphetamines, ecstasy, cocaine) Haemorrhagic transformation of ischaemic stroke
Ischaemic (thrombotic, hypotensive, occlusive)	Hypertension Intracranial arterial atheroma Vasculitis (e.g., temporal arteritis, SLE, PAN, neurosyphilis) Prolonged hypotension (e.g., cardiac arrest) Thrombophilia (hyperviscosity, antiphospholipid syndrome) Drugs (amphetamines, ecstasy, cocaine) Arterial dissection (cervical or vertebral)
Ischaemic (embolic)	Carotid or vertebral atheroma Cardiac: • Atrial fibrillation with left atrial thrombosis • Endocarditis • Ventricular thrombus, e.g., due to MI or ventricular aneurysm • Atrial myxoma Paradoxical: • Venous thrombus can reach the cerebral circulation via an atrial septal defect

MI, *Myocardial infarction*; PAN, *polyarteritis nodosa*; SLE, *systemic lupus erythematosus*.

risk factors for TIA are identical, and the underlying disease processes are very similar, the leading cause being embolism from a distant source. Other causes include thrombotic occlusion of small perforating vessels, low flow through stenosed vessels, vasculitis and haematological conditions such as sickle cell disease. Two or more TIAs occurring closely together (within 1 week) may be due to an unstable plaque and are termed 'crescendo TIA'. Crescendo TIA signifies a high risk of stroke.

Cerebral haemorrhage is usually due to a rupture of perforating arteries or intracerebral vessels; underlying causes include hypertension (causing vessel fragility and aneurysms), cerebral amyloid angiopathy and arteriovenous malformations.

CLINICAL NOTES

DIFFERENTIAL DIAGNOSIS OF STROKE

- Transient ischaemic attack in the first 24 hours
- Trauma
- Drug overdose
- Hypoglycaemia
- Subdural haemorrhage
- Space- occupying lesion
- Epilepsy
- Hemiplegic migraine
- Syncope
- Migraine with aura
- Demyelinating disorders (e.g., multiple sclerosis)
- Infection
- Dementia

HINTS AND TIPS

Amaurosis fugax is a so-called retinal TIA. It is an episode of transient monocular visual loss most frequently resulting from ischaemia.

HISTORY AND EXAMINATION FINDINGS

History

Take a focused history, including a collateral history from family/friends. The history taking should focus on:

- Is this a stroke or a stroke mimic?
- Establish the timing of the event – what was the time of onset? What was the patient doing at the time? Did they wake up with symptoms?
- Consider the lesion's anatomical site and the patient's risk factors.

Symptoms usually develop rapidly (sudden onset is highly suggestive of a stroke), but a stepwise progressive neurological worsening over hours or days can also occur. Established deficit usually abates over time. If there has been gradual neurological deterioration, consider one of the differential diagnoses or hydrocephalus secondary to the stroke (oedema or blood preventing free drainage of cerebrospinal fluid).

Any intracranial artery can be involved. The symptoms and signs will reflect which artery and, therefore, which part of the brain have been involved (summarized in Fig. 20.1). The presence of collateral arteries leads to variation in the presentation.

HINTS AND TIPS

'Time is brain' – stroke is a time-critical diagnosis as the longer the brain is starved of oxygen, the more damage will develop. Timing is also critical when considering interventions such as thrombolysis and thrombectomy.

COMMUNICATION

Taking a history from a patient with a stroke can be challenging. The patient may have receptive or expressive dysphasia and could have visual impairment from homonymous hemianopia. It is important to position yourself where the patient can see you to maximize communication with the patient. A collateral history may be required and is often of great use.

PATIENT SAFETY

FAST is a validated screening tool for the presence of neurological symptoms in patients presenting acutely. It stands for 'face, arm, speech, time' and is mainly used in an out-of-hospital setting for patients in whom a diagnosis of stroke is suspected.

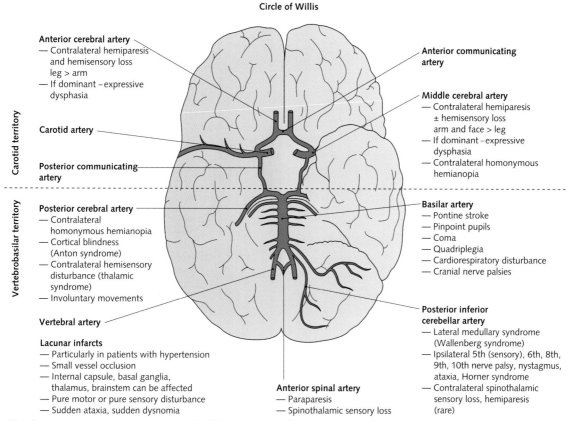

Circle of Willis

Anterior cerebral artery
— Contralateral hemiparesis and hemisensory loss leg > arm
— If dominant – expressive dysphasia

Carotid artery

Posterior communicating artery

Carotid territory

Posterior cerebral artery
— Contralateral homonymous hemianopia
— Cortical blindness (Anton syndrome)
— Contralateral hemisensory disturbance (thalamic syndrome)
— Involuntary movements

Vertebral artery

Vertebrobasilar territory

Lacunar infarcts
— Particularly in patients with hypertension
— Small vessel occlusion
— Internal capsule, basal ganglia, thalamus, brainstem can be affected
— Pure motor or pure sensory disturbance
— Sudden ataxia, sudden dysnomia

Anterior communicating artery

Middle cerebral artery
— Contralateral hemiparesis ± hemisensory loss arm and face > leg
— If dominant – expressive dysphasia
— Contralateral homonymous hemianopia

Basilar artery
— Pontine stroke
— Pinpoint pupils
— Coma
— Quadriplegia
— Cardiorespiratory disturbance
— Cranial nerve palsies

Posterior inferior cerebellar artery
— Lateral medullary syndrome (Wallenberg syndrome)
— Ipsilateral 5th (sensory), 6th, 8th, 9th, 10th nerve palsy, nystagmus, ataxia, Horner syndrome
— Contralateral spinothalamic sensory loss, hemiparesis (rare)

Anterior spinal artery
— Paraparesis
— Spinothalamic sensory loss

Fig. 20.1 Symptoms and signs associated with different strokes. Note that haemorrhagic strokes have symptoms and signs determined by the bleed site. Patients may also develop headaches, loss of consciousness and vomiting because of raised intracranial pressure.

Examination

Clinical examination gives information regarding four important areas in the stroke patient:

- What are the neurological abnormalities, and do they fit with the stroke diagnosis?
- Is there any evidence of an underlying cause?
- Have any complications arisen because of the stroke?
- What immediate treatment is needed?

Fig. 20.2 summarizes this examination approach.

A thorough neurological examination should be performed. The initial Glasgow Coma Scale (GCS) score should be recorded, and any subsequent changes documented. Note that GCS is imperfect in stroke as dysphasia and aphasia reduce the verbal score. Finally, establish if the pattern of neurological deficit fits with disruption of the cerebral vascular supply (see Fig. 20.1).

CLINICAL NOTES

CONTRAINDICATIONS TO THROMBOLYSIS WITH ALTEPLASE

Stroke in last 3 months, prior intracranial haemorrhage, severe stroke

Aortic dissection, arteriovenous malformations

Bleeding diatheses, coagulation defects, oesophageal varices, recent gastrointestinal ulceration

Recent surgery

Postpartum

Recent trauma

Severe hypertension

Hyperglycaemia, hypoglycaemia

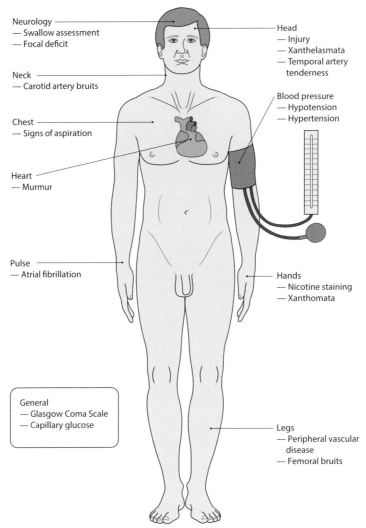

Fig. 20.2 Examining the stroke patient.

STROKE CLASSIFICATION

Numerous different systems are used to classify stroke. The Bamford classification is more commonly used (Table 20.2). One of its advantages is that it gives prognostic estimation.

Complications are prevalent following stroke, both in the short term and during recovery, and are related to the extent of cerebral damage and the degree of neurological deficit. The more common problems, and prophylactic measures, are outlined in Table 20.3.

INVESTIGATIONS

The diagnosis of stroke is clinical. Immediate investigations aim to support this clinical diagnosis, ruling out stroke mimics, access eligibility for interventions such as time-critical thrombolysis and/or thrombectomy, and to offer the best supportive care. The following investigations should be performed for any patient with an acute stroke.

Bedside investigations

- Capillary blood glucose: to rule out hypoglycaemia. Hypoglycaemia may present with stroke-like symptoms or signs, and prolonged severe hypoglycaemia may result in permanent brain injury.

Table 20.2 The Bamford classification of stroke

Category	Percentage of overall strokes	Clinical findings	Percentage at 1 year	
			Deceased	Living independently
Total anterior circulation stroke Middle/anterior cerebral artery territory	20	All of (1) unilateral weakness of two or more of face, arm and leg; with or without sensory deficit; (2) homonymous hemianopia; (3) disturbance of higher cerebral function, e.g., dysphasia, dyspraxia, inattention. If the patient is drowsy, then (2) and (3) are assumed	60	5
Partial anterior circulation stroke	35	Any of the following: (1) two of the components of total anterior circulation stroke; (2) higher cortical function deficit alone; (3) limited sensory or motor deficit	15	55
Lacunar stroke Infarcts involving: basal ganglia, internal capsule, thalamus and pons	20	Pure motor or sensory stroke or mixed affecting two-thirds of the face/arm/leg Sensorimotor stroke affecting two-thirds or more of the face/arm/leg Ataxic hemiparesis Dysarthria – clumsy hand syndrome No disturbance of higher function	10	60
Posterior circulation stroke	25	Brainstem and/or cerebellar deficits (motor deficits of any combination of upper and lower limbs or the whole of the face; sensory deficits in any combination of upper and lower limbs or the whole of the face; or cerebellar signs – ataxia, imbalance, vertigo, diplopia, dysarthria, dysphagia) Isolated homonymous hemianopia	20	60

- Routine bedside observations: blood pressure, pulse and oxygen saturations.
- ECG: this may show atrial fibrillation.

Blood tests

- Full blood count: polycythaemia or thrombocytopenia may cause a stroke; a reactive picture may indicate inflammation (e.g., temporal arteritis).
- Erythrocyte sedimentation rate/C-reactive protein: level elevated in inflammation, vasculitis, infection and malignancy.
- Urea and electrolytes: renal impairment may either be due to or the cause of hypertension. It may also result from reduced oral intake or concurrent sepsis.
- Fasting lipids: hypercholesterolaemia is an important, treatable risk factor for stroke.
- Clotting: to assess the level of anticoagulation if the patient is receiving warfarin or to investigate suspected coagulopathy.
- Arterial blood gas: hypoxia causes cerebral disturbances. Seizure can lead to a raised lactate level.

Imaging

- Chest X-ray: an enlarged heart could indicate hypertension; an enlarged left atrium could suggest this being the point of origin for emboli.
- Head CT: CT findings are often normal in the first few hours following an ischaemic stroke. The accuracy of the investigation increases after about 6 hours. Indications for immediate brain imaging are outlined in red flag: indications for urgent CT brain scan. All patients with possible stroke should have a CT head within 24 hours.
- Brain MRI: this is preferred if a posterior circulation stroke is suspected, as it provides better images of the posterior fossa. It is also helpful in cases of diagnostic uncertainty (especially to exclude tumours). If CT does not show evidence of stroke but clinical suspicion is high, an MRI should be performed.

Further investigations

Further tests may be required depending on the patient and the clinical scenario. The following investigations should be considered, especially in young patients with no obvious risk factors:

Table 20.3 Complications of stroke and measures to prevent them

Complications	Prophylactic measures
Acute	
Cerebral oedema (malignant middle cerebral artery syndrome)	Most common following an MCA territory stroke. Not preventable (avoid overenthusiastic rehydration). Pharmacological measures and surgical decompression can be used to limit space-occupying effects of oedema.
Haemorrhagic transformation of ischaemic stroke	Nonpreventable. Careful assessment of need for anticoagulants. Have a low threshold of repeating brain imaging if any neurological deterioration.
Aspiration pneumonia	Patients should be kept nil by mouth and fed via alternative routes until they can swallow safely (early SALT assessment).
Seizures	Not preventable. Can be treated with antiepileptics such as Levetiracetam. They may also occur later in the illness course as the brain remodels.
Delirium	Early mobilization, frequent orientation, sleep management and hygiene, ensuring patients have glasses or hearing aids, nutrition and hydration, effective pain management, avoidance of constipation, family interaction and cognitive stimulation. Avoid overmedicating patients or treating delirium with benzodiazepines.
Subacute and long term	
Pressure sores	Careful nursing with regular turning on an air mattress.
Contractures and spasticity	Regular skilled physiotherapy.
Falls	Physiotherapy and occupational therapy.
Malnutrition	Feeding via a nasogastric tube or, later, gastrostomy.
Depression and other emotional or psychological problems.	Provision of adequate social and practical support. Psychological support. Antidepressant medication.
Venous thromboembolism	Physiotherapy, VTE prophylaxis (intermitted pneumatic compression devices, pharmacotherapy where indicated).

MCA, *Middle cerebral artery;* SALT, *speech and language therapy;* VTE, *venous thromboembolism.*

- Blood cultures: infective endocarditis.
- Autoantibodies: to investigate the patient for vasculitis (antinuclear antibodies, antineutrophil cytoplasmic antibodies), antiphospholipid syndrome (anticardiolipin antibodies) or cerebral lupus (anti-double-stranded DNA).
- Carotid imaging: to look for carotid stenosis, all patients considered as candidates for carotid endarterectomy (with or without stenting) should have this investigation.
- Cerebral angiography/venography or radiological equivalent: if additional signs or symptoms are suggesting an unusual cause of infarction or haemorrhage, such as venous sinus thrombosis or arterial dissection.
- Echocardiography: if cardiac embolus is suspected, look for atrial enlargement (atrial fibrillation), left ventricular thrombus, vegetations on valves (e.g., in endocarditis) or patent foramen ovale/atrial septal defect which can result in a paradoxical embolus.
- 24- to 48-hour ECG monitoring: paroxysmal atrial fibrillation.
- Syphilis serology: neurosyphilis.

RED FLAG

INDICATIONS FOR IMMEDIATE CT BRAIN SCAN
- Thrombolysis or thrombectomy is considered.
- The patient is taking anticoagulants or has a known bleeding tendency.
- There is uncertainty about the diagnosis (e.g., subdural or subarachnoid haemorrhage).
- There was a severe headache at the onset of symptoms.
- There are progressive or fluctuating neurological signs.
- There is a reduced conscious level (Glasgow Coma Score <13).
- There is papilloedema, neck stiffness or fever.

Management

Patients with established stroke should be admitted to the hospital, ideally to a stroke unit. All patients treated with thrombolysis or thrombectomy need to have access to a high-care stroke facility with stroke physician and neuroradiology support.

Acute treatment

- An ABCDE approach should be instituted.
- Thrombolysis with alteplase or tenecteplase in selected patients with ischaemic stroke is beneficial when given up to 4.5 hours after symptom onset, or up to 9 hours if there is potential to salvage brain tissue as evidenced by CT perfusion or MRI. Brain imaging is required before the commencement of treatment to exclude haemorrhage.
- Thrombectomy should be offered to patients presenting with confirmed anterior circulation stroke within 6 hours of symptom onset or between 6 and 24 hours in proximal anterior circulation stroke with potential to salvage brain tissue.
- Thrombectomy should be considered in patients presenting with confirmed proximal posterior circulation (basilar or posterior cerebral artery) stroke within 24 hours of symptom onset if there is potential to salvage brain tissue.
- Thrombectomy should be offered together with thrombolysis unless contraindicated (see Chapter 34).
- Antiplatelet agents: in acute ischaemic stroke or TIA, aspirin therapy (300 mg daily) should be started immediately and no later than within 24 hours and should be continued for 2 weeks, after which long-term secondary prevention is implemented (see later). In postthrombolysis patients, aspirin therapy is started 48 hours after the intervention. Dual antiplatelets (aspirin with either clopidogrel or ticagrelor) should be considered in any patient presenting within 24 hours of TIA or minor stroke. This is normally continued for 21 days after which aspirin is stopped.
- Anticoagulants: unless contraindicated, patients with cerebral venous sinus thrombosis should be anticoagulated to an international normalized ratio target of 2 to 3.

- Patients with acute arterial dissection should be offered either anticoagulants or antiplatelets.
- Neurosurgical intervention may be indicated for intracerebral haemorrhage or severe middle cerebral artery infarction. Malignant middle cerebral artery syndrome is life-threatening cerebral oedema following an ischaemic stroke (see Table 20.3).

embolism, cerebral venous thrombosis or arterial dissection. The risks and benefits of anticoagulation need to be considered and discussed with the patient.

- High-intensity statins are offered to patients with ischaemic stroke and TIA.
- Antihypertensives are offered to target systolic blood pressure of less than 130 mmHg or 140 to 150 mmHg in patients with severe bilateral carotid artery stenosis.
- Carotid endarterectomy is offered to patients with symptomatic carotid stenosis of 50% to 99% according to the NASCET criteria or more than 70% according to European Carotid Surgery Trial (ECST) criteria.

HINTS AND TIPS

Patients must not drive for 1 month after a single TIA, 3 months after multiple TIAs and 1 month after a stroke provided satisfactory clinical recovery has occurred.

CLINICAL NOTES

PROGNOSIS

Mortality is significantly higher for patients with haemorrhagic stroke than ischaemic stroke. NICE states that 30-day mortality after admission to the hospital for haemorrhagic stroke is 30.5 per 100 patients and 11.9 per 100 patients for ischaemic stroke.

COMMUNICATION

If the patient is unconscious or consciousness is severely impaired, a decision as to the most appropriate degree of intervention should involve relatives/the next of kin. Factors to consider include prognosis, quality of life and if the patient has expressed any wishes in this regard.

● Chapter Summary

- Stroke is described as a focal or global dysfunction of cerebral function lasting longer than 24 hours.
- It is a medical emergency, and you are against the clock to provide the best brain-saving treatment.
- If symptoms last for less than 24 hours, the condition is termed 'transient ischaemic attack' ('TIA').
- The history and examination will point towards the underlying cause and the territory of the brain affected.
- Thrombolysis is considered as a treatment for ischaemic stroke provided the patient presents within 4.5 hours of symptom onset , (or within 9 hours if evidence of salvageable brain tissue on imaging), and meets eligibility criteria.
- Antiplatelet therapy is usually used in patients following a stroke for secondary prevention.
- Patients whose stroke is attributable to atrial fibrillation are generally anticoagulated 14 days post onset of the ischaemic stroke.

UKMLA Conditions
Decreased/loss of consciousness
Stroke
Transient ischaemic attacks

UKMLA Presentations
Decreased/loss of consciousness

Focal neurological deficits 21

INTRODUCTION

Focal neurological deficits or signs describe a nervous system impairment that affects a specific body part. These can include muscle weakness or abnormal sensations resulting from disease occurring anywhere along the central or peripheral nervous system pathways. Many pathological processes can lead to this presentation. The differential diagnosis is approached logically according to the likely anatomical site (the lesion level) and the possible causes at that location (Table 21.1).

HISTORY AND EXAMINATION FINDINGS

History

Despite the vast number of potential underlying diseases, a lesion at a particular point in the pathway between the brain and muscle or skin will always produce the same clinical signs regardless of the cause.

Pattern of deficit

Table 21.2 summarizes characteristic symptoms and signs from a lesion at a specific neurological level. If the neurological abnormalities do not fit with a single localized lesion, consider multiple sclerosis (MS), motor neurone disease, paraneoplastic neuropathy, multisystem disorders (e.g., sarcoidosis or vasculitis) or, rarely, a functional disorder.

Onset

Sudden onset usually indicates a vascular problem such as infarction or haemorrhage. Lesions due to trauma (e.g., enlarging haematoma), MS, infection (e.g., abscess), acute prolapsed disc and myelitis can also develop rapidly (e.g., over hours). An insidious onset, over weeks to months, is more typical of cervical spondylosis, motor neurone disease, neoplasm or myopathy.

Precipitants

Trauma may result in muscular and neurological deficits. Acute myasthenia gravis can be precipitated by intercurrent illness (particularly infection) or drugs (aminoglycosides or penicillamine). The incidence of MS relapses may increase in the postpartum period, and symptoms may be exacerbated by exertion, hot weather or a hot bath (Uhthoff phenomenon).

Progression

Many lesions cause gradually progressive, unremitting disease, including tumours, motor neurone disease, hereditary ataxias, syringomyelia and degenerative brain diseases. Intermittent deficits can be due to transient ischaemic attacks, epilepsy, migraine and myasthenia gravis. MS is characterized by the development of lesions which are dissociated in time and site. Symptoms and signs due to trauma or vascular events may slowly abate with time or remain static following the initial event.

Evidence of cause

The following will aid the diagnosis:

- Family history: e.g., hereditary ataxias, phenylketonuria, neurofibromatosis.
- Drug history: e.g., phenytoin (cerebellar signs), vinca alkaloids and platinum-containing drugs (peripheral neuropathy), penicillamine (myasthenia gravis).
- Dietary history: intake of vitamins B_1, B_6 and B_{12} and folate.
- Alcohol history.
- Preexisting illness: e.g., diabetes, hypertension (cerebrovascular disease), rheumatoid arthritis, tuberculosis or malignancy.
- History of trauma.
- Associated features: e.g., swinging pyrexia and rigors (abscess), vasculitic symptoms (connective tissue disease), anorexia and weight loss (malignancy), symptoms of hypothyroidism or hyperthyroidism.
- Travel history (exposure to infections, e.g., Lyme disease).

Examination

Perform a full neurological examination (see Chapter 2). Try and establish the anatomical site of the lesion(s) (Table 21.1) and what the underlying pathological process could be.

HINTS AND TIPS

Always ask how the patient is affected by the disease and what disability they have because of the neurological deficit.

Table 21.1 Differential diagnosis of sensory and/or motor neurological deficits

Site of lesion	Examples
Muscle (see Chapters 34–36)	*Congenital*
	Dystrophy: Duchenne, Becker, limb-girdle, facioscapulohumeral
	Myotonia: myotonic dystrophy, myotonia congenita (Thomsen disease)
	Acquired
	Drugs: steroids, cholesterol-lowering drugs (statins and fibrates), penicillamine
	Endocrine: Cushing syndrome, thyrotoxicosis, hypothyroidism and hyperparathyroidism
	Infection: viral (influenza, HIV infection), parasitic (toxoplasmosis, trichinosis) and bacterial (*Borrelia* infection, *Clostridium perfringens* infection)
	Inflammation and autoimmune: Guillain–Barré syndrome, polymyositis, dermatomyositis and sarcoidosis
	Metabolic: periodic paralyses, glycogen storage diseases and mitochondrial myopathy
	Toxin: alcohol
	Tumour: sarcoma and paraneoplastic syndromes
Neuromuscular junction (see Chapter 34)	Myasthenia gravis
	Lambert–Eaton myasthenic syndrome
	Clostridium botulinum infection (botulism)
Peripheral nerves (see Chapters 34–37)	*Mononeuropathy (only one nerve involved)*
	Entrapment: carpal tunnel syndrome (median nerve) and meralgia paraesthetica (lateral cutaneous nerve of thigh)
	Stretching: ulnar nerve neuropathy, neuropraxia
	Trauma
	Compression: e.g., by tumour, as in neurofibromatosis, or AVM
	Infarction: e.g., due to vasculitis
	Mononeuritis multiplex/multifocal neuropathy (two or more nerves involved)
	Connective tissue disease: PAN, SLE, RA
	Infection: leprosy, herpes zoster, HIV infection, Lyme disease
	Inflammation: sarcoidosis
	Metabolic: diabetic neuropathy
	Infiltration: amyloidosis
	Tumour: infiltration, paraneoplastic syndrome, neurofibromatosis
	Polyneuropathy (with symmetrical deficit most marked distally)
	Congenital: Charcot–Marie–Tooth disease (hereditary sensorimotor neuropathy), Refsum disease, Friedreich ataxia (spinal cord pathology usually coexists)
	Acquired: Connective tissue disease: PAN, SLE, RA
	Drugs: nitrofurantoin, metronidazole, vinca alkaloids, platinum-containing drugs, isoniazid
	Inflammation: Guillain–Barré syndrome, CIDP, multifocal motor neuropathy
	Metabolic: diabetes, renal failure (uraemic neuropathy), porphyria
	Toxins: alcohol, lead, mercury and arsenic
	Tumour: paraneoplastic syndrome and paraproteinaemias

Table 21.1 Differential diagnosis of sensory and/or motor neurological deficits—cont'd

Site of lesion	Examples
	Infiltration: amyloidosis
	Vitamin deficiency: thiamine (B_1), niacin (B_6), B_{12}, folate
Brachial or lumbar plexus	Compression: cervical rib, thoracic outlet syndrome, after proning or an anaesthetic
	Idiopathic: neuralgic amyotrophy
	Metabolic: diabetes
	Trauma: birth injury (Erb and Klumpke palsies) and, classically, motorbike accidents
	Tumour: malignant infiltration (e.g., Pancoast tumour)
Spinal nerve root	Infection (e.g., pyogenic meningitis, syphilis, CMV infection)
	Prolapsed intervertebral disc and spondylosis
	Spinal stenosis
	Tumour
	Vertebral fracture dislocation
Anterior horn cell (see Chapter 34)	Motor neurone disease (amyotrophic lateral sclerosis)
	Spinal muscular atrophy
	Poliomyelitis
Spinal cord (see Chapter 34)	Degeneration: osteoarthritis (osteophytes may cause spinal stenosis or foraminal stenosis)
	Infection: abscess, HIV infection, TB (Pott disease)
	Inflammation: MS, sarcoidosis, RA (atlantoaxial subluxation)
	Metabolic: Paget disease causing spinal stenosis or compression
	Trauma: direct; prolapsed intervertebral disc; radiotherapy
	Tumour: metastases, neurofibroma, meningioma, glioma, ependymoma
	Vascular: anterior spinal artery occlusion, aortic dissection, aortic aneurysm (emboli), AVM, vasculitis
	Vitamin deficiency: subacute combined degeneration of the spinal cord (vitamin B_{12})
	Other: syringomyelia, spina bifida, motor neurone disease
Cerebellum (see Chapter 34)	*Congenital:* Friedreich ataxia and spinocerebellar ataxias, ataxia telangiectasia
	Acquired
	Endocrine: hypothyroidism
	Infection: abscess, meningoencephalitis, postinfectious encephalitis
	Inflammation: MS
	Toxins: alcohol, lead, anticonvulsants
	Trauma: 'punch-drunk' syndrome
	Tumour: metastases, acoustic neuroma, haemangioblastoma (von Hippel–Lindau disease), paraneoplastic degeneration
	Vascular: infarction, haematoma, AVM
Cerebral hemispheres (see Chapter 34)	Degenerative disease
	Hydrocephalus: primary or secondary
	Infection: abscess, meningitis, encephalitis; HIV infection (e.g., AIDS dementia complex), malaria, rabies, TB, syphilis

Continued

Table 21.1 Differential diagnosis of sensory and/or motor neurological deficits—cont'd

Site of lesion	Examples
	Inflammation: sarcoidosis, SLE, MS
	Metabolic: phenylketonuria, Wilson disease (basal ganglia), other inborn errors of metabolism
	Toxic: alcohol
	Trauma: haematoma, diffuse axonal injury, traumatic brain injury
	Tumour: primary or secondary
	Vascular: infarction, haemorrhage, AVM, aneurysm, thrombosis
	Vitamin deficiency: thiamine (B_1), niacin (B_6), B_{12}

AVM, *Arteriovenous malformation;* CIDP, *chronic inflammatory demyelinating polyneuropathy;* CMV, *cytomegalovirus;* MS, *multiple sclerosis;* PAN, *polyarteritis nodosa;* RA, *rheumatoid arthritis;* SLE, *systemic lupus erythematosus;* TB, *tuberculosis.*

Table 21.2 Symptoms and signs associated with different anatomical lesions

Site of anatomical lesion	Symptoms	Specific signs	Muscle	Reflexes	Sensation
Muscle	Weakness (particularly climbing stairs, getting out of chair) Pain (inflammation)	Myotonia in myotonia dystrophica Calf pseudohypertrophy and Gowers sign in Duchenne muscular dystrophy	Wasting (usually proximal) Tone normal or reduced Power reduced	Usually normal; reduced or absent in severe muscle disease only; downgoing plantar response	Normal
Neuromuscular junction	Diplopia Dysphagia Altered voice Proximal muscle weakness	Fatigable weakness with repetition in myasthenia gravis; Increasing strength with repetition in LEMS	Wasting only if severe Tone normal Power alters with repetition	Normal	Normal
Peripheral nerve	Muscle weakness Sensory disturbance; may be purely sensory, purely motor or mixed	Mononeuropathy and mononeuritis multiplex – signs in distribution of affected nerves; polyneuropathy – signs symmetrical and distal (glove and stocking)	Wasting Fasciculation Reduced tone Reduced power	Reduced or absent	Deficit of all modalities (glove and stocking distribution)
Posterior spinal root	Pain in skin and muscle supplied by that root		Normal	Reduced or absent	Deficit in distribution of affected root
Anterior horn cell	Muscle weakness		Wasting Fasciculation Reduced tone Reduced power in distribution of affected nerve	Reduced or absent	Normal
Spinal cord	Pain at site of lesion; urinary/bowel disturbance/ incontinence; upper or lower limb weakness; sensory disturbance		At level of lesion: wasting, fasciculation, reduced tone, reduced power Below lesion: spasticity, increased tone, reduced power	At level of lesion: reduced or absent Below lesion: increased; upgoing plantar response	Below lesion: ipsilateral posterior column loss (proprioception, vibration sense) contralateral spinothalamic loss (pain and temperature)

Table 21.2 Symptoms and signs associated with different anatomical lesions—cont'd

Site of ana-tomical lesion	Symptoms	Specific signs	Muscle	Reflexes	Sensation
Cerebellum	Unsteadiness Tremor Altered speech Falls Poor coordination	Broad-based gait Falling to side of lesion Intention tremor Past-pointing dysdiadochokinesis Nystagmus Staccato speech	Reduced tone Normal power	Pendular	Normal
Cerebral hemispheres	Determined by site of lesion Weakness Seizures Altered speech Disturbed higher functions	Postural drift Dysphasia Dysarthria Visual disturbance	Increased tone 'Clasp-knife' rigidity Wasting only if disuse Reduced power in pyramidal distribution (flexors stronger than extensors in arms, extensors stronger than flexors in legs)	Brisk Upgoing plantar response	Deficit determined by site of lesion

LEMS, *Lambert–Eaton myasthenic syndrome.*

The anatomical site of the lesion

From the moment you meet the patient, observe the patient carefully. How does the patient shake your hand? Can the patient lift their arm up? Can they let go of your hand (myotonia)? How the patient walks can give clues as to the diagnosis (Table 21.3). Watch how the patient undresses or gets onto the bed. A severe deficit will often become apparent before you start the examination.

The underlying cause

Once the site of the lesion has been identified, think of the differential diagnosis as outlined at the beginning of this chapter.

Look at the patient's face for myotonic facies (myotonic dystrophy), Cushing syndrome (proximal myopathy) or hypothyroidism (myopathy or cerebellar dysfunction). Does the patient have neurofibromatosis (spinal cord or peripheral nerve lesions) or connective tissue disease such as rheumatoid arthritis (entrapment mononeuropathy, mononeuritis multiplex or peripheral neuropathy)?

COMMUNICATION

Often the most important thing for the patient is what the lesion prevents the patient from doing. Assess and distinguish impairment, disability and handicap, and address the problems accordingly.

CLINICAL NOTES

It is important to distinguish three related concepts: 'impairment' refers to a problem of body function or structure (e.g., right arm weakness following stroke); 'disability' refers to an inability to perform an activity (e.g., cannot write); and 'handicap' refers to social function (e.g., cannot work).

Think about what tasks the affected part of the body performs typically and ask the patient to show you how they manage, such as doing up buttons (for peripheral neuropathy), brushing hair or standing up from a chair (for proximal myopathy).

INVESTIGATIONS

The history and examination will guide the choice of investigations. The following tests may be useful.

Bedside investigations

Blood tests

- Full blood count and erythrocyte sedimentation rate: reactive picture in inflammation, infection and neoplasm;

Table 21.3 Abnormalities of gait

Lesion	Gait
Hemiplegia	Foot is plantar flexed; leg is stiff and dragged through a semicircle
Spastic paraplegia	Legs stiff; walk in 'scissor fashion', like 'walking through mud'
Proximal myopathy	Waddling gait; trunk moves to swing legs forward; difficulty in climbing stairs or standing out of a chair
Parkinsonism	Stooped posture, hesitation in starting, shuffling, festinant (accelerating), difficulty turning, poor arm swing and may freeze
Cerebellar dysfunction	Broad based, ataxia with a tendency to fall to the side of the lesion; unable to perform tandem gait (heel to toe)
Dorsal column disease	Stamping; broad based with patient looking at the ground as unable to sense where foot is; clumsy and slaps feet to ground
Foot drop	Stepping; legs lifted high off the ground as no dorsiflexion of the foot
Musculoskeletal disease	Limping; patient avoids weight bearing on affected side because of pain

Table 21.4 Autoantibodies in specific neurological diseases

Autoantibody target	Associated disease
Ganglioside M1	Multifocal motor neuropathy
Ganglioside Q1b	Miller Fisher syndrome
Voltage-gated calcium channel	LEMS
Voltage-gated potassium channel	Autoimmune encephalitis
NMDA receptor	Autoimmune encephalitis
Acetylcholine receptor and muscle-specific kinase	Myasthenia gravis
Aquaporin 4	Neuromyelitis optica
Hu, Ri, Yo	Paraneoplastic neurological syndromes
GAD	Stiff person syndrome

GAD, *Glutamate decarboxylase;* LEMS, *Lambert–Eaton myasthenic syndrome;* NMDA, *N-methyl-D-aspartate.*

raised mean corpuscular volume in vitamin B_{12} deficiency, folate deficiency and alcohol abuse.

- Urea and electrolytes: raised urea and creatinine levels in renal failure, high or low potassium level in periodic paralyses.
- Serum calcium: raised level in sarcoidosis, malignancy.
- Serum glucose or HbA1c: raised level in diabetes mellitus.
- Liver function tests: raised γ-glutamyltransferase level in alcohol abuse, increased alkaline phosphatase level in Paget disease and deranged transaminases in metastases, infection and Wilson disease.
- Thyroid function tests: hyperthyroidism or hypothyroidism.
- Creatine kinase: markedly raised level in muscle inflammation and muscular dystrophies.
- Autoantibodies: in systemic disease (e.g., rheumatoid arthritis, systemic lupus erythematosus and polyarteritis nodosa) and many specific neurological diseases (Table 21.4).
- Serology: HIV infection, herpes and syphilis where appropriate.
- Immunoglobulins: paraproteinaemias.

Cerebrospinal fluid analysis

- The different tests that can be performed on the cerebrospinal fluid are outlined in Table 21.5.

Imaging

- Plain radiographs of the spinal column may demonstrate degenerative and destructive bone lesions and fractures.
- Magnetic resonance imaging (MRI) of the brain and spine is useful in diagnosing and localizing central lesions. It provides greater anatomical detail than computed tomography (CT) and contrast medium can be given to show blood vessels or areas of blood–brain barrier breakdown.
- CT is useful in the acute setting (e.g., for detecting haemorrhage) and provides accurate imaging of bony structures.

Further investigations

- Electromyogram: useful in primary muscle disease (typical changes in myotonia and myasthenia); it also shows denervation (but not its cause).
- Nerve conduction studies: can demonstrate peripheral neuropathies and the site and type of individual nerve lesions.
- Evoked potentials: visual evoked potentials demonstrate previous retrobulbar neuritis in MS. Auditory and somatosensory evoked potential tests may also be performed to look for lesions in these pathways.
- Biopsy: consider if the diagnosis is in doubt despite the history, examination and noninvasive procedures. Muscle, nerve and brain biopsies can be performed to give a definitive histological diagnosis.

Table 21.5 Cerebrospinal fluid analysis and interpretation

Test/result	Interpretation
Opening pressure	Raised in space-occupying lesions, intracerebral haemorrhage, bacterial meningitis, idiopathic intracranial hypertension
Colour	Turbid in bacterial infection, bloody or yellow in intracranial bleed (xanthochromia)
Microscopy	Direct visualization of microorganisms or malignant cells, white cell count (predominately neutrophils in bacterial and lymphocytes in viral infection)
Culture and sensitivity	Infection and organism(s)
PCR	Detection of viral RNA or DNA
Low glucose level (<2/3 of blood glucose level)	Bacterial/TB/fungal/carcinomatous meningitis
Very high protein level (>2 g/L)	GBS, Froin syndrome,[a] TB/fungal meningitis, Behçet syndrome
High protein level (0.4–2 g/L)	Bacterial meningitis, viral encephalitis (can also present with low protein), cerebral abscess, cerebral malignancy
Oligoclonal bands	MS, SLE, neurosyphilis, neurosarcoidosis, Behçet syndrome, SSPE
Lymphocytes	Partially treated bacterial meningitis, viral encephalitis/ meningitis, TB meningitis, CNS vasculitis, Behçet syndrome, HIV-associated, lymphoma/leukaemia, SLE

CNS, *Central nervous system;* GBS, *Guillain–Barré syndrome;* PCR: *polymerase chain reaction;* SLE, *systemic lupus erythematosus;* SSPE, *subacute sclerosing panencephalitis;* TB, *tuberculosis.*
[a]*Raised cerebrospinal fluid protein level and xanthochromia but normal cell count, seen below a block in spinal cord compression.*

● Chapter Summary

- Focal neurological deficits are a disease manifestation along the nerve supply pathway to the tissues.
- The history and examination will help determine the site of the lesion.
- Stroke is the most common cause of focal neurological deficits in the elderly.
- MRI is a more sensitive diagnostic modality in neurological disease than CT.

UKMLA Conditions
Motor neurone disease
Multiple sclerosis
Myasthenia gravis
Stroke

UKMLA Presentations
Altered sensation, numbness and tingling
Diplopia
Facial weakness
Fasciculation
Limb weakness
Neuromuscular weakness

Dizziness and vertigo 22

INTRODUCTION

Dizziness is a nonspecific term that describes disorientation or unsteadiness. Vertigo is the illusion of movement, usually rotation but also swaying or tilting, of a patient or their surroundings. This is often accompanied by nausea, vomiting and postural instability. It results from disease in the labyrinth of the inner ear (the most common cause) or cranial nerve VIII or its connections in the brainstem, including the cerebellum.

Differential diagnoses in the patient with vertigo include labyrinth disorders, cranial nerve VIII disease or brainstem lesions, and are summarized in Table 22.1 and Fig. 22.1. Rarely, vertigo can be a feature of temporal lobe disease (e.g., temporal lobe epilepsy).

Differential diagnoses of dizziness are summarized in Table 22.2.

COMMUNICATION

When a patient presents with vertigo or dizziness, it is vital to establish whether true vertigo is present or not, as these symptoms result from different diseases.

COMMUNICATION

It is important to remember that occasionally patients with vestibular dysfunction will not report vertigo, and patients with presyncope can report a mild spinning sensation.

Table 22.1 Differential diagnoses of vertigo

Location of lesion	Examples
Labyrinth	Middle ear disease (e.g., otitis media)
	Ménière disease
	BPPV
	Labyrinthitis
	Traumatic vertigo
	Perilymphatic fistula
Cranial nerve VIII	Vestibular neuronitis
	Acoustic neuroma
	Ramsay Hunt syndrome: herpes zoster of the geniculate ganglion
	Ototoxic drugs: aminoglycosides such as gentamicin
	Petrous temporal bone disease (e.g., Paget disease)
Brainstem/cerebellum	Vertebrobasilar ischaemia: TIA, posterior circulation stroke (including lateral medullary syndrome), rotational ischaemia Multiple sclerosis: demyelination
	Migraine
	Encephalitis
	Tumour
	Alcohol abuse
	Episodic ataxia (inherited autosomal dominant disorders)
	Syringobulbia

BPPV, *Benign paroxysmal positional vertigo;* TIA, *transient ischaemic attack.*

143

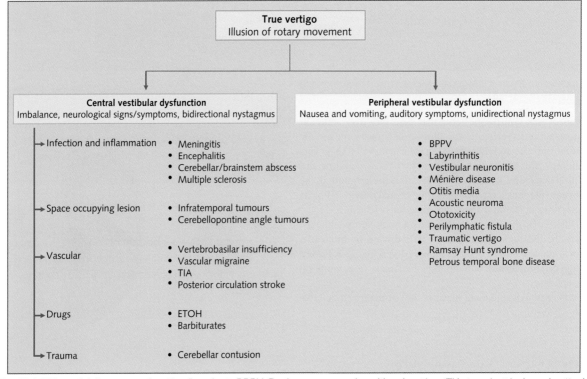

Fig. 22.1 Differential diagnoses of vertigo flowchart. *BPPV*, Benign paroxysmal positional vertigo; *TIA*, transient ischaemic attack.

Table 22.2 Differential diagnosis of dizziness without true vertigo

Causes	Further information
Low cardiac output	See Chapter 28
Nonspecific dizziness – often due to a psychiatric disorder (e.g., anxiety)	See *Crash Course: Psychiatry*
Anaemia	See Chapter 37
Hypoglycaemia	See Chapter 33
Postural hypotension	See Chapter 28
Visual disturbance	See *Crash Course: Neurology and Ophthalmology*
Cerebrovascular disease	See Chapter 34
Pyrexia	See Chapter 38

HINTS AND TIPS

Vertigo is a serious symptom and can significantly affect a person's quality of life and independence. Make sure to establish what effect the diagnosis has on the patient.

HISTORY AND EXAMINATION FINDINGS

History

The history is the basis of the diagnosis of vertigo. It is important to elicit the time course of vertigo and the likely site of the lesion by asking about other auditory and neurological symptoms. Typical features of specific diseases are described in Table 22.3.

Onset and pattern of vertigo

Establish:

- Onset: peripheral lesions generally cause acute severe symptoms; central lesions tend to be gradual onset with less severe vertigo unless caused by ischaemia.
- Duration and recurrence: is it a single episode (e.g., ischaemia) or recurring (e.g., benign paroxysmal positional vertigo (BPPV))? Are the attacks brief (seconds to minutes) or prolonged (hours to days)?
- Aggravating features: is there a relation to specific positions or movements? Is it worse on coughing/sneezing?
- Effect on daily activities (e.g., ability to walk or drive).

Table 22.3 Characteristic features of conditions causing vertigo

Disease	Cause	Length of vertigo	Aural symptoms	Neurological symptoms	Natural history
Ménière disease	Excess endolymphatic fluid (hydrops)	20 minutes to 24 hours Often preceded by sensation of ear fullness	Fluctuating progressive sensorineural deafness Tinnitus	None	Episodic, unilateral then becomes bilateral in 25%–45% Frequency diminishes with duration
Vestibular neuronitis	Possibly viral	Days to weeks Explosive onset	None	None	Spontaneously resolves in weeks
Vestibular labyrinthitis	Viral or bacterial infection, head injury	Symptoms often ease after a few days but permanent hearing loss can occur	None	Hearing loss, tinnitus, nystagmus	Sudden onset of symptoms that tend to get worse as the day goes on
BPPV	Debris within the semicircular canals Can follow head injury and vestibular neuronitis	<1 minute Precipitated by changes in head position	None	None	Episodic attacks Spontaneous resolution over weeks to months May recur after a symptom-free period
Perilymphatic fistula	Rupture of round window membrane Often due to barotrauma Can be spontaneous	Frequent, short-lasting episodes persisting for months to years	Deafness and tinnitus	None	Often resolves with bed rest Can be surgically repaired
Vertebrobasilar insufficiency	Compression of vertebral arteries by osteophytic cervical vertebrae	Seconds Precipitated by neck extension or rotation	None	Dysarthria Diplopia Visual loss Syncope	Episodic attacks
Acoustic neuroma	Schwannoma of vestibular nerve	Gradual onset Progressive	Unilateral deafness and tinnitus	Cranial nerve V and VII palsies Ipsilateral cerebellar signs	Symptoms progress until surgical removal
Central lesions	Tumour Demyelination Vascular migraine	Dependent on underlying disease	Often spared	Usually present and dependent on site of lesion	Tumour/demyelination: symptoms progress until underlying cause treated

BPPV, *Benign paroxysmal positional vertigo.*

CLINICAL NOTES

Vestibular neuronitis is a dysfunction of the branch of the nerve responsible for balance, resulting in dizziness or vertigo without a change in hearing, and often occurs after a viral infection.

Vestibular labyrinthitis occurs when both branches of cranial nerve VIII are affected, resulting in hearing changes and dizziness or vertigo.

Aural symptoms

The presence of aural symptoms suggests that the lesion is peripheral, involving the labyrinth or cranial nerve VIII:

- deafness (fluctuating or progressive)
- tinnitus
- ear discharge or pain
- a sensation of ear 'fullness' (Ménière disease)

Neurological symptoms

Suggest a central lesion or acoustic neuroma:

- Other cranial nerve involvement: facial weakness, facial paraesthesia, visual disturbance, dysarthria, dysphagia.
- Seizures.
- Weakness, paraesthesia, ataxia.

CLINICAL NOTES

History aspects suggesting an underlying cause

- Recent upper respiratory tract infection or ear infection: vestibular neuronitis or labyrinthitis
- Head trauma or recent labyrinthitis: benign paroxysmal positional vertigo
- Direct ear trauma or previous ontological surgery: perilymphatic fistula
- Drug history (e.g., aminoglycosides, furosemide, antipsychotics, anticonvulsants)
- Alcohol history: acute intoxication may cause vertigo
- Recent flying or diving (e.g., barotrauma – perilymphatic fistula)
- Associated headache with photophobia or phonophobia: migrainous vertigo
- Medical history: risk factors for vascular disease (ischaemia), multiple sclerosis and migraine
- Family history of vertigo: inherited episodic ataxia (channelopathies), Ménière disease

Examination

Full neurological examination, ear examination and eye examination should be performed (see Chapter 2). Look for the following:

- Nystagmus: observe the direction of slow and fast phases and whether they change direction or amplitude with the gaze direction. Are there features of a peripheral or central cause (see Chapter 2)?
- Dix–Hallpike manoeuvre: the patient's neck is extended, and the head is turned to one side; the patient is then lowered quickly to a supine position. Reproduction of symptoms of vertigo and horizontal and torsional nystagmus indicates a positive test result. The test is around 80% sensitive for the detection of BPPV.
- Romberg test: the patient stands erect with the feet together and arms outstretched. The patient is then asked to close their eyes. The inability to maintain balance represents a positive test result and indicates a vestibular (labyrinthine) or sensory (proprioceptive) dysfunction. Patients usually fall to the side of the lesion.
- Head impulse test: the patient is asked to fix the gaze on a target; the head is then quickly turned 20 degrees horizontally. Abnormal corrective eye movements suggest a positive test result and a peripheral lesion.

- Unterberger's test: the patient walks in place with their eyes closed; rotation of the patient to one side indicates dysfunction of the labyrinth on that side.
- Focal neurological signs: if present, these suggest a central lesion, acoustic neuroma or Ramsay Hunt syndrome.
- Eyes: papilloedema (tumour with raised intracranial pressure), optic atrophy (demyelination) and ophthalmoplegia (cranial nerve defect, demyelination).
- Ears: otoscopy may reveal otitis media or a herpetic rash.
- Neck movements: are they limited, or do they provoke the symptoms? Rarely, cervical spondylosis can cause 'rotational vertebrobasilar ischaemia' on head turning.

Fig. 22.2 summarizes the examination approach.

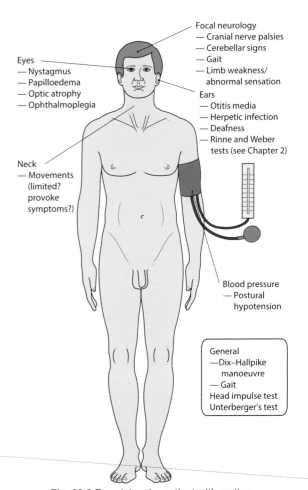

Fig. 22.2 Examining the patient with vertigo.

Remember, benign paroxysmal positional vertigo is diagnosed with the Dix–Hallpike manoeuvre and is treated with the Epley manoeuvre.

INVESTIGATIONS

- Simple tests include routine observations (including lying and standing blood pressure to investigate postural hypotension), blood glucose and ECG. Routine blood tests may reveal infection or evidence of other underlying diseases.
- Imaging: magnetic resonance imaging (MRI) should be performed if a central lesion or acoustic neuroma is suspected.
- Audiometry: this will help distinguish between conductive and sensorineural deafness.
- Caloric tests: normally, running cold and then warm water into the external auditory meatus causes nystagmus with the fast phase away and towards, respectively; where there is disease in the ipsilateral labyrinth, cranial nerve VIII or brainstem, this normal response will be reduced or absent.
- Electronystagmography: a more accurate assessment of the presence and type of nystagmus.

CLINICAL NOTES

INDICATIONS FOR BRAIN IMAGING IN ACUTE VERTIGO

- New-onset headache (raises the possibility of haemorrhage)
- Intact head impulse tests (increased likelihood of central lesion)
- Other cranial nerve symptoms/signs suggesting a central cause
- Nystagmus with features of a central lesion
- Acute deafness (raises the possibility of labyrinthine stroke)

N.B. Significant cardiovascular risk factors should increase the suspicion of a vascular event.

Chapter Summary

- Vertigo can be of peripheral (vestibular labyrinth, semicircular canals, vestibular nerve) or central (cerebral cortex, brainstem, cerebellum) origin.
- Peripheral vertigo is the most common type.
- Benign paroxysmal positional vertigo is the most common disease that leads to vertigo.

UKMLA Conditions
Acoustic neuroma
Benign paroxysmal positional vertigo
BPPV
Ménière disease
Otitis media

UKMLA Presentations
Hearing loss
Tinnitus
Unsteadiness
Vertigo
Dizziness

Back pain and joint pain

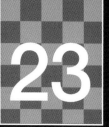

INTRODUCTION

Back pain and joint disease are common problems. Back pain, in particular, affects 8 out of 10 adults at some point in their life and places a considerable burden on health services. Both complaints often present together and can be unspecific and benign but also can manifest through significant underlying disease.

HISTORY AND EXAMINATION FINDINGS

Different types of joint and back pain have many features in common, and examination will provide further additional important clues to the cause.

History

When you are exploring the presenting complaint and determining the characteristics of the pain, remember to consider:

- Site (e.g., level of spine, specific joints) and radiation of pain.
- Time course, including onset, progression and variation throughout the day (e.g., worse in the morning with inflammatory arthritis). Is the pain present at night or waking them from sleep?
- Character (e.g., shooting, arthritis or arthralgia) and severity (what is the loss of function and is it affecting the patient's daily activity?)
- Joint swelling and stiffness. The pattern of distribution and joint deformity (symmetrical or asymmetrical, monoarthritis or polyarthritis).
- Aggravating and relieving features (e.g., pain due to disc prolapse may be worsened on leaning forward; pain due to neoplasia is often unremitting).

Ask about associated features
- Weakness and sensory loss: can this be localized to a single myotome/dermatome (e.g., disc prolapse) or is it more generalized (e.g., cauda equina syndrome)?
- Incontinence (cauda equina syndrome).
- Fever (infection, lymphoma, previous history of TB or TB contact).
- Weight loss (inflammatory disease, neoplasia, chronic infection).
- Pseudoclaudication: leg pain on walking (indicative of spinal stenosis).

- Systemic features (e.g., anaemia, rashes, eye disease, involvement of other systems (e.g., respiratory, gastrointestinal systems)).
- Depression, anxiety and psychosocial factors (Table 23.1).

Other important points to consider
- Age.
- History of trauma.
- Medical history: immune compromise, recent or chronic infection, cancer.
- Previous or current medication (e.g., corticosteroids).
- Family history: inflammatory arthritis.
- Social history: smoking, alcohol, occupation and repeat strain injury (RSI), sport, history of recent travel.
- Sexual history (to exclude reactive arthritis; see Chapter 35).

Determine presence of Red Flag symptoms (Table 23.2)
These warrant urgent medical attention and imaging and consist of signs and symptoms that increase the risk of a serious underlying condition.

- Cauda equina is an orthopaedic emergency and results from compression of lumbar nerve roots. It presents with pain and severe progressive neurological deficit in the legs. It is usually bilateral. Other symptoms include perineal loss of sensation, urinary and bowel incontinence due to sphincteric weakness and urinary retention. It is treated with emergency spinal decompression or with radiotherapy and intravenous steroids if secondary to a malignant compression.
- If presenting red flag symptoms suggest an infective cause, spinal infection/abscess should be excluded. Precipitating factors include long-term use of anticoagulants, intravenous drug use, immunocompromised patients, recent bacteraemias.

CLINICAL NOTES

Remember that with inflammatory causes the pain is worse first thing in the morning, is associated with stiffness, and abates after 30 to 60 minutes of movement (e.g., rheumatoid arthritis). Conversely, mechanical back pain and degenerative arthritis (e.g., osteoarthritis) are often worse with movement and abate at rest.

Table 23.1 Yellow flags: psychosocial factors associated with the development of chronic pain

Factor	Associations
Physical/pain related	Obesity, older age, increased severity of pain, disability, neurological involvement, previous episode of pain
Psychological	Anxiety, depression, emotional distress, somatization
Social	Lack of education, overprotective family
Behavioural	Smoking, poor coping skills, avoidance of activity because of fear of pain, prior inactivity
Occupational	Highly physical employment, dissatisfaction with job, lack of employer flexibility in type of work done
Other	Involvement in litigation

Table 23.2 Red flags for back and joint pain

Factor	Associations
Age >60 or <18 years	Neoplasia more common in the elderly and inflammatory disease more common in the young
Thoracic pain	Neoplastic disease
Nocturnal, constant pain	Malignancy
History of trauma	Vertebral fractures
Systemic symptoms (e.g., weight loss, rashes, objectively unwell with back pain)	Inflammatory, infectious or neoplastic disease
Immunosuppression or history of malignant disease	Infectious disease, neoplasm
Prolonged steroid use	Predisposes to osteoporosis and pathological fractures
Neurological symptoms, including sphincter dysfunction	Cauda equine, nerve root disease, spinal cord compression

CLINICAL NOTES

Chronic arthritis and the associated reduction in function can lead to feelings of helplessness and depression. Assessment of these features is an important part of the history taking in patients with arthritis.

CLINICAL NOTES

Causes of joint pain can be remembered by the mnemonic 'SOFTER TISSUE': *s*epsis, *o*steoarthritis, *f*ractures, *t*endon/muscle, *e*piphyseal, *r*eferred, *t*umour, *i*schaemia, *s*eropositive arthritides, *s*eronegative arthritides, *u*rate, *e*xtraarticular rheumatism (e.g., polymyalgia).

Examination

Examination should start with the affected area of the joint or spine and subsequently be directed by the history. Given a variety of joints can be affected, to make the task easier the general principle of LOOK, FEEL, MOVE can be applied to ensure a complete examination is performed:

- Look: obvious deformities, joint alignment, postural abnormality (kyphosis, scoliosis), swelling or redness, rashes, masses.
- Feel: assess the area for tenderness, inflammation (swelling, heat) and crepitus (joint degeneration). Evaluate any masses fully.
- Move: assess passive and active movement. Is there a reduced range of motion or pain on movement? Is the joint stiff?

Always remember to assess at least the joint above and the joint below the examined area and offer a neurological examination. If particular symptoms occur, examine the systems involved (rectal examination to exclude cauda equina, respiratory examination for lung fibrosis, etc.)

Specific examination findings in the most common joint diseases can be found in Table 23.3.

COMMUNICATION

Be aware that when you are introducing yourself to the patient with rheumatoid arthritis, shaking hands may be painful for the patient.

INVESTIGATIONS

Investigations should be requested according to clinical suspicion elucidated by the history and examination. A list of

Table 23.3 Specific examination findings in common joint diseases (see Chapter 35)

Joint disease	Systemic features	Local features
Rheumatoid arthritis	Symmetrical deforming arthropathy Cervical spine disease Anaemia Eye disease (keratoconjunctivitis sicca, keratitis, scleromalacia perforans)	Swelling of PIP and MCP joints Wasting of small hand muscles Extensor tendons nodules Ulnar deviation of fingers (subluxation of MCP joints) Swan-neck deformity (hyperextension of PIP joints and flexion of MCP and DIP joints) Boutonniere finger deformity (flexion of PIP joints and extension of MCP and DIP joints) Z-thumb Trigger fingers
Osteoarthritis	Most commonly asymmetrical and affecting large weight-bearing joints	Heberden nodes (swelling of DIP joints) Bouchard nodes (swelling of PIP joints) Subluxation of first carpometacarpal joint (square hand)
Ankylosing spondylitis	Most commonly affects spine and sacroiliac joints Reduced chest expansion and lung fibrosis Aortitis Eye iritis	Question mark posture (loss of lumbar lordosis and fixed kyphosis) Limited range of movement in the whole spine but especially in cervical and lumbar regions (Schober test) Tender sacroiliac joints
Septic arthritis	Systemic compromise: fever and rigours; tachycardia; tachypnoea; hypotension	Monoarthritis with swollen, red, hot and extremely tender joint

DIP, *Distal interphalangeal;* MCP, *metacarpophalangeal;* PIP, *proximal interphalangeal.*

investigations that can aid in diagnosis when you are considering joint and back pain follows.

Bedside investigations

Blood tests

- Full blood count: anaemia; raised white cell count in infection and occasionally in rheumatoid arthritis (RA), leucopaenia and thrombocytopenia in systemic lupus erythematosus (SLE), neutropenia in Felty syndrome.
- Erythrocyte sedimentation rate and C-reactive protein: nonspecific markers of inflammation but may be useful in detecting inflammatory arthritis.
- Renal function, liver function, calcium, parathyroid hormone, vitamin D, urate and myeloma.
- Autoantibody screen (see Chapter 36).
- Blood cultures: positive specifically for staphylococcal infections can suggest discitis or spinal abscess (more common in patients with long-standing intravenous lines, catheters and drains).
- Viral serology: if a viral cause for the arthropathy is suspected (e.g., rubella, mumps, infectious mononucleosis, Coxsackie virus).
- Genitourinary testing including for *Chlamydia trachomatis* and *Neisseria gonorrhoea* if indicated.

Joint aspiration (arthrocenthesis) is necessary when you are excluding septic arthritis and diagnosing crystal arthrocentesis. If septic arthritis is suspected, joint aspiration should be performed before antibiotic administration but treatment should never be delayed. Analysis of aspirate should cover:

- Appearance: purulence indicates infection, frank blood indicates haemarthrosis or traumatic tap.
- Microscopy for bacteria, polarized light microscopy for crystals: monosodium urate indicates gout and calcium pyrophosphate indicates pseudogout.
- White cell count: high in inflammatory arthropathies.
- Culture: to diagnose the organism, and their drug sensitivities/resistance.

CLINICAL NOTES

Red, hot, swollen joint that started suddenly and is extremely painful should be treated as septic arthritis until proven otherwise. Even in patients with known rheumatoid problem as they are at higher risk of developing septic joint. Most common joints affected include knee, hip and the shoulder. Treatment is with surgical washout and debridement.

Imaging

Imaging is very useful when you are considering joint disease and back pain. Plain radiographs are readily available and can show specific features characteristic of disease (Table 23.4).

Magnetic resonance imaging (MRI) is now widely used to provide images of soft tissue injury, including ligaments, muscle and intervertebral discs, inflammatory processes such as osteomyelitis and malignancy. It is also a first-line imaging method when spinal cord compression or cauda equina is suspected.

Computed tomography (CT) is used to assess bones and joints, and to further delineate fracture. Other imaging methods to consider include ultrasound scan and more invasive methods such arthroscopy for direct visualization (used for biopsy or foreign body removal).

DIFFERENTIAL DIAGNOSIS

There are many possible causes of joint disease and back pain, and they often occur concurrently. It is important to adopt a systematic approach to ensure correct management.

Table 23.4 Plain radiographic findings in common joint diseases

Disease	Plain radiograph findings
Rheumatoid arthritis	A joint X-ray will show soft tissue thickening, juxtaarticular osteoporosis, loss of joint space, bony erosions and subluxation. Chest imaging may show pleural effusion, pulmonary fibrosis, rheumatoid nodules and rheumatoid pneumoconiosis (Caplan syndrome)
Osteoarthritis	Loss of joint space, marginal osteophytes, subchondral sclerosis and cysts are visible on X-ray
Gout	Soft tissue swelling and punched-out lesions in juxtaarticular bone are common findings in gout
Ankylosing spondylitis	Sacroiliac joint and spine radiograph shows 'bamboo spine' (squaring of the vertebrae and obliteration of sacroiliac joints)
Back pain	Spine and pelvis X-ray is useful for detecting fractures (traumatic and compression fractures), disc space narrowing, degenerative change, spondylolisthesis, and changes of inflammatory disease (e.g., sacroiliitis, squaring of the vertebrae)

Joint disease

A systematic approach to the differential diagnosis of joint disease is illustrated in Fig. 23.1. The most common conditions causing joint pain include:

- RA
- osteoarthritis
- gout
- seronegative arthritides: ankylosing spondylitis, Reiter syndrome (reactive arthritis) and psoriatic arthritis
- septic arthritis
- trauma

Arthritis and arthralgia may also be a feature of the systemic disease, including connective tissue diseases, especially SLE, vasculitis and neoplastic or malignant disease (leukaemia and lymphoma, lung, breast and kidney).

Less common causes include:

- Endocrine and metabolic disease (acromegaly and hyperparathyroidism, haemochromatosis and Wilson disease).
- Other diseases: sarcoidosis, amyloidosis and sickle cell disease.

Back pain

Back pain usually has a mechanical or structural cause (e.g., crush fracture secondary to osteoporosis). This may have a neuropathic element as in the case of spinal stenosis or nerve root compression secondary to a disc prolapse.

Nonmechanical back pain is less common but is important to detect, and includes pain caused by inflammatory conditions, infection and cancer. Back pain may also be referred from other viscera. The causes of back pain are summarized in Table 23.5.

CLINICAL NOTES

The causes of a single hot, red joint is a favourite question. They are:

- septic arthritis – until proven otherwise
- trauma
- gout
- pseudogout
- haemarthrosis
- rheumatoid arthritis

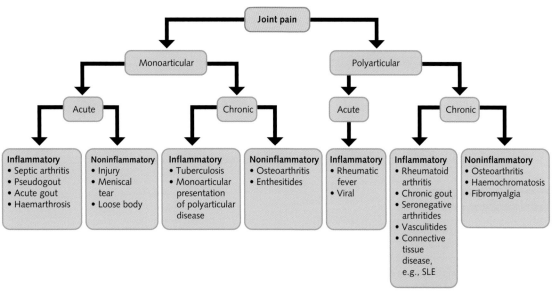

Fig. 23.1 Differential diagnosis algorithm for joint disease. *SLE*, Systemic lupus erythematosus.

Table 23.5 Causes of back pain

Type of pain	Cause	Characteristics
Mechanical back pain (possibly causing neurogenic pain)	Unknown cause/nonspecific pain	Lumbar strain/sprain
	Degenerative disease	
	Disc prolapse	Facet joint arthritis
	Spinal fracture	
	Spinal stenosis	Pathological fracture (e.g., due to neoplasia or osteoporosis) Traumatic fracture
	Spondylolysis and spondylolisthesis	

Continued

Table 23.5 Causes of back pain—cont'd

Type of pain	Cause	Characteristics
Nonmechanical pain	Neoplastic infiltration	Myeloma Metastatic carcinoma Direct invasion of retroperitoneal tumour Lymphoma/leukaemia Spinal cord tumours
	Infection	Osteomyelitis Discitis Spinal abscess (very common in drug users)
	Inflammatory conditions	Ankylosing spondylitis Reactive arthritis Enteropathic arthritis Sacroiliitis
	Paget disease	
Referred pain from visceral disease	Pelvic	Prostatitis Endometriosis Pelvic inflammatory disease
	Renal	Calculi Neoplasia Pyelonephritis
	Gastrointestinal	Pancreatitis Ulcer disease
	Aortic aneurysm	
Other	Fibromyalgia	

● Chapter Summary

- When assessing a patient with joint or back pain, the history and examination are crucial in assessing the cause of the symptoms.
- Because there is a wide range of conditions affecting these systems, it is important to maintain a systemic approach and repeat steps if necessary.
- Remember it is important to assess red flag symptoms and rule out a sinister cause of pain and direct your investigations and management by the clinical picture obtained.

UKMLA Conditions
Acute joint pain/stiffness
Bone pain
Chronic joint pain/stiffness
Crystal arthropathy
Osteoarthritis
Pathological fracture
Reactive arthritis
Rheumatoid arthritis
Septic arthritis
Spinal fracture

UKMLA Presentations
Back pain
Immobility
Muscle pain/myalgia

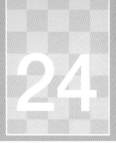

Skin lesions and rash   24

INTRODUCTION

Rashes and skin lesions can be diverse and misleading. This chapter will focus on the most common presentations for which appropriate history taking, examination and investigations can lead to the establishment of accurate differential diagnosis and management.

HISTORY AND EXAMINATION FINDINGS

History

The following should be assessed when you are taking the history of a patient with skin lesions:

- Rash: its character, onset, initial site of origin and progression, evolution of lesions and duration.
- Aggravating and relieving factors: physical or chemical agents; cold (cold urticaria or cryoglobulinaemia) and heat (worsens seborrhoeic conditions and superficial skin conditions).
- Timing of change in skin lesions (e.g., moles and their malignant transformation).
- Precipitants: stress may lead to alopecia or eczema.
- Associated hair and nail abnormalities.
- Possible infective agents: foreign travel and close contacts (tropical infections), pets (papular urticaria or animal scabies), farm animals (poxvirus, ringworm).
- Chemical exposure: at home or work (ask about occupation), acting as antigens or direct irritants. Ask about soap and laundry detergent.
- Foods: nuts and shellfish.
- Light exposure: eruption in skin-exposed areas (herpes simplex, systemic lupus erythematous and vitiligo).
- Current and past medication. Have any drug therapies been started or altered recently?
- General health and medical history.
- Family history: important in eczema, psoriasis, inherited skin disorders.
- Patient's concerns and explanation for rash.

Systemic symptoms should also be assessed:

- Itching (Table 24.1): atopy or urticaria, scabies, eczema, dermatitis herpetiformis, lichen planus, psoriasis.
- Pain: inflammatory conditions, skin tumours.
- Any other constitutional symptoms.

Table 24.1 Possible causes of generalized and localized itching

Generalized itching	Localized itching
Uraemia	Scabies and other mite infestations
Cholestasis	Contact eczema
Lymphoma	Dermatitis herpetiformis (associated with coeliac disease)
Iron deficiency anaemia	Urticaria ('nettle rash')
Hypothyroidism and hyperthyroidism	Lichen planus
Pregnancy	Prickly heat
Carcinoma	Winter itch
Allergies (e.g., atopic eczema)	Aquagenic pruritus
Morphine ingestion	Old age
Diabetes mellitus	Pruritus ani
Multiple sclerosis	Pruritus vulvae
Syphilis	
Intestinal parasites	

COMMUNICATION

Skin diseases affecting exposed areas such as the face can have a devastating effect on patients that is often disproportionate to the severity of the disease. Careful questioning of the patient's concerns and appropriate reassurance that the condition can be treated are important aspects of managing dermatological problems.

Examination

Always examine the entire skin, remembering to maintain dignity of the patient. Ask for a chaperone and use a room with good light. Look in the mouth (lesions seen, e.g., with lichen planus, herpes virus infection and infective exanthemata), behind the ears, on the scalp and between finger web spaces. Look at the distribution of lesions and their characteristics:

Table 24.2 Terms and characteristics of dermatological lesions

Term	Characteristics
Alopecia	Hair loss
Blister or bulla	Vesicle >1 cm in diameter
Crust	Dried exudate on skin surface
Cyst	Epithelium-lined cavity containing fluid or semisolid material
Erythema	Area of reddened skin that blanches with pressure
Fissure	Linear crack in epidermis
Indurated	Hard and thickened
Köbner phenomenon	Skin lesions occurring at sites of external injury
Lichenification	Thickened skin with exaggerated skin markings
Macule	Circumscribed change in the skin colour ≤1 cm in diameter. It is not elevated above the surface
Nodule	Solid elevated skin lesion >1 cm in diameter
Papule	Solid raised palpable area ≤1 cm in diameter
Patch	Macule >1 cm across
Petechiae	Pinpoint haemorrhages
Plaque	Palpable plateau-like elevation of skin
Purpura	Area of reddened skin caused by extravasation of blood that does not blanch with pressure
Pustule	Circumscribed, pus-filled lesion
Scale	Flake of hard skin
Scar	Connective tissue replacement following loss of dermal tissue
Ulcer	Irregularly shaped break in surface continuity of epithelium
Vesicle	Fluid-filled lesion <1 cm in diameter
Wheal	Raised, palpable lesion with pale centre

- If widespread and symmetrical, suspect systemic disease.
- If only areas exposed to the sun are involved, suspect light sensitivity.

Describe the type of lesions (Table 24.2) and their site, distribution, size, shape and colour. Palpate the lesion and examine surrounding skin. Describe the border and its surface. Always remember to examine lymph nodes in the adjacent area.

INVESTIGATIONS

The history and examination may be enough to determine the diagnosis. If the patient is not unwell, it may be possible to examine the patient for skin changes over time, thereby allowing the development of lesions. Make sure clinical photography is completed to document the progress. Otherwise the following investigations can be considered:

- Blood tests: full blood count, urea and electrolytes, bacterial and viral titres with immunological tests for tropical diseases if appropriate, and blood cultures.
- Skin scrapings and nail clippings (e.g., fungal infection).
- Examination of the skin under ultraviolet light (e.g., fungal/bacterial infections, tuberous sclerosis, porphyria).
- Microscopy and culture, and virology of fluid-containing lesions.
- Allergy testing.
- Skin biopsy.
- Investigations for suspected systemic diseases or malignancy suggested by the history and examination or initial investigations.

DIFFERENTIAL DIAGNOSIS

Differential diagnosis when considering skin disease can be difficult given the diversity of presentations. The most commonly seen lesions are described next.

Pigmented lesions

- Freckles (ephelides): flat, brown spots arising on sun-exposed areas.
- Lentigines: similar to freckles but often larger, and not affected by sunlight, although they may develop because of sun exposure.
- Seborrhoeic keratosis: benign, beige/brown plaques, with a velvety or warty surface (Fig. 24.1).
- Melanocytic naevus (mole): there are many subtypes, including the blue naevus (small, slightly elevated blue-black lesions) and dysplastic naevus (usually a larger naevus, >5 mm, with an irregular, blurred border and mixed pigmentation and texture).
- Melanoma: flat or raised pigmented lesion with possibly a recent change in appearance (Fig. 24.2; see Chapter 36 for malignant melanoma). It has various colours and typically irregular borders.
- Melasma: well-demarcated patches of increased pigmentation with an irregular border, usually on the face and predominantly in women, associated with pregnancy.

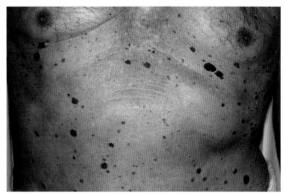

Fig. 24.1 Seborrheic keratosis. Benign raised warty lesions. (Reprinted with permission from Bolognia JL, et al. *Dermatology,* 3rd Edition.)

CLINICAL NOTES

Remember to use the ABCDE approach to examine a skin lesion for potential neoplastic characteristics:

- A: asymmetry
- B: irregular border
- C: variable colour
- D: diameter greater than 7 mm
- E: evolving with time

Scaly lesions

- Psoriasis: silvery, scaled, well-demarcated plaques on skin, usually over the extensor surfaces. It can also be pustular or guttate (widespread, small, round lesions) and involve the nails.
- Atopic dermatitis/eczema: dry, pruritic skin on the face, neck, wrists and on the flexures, most common in children. Over time the excoriated areas may become lichenified.
- Seborrhoeic dermatitis: greasy plaques with yellowish scale affecting the face, scalp, armpits, groin and trunk. Can be infected (Fig. 24.3).
- Lichen simplex chronicus: long-term rubbing or scratching in response to itch, causing pigmented, lichenified skin lesions with exaggerated markings.
- Tinea: fungal infection causing ring-shaped lesions with a scaly border and central healing, or scaly inflamed patches with a distinct border. Can appear anywhere on the skin (Fig. 24.4).

- Pityriasis versicolor: scaly, hypopigmented macules or patches usually on the chest or back (Fig. 24.5).
- Pityriasis rosea: oval, pink/red, scaly lesions following the skin tension lines of the trunk preceded by a herald patch.
- Discoid lupus erythematosus: well-defined red patches, usually on the face. There is scaling, follicular plugging, atrophy and telangiectasia of involved areas. The patches may thicken and often leave scars (Fig. 24.6).
- Exfoliative dermatitis: widespread skin erythema (erythroderma) with scaling or peeling.
- Actinic (solar) keratoses: small, pink lesions that are rough, crusted and scaly in texture. They are due to sun damage, and are considered to be premalignant.
- Bowen disease (intraepidermal squamous cell carcinoma): small, well-demarcated, slightly raised, pink-to-red, scaly plaques.
- Intertrigo: rash in body/skin folds due to excess moisture and often infection, causing fissuring, erythema and superficial denudation.

CLINICAL NOTES

'Dermatitis' and 'eczema' are interchangeable terms (although 'eczema' is commonly used to refer to the atopic form). There are several types, and they may exist simultaneously.

Vesicular lesions

- Herpes simplex: recurrent, small, grouped vesicles on an erythematous base, especially around the oral and genital areas.

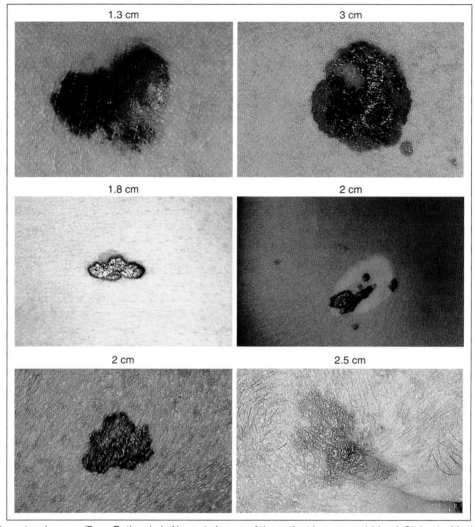

Fig. 24.2 Malignant melanoma. (From Rothrock J. *Alexander's care of the patient in surgery.* 14th ed. St. Louis, Mosby; 2011.)

- Herpes zoster (shingles): vesicular lesions in a dermatomal distribution, usually preceded by pain and general malaise (Fig. 24.7).
- Pompholyx (dyshidrotic eczema): small, intensely pruritic vesicles or bullae on the palms, soles and sides of fingers.
- Dermatitis herpetiformis: pruritic papulovesicular lesions mainly on the elbows, knees, buttocks, shoulders and scalp. It is associated with gluten-sensitive enteropathy.
- Miliaria (heat rash): superficial, aggregated, small vesicles, papules or pustules on covered areas of the skin.
- Scabies: pruritic vesicles and pustules especially between the fingers with characteristic burrows (Fig. 24.8).

Weepy or pustular lesions

- Impetigo: vesiculopustular lesions with thick, golden-crusted exudate, associated with group A streptococci or *Staphylococcus aureus*.
- Acne vulgaris: the most common skin condition, characterized by open and closed comedones and frequently accompanied by cysts, papules and pustules. It ranges from mild, purely comedonal to pustular inflammatory acne. Scarring can occur.
- Acne rosacea: papules, pustules and erythema over the forehead, cheeks and nose, with telangiectasia and a tendency to flush easily. Hyperplasia of the soft tissue of the nose (rhinophyma) may occur.

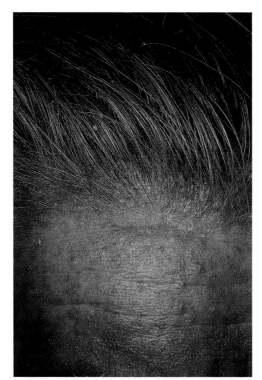

Fig. 24.3 Seborrheic dermatitis. Red, scaly rash on face. (Reprinted with permission from *Dermatology,* 3rd Edition. Bolognia et al.)

Fig. 24.5 Pityriasis versicolour and its hypopigmented lesions. (Reprinted with permission from *Dermatology,* 3rd Edition. Bolognia et al.)

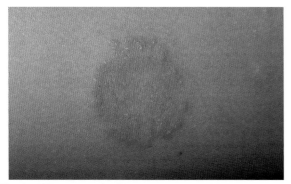

Fig. 24.4 Tinea corporis. Characteristic ring with central healing. (Reprinted with permission from *Dermatology,* 3rd Edition. Bolognia et al.)

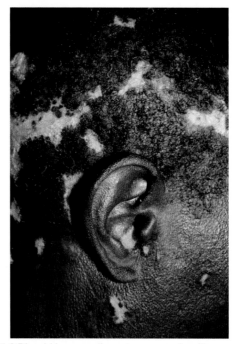

Fig. 24.6 Discoid lupus erythematous on scalp with associated scaring alopecia. (Reprinted with permission from *Dermatology,* 3rd Edition. Bolognia et al. Courtesy Joyce Rico.)

- Folliculitis: infection of the hair follicles causing pustular, erythematous lesions (Fig. 24.9).

Figurate erythema

These are lesions that look like rings or arcs:

- Urticaria: eruptions of evanescent (short-lasting) wheals or hives

- Erythema multiforme: erythematous lesions in a symmetrical distribution, initially over the extensor surfaces of the limbs, spreading to the trunk (Fig. 24.10). Palms, soles and mucous membranes may be involved. Lesions start as macules which evolve to become papular, urticarial, bullous or purpuric.
- Erythema migrans: an enlarging red patch or ring around an initial papule. The centre may clear or become

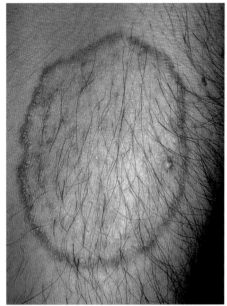

Fig. 24.7 Herpes zoster with vesicular lesion. (Reprinted with permission from *Dermatology,* 3rd Edition. Bolognia et al.)

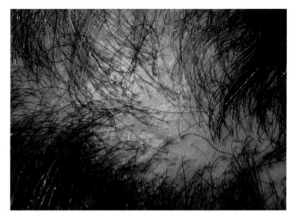

Fig. 24.9 Folliculitis on scalp. (Reprinted with permission from *Dermatology,* 3rd Edition. Bolognia et al.)

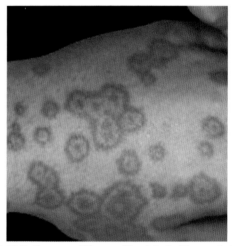

Fig. 24.10 Erythema multiforme. (Reprinted with permission from *Dermatology,* 3rd Edition. Bolognia et al.)

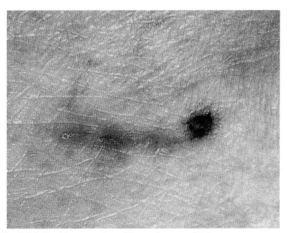

Fig. 24.8 Scabies causing skin erythema with burrows. (Reprinted with permission from *Dermatology,* 3rd Edition. Bolognia et al.)

indurated, vesicular or necrotic. It is a feature of Lyme disease (Fig. 24.11).

Bullous lesions

- Pemphigus: relapsing crops of flaccid bullae appearing on normal skin, which rupture easily leaving erosions and ulcerations. Mucous membrane (especially oral)

involvement is usually the first sign. There may be superficial exfoliation after slight pressure (Nikolsky sign).
- Bullous pemphigoid: tense blisters, typically in flexural areas. They may be preceded by urticarial or eczematous lesions.
- Porphyria cutanea tarda: blistering on sun-exposed areas.

Papular and nodular lesions

- Hyperkeratotic: warts, corns, seborrhoeic keratoses.
- Purple: lichen planus (see Chapter 36); Kaposi sarcoma – malignant skin lesions with dark plaques or nodules on cutaneous or mucosal surfaces, common in people with HIV infection.

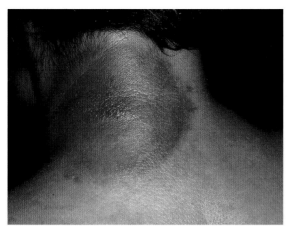

Fig. 24.11 Erythema migrans of Lyme disease. (Reprinted with permission from *Dermatology,* 3rd Edition. Bolognia et al.)

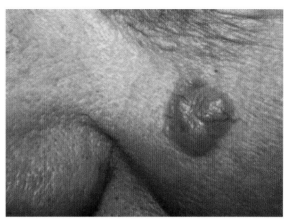

Fig. 24.12 Basal cell carcinoma. (Courtesy Stanley J. Miller, MD.)

- Flesh coloured and umbilicated: molluscum contagiosum – a viral infection causing single or multiple, rounded, dome-shaped, waxy papules, which are umbilicated and contain a caseous plug; keratoacanthoma – a rapidly growing, usually benign skin tumour with a crater topped with keratin debris.
- Pearly: basal cell carcinoma (Fig. 24.12; see Chapter 36).
- Small, red and inflammatory: acne, miliaria, candidiasis, intertrigo, scabies, folliculitis.
- Photodermatoses.

Painful erythema, oedema and vesiculation on sun-exposed surfaces. Causes include drugs (e.g., amiodarone, phenothiazines and sulphonamides), polymorphic light eruption and systemic lupus erythematous.

Maculopapular lesions

- Morbilliform drug eruptions, most commonly due to antibiotics and antiepileptics.
- Exanthemata due to viral (e.g., measles) or bacterial infection (e.g., scarlet fever).
- Secondary syphilis.

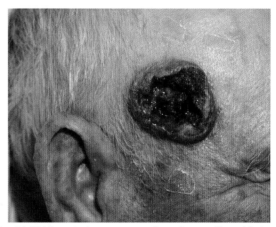

Fig. 24.13 Ulcerated squamous cell carcinoma. (From Marks JG, Miller JJ. *Lookingbill and Marks' Principles of Dermatology*, 5th ed. Philadelphia, Saunders Elsevier. 2013, p 52, Fig. 5.10.)

Ulcerated lesions

- Decubitus ulcers: bed sores or pressure sores.
- Skin cancers commonly ulcerate (Fig. 24.13; squamous cell carcinoma most commonly).
- Parasitic infections (e.g., leishmaniasis).
- Syphilis: primary chancre.
- Venous or arterial insufficiency.
- Neuropathic ulcers: particularly in diabetes.

Petechial and purpuric lesions

- Thrombocytopenia: primary or secondary.
- Coagulation disorders (e.g., disseminated intravascular coagulation).
- Vascular disorders (e.g., vasculitis).

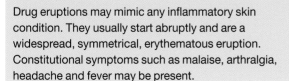

> **HINTS AND TIPS**
>
> Drug eruptions may mimic any inflammatory skin condition. They usually start abruptly and are a widespread, symmetrical, erythematous eruption. Constitutional symptoms such as malaise, arthralgia, headache and fever may be present.

Miscellaneous lesions

- Candidiasis: superficial, denuded, red areas with or without satellite vesicopustular lesions. There are whitish, curd-like concretions on the oral and vaginal mucous membranes.

- Staphylococcal scalded skin syndrome: widespread erythematous blistering skin lesions due to release of staphylococcal toxins.

● Chapter Summary

- The wide array of skin lesions sometimes makes it very difficult for an inexperienced eye to correctly identify the underlying disease.
- There are therefore specific characteristics that dermatology describes to aid in correct diagnosis and therefore optimal management.
- Remember that history and examination are crucial in directing the clinical train of thought.
- Appropriate description of lesions, including their progression and associated features, is pivotal in understanding disease processes.
- Make sure the patient is assessed in a systemic way and that the psychological impact of the condition is elucidated.

UKMLA Conditions
Arterial ulcers
Atopic dermatitis and eczema
Basal cell carcinoma
Contact dermatitis
Cutaneous fungal infections
Cutaneous warts
Folliculitis
Malignant melanoma
Pressure sores
Psoriasis
Scabies
Squamous cell carcinoma
Urticaria

UKMLA Presentations
Acute rash
Chronic rash
Pruritis
Skin ulcers

INTRODUCTION

Lumps and bumps are extremely common presenting patient complaints. A lump can also be identified by the clinician on examination. Aetiologically, lumps generally fall into one of the following categories:

- congenital or acquired
- inflammatory (either acute or chronic)
- traumatic
- neoplastic (primary or secondary and malignant or benign)
- other (e.g., metabolic, degenerative, hormonal)

A detailed history, examination and subsequent investigations will help in determining the differential diagnosis, and therefore management for a mass found. Management can range from simple explanation, reassurance and monitoring to urgent referral for surgery.

HISTORY AND EXAMINATION FINDINGS

A methodological approach to history taking and examination with particular emphasis on mass inspection is crucial in determining the potential cause.

It is important to determine where was the lump found. Common places include the neck, breast, axilla, scrotum and perianal area, and skin. To a clinician the site will give important clues regarding the anatomical origin of the lump and potential underlying disease.

Important questions to ask about the lump include:

- When was the lump first noticed?
- Has it developed with time?
- Is it tender?
- Are there any other lumps or associated symptoms?

Enquire about past medical history as previous illness could itself be a cause of a lump. Ask if there is a history of any other lumps, history of trauma or foreign travel.

The examination should focus on describing the lump. It is important to try to establish an anatomical plane of the swelling as it may be arising from the skin, subcutaneous tissue, tendon, muscle, bone or internal organ.

Inspection and palpation will help further characterize the swelling. These can be remembered by the S's:

- Site: should be described anatomically (e.g., lump in the breast). If it is difficult to describe, neighbouring structures should be identified.
- Size: needs to be measured with a diagram recording the position, dimension and shape.
- Shape: certain lumps can have a characteristic shape (e.g., two-lobed thyroid).
- Surface: comment on regularity, whether it is uniform or smooth or irregular. Margins as well- or ill-defined, smooth and regular or irregular.
- Surroundings: examine around the lump, its regional lymph nodes or, if it is a lymph node, its draining area.
- Structure (consistency): the lump may be solid or gaseous, soft, fluctuant or firm. Fluid lumps can be transilluminated, and they are compressible with displacement of the fluid in two planes.
- Stability: describe if the lump is mobile or fixed to surrounding/underlying structures.
- Sound: auscultate the swelling looking for bruits (aneurysm) or bowel sounds (hernia).
- Secretion: look for evidence of discharge or a punctum (sebaceous cyst).
- Sensation: feel the lump for temperature (may be raised over inflamed lumps), tenderness and pulsation (distinguish between expansile and transmitted pulsation).
- Sign of emptying or indentation: examine if the lump decreases in size or disappears when compressed or remains indented.

It is extremely important to keep a good record of the examined lump to ensure an appropriate timeline, and monitor any changes or developments. A diagram should be drawn of the findings or a picture can be kept in the records with appropriate patient consent.

HINTS AND TIPS

Remember to always examine the corresponding area of the patient on the opposite side of the body.

CLINICAL NOTES

A sebaceous cyst can be differentiated from lipoma by the presence of a punctum on its surface.

INVESTIGATIONS

Often diagnosis of a lump can be made clinically and does not require investigating. When, however, this is not adequate, several tests can be helpful:

- Ultrasound scan or Doppler studies are useful for fluid-filled lumps or to determine heterogeneity of a swelling.
- Excision biopsy for histology.
- Aspiration or fluid for microscopy and culture, and cytology.
- Fine-needle aspiration is used in solid masses for cytology.
- Blood tests, if the lump is thought to be inflammatory.
- CT and MRI scans are best in determining the characteristics of a lump, surrounding anatomy or investigating the presence of other masses (CT is best for bones; MRI for soft tissues).

DIFFERENTIAL DIAGNOSIS

The features of the lump, its anatomical position and its origin will determine the most likely diagnosis. Table 25.1 describes the most common differential diagnoses based on anatomical location.

Localized lymphadenopathy

'Localized lymphadenopathy' describes a lymph node that is abnormal in size, consistency or number. As a general rule, in adults abnormal size is defined as a short axis of the node of longer than 10 mm. There is a regional variation between lymph nodes, however, and a specific enlarged lymph node should be investigated based on individual criteria.

Localized lymphadenopathy is most commonly caused by a local site of infection (e.g., an abscess on the upper limb will cause localized lymphadenopathy in the same area).

Generalized lymphadenopathy

This is when more than two noncontiguous lymph node groups are found to be enlarged. Lymph nodes can increase in size depending on age, location and their current immune activity. Most generalized lymphadenopathy is caused by benign conditions such as bacterial or viral infections. Lymphoma, malignancy (e.g., acute leukaemia), HIV infection, tuberculosis (Fig. 25.1) or autoimmune disorders (e.g., systemic lupus erythematosus, sarcoidosis) can also be the cause.

Constitutional symptoms of fever, night sweats and malaise should always raise suspicion. Supraclavicular and infraclavicular lymph nodes are suggestive of malignancy. Firm, nontender nodes increase the risk of malignancy.

Table 25.1 Anatomical distribution of lumps and their most likely causes

Location	Differential diagnosis
Neck lump	Anterior triangle: • pharyngeal pouch • thyroid disease • branchial cyst • parotid gland swelling • lymphadenopathy Posterior triangle: • carotid body tumour • carotid artery aneurysm • cystic hygroma • cervical rib • lymphadenopathy Midline swelling: • thyroglossal cyst • lymphadenopathy
Breast lumps	Simple cysts Breast abscess Fibroadenomata (mobile lump) Fibroadenosis (lumpy breast) Fat necrosis Breast cancer
Axilla	Breast cancer Metastatic disease Hidradenitis suppurativa Sebaceous cyst Lipoma
Groin and scrotum	Hernias (inguinal or femoral) Epididymal cyst Epididymo-orchitis Hydrocele Haematocele Sebaceous cyst Psoas muscle abscess Femoral artery aneurysm Saphena varix Cancer
Abdomen	Enlarged abdominal organs (e.g., liver or spleen) Fibroids Abdominal cancer Abdominal aortic aneurysm Pregnancy
Other	Epitrochlear lymph nodes: characteristic of Hodgkin disease Supraclavicular lymph node (Virchow node): strongly suggestive of abdominal malignancy (most likely gastric) Neurofibromas (multiple cutaneous/subcutaneous/intramuscular lumps with café-au-lait spots and axillary freckling)

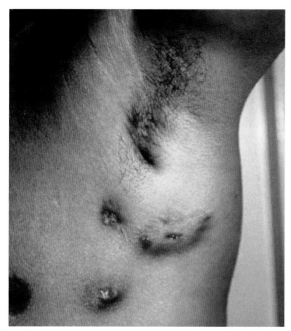

Fig. 25.1 Cutaneous tuberculosis. Lumps can be superficial but can also infiltrate deeper tissues. (Reprinted with permission from Bolognia JL, et al. *Dermatology*, 3rd Edition. Figure taken from Bolognia JL, Jorizzo JL, Schaffer JV. *Scrofuloderma Dermatology*: 2-Volume Set, 3rd Edition Expert Consult Premium Edition – Enhanced Online Features and Print. Elsevier, Figure 75.15.)

Investigations should be directed by the history and examination, and can include:

- Simple blood tests (e.g., full blood count, blood film and inflammatory markers)
- Infection swabs for primary disease
- Viral titres (e.g., hepatitis, Epstein – Barr virus)
- Imaging (chest radiograph, ultrasound scans, CT/MRI scan)

Management is directed by the diagnosis. The most important aspect concentrates on eliminating a serious underlying cause. Patients are advised to monitor the condition and seek help if symptoms persist or lymph nodes enlarge or multiply. As a general rule, the presence of any of the following should raise suspicion for further investigations or referral:

- Presence for more than 6 weeks
- Lymph nodes greater than 2 cm or increasing in size
- Widespread nature
- Associated constitutional symptoms or splenomegaly

Treatment is of the underlying condition and determines the prognosis.

Splenomegaly

The spleen plays an important role in immunity, and acts as a large lymph node. It has usually reached twice its original size by the time it is palpable. Splenomegaly most commonly presents as left upper quadrant mass, abdominal pain or early satiety if the spleen compresses the stomach.

The presence of splenomegaly should raise suspicion of a potentially serious underlying condition and should be investigated. Specific tests to consider include bone marrow, liver and lymph node biopsy.

The causes of splenomegaly include:

- Haematological causes: leukaemia, lymphoma, haemolytic anaemia, myelofibrosis, polycythaemia vera.
- Infections: tuberculosis, malaria, schistosomiasis, viral hepatitis, infective endocarditis, leishmaniasis.
- Tumours and cysts: abscess, splenic metastases, haemangioma.
- Connective tissue disorder: systemic lupus erythematosus, Felty syndrome.
- Congestive splenomegaly: heart failure, cirrhosis, portal and splenic vein obstruction, Budd–Chiari syndrome.

If massive splenomegaly is present, chronic myeloid leukaemia, myelofibrosis, leishmaniasis and malaria should be suspected.

Management is with treatment of the underlying condition. Splenectomy can be considered.

CLINICAL NOTES

In the patient presenting with subcutaneous nodules, think of systemic cause:

- rheumatoid nodules
- rheumatic fever
- polyarteritis
- xanthelasmata
- tuberous sclerosis
- neurofibromatosis
- sarcoidosis

Chapter Summary

- Lumps are one of the most common presenting complaints of patients. They can be signs of local infection or manifest themselves as features of a serious underlying condition.
- The most important aspects in determining the origin of a lump and establishing the differential diagnosis are thorough history taking and clinical examination.

UKMLA Conditions
Breast cyst
Breast lump

UKMLA Presentations
Lump
Lump in groin
Lymphadenopathy
Neck lump
Organomegaly
Scrotal/testicular pain and/or Lump/swelling
Skin or subcutaneous lump
Vulval/vaginal lump

Excessive bruising and bleeding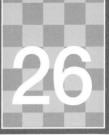

26

INTRODUCTION

Excessive bruising and bleeding (prolonged, spontaneous or following an insignificant injury) arise when there is abnormal haemostasis; this may occur because of abnormalities of the coagulation pathway, abnormalities of platelet number or function or abnormalities of the blood vessel (e.g., fragility of the vessel wall).

HISTORY AND EXAMINATION FINDINGS

History

It is important to maintain a general approach with a specific focus on the characteristics of bleeding. When you are concentrating on history, certain points should be emphasized and these include:

- The pattern and extent of bleeding and bruising.
  - Platelet abnormalities (deficiency or dysfunction) cause skin or mucosal purpura and haemorrhage. There is prolonged bleeding following minor procedures or trauma.
  - Vessel wall abnormalities cause petechiae and ecchymoses due to bleeding from small vessels. These are usually in the skin but are also in mucous membranes.
  - Coagulopathies cause haemarthrosis, muscle haematomas, postoperative or traumatic bleeding and palpable ecchymoses. If inherited they present early in life.
- The underlying cause:
  - Bleeding and bruising: determine whether it is within the spectrum of normal (e.g., related to trauma or recent haemostatic abnormality).
  - Liver disease: intrinsic liver disease (coagulopathy) or biliary obstruction may cause reduced platelet function and vitamin K deficiency.
  - Drug history: blood thinning medication, including antiplatelets, anticoagulants, steroids or previous chemotherapy.
  - Symptoms of underlying bone marrow failure (e.g., recurrent infection, symptoms of anaemia).

- Hyperextensibility of the skin or joints: Ehlers–Danlos syndrome, pseudoxanthoma elasticum.
- Known AIDS or risk factors for HIV infection.
- Have complications occurred?
  - Evaluate the severity of bleeding.
  - Establish symptoms of anaemia.
  - Musculoskeletal symptoms (muscle and joint pain, and deformity).

Examination

The examination should be approached similarly to history taking. Fig. 26.1 summarizes the examination approach. Features to concentrate on include:

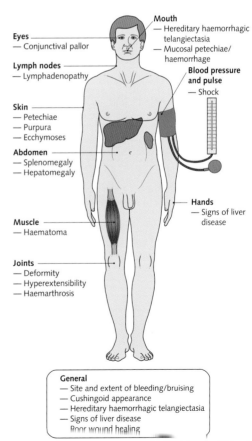

Eyes
— Conjunctival pallor

Lymph nodes
— Lymphadenopathy

Skin
— Petechiae
— Purpura
— Ecchymoses

Abdomen
— Splenomegaly
— Hepatomegaly

Muscle
— Haematoma

Joints
— Deformity
— Hyperextensibility
— Haemarthrosis

Mouth
— Hereditary haemorrhagic telangiectasia
— Mucosal petechiae/ haemorrhage

Blood pressure and pulse
— Shock

Hands
— Signs of liver disease

General
— Site and extent of bleeding/bruising
— Cushingoid appearance
— Hereditary haemorrhagic telangiectasia
— Signs of liver disease
— Poor wound healing

Fig. 26.1 Examining the patient with bruising and bleeding.

- The pattern and extent of bruising and bleeding.
- The sites and types of lesions (petechiae are smaller than 2 mm, characterized by pinpoint bleeding into skin or mucosa; purpura denotes bruises between 2 mm and 1 cm; ecchymosis refers to anything larger than 1 cm).
- Whether there are signs suggestive of a specific underlying cause (e.g., liver disease).
- How severe the bleeding has been and if there are complications.
- Look for evidence of anaemia, which may be due to chronic bleeding or an acute haemorrhage. Look for joint deformities (haemarthrosis) or muscle mass (haematoma).

INVESTIGATIONS

When an abnormality of haemostasis is suspected, a full blood count (FBC) and simple coagulation assays should be performed first. More specific tests to diagnose the underlying cause can then be considered. Fig. 26.2 summarizes the normal coagulation pathway.

An algorithm for investigating the patient with bruising and bleeding is given in Fig. 26.3.

Common blood tests are described later and summarized in Table 26.1. FBC and blood film may detect lymphoma,

leukaemia, thrombocytopaenia or abnormal platelet levels. Checking renal function may detect an abnormal urea level that can cause platelet dysfunction. Liver function tests will detect a hepatic cause of abnormal bleeding, such as alcohol abuse or acquired platelet disorders.

Recommended coagulation studies include:

- Prothrombin time (PT): measures the extrinsic system (tissue factor and factor VII) and the final common pathway. It is prolonged in liver disease and with warfarin therapy and is generally expressed as the international normalized ratio (INR).
- Activated partial thromboplastin time (APTT): measures the intrinsic system (factors VIII, IX, XI and XII) and the common pathway (fibrinogen, prothrombin and factors V and X). It is prolonged with unfractionated heparin therapy (not low-molecular-weight heparins) and deficiency of factors such as factor VIII (haemophilia A) and factor IX (haemophilia B, Christmas disease), and measures overall competence of the coagulation system.
- Thrombin time (TT): measures the rate of clot formation and therefore the activity of thrombin and fibrinogen in the common pathway. It is prolonged in disseminated intravascular coagulation (DIC) or other conditions causing fibrinogen deficiency (e.g., liver disease).

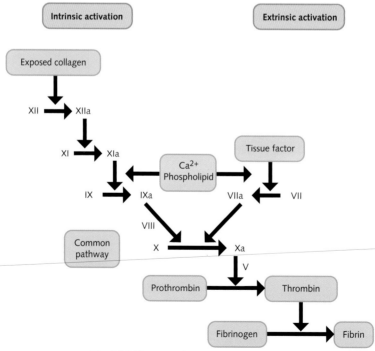

Fig. 26.2 The normal coagulation pathway.

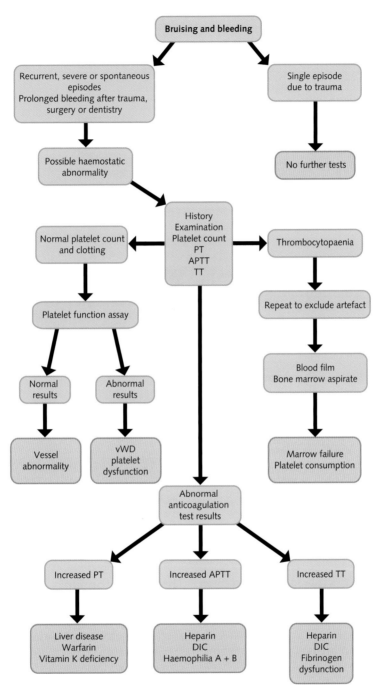

Fig. 26.3 Algorithm for investigating the patient with bruising or bleeding. *APTT*, Activated partial thromboplastin time; *DIC*, disseminated intravascular coagulation; *PT*, prothrombin time; *TT*, thrombin time; *vWD*, von Willebrand disease.

Table 26.1 Summary of the common clotting tests in bleeding disorders

	Platelet count	PT	APTT	TT
Haemophilia A	Normal	Normal	Prolonged	Normal
Haemophilia B	Normal	Normal	Prolonged	Normal
vWD	Normal	Normal	Prolonged/normal	Normal
DIC	Low	Prolonged	Prolonged	Prolonged
Liver disease	Low	Prolonged	Prolonged	Prolonged
Warfarin	Normal	Grossly prolonged	Prolonged	Normal
Heparin	Normal	Mildly prolonged	Prolonged	Prolonged
DOAC	Normal	Prolonged/normal	Prolonged	Prolonged/normal

APTT, *Activated partial thromboplastin time;* DIC, *disseminated intravascular coagulation;* DOAC, *direct oral anticoagulant;* PT, *prothrombin time;* TT, *thrombin time;* vWD, *von Willebrand disease.*

- The levels of fibrin degradation products, including D-dimers. The levels will be grossly elevated in DIC and may be raised in other conditions, including malignancy, renal disease and sepsis.

If these tests do not show an abnormality, most common bleeding disorders would have been excluded. Further tests to elucidate the nature of the problem include:

- Platelet function analyser (PFA), which measures platelet adhesion and aggregation and has replaced the bleeding time test. It is useful in the diagnosis of von Willebrand disease (vWD) and other inherited disorders of platelet function.
- Bleeding time measures the interaction between platelets and the vessel wall. It is nonspecific and therefore has now been largely replaced by the PFA.
- Fibrinogen levels, which are usually measured if the APTT and the PT are deranged, and are altered in inherited fibrinogen disorders, liver disease or acute bleeding.
- Specific factors assay.
- Genetic analysis.

HAEMORRHAGIC SHOCK

This is a medical emergency and needs immediate management. If left untreated it will lead to multiorgan dysfunction and death. A haemorrhagic shock is a form of hypovolaemic shock. Depending on the degree of blood loss the patient can present with different signs and symptoms (see Fig. 26.4 for classifications of haemorrhagic shock). Management focuses on the identification and treatment of the underlying cause and volume replacement. Temporalizing measures that aim to minimize ischaemic damage include rapid resuscitation with blood products. Tranexamic acid (antifibrinolytic) can be helpful in overt bleeding and is recommended in bleeding trauma patients.

RED FLAG

Young fit and healthy patients have much higher physiological reserves than frail patients and as such, they may not show typical signs and symptoms of severe blood loss until their compensatory mechanisms have been saturated, at which point the deterioration will be quick and may be catastrophic. Often the only sign may be tachycardia.

DIFFERENTIAL DIAGNOSIS

The differential diagnosis for bleeding disorders can be based on a possible underlying abnormality. This can include platelets, coagulation cascade or vessel wall disease.

Platelet abnormality

Thrombocytopaenia

This is described as a platelet count below 150×10^9/L. It can have a variety of causes:

- Reduced production: bone marrow failure (e.g., myelodysplastic syndrome), drugs (commonly cytotoxic medication), chemotherapy or radiotherapy, viral infections, hereditary syndromes (e.g., Fanconi anaemia).
- Decreased survival: immune thrombocytopaenic purpura, DIC, thrombotic thrombocytopaenic purpura, haemolytic uraemic syndrome, systemic lupus erythematosus, HIV and hypersplenism.
- Abnormal distribution: splenic pooling in splenomegaly.
- Dilutional: massive transfusion.

A summary of the four stages of shock as characterized by the physiological, neurological and cellular responses to the mismatch between falling oxygen delivery (eDO_2) and metabolic rate (VO_2).

	Stage 1	Stage 2	Stage 3	Stage 4
Blood loss (mL)	<750 <15%	750–1500 15%–30%	1500–2000 30%–40%	>2000 >40%
Heart rate (bpm)	<100	>100	>120	>140
Blood pressure	Normal	Reduced	Reduced	Reduced
Respiratory rate (breaths/minute)	14–20	20–30	30–40	>35
Urine output (mL/hour)	Normal >30	Oliguria 20–30	Oliguria 5–15	Anuria
Neurological status	Normal	Agitated	Confused	Lethargic
ATP status	Supply= demand	Supply= demand	Supply< demand	Supply<< demand

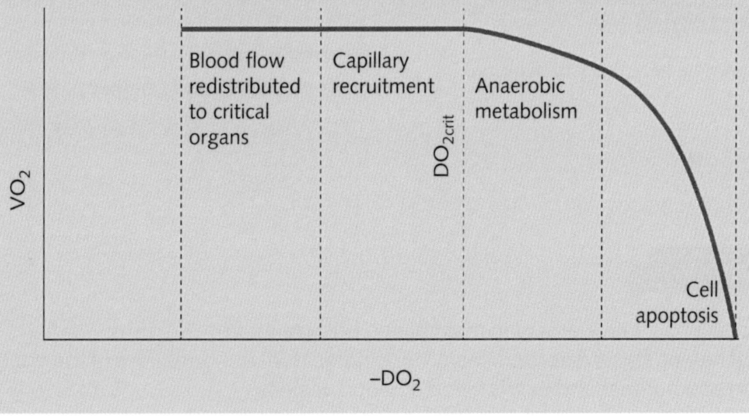

Fig. 26.4 Stages of haemorrhagic shock. Haemorrhagic and severe hypovolaemic shock can be rapidly fatal unless identified and resuscitated quickly. (From Kalla M, Green P, Herring N. *Physiology of shock and volume resuscitation*. MPSUR. 0263-9319. Elsevier; 2019.)

- Factitious: isolated thrombocytopaenia may be related to aggregation caused by EDTA (ethylenediaminetetraacetic acid) used in FBC bottles.

> **HINTS AND TIPS**
>
> Heparin is the most common drug-related cause of thrombocytopaenia in hospitalized patients. Heparin-induced thrombocytopaenia is a procoagulant state.

Platelet dysfunction

- Hereditary: Glanzmann thrombasthenia, vWD.
- Acquired: medication (aspirin, heparin, clopidogrel), chronic kidney disease, myeloproliferative and myelodysplastic syndromes, multiple myeloma and paraproteinaemia.

Coagulation abnormality

Coagulopathies may be due to vitamin K deficiency, factor deficiency (which can be specific or combined, inherited or acquired) or acquired clotting factor inhibitors.

Vitamin K deficiency

Prothrombin and factor VII, IX and X are dependent on vitamin K. Deficiency may be caused by:

- Malabsorption: bowel disease such as coeliac disease or biliary obstruction (vitamin K is fat-soluble).
- Antagonist drugs: coumarins (warfarin).

Factor deficiency

- Hereditary: haemophilia A (factor VIII), haemophilia B (factor IX), vWD (von Willebrand factor).
- Acquired: liver disease (decreased production of clotting factors as synthetic function fails), DIC (massive consumption of clotting factors resulting in deficiency).

Acquired factor inhibitors

These are most commonly directed against factor VIII:

- Postpartum.
- Autoimmune disease: systemic lupus erythematosus and rheumatoid arthritis.
- Malignancy.

Vessel wall abnormalities

Vessel wall abnormalities may be hereditary or acquired.

Hereditary

- Hereditary haemorrhagic telangiectasia (Osler–Weber–Rendu disease).
- Connective tissue disease: pseudoxanthoma elasticum, Ehlers–Danlos syndrome.

Acquired

- Trauma.
- Physiological: senile purpura.
- Drugs: corticosteroids.
- Infections: meningococcal septicaemia (damage due to endotoxin and inflammation).
- Vitamin deficiency: scurvy (vitamin C).
- Endocrine: Cushing syndrome.

HINTS AND TIPS

Von Willebrand factor is necessary for platelet adhesion and prevents degradation of factor VIII. Von Willebrand factor deficiency causing von Willebrand disease may therefore cause bleeding consistent with both platelet abnormalities and coagulopathy.

● Chapter Summary

- Haemostasis is an important element in maintaining body function.
- The aetiology of haemostasis disorders mainly originates from abnormalities in the coagulation cascade, platelet function and number and dysfunction of blood vessels.
- Apart from causing severe excessive bruising and bleeding clotting abnormalities can also be a manifestation of a sinister underlying condition, such as a malignancy.
- Simple blood tests, including FBC and coagulation screen, can elucidate the disease involved, but more specific tests are also available in more complicated cases.

UKMLA Conditions
Epistaxis
Haemophilia
Leukaemia
Lymphoma
Multiple myeloma
Myeloproliferative disorders

UKMLA Presentations
Bruising
Epistaxis
Purpura

Pain 27

INTRODUCTION

Pain is a common presenting symptom for which there can be many causes. Whilst it is important to identify any physical cause for pain, it must be remembered that there may be psychosocial factors which also contribute.

HISTORY AND EXAMINATION FINDINGS

The type and location of pain a patient presents with will help guide your history and examination. Pain can be acute, which is self-limiting provoked by a specific disease or injury, or chronic which is often defined as continuing greater than 12 weeks. Pain can be broadly divided into *somatic* (originating from peripheral tissues such as skin, muscle, joints, bones), *visceral* (originating from internal organs) or *neuropathic* (originating from the nervous system). Table 27.1 gives a further overview of different types of pain. It is important to remember that patients may present with more than one type of pain, separating the history and examination of each type of pain is important to identify each cause and appropriate treatment. Earlier chapters cover specifics of chest, abdominal, back and joint pain as well as headaches.

History

Site and radiation

Where the pain starts is often key to allow you to focus your history and examination. Is there a specific location they can point to or is the pain more generalized? Does the pain move location or originate in one place and radiate elsewhere? Consider central chest pain as an example – is this sudden onset central which radiates to the jaw/arm and could be cardiac in

Table 27.1 Key factors in different types of pain

Type	Onset	Description	Duration	Timeline	Analgesia
Acute	Quick		Short	Gradually reduces as contributing factor resolves	Usually responsive to simple analgesia
Chronic	Variable		Long	Fluctuates	Variable response
Somatic	Quick	Localized pain. Initially sharp, then ache or burning	Variable depending on stimulus	Variable depending on stimulus	Responsive, often to simple analgesia. Nonpharmacological treatments may be beneficial
Visceral	Variable	Poorly localizing. Constant, sharp or aching	Variable depending on stimulus	Variable depending on stimulus	Often responsive, may require adjuncts (e.g., antispasmodics)
Neuropathic	Variable	Burning, sharp, electric shock, radiates	Long	Variable – often longstanding and progressive	Poorly responsive to standard analgesia. Requires neuropathic agents

nature, or is this epigastric in onset which radiates to central chest and could indicate gastric reflux? When considering where the pain radiates to, does this follow a dermatomal pattern? A commonly seen example is 'sciatica' when pain originates from the spine/buttock and radiates down the back of the leg following an L5/S1 dermatomal pattern.

Character

What does the pain feel like? Is it sharp or aching (often somatic), cramping or pressure-like (often visceral), burning or electric shock-like (often neuropathic)? Does the sensation change over time? Is there a constant pain that builds into a different type of pain? It is important to distinguish whether this is a new acute pain or a chronic longstanding pain as the management may differ. In those with longstanding pain, is this a breakthrough of their background pain or a different sensation? This allows you to identify any new pains, triggers or up-titrate analgesia as required.

Onset and timeline

It is important to ascertain when the pain began and how it has changed over time. Is this a new pain? If so, when did they first notice it and how has it changed? This can help you identify any possible triggers (e.g., injury, change in medication, occupational/home changes, food) or when the pain began compared to other symptoms. Did the pain begin suddenly or build gradually over time? These subtle differences in a pain history are often key for diagnosis.

COMMUNICATION

Using open questions such as 'can you tell me about the pain' or 'can you describe your pain' often allows the patient to answer many elements of 'SOCRATES' themselves, following which you can ask more specifics as needed.

Associated features

- Respiratory: cough/sputum (infection, costochondritis, malignancy), shortness of breath (pulmonary embolism, pleural effusion).
- Cardiac: shortness of breath/orthopnoea/paroxysmal nocturnal dyspnoea/peripheral oedema (heart failure, valvular disease), grey/clammy (MI, PE), exertional (angina, arrhythmia).
- Neurological: visual disturbance (migraine), weakness or sensory changes (vertebral disc prolapse, spinal cord compression/cauda equina), neck stiffness (meningitis).

- Abdominal: haematemesis or melaena (upper GI bleed), PR bleeding (lower GI bleed), change in bowel habits (inflammatory bowel disease (IBD), irritable bowel syndrome (IBS), diverticulitis, malignancy), tenesmus (IBD), nausea or vomiting (gastritis, bowel obstruction).
- Other: injury (bruising, fracture, wounds), rash (meningitis, sepsis, underlying condition), weight loss (IBD, malignancy). Consider mood, sleep and effect on activities of daily living.

Exacerbating and relieving factors

- Precipitating factors: injury (accident, heavy lifting, muscular strain), exercise, specific movement, cough, change in position (sitting, standing, lying, bending), time of day, food, medications (new or changes), underlying conditions.
- Relieving factors: has any analgesia been tried and was it helpful? Other adjuncts (heat, cold, topical gels)? Change in position, rest, opening bladder or bowels.

Severity

A common approach is to ask the patient to grade how severe the pain is on a scale of 1 to 10. Another approach is to use visual aids. It is important to identify how bad the pain is at its worst, best and current level, as well as to reassess following any interventions.

Examination

Your examination will be guided by the history. It is important to ensure the patient is as comfortable as possible before beginning your examination. Key examinations for chest, abdominal, back, joint pain and headaches are covered in the relevant chapters.

HINTS AND TIPS

Remember in examinations, warn the patient of where and how you are completing an examination and starting with gentle initial examination (e.g., soft palpation of the abdomen or patient-initiated limb movements) prior to further examination allows you identify areas of pain without causing undue pain to the patient.

INVESTIGATIONS

History and examination alone may be enough to identify causes of pain in those with an injury or musculoskeletal pain.

In the majority of cases (such as chest or abdominal pain), further investigations are often warranted.

Investigations which may be considered:

- Blood tests: to look for and rule out any causes (e.g., CRP in infection, troponin for myocardial infarctions, amylase in pancreatitis, etc.) or to ensure appropriate treatment (renal and liver function).
- Bedside tests: ECG, urine dip.
- X-ray: fractures, malignancy, arthritic changes, pleural effusions, pneumonia.
- CT scanning: intraabdominal, neurological, respiratory causes.

The relevant presentation or diagnosis chapter will cover specific conditions and their investigations.

THE WHO PAIN LADDER

The initial aim of pain management should be to treat any underlying cause if possible. If the cause cannot be reversed or whilst it is being investigated, the World Health Organization (WHO) pain ladder helps guide analgesia use and is a good place to start (see Fig. 27.1). The basic principle of the ladder is to start with simple analgesia and then move in a stepwise approach to weak then stronger opioids. However, clinical judgement remains important as there are times when you may need to start higher up the pain ladder (e.g., in an acute MI) to adequately control the pain. In general, the initial steps of the ladder have fewer side effects to stronger medications such as opioids. Naloxone is an opioid antagonist, which is used in reversing opioid toxicity (see Chapter 39 for more details). Caution should be exercised in end-of-life care, where naloxone use is extremely rare and often only if severe respiratory depression is present, as it will result in reversal of analgesia leading to severe pain, which may be more difficult to control.

CLINICAL NOTES

It is often best to prescribe medication regularly, with as required (PRN) medication alongside, to ensure pain control between doses. Remember to review PRN's used and up-titrate regular medications to incorporate these doses if the type of analgesia is felt to be effective.

HINTS AND TIPS

Use caution in prescribing analgesia, consider:

- *Age* – the elderly are more at risk of opioid toxicity and may have the other risk factors discussed later.
- *Weight* – paracetamol dosing needs to be reduced in those with low weight (<50 kg).
- *Renal function* – nonsteroidal antiinflammatory drugs (NSAIDs) are general avoided in those with or at risk of renal disease. Morphine, codeine and neuropathic agents will require dose reductions, slow up-titration and regular reassessment depending on estimated glomerular filtration rate (eGFR). Oxycodone is often used as an alternative to morphine-based analgesia in renal impairment.
- *Liver function* – NSAIDs, codeine and tramadol should be used with caution in severe hepatic failure. Paracetamol and neuropathic agents will require dose reduction and morphine-based analgesia may require increased dose intervals and slow up-titration.
- *Underlying medical conditions* – consider the side effects of analgesic agents on underlying conditions (e.g., NSAIDs with gastro-oesophageal reflux disease, opioids in those with chronic respiratory failure).

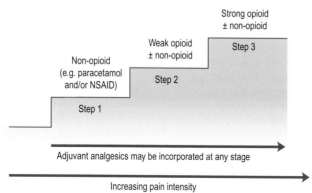

Fig. 27.1 The WHO analgesic pain ladder. *NSAID*, Nonsteroidal antiinflammatory drug. (From Knaggs RD, Hobbs GJ, Whittlesea C, Walker R. *Clinical Pharmacy and Therapeutics*, 5th ed. Elsevier; 2012.)

It is important to remember:

- Nonpharmacological treatments: heat, ice, relaxation, TENS.
- adjuvant analgesia: NSAIDs, neuropathic agents, steroids, benzodiazepines.
- Cause-specific treatments: radiotherapy in malignancy, bisphosphonates for bone metastases, neural blockade of nerve pain, chest drain of pleural fluid.

It is important to reassess response to analgesia and escalate as appropriate. Encourage patients to record analgesia usage, particularly when using opioids, to allow appropriate review and escalation of analgesia. Patients will often require analgesia for 'breakthrough pain', which may be associated with a trigger (e.g., movement). The dose for breakthrough analgesia is usually one-sixth of the *total daily* opioid dose. If using regular immediate-release preparations ('top-up' doses), this should be incorporated into their long-acting analgesic agents. Neuropathic pain often does not respond to simple analgesia or opiates and neuropathic agents (gabapentin, pregabalin, amitriptyline) are often used instead. Table 27.1 gives an overview of typical responses to analgesia. If pain is difficult to control or complex, seek specialist advice from services such as acute or chronic pain teams and palliative care as appropriate.

CLINICAL NOTES

Consider the best route for pain control. If the patient has bowel obstruction or is nil by mouth, nonoral routes of medication need to be used (e.g., intravenously (IV), subcutaneously (SC)).

Remember – if changing route (oral to IV/SC) or preparation (i.e., codeine to morphine, morphine to oxycodone), the doses are not equivalent and you will need to ensure correct conversion to the appropriate form.

CHRONIC PAIN

Chronic pain, as described earlier, can be secondary to an underlying condition (such as endometriosis, IBS, sciatica and arthritis) or primary chronic pain where there is no clear underlying condition or the impact of the pain is disproportionate to the injury/disease process (e.g., fibromyalgia, complex regional pain syndrome, chronic primary musculoskeletal pain and chronic primary visceral pain). Management of chronic pain should include a patient-centred assessment (discussion of triggers, developing a support plan and advice on flare-ups) and may include exercise programmes, psychological therapy, acupuncture and pharmacological management (e.g., amitriptyline, citalopram, duloxetine, fluoxetine, paroxetine and sertraline). Conventional analgesics (paracetamol, NSAIDs, opioids) are not recommended by NICE for chronic pain management.

CLINICAL NOTES

Fibromyalgia, or fibromyalgia syndrome (FMS), is characterized by widespread, persistent pain which is associated with fatigue, sleep and cognitive disturbance and is classified as a cause of chronic primary pain. Drug treatments and surgical interventions are often ineffective. See Chapter 35 for further information on fibromyalgia. For further reading, see the Royal College of Physicians 2022 UK guidelines on diagnosis of FMS.

PALLIATIVE CARE

Pain management is a key factor in palliative care and may be complex with multiple causes. Alongside pain, agitation/anxiety, nausea and vomiting and respiratory secretions are often prominent and distressing symptoms in end-of-life care. Continuous subcutaneous infusions (CSCI), via syringe drivers, prescribed over 24 hours, are often used to provide continuous control of symptoms in those unable to take or absorb oral medications and to prevent regular intramuscular injections or intravenous access being needed. For those receiving end-of-life care, individuals are often prescribed 'anticipatory medications' to manage symptoms which are likely to occur, see Table 27.2.

Table 27.2 Examples of commonly used 'anticipatory medications'

Symptom	Medication (usually PRN, subcutaneous administration)
Pain	Morphine sulphate Oxycodone
Agitation/anxiety	Midazolam
Nausea and vomiting	Hyoscine butylbromide Glycopyrronium
Respiratory secretions	Levomepromazine Haloperidol Cyclizine

Chapter Summary

- Pain can be a symptom related to an acute event or a manifestation of disease of different systems, including respiratory, cardiovascular, intraabdominal and neurological.
- Careful history taking and examination will help identify the cause and guide investigations.
- Treat the underlying cause of the pain where possible and use the WHO pain ladder to help guide analgesia.
- Pain lasting greater than 12 weeks is often defined as chronic pain. It can be primary (as in fibromyalgia) or secondary to an underlying condition.
- Pain control is a key aspect in palliative care. Syringe drivers and anticipatory medications are often used in end-of-life care.

UKMLA Presentations
Acute abdominal pain
Acute and chronic pain management
Acute joint pain/swelling
Back pain
Bone pain
Chest pain
Chronic abdominal pain
Chronic joint pain/stiffness
End-of-life care/symptoms of terminal illness
Facial pain
Fibromyalgia
Loin pain
Muscle pain/myalgia
Nausea
Neck pain/stiffness
Pain on inspiration
Pelvic pain

Diagnoses

ISCHAEMIC HEART DISEASE

General overview

Ischaemic heart disease (IHD) is a condition that falls under the umbrella term of 'cardiovascular disease' (CVD). CVD is responsible for a quarter of all deaths in the United Kingdom, with IHD being the biggest contributor, accounting for more than 66,000 deaths each year. The term covers a group of clinical syndromes, including angina pectoris and acute coronary syndrome (ACS), which includes unstable angina, non-ST elevation myocardial infarction (NSTEMI) and ST-elevation myocardial infarction (STEMI). The commonest underlying disease is atherosclerosis of the coronary arteries. More rarely, CVD can result from coronary artery spasm, emboli, coronary ostial stenosis, aortic stenosis, hypertrophic obstructive cardiomyopathy (HOCM), arrhythmias causing decreased coronary perfusion pressures and anaemia.

The prevalence of CVD has a geographical variation, reflecting both genetic and lifestyle factors. It is estimated that 1 in 8 men and 1 in 14 women die of CVD each year in the United Kingdom. Prevalence is age dependent and is highest in those older than 75 years.

Risk factors

Multiple factors are involved in the cause of CVD. The disease results from an interaction of genetic, lifestyle and environmental factors. Risk factors for developing CVD are summarized in Table 28.1. Typically, risk factors are divided into modifiable and nonmodifiable. All modifiable risk factors should be addressed as part of the assessment in patients with suspected CVD.

> **HINTS AND TIPS**
>
> The description of symptoms in ischaemic heart disease is very variable. Patients often use words such as 'heaviness', 'tightness' or 'restriction' rather than 'pain'.

Pathophysiology

Atherosclerosis is a slowly progressive focal proliferation of connective tissue within the arterial intima that begins as early as the second decade of life. It is linked to high lipid levels. Low-density lipoprotein (LDL) is the main atherogenic lipid,

although the principal constituent of atherosclerotic plaques is collagen synthesized by smooth muscle cells.

The initial process involves endothelial dysfunction in association with high circulating cholesterol levels, inflammation and shear forces. Macrophages enter the arterial wall between endothelial cells, taking up lipids and forming foam cells. The accumulation of lipid-laden macrophages in the subendothelial zone leads to the formation of fatty streaks. Toxic products released from the macrophages result in platelet adhesion and smooth muscle cell proliferation and thrombus formation. Subsequently, an atherosclerotic plaque surrounded by a fibrotic cap is formed. Progressive enlargement of these lesions leads to segmental narrowing of the lumen, which, when sufficient to be flow-limiting on exercise, causes stable exertion-associated angina.

Atherosclerotic plaques are liable to rupture, resulting in sudden thrombosis, and ACS. Factors associated with plaque disruption and consequent thrombosis include a large lipid core, a high monocyte density and low smooth muscle cell density.

Clinical features

CVD clinically presents in broadly two categories: stable angina and ACS. Stable angina is due to a predictable mismatch between the oxygen supply and demand of cardiac myocytes (cardiac ischaemia). This is brought on by exertion and relieved by rest. Symptoms include central chest pain, heaviness or discomfort commonly radiating to the jaw or arm, and may be associated with shortness of breath, sweating, nausea or faintness (see Chapter 4). ACS presents with the same symptoms but, unlike stable angina, occurs suddenly and is often a result of atherosclerotic plaque rupture.

Investigations

Although stable angina and ACS present with similar symptoms, they are investigated differently. ACS is a medical emergency and requires urgent inpatient diagnosis. Stable angina is commonly managed in primary care with diagnostic investigations arranged as an outpatient.

Electrocardiogram

A normal ECG (Fig. 28.1) does not exclude a diagnosis of stable angina or ACS. The ECG may show signs of an old myocardial infarction (MI) (Q waves) (Fig. 28.2) or left ventricular

Table 28.1 Major risk factors for coronary artery disease

Type	Risk factors	Importance
Nonmodifiable	Age	Prevalence rises steeply with age.
	Male sex > female sex	70% of deaths in men occur in those younger than 75 years. On average, women develop CVD 10–15 years later than men. The difference diminishes with increasing age.
	Family history	A family history in first-degree relatives increases the risk of developing CVD. A small proportion of cases are associated with familial hypercholesterolaemia.
	Ethnicity	Increased risk in people of South Asian and African Caribbean origin.
Modifiable	Smoking	Smoking accounts for more than 20% of CVD, with mortality from CVD 60% higher in smokers. Passive smoking increases the risk by around 25%.
	Poor nutrition	Increased risk with diet high in saturated fat, salt and sugar.
	Hyperlipidaemia	Increased risk with high levels of serum total cholesterol and low-density lipoprotein (LDL) cholesterol. High-density lipoprotein (HDL) cholesterol is protective.
	Hypertension	Both systolic and diastolic hypertension increase risk.
	Diabetes	Risk increased by two to three times.
	CKD	Increases risk of and is associated with adverse outcomes in patients with CVD.
	Left ventricular hypertrophy	
	Infrequent exercise	
	Obesity	In addition to being an independent risk factor for CVD, obesity also increases the likelihood of developing hypertension, hyperlipidaemia and diabetes mellitus.
Other	Social deprivation	

CKD, *Chronic kidney disease*; CVD, *cardiovascular disease*.

hypertrophy. The correlation between ECG changes and the territory of an MI is outlined in Table 28.2. Comparison with an old ECG is very useful.

Exercise tolerance test

Also known as exercise ECG, an exercise tolerance test helps determine exercise performance and is an independent indicator of prognosis. It is contraindicated in ACS, severe aortic stenosis, HOCM, severe pulmonary hypertension and significant rhythm disturbances. The sensitivity for CVD is 78% and the specificity is 70%. The test should be terminated if there is chest pain, ST elevation, more than 2 mm of ST depression, a fall in BP or arrhythmia.

Echocardiography

Echocardiography allows visualization of cardiac structures and assessment of their function. It is a useful tool to identify valvular heart disease, ventricular dysfunction, structural abnormalities of the heart or pericardial disease.

Echocardiography can be transthoracic (transducer probe is placed in the intercostal spaces) or transoesophageal (ultrasound probe is passed into the oesophagus). A transoesophageal echocardiogram is an invasive procedure but allows better visualization of the posterior structures of the heart, and the test of choice to look for vegetations on the valves.

CT coronary angiography/cardiac MRI

CT coronary angiography allows noninvasive assessment of the coronary arteries. CT scans can be used in CVD risk stratification through measurement of possible atherosclerosis expressed as calcium score, or as a noninvasive method for assessing coronary artery patency. Cardiac MRI can assess the structure of the heart and/or myocardial blood flow.

Functional stress tests

Stress echocardiogram

This is a noninvasive functional test of the myocardium used to identify areas of inducible ischaemia with stress (dobutamine). Areas of inducible ischaemia can be used as targets to improve revascularization.

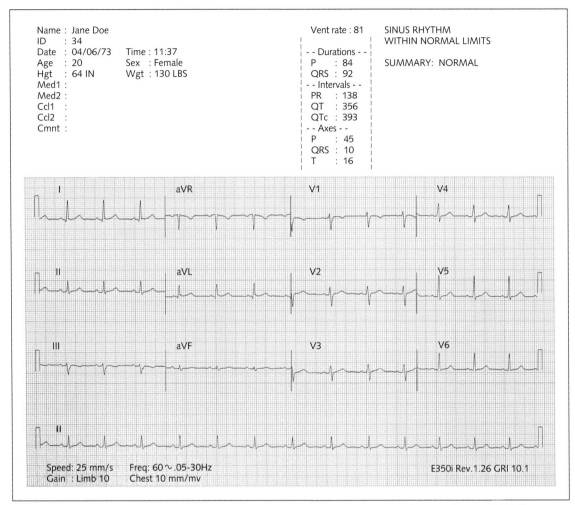

Fig. 28.1 A normal ECG with a rhythm strip. (From Shiland BJ. *Medical Assistant: Cardiopulmonary Systems, Vital Signs, Electrocardiography and CPR – Module D*, 2nd ed. Elsevier; 2016.)

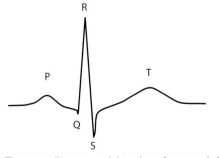

Fig. 28.2 Electrocardiogram, serial tracing of a normal single heartbeat. The QRS complex represents the ventricular contraction. (From Rifai N, Jaffe AS, Chiu RWK, et al. *Tietz Textbook of Laboratory Medicine*, 7th ed. Elsevier; 2023.)

Nuclear imaging

Radioactive isotopes (e.g., thallium, technetium myocardial perfusion (MIBI) scan or multigated acquisition (MUGA) scan) can also be used to assess myocardial structure, function and look for inducible ischaemia. The isotope is taken up by healthy myocardium, whereas areas of infarction show up as 'cold spots'.

Coronary angiography

Coronary angiography allows visualization of the coronary arteries and measurement of intracardiac pressures, blood oxygen saturation in different cardiac chambers and cardiac output. It is used as a guide to decide on further management (i.e., medical therapy, coronary angioplasty or coronary artery bypass surgery).

Table 28.2 Correlation between myocardial infarction territory, electrocardiogram leads in which changes are seen and the artery involved

MI territory	Leads	Artery
Anterior	• ST elevation ± Q waves in leads $V_1–V_6$ ± I and aVL • Reciprocal ST depression in leads II, III and aVF (inferior leads)	Left anterior descending artery
Anteroseptal	• ST elevation in leads $V_1–V_4$	Left anterior descending and right coronary arteries
Posterior	• Reciprocal changes in leads $V_1–V_4$ (anteroseptal leads)	Right coronary artery Left circumflex coronary artery
Inferior	• ST elevation in leads II, III and aVF • Reciprocal ST depression in lead aVL	Dominant right coronary artery (80%) Any of the other coronary arteries
Lateral	• ST elevation in leads I, aVL, V_5 and V_6 (lateral leads) • Reciprocal ST depression in leads III and aVF (inferior leads)	Left anterior descending artery Right or left circumflex artery

MI, *Myocardial infarction.*

The mortality from the procedure is approximately 1 in 1000. Complications include:

- Haemorrhage and haematoma at the site of arterial puncture
- Emboli into arteries resulting in coronary or peripheral ischaemia
- Stroke
- Arrhythmias
- Coronary artery dissection

CLINICAL NOTES

CARDIAC SYNDROME X

Cardiac syndrome X is cardiac ischaemia in the presence of normal coronary arteries. It is thought to be due to abnormalities of small coronary vessels resulting in a reduction of coronary flow reserve and is therefore also referred to as 'microvascular angina'.

Treatment

As for all chronic diseases, optimal management includes patient education, lifestyle changes, medication and procedural interventions. Noncoronary causes of angina should be sought and treated (e.g., valvular heart disease and anaemia).

Lifestyle changes

Ask about possible risk factors and address those that are present. Weight loss, smoking cessation, exercise and a healthy diet should all be encouraged. Exercise may improve the collateral circulation in the heart. Factors precipitating angina (e.g., cold weather or extremes of emotion) should be avoided. All patients should be provided with a sublingually administered nitrate, for relief of acute attacks or prophylactic use before exercise.

HINTS AND TIPS

Patients with stable angina should be advised to seek urgent medical help if their symptoms have not resolved 5 minutes after taking the second dose of a short-acting nitrate such as glyceryl trinitrate.

Drug agents

Antiplatelet drugs

These inhibit platelet aggregation and thrombus formation in arterial circulation. Aspirin should not be prescribed for primary prevention of CVD unless the patient is at high risk of stroke or MI as assessed by the QRISK assessment tool.

Antiplatelets should be prescribed for secondary prevention in patients with ACS, angina, peripheral arterial disease, MI, cardiac stents, and stroke and transient ischaemic attack (TIA) (normally aspirin 75 mg/day).

CLINICAL NOTES

QRISK

- Used in patients <85 years old who do not already have CVD or suffer from inherited lipid disorders.
- The scoring system incorporates numerous variables and estimates a 10-year risk of developing CVD expressed as a percentage.

Nitrates

Nitrates cause peripheral vasodilation that is most marked in the veins. This reduces venous return and preload, thereby decreasing cardiac output and oxygen demand, resulting in relief of angina. Nitrates are converted to the active molecule nitric oxide, which results in an increase in the level of intracellular cyclic guanosine monophosphate in smooth muscle. This stimulates calcium-binding processes and reduces the amount of free calcium available to trigger muscle contraction.

Short-acting nitrates are the mainstay of relief of acute angina and, when combined with rest, they normally relieve the pain in minutes. If the pain continues, then this should be a warning sign to patients.

Adverse effects are normally due to arterial dilation and include headaches, flushing, hypotension and, rarely, fainting. Patients may become tolerant to nitrates, reducing their effectiveness.

β-Blockers

β-Blockers improve the oxygen supply and demand balance by lowering heart rate and BP, decreasing end-systolic stress and contractility and prolonging diastole, permitting greater coronary flow.

Cardioselective β-blockers are those acting primarily on the β_1-adrenergic receptor located mainly in the heart and in the kidneys. These include atenolol, bisoprolol, esmolol and metoprolol. Contraindications include asthma, hypotension, marked bradycardia, second- and third-degree heart block, severe peripheral arterial disease and uncontrolled heart failure.

Calcium channel blockers

Calcium antagonists inhibit the influx of calcium into the myocyte during the action potential and relax peripheral vascular smooth muscle. They relieve angina by a combination of reduced afterload (and hence myocardial oxygen demand) plus reduced heart rate and increased coronary vasodilation. They are especially useful if there is a degree of coronary artery spasm. Dihydropyridines such as nifedipine can cause reflex tachycardia secondary to peripheral vasodilatation, and therefore may be combined with a β-blocker.

Side effects include headache, flushing, dizziness, constipation and gravitational oedema.

CLINICAL NOTES

TREATMENT OF STABLE ANGINA

β-blocker and calcium channel blocker are first-line treatments for angina. Second-line therapies include long-acting nitrates, ivabradine, nicorandil and ranolazine.

Potassium channel activators

Nicorandil has arterial and venous vasodilating properties and is useful in patients refractory to treatment with other antianginal agents.

Angiotensin-converting enzyme inhibitors

Unless contraindicated, angiotensin-converting enzyme (ACE) inhibitor therapy should be started in patients with stable angina and left ventricular dysfunction and/or diabetes. Angiotensin receptor blockers (ARBs) have similar benefits and are used where ACE inhibitors are not tolerated, e.g., bradykinin-related cough.

Lipid-lowering drugs

Statins (3-hydroxy-3-methylglutaryl coenzyme A reductase inhibitors) are the mainstay of lipid-lowering therapy. They may also help to stabilize atherosclerotic plaques and reduce the frequency of acute cardiac events. Most patients with CVD should be taking a statin even if their cholesterol level is within the normal range. Atorvastatin 20 mg daily should be offered to patients with a CVD risk of 10% or more.

CLINICAL NOTES

Non-HDL cholesterol is used as a guide to starting statin treatment.

Revascularization

Revascularization should be considered in patients with stable angina in whom symptoms are not controlled by medical management. This can be achieved by percutaneous coronary intervention (PCI) or coronary artery bypass graft (CABG). The choice of procedure depends on clinical assessment and patient preference.

PCI involves the use of a balloon catheter to widen the coronary artery. Bare metal or drug-eluting stents are usually used after dilation to reduce rates of restenosis.

CABG is a surgical technique where vessels are harvested from another part of the body and used to replace the stenosed coronary artery. A bypass procedure using one or both of the internal mammary arteries is preferred to the traditional vein graft as it results in better patency and flow.

In all patients who have undergone revascularization, lifelong aspirin therapy is started. Patients with stents should be receiving dual antiplatelet therapy (usually aspirin and clopidogrel). This is continued for at least 1 month in the case of bare-metal stents and 6 months for drug-eluting stents.

ACUTE CORONARY SYNDROMES

ACS is a term that encompasses a range of diagnoses, including STEMI, NSTEMI and unstable angina. It is a medical emergency. Most commonly it results from atherosclerotic plaque rupture, leading to a sudden reduction of blood flow to the myocardium with or without the formation of emboli. Presenting symptoms include severe pain in the chest, jaw, arms and/or back that may be associated with sweating, breathlessness and nausea and vomiting (see Chapter 4). Despite uniform clinical features, the underlying disorders differ: STEMI is usually a result of a large territory myocardial damage, NSTEMI is a consequence of a relatively smaller injury, and angina is caused by narrowing, but not complete obstruction, of the coronary arteries. Angina is termed unstable if it is not relieved by rest or medical treatment.

ACS is common with one heart attack patient being admitted to a UK hospital every 5 minutes. Around 60% of patients present with a STEMI and around 40% present with an NSTEMI and/or unstable angina.

Risk scoring

All patients who present with ACS should undergo risk stratification. This allows the identification of patients who are most likely to benefit from an early therapeutic intervention such as PCI or CABG. Individuals at increased risk of adverse future events are identified with established scoring systems such as the Global Registry of Acute Cardiac Events (GRACE) score. The GRACE score is validated as a prognostic tool to predict mortality and cardiovascular events risk in hospital and at 6 months.

ST-elevation myocardial infarction

General overview

Most STEMIs are caused by an occlusive intracoronary thrombus overlying an ulcerated or fissured stenotic plaque. Underlying most cases there is a dynamic interaction between severe coronary atherosclerosis, an acute atheromatous plaque change, superimposed thrombosis, platelet activation and vasospasm. The microscopic changes of acute MI follow a predictable sequence (Table 28.3). Almost 50% of myocardial tissue that lies in the area of ischaemia dies within 1 hour of occlusion,

Table 28.3 Changes induced by acute myocardial infarction

Time after onset of symptoms	Macroscopic changes	Microscopic changes
Up to 18 hours	None	None
24–48 hours	Pale oedematous muscle	Oedema, acute inflammatory cell infiltration, necrosis of myocytes
3–4 days	Yellow rubbery centre with haemorrhagic border	Obvious necrosis and inflammation, early granulation tissue
3–6 weeks	Silvery scar becoming rough and white	Dense fibrosis

and more than 60% within 3 hours; thus restoration of coronary blood flow is a key treatment goal.

Clinical features

Patients commonly present with acute-onset chest, jaw, back or arm pain (see Chapter 4), although occasionally ACS may be silent. Associated features include nausea, vomiting, sweating, palpitations, dyspnoea, syncope and/or pulmonary oedema. The patient will often be distressed.

Investigations

The hyperacute ECG changes consist of tall, pointed T waves and subsequent ST elevation (Fig. 28.3). This is followed by T-wave inversion, decreasing R-wave voltage and the development of Q waves. After weeks or months, the T wave may become upright again, but the Q waves will remain (Fig. 28.4). The site of the infarction may be deduced from the affected leads on the ECG (Table 28.2). Reciprocal ECG changes with ST depression in leads opposite the site of infarction may also be present.

Cardiac biomarkers are intracellular molecules which leak out of infarcted myocardium into the bloodstream (Fig. 28.5):

* Elevated troponin I or troponin T concentrations are highly reliable markers of myocardial damage. Serum levels increase within 3 to 12 hours of the onset of pain and peak at 24 to 48 hours. They remain elevated for 1 to 2 weeks.
* Myocardial muscle creatine kinase (CK-MB) levels increase within 3 to 12 hours and peak at 24 hours. They remain elevated for 48 to 72 hours.
* Aspartate aminotransferase and lactate dehydrogenase were formerly used to assess MI as their levels remain elevated for several days. Their use is now largely obsolete.

Acute management

Follow the ABCDE approach. The aim of treatment is to prevent ischaemia and alleviate pain and anxiety. All patients should be assessed for eligibility for reperfusion therapy (PCI

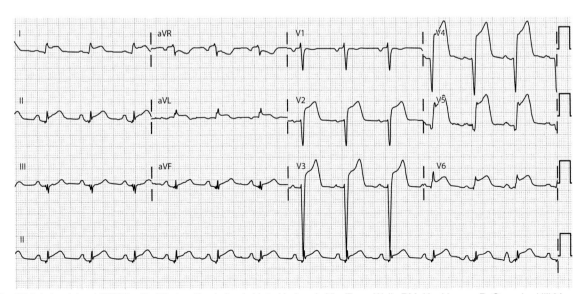

Fig. 28.3 Anterolateral STEMI with ST-elevation in leads V_2 to V_6, I and aVL. (From Walls RM, Hockberger R, Gausche Hill M. *Rosen's Emergency Medicine: Concepts and Clinical Practice, 2-Volume Set, 10th ed.* Elsevier; 2023.)

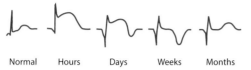

Normal   Hours   Days   Weeks   Months

Fig. 28.4 Progressive electrocardiogram changes in myocardial infarction.

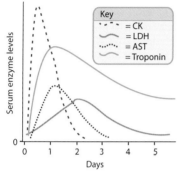

Key
- - - = CK
⌒ = LDH
········· = AST
⌒ = Troponin

Serum enzyme levels

Days

Fig. 28.5 The pattern of serum markers after acute myocardial infarction. *AST*, Aspartate aminotransferase; *CK*, creatine kinase; *LDH*, lactate dehydrogenase.

or fibrinolysis). Pain can be managed with sublingually or buccally administered glyceryl trinitrate (GTN) and intravenous opioids. In addition to providing analgesia, morphine compounds also reduce cardiac workload by vasodilation and reduced sympathetic activation. Antiemetics should be administered with opiates. Aspirin (300 mg) should be given as soon as possible.

Coronary angiography with follow-on PCI is superior to fibrinolysis if the patient presents within 12 hours of the onset of symptoms and it can be delivered within 120 minutes of the time when fibrinolysis could have been given or if it has been more than 12 hours but there is evidence of continuing myocardial ischaemia or cardiogenic shock. If stenting is indicated, drug-eluting stents are the first-line choice. If a delay to PCI is expected, fibrinolysis should be offered (see Table 28.4 for contraindications to thrombolytic therapy). Patients undergoing PCI should be offered prasugrel if they are not already taking an oral anticoagulant or clopidogrel if they are already taking an oral anticoagulant, as part of dual antiplatelet therapy (DAPT). Patients not treated with PCI should receive ticagrelor as part of DAPT.

Non-ST elevation myocardial infarction and unstable angina

General overview
NSTEMI is diagnosed in patients who fit the criteria for MI but do not have persistent ST elevation on ECG, whereas unstable

Table 28.4 Contraindications to thrombolytic therapy

Contraindications	Relative contraindications
Stroke in last 3 months or severe stroke	Pregnancy or postpartum
Active bleeding	Recent retinal laser treatment
Known bleeding disorder	Noncompressible punctures
Dissecting aneurysm	Traumatic resuscitation
Recent major surgery, trauma or head injury	Severe hypertension

SBP, Systolic blood pressure.

angina is diagnosed in patients without elevated biomarker values.

Clinical features
The history and clinical features are the same as those for STEMI. Patients with stable angina may note that their pain is no longer relieved fully by GTN, that it is increasing in intensity or that it is occurring at rest.

Investigations
Investigations are the same as those for STEMI. The ECG may show ST-segment depression, T-wave flattening, biphasic changes or inversion (Fig. 28.6). The initial ECG may be normal, and serial ECGs are needed to demonstrate the dynamic ischaemia.

HINTS AND TIPS

Old ECGs are invaluable in assessing patients with chest pain, allowing comparison.

Acute management
The initial emergency management of NSTEMI and unstable angina is identical to that of STEMI: aspirin (300 mg), morphine and nitrates. Antithrombin therapy with fondaparinux should be offered unless undergoing immediate angiography, in which case prasugrel or ticagrelor (no separate indication for ongoing oral anticoagulation) or clopidogrel (separate indication for ongoing oral anticoagulation) are given as part of DAPT. Immediate angiography +/– PCI should be offered to all unstable patients. Clinical instability is defined as pain despite treatment, haemodynamic instability, left ventricular failure and/or dynamic ECG changes. Angiography +/– PCI within 72 hours should be offered to those with predicted 6-month mortality of >3%, as per GRACE score, or those less at risk if they suffer subsequent ischaemia. Ticagrelor or

Boston University Hospital

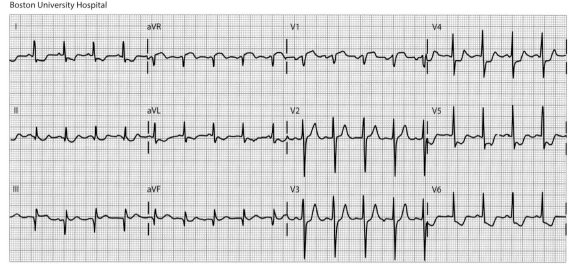

Fig. 28.6 NSTEMI. Between 1 and 3 mm of marked ST-segment depression is seen in leads I, aVL, and V_4 to V_6. (From Wing EJ, Schiffman FJ. *Cecil Essentials of Medicine*, 10th ed. Elsevier; 2021.)

clopidogrel are given as part of DAPT in patients without indication for PCI.

Subsequent inpatient management of patients with ACS: cardiac rehabilitation and secondary prevention

Long-term drug treatment—All patients should have their cardiovascular risks assessed and modified. Daily use of aspirin is continued indefinitely after MI. It reduces the risk of reinfarction and death by 25%. There is no clear benefit of oral anticoagulation over antiplatelet therapy, although it may be considered for patients with left ventricular aneurysm, atrial fibrillation (AF) or echocardiographically proven left ventricular thrombus. If aspirin is contraindicated, clopidogrel monotherapy should be considered.

DAPT therapy started in the acute stage is continued unless there is a separate indication for anticoagulation in which case aspirin and clopidogrel is the combination of choice that is taken alongside an oral anticoagulant. DAPT is normally continued for up to 12 months.

Unless contraindicated, treatment with a β-blocker (reduces mortality and reinfarction rates), ACE inhibitor (reduces the risk of death and heart failure) and a statin (statins have anti-inflammatory plaque-stabilizing effects) should be started in addition to DAPT. Calcium channel blockers such as diltiazem, verapamil or amlodipine can be used in patients in whom β-blockers are contraindicated. In patients with signs of heart failure or left ventricular systolic dysfunction, aldosterone antagonist therapy should be started. Use of β-blockers is

continued for at least 12 months in patients without left ventricular systolic dysfunction, and indefinitely in those with left ventricular systolic dysfunction. ACE inhibitors are given lifelong.

Other management—All patients who have had an MI should undergo a left ventricular function assessment, most commonly done by the use of echocardiography. In patients managed conservatively ischaemia testing prior to discharge should be considered. Cardiac rehabilitation programmes of exercise, stress management and health information sessions should be offered to all patients following an acute MI. People should be advised regarding lifestyle modifications: eating a Mediterranean-style diet, physical activity for 20 to 30 minutes per day, smoking cessation and alcohol consumption (maximal intake of 14 units per week). Overweight patients should be offered weight management advice.

Complications of myocardial infarction

Patients who suffered an MI remain at a high risk of dying even with immediate intervention. A summary of complications that may occur as a result of MI is given in Table 28.5.

Cardiac failure and cardiogenic shock

Overt left ventricular failure after MI is associated with a poor prognosis. Cardiogenic pulmonary oedema is a common finding (Table 28.6). The management of heart failure is described later in this chapter.

Cardiogenic shock is described as secondary to pump failure, inadequate end-organ perfusion and subsequent tissue hypoxia. MI-related cardiogenic shock occurs as a result of damage to the myocardium leading to mechanical insufficiency. Other causes

Table 28.5 Complications of myocardial infarction

Complication	Interval	Mechanism
Sudden death	Usually within hours	Often ventricular fibrillation
Arrhythmias	First few days	–
Persistent pain	12 hours to a few days	Progressive myocardial necrosis (extension of myocardial infarction)
Angina	Immediate or delayed (weeks)	Ischaemia of noninfarcted muscle
Cardiac failure	Variable	Ventricular dysfunction following muscle necrosis; arrhythmias
Mitral incompetence	First few days	Papillary muscle dysfunction, necrosis or rupture
Pericarditis	2–4 days	Transmural infarct with inflammation of the pericardium
Cardiac rupture and ventricular septal defects	3–5 days	Weakening of wall following muscle necrosis and acute inflammation
Mural thrombus	1 week or more	Abnormal endothelial surface following infarction
Ventricular aneurysm	4 weeks or more	Stretching of newly formed collagenous scar tissue
Dressler syndrome	Weeks to months	Autoimmune
Pulmonary emboli	1 week or more	Deep vein thrombosis in lower limbs
Late ventricular arrhythmias	–	–

Table 28.6 Killip classification for assessment of heart failure

Class	Features
1	No crepitations or third heart sound
2	Mild to moderate heart failure signs and symptoms (crepitations over less than 50% of lung fields, third heart sound, jugular venous distension)
3	Overt pulmonary oedema
4	Cardiogenic shock

of shock include hypovolaemia, vasovagal reactions, drugs or arrhythmias. Ventricular and valvular function should be evaluated by echocardiography. Inotropic agents are of value: dobutamine or milrinone are positive inotropes that enhance cardiac contractility.

Cardiac rupture

Free wall rupture, if acute, is usually fatal within minutes. If subacute, there is haemodynamic deterioration with hypotension and signs of cardiac tamponade. Cardiac tamponade is life-threatening and requires immediate surgical management.

Postinfarction ventricular septal defects (VSDs) are rare but associated with high mortality without prompt surgical repair. They should be suspected if there is clinical deterioration and a loud pansystolic murmur at the left sternal edge.

Mitral regurgitation

The development of mitral regurgitation is a poor prognostic factor. It usually occurs within the first week after MI. Mortality without surgical intervention is high.

Pericarditis

This usually develops within 24 to 96 hours after an MI, causing pain that is sharp in nature and varies with posture and respiration. Treatment is with nonsteroidal antiinflammatory drugs (NSAIDs) or colchicine if NSAIDs are contraindicated. Dressler syndrome is a form of secondary pericarditis that occurs up to 3 months after MI. Clinical features include fever, leucocytosis, pericarditis and serositis. Treatment is as for pericarditis.

Arrhythmias and conduction disturbances

These are extremely common in the early period following MI. Often, the arrhythmias are not hazardous in themselves but are a manifestation of a serious underlying disorder such as continuing ischaemia, vagal overactivity or electrolyte disturbance, particularly potassium and magnesium. Arrhythmias can also occur following reperfusion. The management of arrhythmias is covered in detail later in this chapter.

Ventricular arrhythmias—Ventricular arrhythmias may present as ventricular ectopics, ventricular tachycardia (VT) or ventricular fibrillation (VF).

Ventricular ectopics are almost universal on the first day and require no treatment if the patient is asymptomatic. Short episodes of VT may be well tolerated and require no treatment. More prolonged episodes may cause hypotension and heart failure. VF is rapidly fatal if not treated. If VF occurs, immediate defibrillation should be performed as part of the advanced life support protocol.

When arrhythmias occur late in the course of MI, they are likely to recur and are associated with a high risk of death. If it is probable that the arrhythmia is induced by ischaemia, revascularization should be considered. If this is unlikely, anti-arrhythmic agents (e.g., β-blockers and amiodarone) and electrophysiologically guided treatment may be given. In some cases, an implantable defibrillator is indicated.

Supraventricular arrhythmias—Atrial fibrillation (AF) complicates 15% to 20% of MIs, and is often associated with severe left ventricular damage and heart failure; it is usually self-limiting. If the heart rate is fast, bisoprolol or digoxin is effective in slowing the rate, but amiodarone is more efficacious in terminating the arrhythmia.

Other supraventricular arrhythmias are rare but are also usually self-limiting. They may respond to carotid sinus massage. Adenosine or β-blockers may be effective and direct current (DC) cardioversion should be used if the arrhythmia is associated with haemodynamic instability.

Sinus bradycardia and heart block—Sinus bradycardia and atrioventricular (AV) block are common after an inferior MI related to the right coronary artery (which supplies the AV node). The bradycardia may respond to atropine, although patients may go on to need a permanent pacemaker. Heart block with anterior MI is ominous because it indicates a large infarct. The development of left bundle branch block (LBBB) or bifascicular block (altered transmission between two of the three bundle branches of the conduction pathway) may presage complete heart block and is an indication for temporary pacemaker insertion. If a complete heart block does occur and persists, a permanent pacemaker will be needed.

CARDIAC ARREST

General overview

Cardiac arrest or cardiorespiratory arrest occurs secondary to an acute loss of cardiac function leading to circulatory collapse. It is a critical medical emergency that, unless treated immediately, results in death, with mortality increased by 10% every minute without cardiorespiratory resuscitation (CPR). Even with treatment survival is poor with less than 1 in 10 and only 7% to 8% of patients surviving to hospital discharge. Risk factors are many but some of the more common include IHD, CAD, cardiac dysfunction (left ventricular failure, cardiomyopathy), dysrhythmias including long QT syndrome, and medical emergencies (major haemorrhage, thromboembolism, polytrauma).

Four rhythm disturbances lead to a cardiac arrest:

- Pulseless VT
- VF
- Asystole
- Pulseless electrical activity (PEA)

VT and VF are shockable rhythms that respond to defibrillation. Asystole and PEA are nonshockable rhythms that should not be treated with defibrillation.

Management

The chain of survival is a sequence of time-sensitive actions that when properly executed significantly increase the chances of surviving a cardiac arrest (Fig. 28.7). Resuscitation and defibrillation are delivered according to specific guidelines produced by the RESUS council. These outline the approach to an unresponsive patient suspected of suffering a cardiac arrest. Fig. 28.8 shows the RESUS adult advanced life support guideline which includes advice on identifying and treating potentially reversible causes of cardiac arrest (four Hs and four Ts), drug delivery, possible considerations and postreturn of spontaneous circulation (ROSC) care.

ARRHYTHMIAS

General overview

An arrhythmia is a disturbance of normal sinus cardiac rhythm. Arrhythmias are very common, often intermittent, but can cause cardiac compromise. They are commonly secondary to CVD. Other causes include drugs (prescribed or illicit),

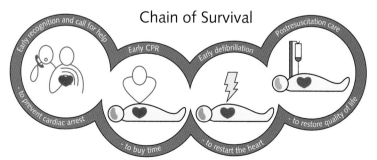

Fig. 28.7 Chain of survival. (From Dinsmore J, Zoumprouli A. *Lee's Synopsis of Anaesthesia*, 15th ed. Elsevier; 2022.)

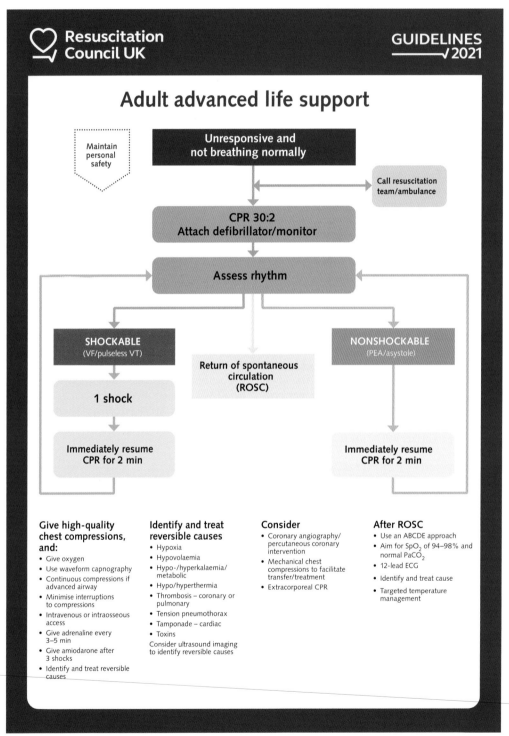

Fig. 28.8 RESUS council adult advanced life support algorithm 2021. (Resuscitation Council UK, 2021.) *CPR*, Cardiorespiratory resuscitation; *VF*, ventricular fibrillation; *VT*, ventricular tachycardia; *PEA*, pulseless electrical activity.

cardiomyopathy, myocarditis, thyroid dysfunction and electrolyte disturbances.

Arrhythmias may present with palpitations (see Chapter 7), dizziness, angina, shortness of breath (see Chapter 5), syncope, cardiac arrest or sudden death; they may also be asymptomatic. The history-taking should focus on symptoms and possible underlying causes.

Supraventricular arrhythmias

Sinus tachycardia

This is defined as a heart rate of more than 100 bpm originating from the sinoatrial (SA) node (sinus rhythm). It can be entirely physiological (e.g., during exercise) but may be pathological. Causes include anaemia, pulmonary embolism, pain, fever, sepsis, thyroid toxicosis, hypovolaemia, anxiety and heart failure. Treating the underlying cause should resolve the tachycardia. Rarely patients have idiopathic inappropriate sinus tachycardia, which is thought to be due to abnormal autonomic tone.

Atrial fibrillation

Aetiology and pathophysiology

AF is the most common sustained cardiac arrhythmia. It is an irregular, chaotic atrial rhythm at a rate of 300 to 600 bpm with a transmitted ventricular rate usually around 160 to 180 bmp. AF is triggered by rapidly firing foci, usually localized to the pulmonary veins. It is transmitted to the ventricles via the AV node at different intervals, leading to an irregular heart rate, dependent on the speed of AV node conduction and how refractory the AV node is. The incidence rises with age and is higher in men. It may be idiopathic, secondary to chronic heart disease or a response to acute illness. Different patterns are described in Table 28.7. Permanent AF is often a result of tissue fibrosis and structural remodelling. Causes can be divided into cardiac and noncardiac (Table 28.8).

Clinically, there is an irregularly irregular pulse, and the apical rate can be greater than the rate at the radial artery since the pulse volume varies. The first heart sound is of variable intensity. The ECG shows absent P waves and irregular narrow QRS complexes (unless there is an associated bundle branch block) (Fig. 28.9).

Complications

The most common complication associated with AF is stroke and thromboembolic disease. Poor synchronization of atrial contraction and the resultant stagnation of blood in the atria leads to thrombus formation. The thrombus can embolize to anywhere in the systemic circulation, but stroke and ischaemic gut are the most common presentations. Patients with

Table 28.7 Classification of AF

Type	Features
Paroxysmal AF	• Episodes of >30 s duration but <7 days • Self-limiting/terminating
Persistent AF	• 7 days duration not requiring treatment • <7 days but needing cardioversion
Permanent AF	• Does not respond to cardioversion • Initially responds to cardioversion but relapses within 24 hours • AF for >1 year where cardioversion is not indicated or attempted

Table 28.8 Causes of AF

Cause	Conditions
Cardiac	• CVD • Hypertension • Rheumatic valve disease • Congestive cardiac failure • Preexcitation syndromes (e.g., Wolff–Parkinson–White syndrome) • Pericarditis • Congenital heart disease • Cardiomyopathy • Atrial myxoma • Infiltrative cardiac disease (e.g., sarcoidosis, amyloidosis)
Noncardiac	• Electrolyte disturbances • Hyperthyroidism • Infection (including endocarditis) • Drugs (e.g., thyroxine, salbutamol) • Pulmonary embolism • Diabetes • Excess alcohol or caffeine consumption • Smoking • Obesity

AF, Atrial fibrillation; CVD, cardiovascular disease.

AF (and atrial flutter, see later) should have their risk of stroke calculated with the CHA_2DS_2-VASc score (Table 28.9) to allow a reasoned decision regarding anticoagulation. Direct-acting oral anticoagulants (DOACs) (apixaban, dabigatran, edoxaban, rivaroxaban) should be offered to patients with a score of 2 or more and considered for men with a score of 1. If DOACs are contraindicated warfarin is the next-line treatment. If anticoagulation is contraindicated, dual therapy with aspirin and clopidogrel may be appropriate (see Chapter 20), alternatively left atrial appendage occlusion can be considered.

Other complications of AF include heart failure (a result of a reduction in cardiac output), and tachycardia-induced cardiomyopathy.

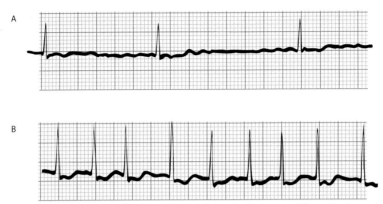

Fig. 28.9 Electrocardiograms of atrial fibrillation with a slow ventricular rate (A) and fast ventricular rate (B).

Table 28.9 CHA$_2$DS$_2$-VASc score for stroke risk with atrial fibrillation

Feature	Score
Congestive heart failure	1
Hypertension history	1
Age 65–74 years	1
Age ≥75 years	2
Diabetes	1
Previous stroke/TIA/thromboembolism	2
Vascular disease history	1
Female sex	1

A score of 1 or higher in men and 2 or higher in women is generally taken as an indication for starting anticoagulation.
TIA, Transient ischaemic attack.

Management

Underlying causes should be treated. Management of AF involves rate and rhythm control. NICE recommends rate control as a first-line treatment except in patients:

- with AF with a reversible cause;
- with heart failure primarily caused by AF;
- with new-onset AF;
- with atrial flutter, suitable for ablation;
- who are more suitable for rhythm control (based on clinical judgement).

The ventricular rate can usually be controlled with a standard β-blocker (a β-blocker other than sotalol) or a rate-limiting calcium channel blocker (diltiazem or verapamil). Digoxin monotherapy can be considered in sedentary patients or those who cannot take other rate-limiting agents. Other classes of drugs may sometimes be required. If the AF is of recent onset, electrical DC cardioversion or pharmacological cardioversion with amiodarone or flecainide may be attempted. After more than 48 hours of AF, the patient should be fully anticoagulated for at least 3 weeks before cardioversion to prevent embolization to distant sites. If pharmacological management is unsuccessful or not possible left atrial ablation with radiofrequency or cryoballoon/laser balloon ablation should be considered.

> **HINTS AND TIPS**
>
> Calcium channel blockers are contraindicated in patients presenting with acute decompensated heart failure.

Atrial flutter

This is due to a regular circus movement of continuous atrial depolarization. As the AV node cannot conduct that fast, it is usually transmitted with a degree of block (e.g., 2:1, 3:1).

The causes and treatments are similar to those for AF.

The ECG shows a sawtooth appearance to the baseline at rates of up to 350 bpm due to flutter or F waves (Fig. 28.10). The ventricular rate is usually divisible into this (e.g., 150 bpm in 2:1 block or 100 bpm in 3:1 block).

Paroxysmal supraventricular tachycardia

SVT is generally divided into AV reentry tachycardia (AVRT), AV nodal reentry tachycardia (AVNRT) and atrial tachycardia. It is caused by either abnormalities of impulse initiation or disorders of impulse conduction (the presence of an accessory pathway between the atria and ventricles, reentrant tachycardias). SVT is usually paroxysmal. In reentrant tachycardias, one pathway is fast- and the other slow-conducting. This leads to antegrade or retrograde conduction and the formation of a reentrant circuit. The result is premature atrial contraction and ventricular depolarization

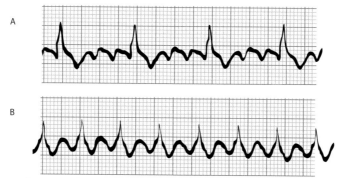

Fig. 28.10 Electrocardiograms of atrial flutter. (A) Atrial flutter with 4:1 block. (B) Atrial flutter with 2:1 block.

giving rise to a fast ventricular rate. The refractory period for an accessory pathway may be shorter than the AV node, leading to ventricular rates exceeding 200 bpm.

Atrioventricular reentry tachycardia

This condition is due to a reentry accessory circuit not involving the AV node. Patients tend to present at a younger age, as these pathways are often congenital. AVRTs frequently settle with fle-cainide but may require accessory pathway ablation to cure the condition. Wolff–Parkinson–White syndrome is an example of a congenital AVRT.

Atrioventricular nodal reentry tachycardia

This is the commonest cause of narrow complex tachycardia. By definition, the reentry is through the AV node. The pre-dominant symptom is palpitations. The condition is commonly benign and may require no treatment beyond the termination of the tachycardia (see later).

CLINICAL NOTES

NARROW COMPLEX TACHYCARDIA TREATMENT: VAGAL STIMULATION

In haemodynamically stable patients, vagal stimulation can be tried initially. This can be achieved in the following ways:

- Valsalva manoeuvre: blowing against resistance (the closed glottis) for approximately 15 s. The tachycardia usually terminates in the relaxation (parasympathetic) phase.
- Carotid sinus massage: massage of the carotid artery at the level of the thyroid cartilage. Do not perform the manoeuvre on both sides simultaneously.

HINTS AND TIPS

Adenosine can be administered intravenously to reveal the underlying rhythm in supraventricular tachycardias by temporary blocking of the AV node. Fast administration of intravenous adenosine can cause very unpleasant but short-acting side effects to awake patients (impending doom, headache, flushing, pain, dizziness, paraesthesia, throat discomfort). Ensure patients are warned of these prior to administration of the drug.

Ventricular tachycardia

VT is a broad complex (wide QRS complexes >120 ms) tachy-cardia defined as three or more consecutive ventricular extra-systoles with a rate greater than 120 bpm (Fig. 28.11). Common causes include CVD, cardiomyopathy, aortic stenosis, myocar-dial ischaemia and electrolyte disturbances. Sustained VT is that lasting longer than 30 s.

HINTS AND TIPS

DC cardioversion is poorly tolerated in an awake patient and sedation or general anaesthesia should be offered to conscious patients needing the intervention.

RED FLAG

Stable patients with VT can quickly deteriorate and become critically unwell. Placing the patient on a cardiac monitor with regular observations is essential and will often require management on high dependency or coronary care unit.

Torsades de pointes

This is a special form of polymorphic VT, associated with a prolonged QT interval. QRS complexes are of variable amplitude, appearing as if they were twisting around the baseline (Fig. 28.12). Torsades de pointes may progress to VF. Treatment is with intravenously administered magnesium sulphate but the condition is often refractory to this. Antiarrhythmics may further prolong the QT interval and worsen the condition. Temporary overdrive pacing may be effective.

Ventricular fibrillation

VF is a medical emergency and is the most common arrhythmia in cardiac arrest. Electrical activity in the ventricles becomes completely desynchronized, leading to mechanical pump failure. Patients should be treated according to the adult advanced life support algorithm (Fig. 28.8) for VF/VT (Fig. 28.13).

Management of tachycardias

See Fig. 28.14 for RESUS council tachycardia algorithm 2021 outlining the approach to a patient with tachycardia.

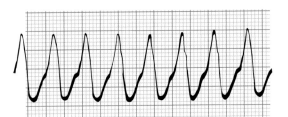

Fig. 28.11 Electrocardiogram of ventricular tachycardia.

Bradycardias

Sinus bradycardia

Sinus bradycardia is defined as a resting pulse rate of less than 60 per minute. For notes on sinus bradycardia, see Chapter 7.

Sick sinus syndrome

This is due to irreversible dysfunction of the sinus node and can lead to periods of sinus bradycardia with asystole, and tachycardia. Dual-chamber pacemakers are recommended as a treatment option, although they will function as an atrial pacemaker only if there is no AV conduction defect.

Heart block

This refers to aberrant conduction through the heart and has three forms: first-, second- and third-degree block. As the 'degree of block' increases, so does the seriousness of the problem.

First-degree heart block—The ECG shows a prolonged PR interval (more than 0.2 s) (Fig. 28.15). All impulses are conducted to the ventricles.

Second-degree heart block—Only some of the atrial impulses are conducted via the AV node. In Wenckebach (Mobitz type I) heart block, there is progressive widening of the PR interval, culminating in nonconduction through the AV node. The cycle then repeats (Fig. 28.16). Mobitz type II heart block is an intermittent failure of AV conduction (Fig. 28.17). This is the more serious of the two because the block is below the AV node in the bundle of His, which may lead to a third-degree block.

Third-degree (complete) heart block—This is complete dissociation between atrial and ventricular contraction (Fig. 28.18).

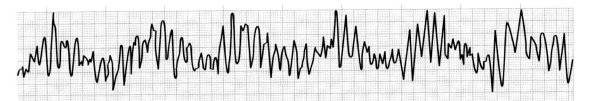

Fig. 28.12 Torsades de pointes with the classic spiralling of QRS complexes around the baseline. (From Walls RM, Hockberger R, Gausche-Hill M. *Rosen's Emergency Medicine: Concepts and Clinical Practice*, 2-Volume Set, 10th ed. Elsevier; 2023.)

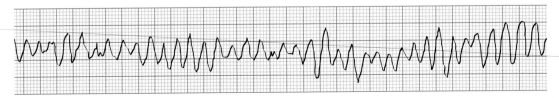

Fig. 28.13 Electrocardiogram of ventricular fibrillation. Coordinated activity of the ventricles ceases. The electrocardiogram shows irregular waves of no defined shape. In this trace there are short periods suggestive of ventricular flutter.

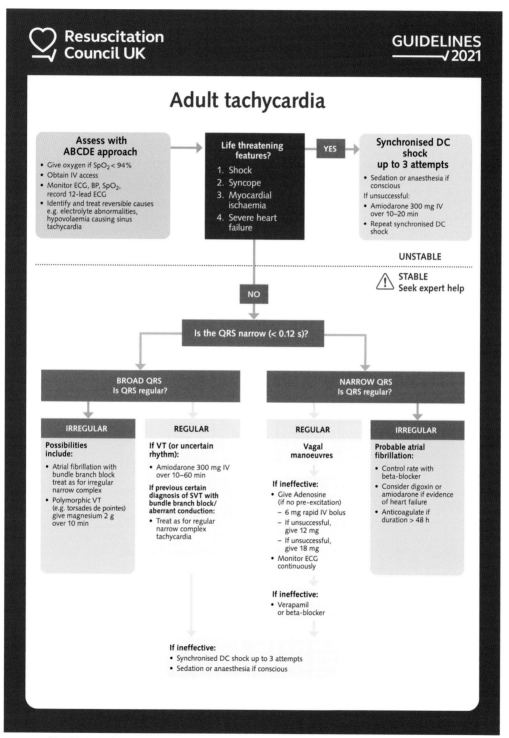

Fig. 28.14 RESUS council tachycardia algorithm 2021. (Resuscitation Council UK, 2021.)

SA impulses are not propagated to the ventricles. The ventricular rate assumes a slow escape rhythm with a rate between 30 and 50 bpm.

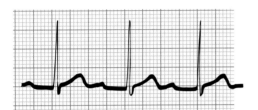

Fig. 28.15 Electrocardiogram of first-degree heart block.

Management of bradycardia

See Fig. 28.19 for RESUS council bradycardia algorithm 2021 outlining the approach to a patient with bradycardia.

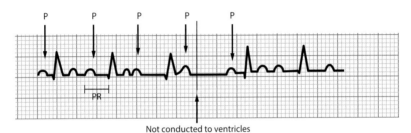

Not conducted to ventricles

Fig. 28.16 Electrocardiogram of Wenckebach heart block.

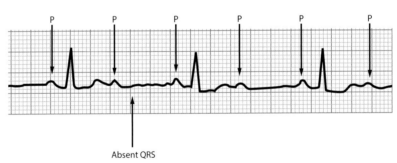

Absent QRS

Fig. 28.17 Electrocardiogram of Mobitz type II heart block showing two P waves for each QRS complex (i.e., 2:1 block).

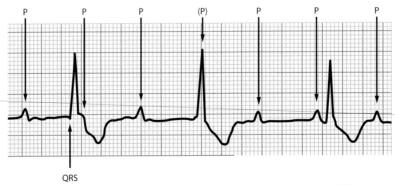

QRS

Fig. 28.18 Electrocardiogram of complete heart block. No relationship between atria (P) and ventricles (QRS).

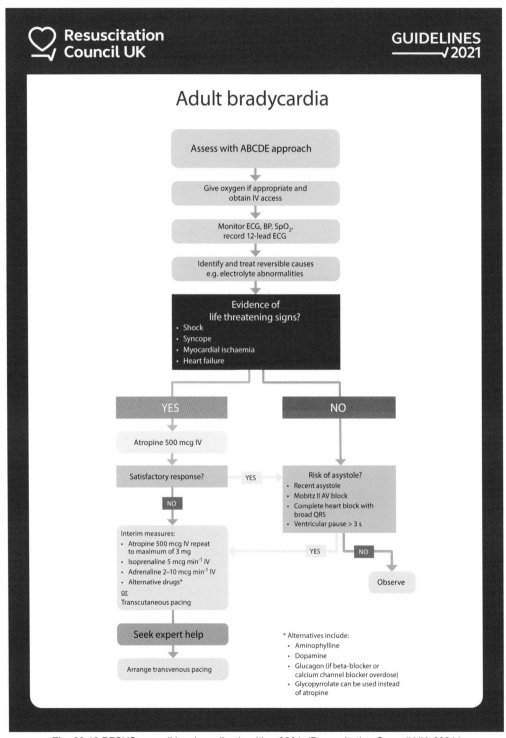

Fig. 28.19 RESUS council bradycardia algorithm 2021. (Resuscitation Council UK, 2021.)

Antiarrhythmic drugs

Antiarrhythmics are classified according to the site of their action (supraventricular, ventricular or both) and their effects on the action potential (Vaughan Williams classification; Table 28.10 and Fig. 28.20). Examples of antiarrhythmic drugs are given next.

Supraventricular arrhythmias

Adenosine

Adenosine is used for terminating SVT. It is a purine nucleoside that causes transient AV block. It has a short half-life (<10 s). Side effects include flushing, arrhythmia, chest pain and bronchospasm. Contraindications include asthma, decompensated heart failure and prolonged QT syndromes.

Verapamil

Verapamil is an L-type calcium channel blocker and an alternative to adenosine. It is negatively inotropic and interferes with electrical conduction. Side effects include flushing, headache, dizziness and constipation. Contraindications include bradycardia, severe left ventricular dysfunction, cardiogenic shock and second and third-degree heart block.

Digoxin

Digoxin is a purified cardiac glycoside (derived from foxgloves) that increases cardiac contractility (positive inotropic effect) and reduces AV conduction. Its mechanism of action is thought to work through binding to the Na^+/K^+-ATPase of cardiac myocytes, altering Na^+ and Ca^{2+} balance. Its main role is in the treatment of AF, atrial flutter and heart failure. Side effects include arrhythmias, blurred or yellow vision and dizziness. It is contraindicated in VT, VF and intermittent complete and second-degree heart block.

Supraventricular and ventricular arrhythmias

Amiodarone

Amiodarone is effective in both supraventricular and ventricular arrhythmias, with little deleterious effect on haemodynamics. Although it is classified as a class III antiarrhythmic, it also has class Ia, II and IV properties. It has a prolonged half-life of several weeks. It may therefore take some weeks to achieve steady-state plasma concentration.

It is an iodine-containing compound, and side effects include hypothyroidism, hyperthyroidism and liver dysfunction. TFTs and liver function test (LFT) results should be checked at the baseline and every 6 months. It may cause pulmonary fibrosis, corneal microdeposits (which are reversible on stopping treatment) and photosensitivity.

β-Blockers

β-Blockers act mainly by attenuating the effects of the sympathetic nervous system on automaticity and conductivity within the heart. Sotalol is a β-blocker that also has class III actions. β-Blockers are

Table 28.10 The Vaughan Williams classification of antiarrhythmic drugs

Class	Features
Ia, Ib, Ic	Membrane sodium channel blockers (e.g., quinidine, lidocaine and flecainide, respectively)
II	Antisympathetic nervous system (β-blockers)
III	Potassium channel blockers (amiodarone, bretylium, sotalol)
IV	Calcium channel blockers (excluding dihydropyridines, e.g., nifedipine)
V	Other (adenosine, digoxin, magnesium sulphate)

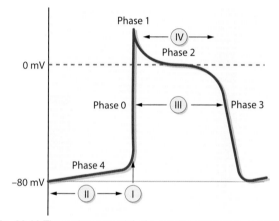

Fig. 28.20 The action potential of a cardiac cell that is capable of spontaneous depolarization (SA or AV nodal, or His–Purkinje) indicating phases 0–4. The modes of action of antiarrhythmic drugs of classes I, II, III and IV are indicated in relation to these phases. (From Brown MJ, et al. *Clinical Pharmacology*, 12th ed. Elsevier; 2019.)

contraindicated in cardiogenic shock and marked bradycardia. They should be used cautiously in patients with asthma.

Flecainide

Flecainide is used to treat a variety of arrhythmias, including AF, SVT and VT. It works by prolonging the action potential. Side effects include arrhythmia, dizziness and dyspnoea. It is contraindicated in known structural heart disease and left ventricular dysfunction. It should not be used to control arrhythmias in an acute setting,

Ventricular arrhythmias

Lidocaine

Works by blocking Na+ and K+ channels. Side effects include bradycardia, convulsions, hypotension and respiratory depression. It is contraindicated in AV block, severe myocardial depression and SA disorders.

Magnesium

Magnesium sulphate is indicated as an emergency treatment for arrhythmias. It is also the treatment of choice for torsades de pointes.

CARDIAC FAILURE

General overview

Cardiac failure occurs when the heart is unable to maintain sufficient cardiac output to meet the demands placed on it by the body. It is a direct consequence of an underlying disorder such as CVD, valvular dysfunction or cardiomyopathy. The problem is usually one of failure of the myocardium, although excess preload and afterload plus rhythm disturbances and increased demand beyond that of a normal heart's capacity are possible. Failure can be systolic (impairment of contraction), diastolic (impairment of relaxation) or both. The incidence rises with age, and almost one million people in the United Kingdom have heart failure. Prognosis is poor, with almost 50% 5-year mortality. It is classified by time course (acute or chronic), its severity (Table 28.11), or ejection fraction (EF).

CLINICAL NOTES

HEART FAILURE CLASSIFIED BY LEFT VENTRICULAR EJECTION FRACTION

- Heart failure with preserved EF: left ventricular ejection fraction (LVEF) >50% + symptoms of heart failure (about 50% of heart failure diagnosis).
- Heart failure with mildly reduced EF: LVEF 41% to 49%.
- Heart failure with reduced EF: LVEF ≤40%.
  Heart failure due to right ventricular dysfunction can also occur. Although left ventricular-induced pulmonary hypertension is the most common cause it can also develop as a result of valve disease, MI or cardiomyopathy.

Aetiology

The most common cause of heart failure is cardiovascular disease. Pathophysiology is often unmasked when a heart with reduced reserve is unable to cope with the often seemingly minor stresses placed on it. Causes include:

- CVD
- Hypertension
- Valvular heart disease
- Tachyarrhythmias (e.g., AF, atrial flutter)
- Cardiomyopathies (e.g., HOCM, Duchenne muscular dystrophy)
- Pericardial disease (e.g., constrictive pericarditis)
- Congenital heart disease

Table 28.11 The New York Heart Association classification of heart failure

Class	Features
I	No limitation of physical activity
II	Slight limitation of physical activity, breathless/fatigue/palpitations on ordinary physical activity
III	Marked limitation of physical activity, breathless/fatigue/palpitations on less than ordinary physical activity
IV	Inability to perform any physical activity without discomfort

Heart failure can also occur in seemingly normal hearts. This is a result of cardiac inability to maintain an increased cardiac output in the face of grossly elevated requirements. The following conditions cause this form of cardiac decompensation:

- Thyrotoxicosis
- Anaemia
- Pregnancy
- Sepsis
- Liver failure
- AV shunts
- Paget disease
- Volume overload (e.g., end-stage chronic kidney disease, nephrotic syndrome)
- Drugs and toxins (e.g., alcohol, cocaine, negatively inotropic drugs)

Clinical features

Heart failure used to be described as left-sided (left-ventricular), right-sided (right-ventricular) or congestive (bi-ventricular); however, these terms can be misleading and are no longer used. With that said, patients often present with different predominate symptoms depending on whether the primary dysfunction localizes to the pulmonary (left) or systemic (right) circulations (Table 28.12).

CLINICAL NOTES

USEFUL INVESTIGATIONS

- N-terminal pro-B-type natriuretic peptide (NT-pro-BNP): if within normal range chronic heart failure is unlikely. Note that different guidelines suggest different levels as normal.
- Echocardiography: key test to identify structural abnormalities and assess ventricular and valvular function.
- CXR: cardiomegaly, evidence of fluid overload (alveolar oedema, 'bat's wings shadowing', prominent upper lobe vessels, Kerley B lines, pleural effusions).

Table 28.12 Heart failure signs and symptoms characteristic for the pulmonary and systemic circulations

Characteristic left-sided features

Signs:
- Exertional breathlessness (most common)
- Orthopnoea
- Paroxysmal nocturnal dyspnoea
- Wheeze ('cardiac asthma')
- Nocturnal cough
- Fatigue

Symptoms:
- Tachypnoea, tachycardia, low volume pulse or pulsus alternans (alternating large- and small-volume pulse), third heart sound ('S3 gallop'), functional mitral regurgitation, peripheral cyanosis

Characteristic right-sided features

Signs:
- Swollen ankles
- Wasting
- Nausea
- Abdominal discomfort (engorged liver)
- Anorexia
- Fatigue

Symptoms:
- Raised JVP, pitting oedema, smooth hepatomegaly, liver tenderness, ascites, functional tricuspid regurgitation, right ventricular third heart sound, hepatojugular reflux

Acute heart failure

Acute heart failure is a medical emergency and in the case of acute left ventricular failure usually presents with severe dyspnoea secondary to pulmonary oedema. Patients will be sitting up, distressed, pale and sweaty and may be coughing up pink frothy sputum. Key treatment goals in acute heart failure include patient stabilization, symptom relief and adequate organ perfusion. Use the ABCDE approach. Ensure:

- The patient is sitting upright.
- Oxygen is administered to hypoxic patients to maintain oxygen saturations of >94% unless the patient is at risk of hypercapnic respiratory failure, where the target range is usually 88% to 92%. Remember that oxygen is used to treat hypoxaemia and not breathlessness.
- Diuresis is commenced with furosemide. Furosemide also causes vasodilation.
- Ensure close fluid balance monitoring.

Routine use of nitrates, opiates or sodium nitroprusside in people with acute heart failure is not recommended. If intravenous nitrates are used, then this should be administered in at least a level 2 setting. Nitrates are vasodilators and work by reducing preload. Routine use of respiratory support with continuous positive airway pressure to improve oxygenation or noninvasive positive pressure ventilation in people with acute heart failure and cardiogenic pulmonary oedema is not recommended. Consider using such support in patients with severe dyspnoea and acidaemia or those that failed to respond to pharmacological therapy. Invasive ventilation should be considered in patients who are deteriorating despite treatment.

Treat other conditions that may compromise cardiac function (e.g., arrhythmias).

Intravenous inotropic agents may be of value if there is refractory hypotension. Drugs used include milrinone or enoximone (phosphodiesterase inhibitors) and dobutamine (β-agonist). If pulmonary congestion is dominant, dobutamine is preferred. It has vasodilating properties and so may lower the BP. It can be combined with noradrenaline if needed.

In cases of pulmonary oedema refractory to diuresis, haemofiltration can be used as a way of fluid removal.

Intraaortic balloon counterpulsation in primary cardiac failure may be available to support the heart while therapy is planned.

Chronic heart failure

The underlying cause of heart failure should be sought and treated appropriately. Exacerbating factors such as anaemia and hypertension should be treated. Patients should be advised to maintain an optimal weight, avoid excessive salt intake and alcohol consumption and stop smoking. Annual vaccinations for influenza and a one-off pneumococcal vaccination should be offered.

Management

Heart failure with reduced ejection fraction (HFrEF)

First-line treatment is ACE inhibitors and β-blockers. ARBs are an alternative. In patients who continue to have symptoms despite maximized therapy mineralocorticoid receptor antagonists (MRAs) are added. Further treatments are described later.

Heart failure with preserved ejection fraction (HFpEF)

These patients are normally started on a low/medium dose of a loop diuretic and β-blockers can be effective. There is no evidence of benefit from other medications used in HFrEF.

Drug treatment for HFrEF

Renin angiotensin system (RAS) blockade

The renin–angiotensin–aldosterone system is activated in heart failure, and ACE inhibitors reduce angiotensin-mediated vasoconstriction, reducing afterload, and decreasing aldosterone-mediated salt and water retention. This improves cardiac function. In heart failure, ACE inhibitors reduce both morbidity and mortality. Side effects include cough, first-dose hypotension, hyperkalaemia and worsening renal function. Contraindications include bilateral renal artery stenosis and severe renal impairment. Commonly used drugs include ramipril, enalapril, perindopril and lisinopril. ARBs, for example, candesartan, valsartan, losartan, can be used in patients intolerant to ACE inhibitors.

Sacubitril/valsartan—A new class of drugs called angiotensin receptor neprilysin inhibitors. It is a combined medication that consists of sacubitril (a neprilysin inhibitor – inhibits the breakdown of natriuretic peptides promoting diuresis, natriuresis and vasodilation) and valsartan (an ARB). It is recommended in preference to ACEi/ARB in patients with NYHA class II–IV heart failure and left ventricular ejection fraction (LVEF) ≤35%. Side effects include electrolyte imbalance, renal impairment, anaemia and gastritis. It should not be taken concomitantly with an ACE inhibitor or ARB.

β-Blockers

For many years it was believed that these were contraindicated in heart failure because the sympathetic nervous system was compensating for the failing heart and blocking this was deleterious. This remains true in the acute setting, where the negatively inotropic and chronotropic effects of β-blockade can be harmful. However, β-blockers are recommended in patients with chronic heart failure and left ventricular dysfunction.

They reduce morbidity and mortality associated with heart failure. The β-blockers currently licensed for use in heart failure are carvedilol, bisoprolol and nebivolol.

Mineralocorticoid receptor antagonists

Also known as aldosterone antagonists. Aldosterone may act directly as a deleterious growth factor on myocytes, in addition to its salt- and water-retaining effects. These are recommended in patients with heart failure and reduced LVEF. Examples of drugs include spironolactone and eplerenone. They reduce mortality and risk of hospitalization associated with heart failure.

Sodium-glucose co-transporter 2 (SGLT2)—

Class of drugs usually used for the treatment of diabetes are now recommended by the European Society of Cardiology in addition to ACE inhibitors, β-blockers, MRAs for the management of patients with heart failure and reduced LVEF. Dapagliflozin and empagliflozin have been found to reduce the risk of cardiovascular death and worsening of heart failure and should be used regardless of their diabetic status.

Diuretics

Loop diuretics, commonly furosemide and bumetanide, are very effective at reducing symptoms in patients with heart failure in both acute and long term care. They have beneficial effects on clinical outcomes and reduce mortality. Side effects include hypovolaemia, renal impairment, electrolyte disturbances (hypokalaemia, hypomagnesaemia, hyponatraemia, hypocalcaemia) and, rarely, ototoxicity. Contraindications to their use include severe hypokalaemia and hyponatraemia.

Hydralazine in combination with a nitrate

This should be considered second-line treatment in patients with chronic NYHA class III–IV heart failure with reduced ejection fraction, especially if they are of black African or Caribbean heritage.

Digoxin

Recommended in patients with worsening or severe heart failure due to left ventricular dysfunction refractory to treatment with first- and second-line drugs.

Ivabradine

This is an option in patients with NYHA class II–IV stable chronic heart failure who have LVEF of 35% or less, are in sinus rhythm with a heart rate of 75 bpm or more and are already taking standard therapy (unless contraindicated).

Nondrug therapy

Implantable cardioverter defibrillator and cardiac resynchronization therapy

Implantable cardioverter defibrillator (ICD) insertion is recommended for people with previous serious ventricular arrhythmias without a treatable cause or people who have a familial cardiac condition with a high risk of sudden death (e.g., hypertrophic cardiomyopathy, long QT syndrome, Brugada syndrome). In patients with heart failure, ICD placement or cardiac resynchronization therapy (CRT) is recommended in patients with LVEF ≤35% and dyssynchrony. CRT, also called biventricular pacing, refers to devices that apart from standard right atrial and right ventricular wires also have a left ventricular pacemaker.

Left ventricular assist devices

Left ventricular assist devices are mechanical circulatory devices that can be used to partially or completely replace the function of the failing heart. Their most common clinical indication is after cardiac surgery, where the device allows the heart to recover.

Transplantation

Heart transplantation can be performed as a treatment for chronic heart failure. The extent of the surgery and postoperative immunosuppression means that only a select group of patients are suitable for transplantation. The current prognosis for heart transplantation is very good with 70% of recipients alive at 5 years.

HYPERTENSION

General overview

Hypertension is one of the most important modifiable risk factors for CVD such as stroke, MI and renal disease and, as such, premature morbidity and mortality in the world.

Hypertension is defined as systemic arterial BP persistently above or equal to 140/90 mmHg. The prevalence of hypertension differs depending on BP cut-off points, age, sex and race but figures suggest that one in four adults suffers from hypertension in the United Kingdom. It increases with age and is more common in men and those of African or Black Caribbean origin. Systolic hypertension is more prevalent in older people; this results from progressive stiffening and loss of compliance of larger arteries. Diastolic hypertension is more common in people younger than 50 years.

The risk of morbidity and mortality rises continuously with increasing BP. When diagnosing hypertension, if the reading is 140/90 mmHg or greater in the clinic, the patient should be offered ambulatory BP monitoring to confirm the diagnosis. BP between 140/90 and 155/99 mmHg is termed stage 1 hypertension and BP between 160/100 and 180/120 mmHg is termed stage 2 hypertension. Stage 3 hypertension or severe hypertension is systolic BP of 180 mmHg or higher or diastolic BP of 120 mmHg or higher. These are arbitrary cut-off points that are influenced by age, the presence of end-organ damage or established CVD, and other cardiovascular risk factors (e.g., diabetes mellitus). Approximately 95% of all hypertensive patients have essential or primary hypertension and have no underlying disease (i.e., no identifiable cause). Secondary hypertension can be the result of a range of different pathological processes.

> **RED FLAG**
>
> ### MALIGNANT HYPERTENSION
>
> BP of 180/120 mmHg or higher with evidence of end-organ damage such as retinal haemorrhages/papilloedema. This is a medical emergency.
>
> Treatment is normally given orally with β-blockers or calcium antagonists to reduce diastolic BP to 100 to 110 mmHg within the first 24 hours. Intravenous antihypertensive drugs such as nitroprusside, GTN or labetalol are used when more rapid reduction is necessary or when the oral route is unavailable. Over the next few days, further antihypertensives should be given to lower BP further.
>
> Very rapid falls in BP should be avoided because the reduction in cerebral perfusion may lead to cerebral infarction, blindness, worsening renal function and myocardial ischaemia. Patients with untreated malignant hypertension have 90% mortality at 1 year.

CLINICAL NOTES

MECHANISMS INVOLVED IN THE DEVELOPMENT OF ESSENTIAL HYPERTENSION

- Obesity: there is a continuous linear relationship between excess body fat and blood pressure levels.
- Alcohol: increased alcohol consumption is related to higher blood pressure.
- Dietary sodium: salt restriction may reduce systolic blood pressure by 3 to 5 mmHg in hypertensives and is most clear-cut in older people and those with severe hypertension.
- Genetics: defects in the renin–angiotensin–aldosterone axis, problems with sodium handling and increased sympathetic nervous system activation.

CLINICAL NOTES

CAUSES OF SECONDARY HYPERTENSION

A definite underlying cause of hypertension is more common in younger people, and should be looked for specifically in those younger than 35 years:

- Renal: renal artery stenosis, fibromuscular dysplasia, chronic glomerulonephritis, chronic pyelonephritis, obstructive uropathy and polycystic kidney disease.
- Endocrine: hyperaldosteronism, phaeochromocytoma, hyperparathyroidism, Cushing disease and acromegaly.
- Respiratory: obstructive sleep apnoea.
- Pregnancy-induced hypertension and preeclampsia: associated with oedema and proteinuria.
- Congenital: coarctation of the aorta.
- Drugs: oestrogen-containing oral contraceptive pill, NSAIDs, steroids, sympathomimetics, carbenoxolone and liquorice.

Clinical features

Patients with hypertension are usually asymptomatic. However, symptoms can be associated with complications resulting from end-organ damage. The following symptoms may occur:

- Headaches.
- Dyspnoea.
- Symptoms of cardiac failure.

- Angina pectoris or MI.
- TIA or stroke.
- Visual disturbance.
- Hypertensive emergency: hypertensive encephalopathy. This requires immediate management with antihypertensives such as intravenously administered labetalol.

The clinical approach to the patient with hypertension is summarized in Table 28.13, and the examination approach in Fig. 28.21. Complications or an underlying cause should be sought.

Investigations

An algorithm for the investigation of the patient with hypertension is given in Fig. 28.22. Further investigations to look for a secondary cause are warranted in young patients, i.e., those under 40 years, in patients with severe hypertension, those who have treatment-resistant disease or where there is worsening of previously stable hypertension, as they are more likely to have a secondary cause. These investigations include 24-hour urinary catecholamine and metanephrine measurements for phaeochromocytoma, renin:aldosterone ratio to look for evidence of hyperaldosteronism, and renal tract ultrasound scan for structural abnormalities; renal artery imaging, e.g., magnetic

Table 28.13 Clinical evaluation of the patient with hypertension (look for the five Cs)

Causes of hypertension	Drugs causing hypertension? Paroxysmal features? (phaeochromocytoma) Renal disease, history of renal disease or family history of renal disease? General appearance? (Cushing syndrome) Radiofemoral delay? (coarctation) Kidney(s) palpable? (polycystic, hydronephrosis, neoplasm) Abdominal or loin bruit? (renal artery stenosis)
Contributory factors	Overweight? Alcohol intake?
Complications	Cerebrovascular disease Left ventricular hypertrophy or cardiac failure Ischaemic heart disease Fundal haemorrhages and exudates (accelerated phase)
Contraindications to drugs	Gout, diabetes (thiazides) Asthma, heart block (β-blockers) Heart failure, heart block (verapamil)
Cardiovascular risk	Assessment of other cardiovascular risk factors

resonance imaging of renal arteries. Further investigations depend on clinical suspicion (e.g., aortography for coarctation of the aorta).

> **HINTS AND TIPS**
>
> Many patients find visiting their doctor stressful and will often have a raised blood pressure – white-coat hypertension. A diagnosis of hypertension can therefore be made only after ambulatory or home blood pressure monitoring.

Management

Fig. 28.23 summarizes current NICE-recommendations for the clinical management of adult hypertension. Treatment of the underlying condition may be indicated in cases of secondary hypertension (e.g., treatment of an endocrine condition or surgical correction of aortic coarctation). Patients should be educated about lifestyle modifications which can reduce the risk of CVD (diet and exercise, caffeine and alcohol intake, dietary sodium, smoking).

In hypertension, as in many chronic disorders, drugs are best added stepwise until control has been achieved. Monotherapy controls BP in only 30% to 50% of individuals, and most patients need two or more drugs. In uncomplicated mild hypertension, drugs may be substituted rather than added. See Table 28.14 for NICE-recommended BP targets.

Drug treatment

Angiotensin-converting enzyme inhibitors

ACE inhibitors act by inhibiting the renin–angiotensin–aldosterone axis with an increase in the level of vasodilating bradykinin. They are more effective in patients with higher renin levels, and so are best used in young white patients. These are treatment of choice in systemic sclerosis or in scleroderma renal crises. A serious side effect is an angioedema.

Angiotensin II receptor blockers

These block the renin–angiotensin system, producing effects similar to ACE inhibitors. They do not affect bradykinin production, and so are useful for people who develop a chronic cough with ACE inhibitors.

Calcium channel blockers

These are effective as monotherapy in 50% of patients, and amlodipine has become the most common antihypertensive worldwide. Side effects include flushing, headache, constipation and diuretic-resistant oedema (generally dependent ankle oedema).

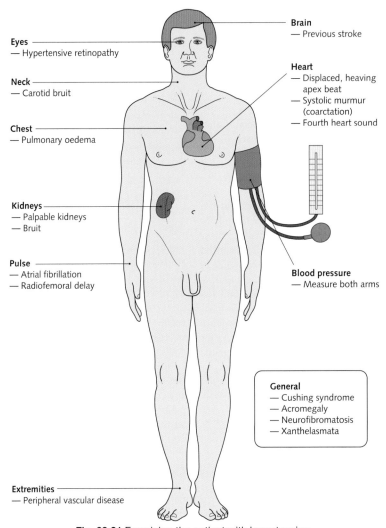

Brain
— Previous stroke

Eyes
— Hypertensive retinopathy

Neck
— Carotid bruit

Heart
— Displaced, heaving apex beat
— Systolic murmur (coarctation)
— Fourth heart sound

Chest
— Pulmonary oedema

Kidneys
— Palpable kidneys
— Bruit

Pulse
— Atrial fibrillation
— Radiofemoral delay

Blood pressure
— Measure both arms

General
— Cushing syndrome
— Acromegaly
— Neurofibromatosis
— Xanthelasmata

Extremities
— Peripheral vascular disease

Fig. 28.21 Examining the patient with hypertension.

Thiazide diuretics

Thiazides mainly affect the BP by lowering body sodium stores. Initially, BP falls because of a decrease in blood volume, venous return and cardiac output. Gradually, the cardiac output returns to normal, but the hypotensive effect remains because the peripheral resistance decreases. Side effects include impaired glucose tolerance and gout. Thiazides are contraindicated in Addison disease, hypercalcaemia, hyponatraemia and refractory hypokalaemia. Women tolerate thiazides better than men, and the drug is more effective in the elderly. Other diuretics, such as spironolactone, can be considered in the treatment of resistant hypertension.

β-Blockers

β-Blockers may be considered in young patients or in treatment-resistant hypertension. β-Blockers initially produce a fall in BP by decreasing cardiac output. With continued use, the cardiac output returns to normal but the BP remains low because the peripheral resistance is reset at a lower level and renin levels are reduced.

α-Adrenergic receptor blockers

α-Blockers such as doxazosin reduce both arteriolar and venous resistance and maintain high cardiac output. They can be considered in resistant hypertension.

Central acting agents

Methyldopa stimulates α_2 receptors in the medulla and reduces sympathetic outflow. In 20% of patients it causes a positive Coombs test result and, rarely, haemolytic anaemia. Drug-induced hepatitis with fever may also occur.

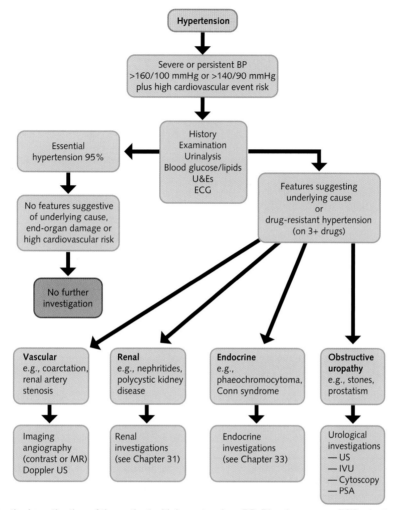

Fig. 28.22 Algorithm for the investigation of the patient with hypertension. *BP*, Blood pressure; *ECG*, electrocardiogram; *IVU*, intravenous urogram; *MR*, magnetic resonance; *PSA*, prostate-specific antigen; *U&Es*, urea and electrolytes; *US*, ultrasonography.

Vasodilators

Minoxidil is a potent vasodilator and decreases peripheral resistance. It can be used in the treatment of severe hypertension in addition to a diuretic and a β-blocker. Side effects include reflex tachycardia, fluid retention and hypertrichosis.

Management of hypertension in pregnancy

Orally administered methyldopa is safe. β-Blockers are effective and safe in the third trimester; labetalol is used relatively frequently but may cause intrauterine growth retardation when administered earlier in pregnancy. Hydralazine may also be used. Its side effects include drug-induced lupus.

VALVULAR HEART DISEASE

General overview

Valvular heart disease can affect any of the four heart valves. It is a common condition that may be congenital or acquired. Clinically, most heart valve abnormalities are asymptomatic and discovered only by the presence of a heart murmur on careful auscultation of the precordium. Heart murmurs are due to vibration caused by turbulent blood flow within the heart. The commonest causes are left-sided valvular heart disease and tricuspid regurgitation. Nonvalvular causes include:

- Innocent 'flow' murmurs, especially in children

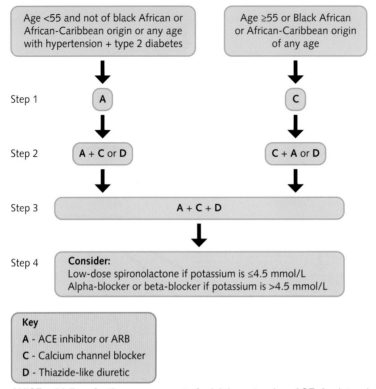

Step 1

Step 2

Step 3

Step 4

Fig. 28.23 Summary of NICE guidelines for the management of adult hypertension. *ACE,* Angiotensin-converting enzyme.

Table 28.14 NICE recommended BP targets

Patient characteristics	BP target
Age <80 years	Clinic BP <140/90 mmHg ABPM/HBPM <135/85 mmHg
Age ≥80 years	Clinic BP <150/90 mmHg ABPM/HBPM <145/85 mmHg

ABPM, Ambulatory BP monitoring; HBPM, home BP monitoring.

- High cardiac output states (e.g., pregnancy, anaemia, thyrotoxicosis and fever)
- Congenital heart disease (e.g., atrial septal defect (ASD), VSD, patent ductus arteriosus (PDA) and coarctation of the aorta).

The classification of heart murmurs includes ejection systolic murmurs, pansystolic murmurs, diastolic murmurs and continuous murmurs.

Mitral stenosis

The mitral valve separates the left atrium and left ventricle. The most common cause of mitral stenosis is rheumatic fever, although only approximately half of all patients report this history. Other causes include systemic lupus erythematosus, rheumatoid arthritis, congenital defects and infective endocarditis. Mitral stenosis is four times more common than mitral regurgitation after rheumatic fever and is more common in women than in men.

Progressive stenosis of the mitral valve, via thickening of the cusps and fusion of the commissures, results in a pressure gradient between the left atrium and the left ventricle. As the stenosis worsens, ventricular filling becomes impaired, and this is compounded by fibrosis of the subvalvular apparatus leading to left atrial dilatation and hypertrophy, AF and thrombus formation. Pulmonary congestion ensues as left atrial pressure rises, and an increase in pulmonary artery pressure may lead to right ventricular dilatation and tricuspid regurgitation.

Clinical features

Dyspnoea on exertion is an early symptom and may progress to orthopnoea and paroxysmal nocturnal dyspnea. Breathlessness often worsens considerably with the onset of AF (loss of atrial systole) and is commonly accompanied by palpitations. Cough and haemoptysis may occur because of bronchitis, pulmonary infarction, pulmonary congestion and bronchial vein rupture. Fatigue and cold extremities are late symptoms, probably secondary to a low cardiac output. Chest pain occurs in a few people and may be due to coronary artery embolism or severe pulmonary hypertension. On auscultation, there will be a loud

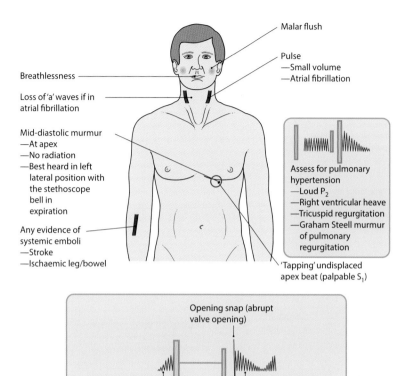

Malar flush

Pulse
—Small volume
—Atrial fibrillation

Breathlessness

Loss of 'a' waves if in
atrial fibrillation

Mid-diastolic murmur
—At apex
—No radiation
—Best heard in left
  lateral position with
  the stethoscope
  bell in
  expiration

Assess for pulmonary
hypertension
—Loud P$_2$
—Right ventricular heave
—Tricuspid regurgitation
—Graham Steel murmur
  of pulmonary
  regurgitation

Any evidence of
systemic emboli
—Stroke
—Ischaemic leg/bowel

'Tapping' undisplaced
apex beat (palpable S$_1$)

Opening snap (abrupt
valve opening)

Presystolic accentuation
(only present in sinus
rhythm as is caused by atrial systole)

S$_1$ S$_2$

Mid-diastolic rumble
(longer, the tighter
the stenosis)

Fig. 28.24 Mitral stenosis.

S$_1$ opening snap followed by a mid-diastolic rumbling murmur, heard best in expiration with the patient in the left lateral position with the bell of the stethoscope. A summary of the clinical signs of mitral stenosis is given in Fig. 28.24.

Management

Maintenance of sinus rhythm confers haemodynamic benefit as ventricular filling is improved (see AF management). The risk of emboli is greater with a large left atrium or left atrial appendage. It may be necessary to add other drugs which will control cardiac rate, such as β-blockers or calcium channel blockers. Dyspnoea can be alleviated by diuretics.

If symptoms persist, the patient should be considered for percutaneous mitral commissurotomy or mitral valve replacement. If the valve is not calcified and the leaflets are pliable, balloon valvuloplasty may be attempted.

Mitral regurgitation

The incidence of mitral regurgitation is equal in men and women. Mitral regurgitation is usually secondary to rheumatic fever, floppy prolapsing mitral valve leaflets, papillary muscle dysfunction, rupture after an inferior MI, cardiomyopathy or ventricular dilatation or dysfunction. Less common causes include congenital malformations, which may be associated with an ostium primum ASD, infective endocarditis, rupture of the chordae tendineae, cardiomyopathy, rheumatoid arthritis or left atrial tumour interfering with mitral valve closure.

The circulatory changes depend on the speed of onset and severity of mitral regurgitation. Acute regurgitation (e.g., due to papillary muscle rupture) may lead to acute pulmonary oedema, whereas chronic regurgitation allows compensatory left ventricular and atrial dilatation.

Clinical features

Progressive exertional dyspnoea, palpitations and fatigue are common, with symptoms of pulmonary oedema if severe. AF, systemic emboli and chest pain are less common than in mitral stenosis. The murmur is a pansystolic murmur at the apex, radiating to the axilla. A summary of the clinical signs of mitral regurgitation is given in Fig. 28.25.

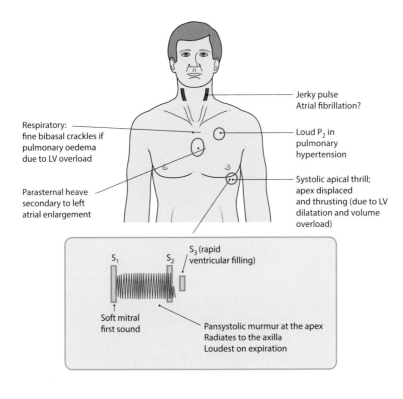

Fine bibasal crackles if pulmonary oedema due to LV overload

Fig. 28.25 Mitral regurgitation. *LV,* Left ventricular.

Management

Diuretics are used for pulmonary congestion, and vasodilators are helpful in acute regurgitation.

Mitral valve replacement is indicated if symptoms are severe and uncontrolled by medical treatment, or if pulmonary hypertension develops. Good results are achieved if left ventricular function is preserved, and early referral may allow repair of the valve rather than replacement.

Mitral valve prolapse

This is due to prolapse of the mitral valve leaflets into the left atrium during ventricular systole. It may affect up to 5% of the population and is three times commoner in women. Mitral valve prolapse is associated with Turner syndrome, Marfan syndrome, osteogenesis imperfecta, PDA and ASDs. The condition is often asymptomatic and found incidentally. An apical mid-systolic click is heard, associated with a late systolic murmur if the valve is regurgitant. It may be associated with palpitations and atypical chest pain. Systemic emboli and syncope are rare.

The ECG may show inferolateral ST/T segment changes. The commonest rhythm disturbance is ventricular extrasystoles. Treatment involves symptomatic management and mitral valve repair or replacement.

Aortic stenosis

The commonest cause of aortic stenosis in individuals younger than 65 years is a calcified bicuspid valve, and this is more common in men. In younger patients, the cause may be congenital or due to rheumatic fever. In patients older than 65 years, the condition is usually due to senile calcific aortic stenosis, which is commoner in women. Aortic stenosis tends to progress gradually, obstructing the left ventricular outflow, with resultant hypertrophy. Ventricular dilatation and heart failure are late complications. Conduction defects may result from calcification extending into the ventricular system.

Clinical features

Initially, the patient may be asymptomatic. Classically late symptoms include angina pectoris, exertional dyspnoea and syncope. Sudden death may occur; it is thought that this is probably secondary to ventricular dysrhythmias. On auscultation, there is an ejection systolic murmur radiating to the carotids. Occasionally the stenosis is so severe that minimal flow causes no murmur. A fourth heart sound indicates left ventricular hypertrophy. A summary of the clinical signs in aortic stenosis is given in Fig. 28.26.

Aortic sclerosis is a distinctly different condition secondary to senile degeneration of the aortic valve. Clinically it does result in an ejection systolic murmur, but this does not radiate to the carotid artery nor does it cause a change in the character of the pulse.

Management

Valve replacement is indicated for severe stenosis because of the risk of sudden death, or if the stenosis is symptomatic. Valve replacement surgery can be either open or using transcatheter aortic valve implantation. Drugs do not alter the progression of the disease, although diuretics and ACE inhibitors can be given for heart failure. Many cardiovascular drugs are contraindicated in aortic stenosis: these are predominantly vasodilating medications, which by decreasing systemic vascular resistance increases the gradient across the valve, and therefore the work the ventricle has to perform.

Aortic regurgitation

Aortic regurgitation can be caused by abnormalities of either the aortic valve or the aortic root. Cusp malformation (e.g., bicuspid valve) and cusp erosion (e.g., infective endocarditis) are the most common causes.

Other causes include:

- Cusp distortion (e.g., senile calcification and rheumatic fever)
- Loss of support (e.g., VSD)
- Aortic wall disease due to inflammation (e.g., syphilis)
- Aortic wall disease due to dilatation (e.g., hypertension with or without dissection)
- Ankylosing spondylitis
- Reiter syndrome
- Psoriatic arthropathy

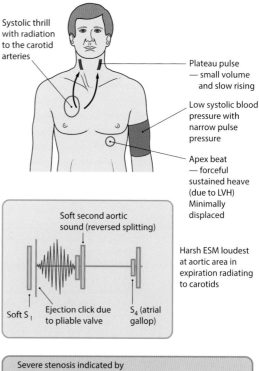

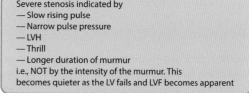

Fig. 28.26 Aortic stenosis. *ESM*, Ejection systolic murmur; *LV*, left ventricle; *LVF*, left ventricular failure; *LVH*, left ventricular hypertrophy.

Clinical features

The patient is usually asymptomatic until the ventricle fails, giving rise to symptoms of heart failure. Angina rarely occurs. Clinical signs in aortic regurgitation are given in Fig. 28.27. The pulse has a sharp rise and fall (collapsing or 'water hammer') with a wide pulse pressure. Other manifestations include visible pulsation in the nail bed (Quincke sign), visible arterial pulsation in the neck (Corrigan sign), head bobbing (de Musset sign), pistol shot femoral artery sound (Traube sign) and a diastolic murmur following distal compression of the artery (Duroziez sign). Aortic regurgitation murmur is best heard in the aortic area in expiration, with the patient sitting forward.

Management

Valve replacement is indicated for symptomatic patients. Diuretics and ACE inhibitors may be given to control symptoms of

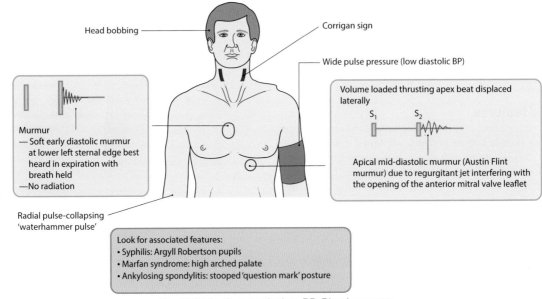

Head bobbing

Corrigan sign

Wide pulse pressure (low diastolic BP)

Volume loaded thrusting apex beat displaced laterally

S_1 S_2

Murmur
— Soft early diastolic murmur at lower left sternal edge best heard in expiration with breath held
—No radiation

Apical mid-diastolic murmur (Austin Flint murmur) due to regurgitant jet interfering with the opening of the anterior mitral valve leaflet

Radial pulse-collapsing 'waterhammer pulse'

Look for associated features:
• Syphilis: Argyll Robertson pupils
• Marfan syndrome: high arched palate
• Ankylosing spondylitis: stooped 'question mark' posture

Fig. 28.27 Aortic regurgitation. *BP*, Blood pressure.

heart failure. The prognosis is good while the ventricular function is preserved, but death usually occurs within 2–3 years after the onset of ventricular failure.

Tricuspid regurgitation

This may be functional, secondary to right-sided heart failure, most commonly caused by pulmonary hypertension. It may also be rheumatic in association with mitral valve disease, or due to endocarditis in intravenous drug users.

Clinical features include fatigue, oedema, ascites and hepatic pain as the liver capsule is stretched. On examination there may be giant 'v' waves in the JVP. There may be a right ventricular heave. A pansystolic murmur will be audible at the lower sternal edge, best heard on inspiration. The clinical findings of tricuspid regurgitation are summarized in Fig. 28.28.

Management includes treating any underlying cause, followed by management of the consequences of right-sided heart strain (see management of heart failure). Valve replacement is an option but is high risk if pulmonary hypertension is present.

Pulmonary valve lesions

Pulmonary valve lesions are the least common. Pulmonary stenosis is often congenital (e.g., associated with Noonan syndrome). It is also one of the features of the tetralogy of Fallot. Pulmonary regurgitation can be caused by any cause of pulmonary hypertension and causes a Graham Steell murmur (high-pitched early diastolic murmur best heard at the left sternal edge in inspiration).

HINTS AND TIPS

Left-sided heart murmurs are loudest in expiration and right-sided murmurs are loudest in inspiration because of increased blood flow across the valves.

HINTS AND TIPS

There are four things to remember when you are describing a murmur:

1. Where is it loudest on the precordium?
2. Where is it in the cardiac cycle?
3. What happens on inspiration and expiration?
4. Where does it radiate to?

MISCELLANEOUS CONDITIONS

Pericardial disease: pericarditis and pericardial effusion

Pericarditis is inflammation of the pericardium which may be primary or secondary to systemic disease. Common causes include viruses, bacteria, MI, autoimmune disorders, drugs (e.g., hydralazine).

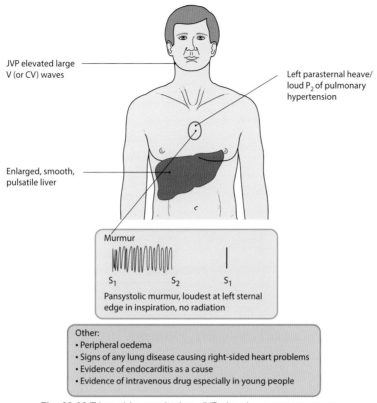

JVP elevated large V (or CV) waves

Left parasternal heave/ loud P_2 of pulmonary hypertension

Enlarged, smooth, pulsatile liver

Murmur

S_1 S_2 S_1

Pansystolic murmur, loudest at left sternal edge in inspiration, no radiation

Other:
• Peripheral oedema
• Signs of any lung disease causing right-sided heart problems
• Evidence of endocarditis as a cause
• Evidence of intravenous drug especially in young people

Fig. 28.28 Tricuspid regurgitation. *JVP*, Jugular venous pressure.

Clinical features

Patients usually present with dull, sharp or burning retrosternal chest pain that is classically relieved by sitting up and leaning forward. It may radiate to the left arm, neck or shoulders. It is worse on lying flat, with inspiration and coughing. There may be a 'scratchy' pericardial friction rub on auscultation. Pericardial effusion may be present. If left untreated pericarditis can lead to the development of cardiac tamponade which is a medical emergency as increased intrapericardial pressure reduces filling pressures and critically compromises cardiac output. Those patients may present with the Beck triad of signs characteristic of cardiac tamponade (hypotension with narrow pulse pressure, elevated systemic venous pressure with jugular venous distension and muffled heart sounds).

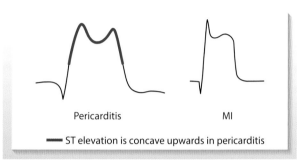

Pericarditis   MI

— ST elevation is concave upwards in pericarditis

Fig. 28.29 ST elevation characteristic for pericarditis versus that of myocardial infarction (MI). (From Kumar P, Clark ML. *Clark's Cases in Clinical Medicine,* 4th ed. Elsevier; 2021.)

Management

The underlying cause should be treated. NSAIDs relieve pain.

Clinical features of an associated pericardial effusion include signs of bi-ventricular heart failure. Pericardial tamponade is managed with pericardiocentesis.

Constrictive pericarditis

This is usually idiopathic or secondary to an infection, most commonly tuberculosis, although it may follow any cause of pericarditis. The heart is encased within a nonexpansile, thickened, fibrotic pericardium. Clinically the signs are of right-sided heart strain with ascites, hepatomegaly and a raised JVP. There may be pulsus paradoxus and hypotension, and auscultation reveals a pericardial 'knock' due to an abrupt end to ventricular filling. The CXR may show pericardial calcification. Management is by pericardiectomy (pericardial stripping) if constriction is severe.

Cardiomyopathy

Cardiomyopathy is a disorder of the heart muscle. There are four major types of cardiomyopathy: hypertrophic, dilated,

Table 28.15 Causes of cardiomyopathy

Cause	Examples
Toxic	Alcohol, cyclophosphamide, corticosteroids, lithium, phenothiazines
Metabolic	Thiamine deficiency, pellagra, obesity, porphyria, uraemia
Endocrine	Thyrotoxicosis, acromegaly, myxoedema, Cushing disease, diabetes mellitus
Collagen diseases	Systemic lupus erythematosus, polyarteritis nodosum
Infiltrative	Amyloidosis, haemochromatosis, neoplasia, sarcoidosis, mucopolysaccharidosis, Whipple disease
Infective	Viral, rickettsial, mycobacterial
Genetic	Hypertrophic cardiomyopathy, muscular dystrophies
Fibroplastic	Endomyocardial fibrosis, Löffler endomyocardial disease, carcinoid
Miscellaneous	Ischaemic heart disease, pregnancy

restrictive and arrhythmogenic. Table 28.15 gives examples of the causes.

Hypertrophic obstructive cardiomyopathy

HOCM is an autosomal dominant genetic disorder, although most cases occur sporadically. There is asymmetrical left ventricular hypertrophy, usually of the intraventricular septum, associated with mitral dysfunction and impaired diastolic filling. Patients are at an increased risk of left ventricular outflow tract obstruction and tachyarrhythmias.

Symptoms of HOCM include breathlessness, angina, palpitations and syncope. On examination there is a jerky pulse, the apex beat has a double impulse, third and fourth heart sounds may be present and there is a harsh ejection systolic murmur best heard at the left sternal edge when the patient is upright or performing a Valsalva manoeuvre.

ECG shows left ventricular hypertrophy and sometimes AF, LBBB or ventricular ectopics. The classic echocardiography finding is asymmetrical septal hypertrophy and systolic anterior movement of the mitral valve. Cardiac catheterization shows a small left ventricular cavity with obliteration in systole. There is a systolic outflow tract gradient within the ventricle.

HOCM may be complicated by AF, systemic emboli, heart failure and sudden death.

Management focuses on symptom control and prevention of complications. Antiarrhythmics or radiofrequency catheter ablation are used for rhythm control. β-Blockers or verapamil help with symptoms and are useful for angina and left ventricular dysfunction. If HOCM is refractory to medical treatment, patients can be considered for a dual-chamber pacemaker, septal myomectomy, myotomy or cardiac transplantation. Patients' first-degree relatives should be screened as HOCM is a risk factor for sudden death in young people.

Dilated cardiomyopathy

This is characterized by poorly contracting dilated ventricles that have a left ventricular wall with normal thickness. Causes include CVD, alcohol, infiltrative disorders, collagen diseases, infection, toxins, metabolic abnormalities and pregnancy.

There are usually signs and symptoms of bi-ventricular cardiomegaly and AF. Patients may have permanent tachycardia with a low BP. The apex beat may feel diffuse, with an S_3 gallop rhythm and potential mitral and/or tricuspid valve regurgitation. More dangerous arrhythmias and conduction defects occur. Echocardiography shows a globally hypokinetic and dilated heart.

Management includes treatment of the underlying condition. Heart failure treatment should be initiated with antiarrhythmics and anticoagulants where appropriate. The prognosis is variable. Patients should be considered for cardiac transplantation. Without transplantation, 5-year mortality is 25%.

Restrictive/infiltrative cardiomyopathy

This is due to endomyocardial stiffening with normal left ventricular size and function. Causes include fibroplastic and infiltrative conditions as shown in Table 28.15. Amyloidosis is the leading cause in the United Kingdom. In restrictive cardiomyopathy diastolic function is impaired and clinical features include those of right-sided heart strain. The ECG may show small voltage complexes. The differential diagnosis includes constrictive pericarditis. A myocardial biopsy may be indicated.

Arrhythmogenic right ventricular dysplasia/cardiomyopathy

Arrhythmogenic right ventricular dysplasia is a rare, genetic disorder of desmosomal function leading to fibrofatty deposits and inflammatory changes. It predominately affects the right side of the heart. The most common presentation is with symptomatic arrhythmias, syncope or sudden death. Management includes standard heart failure treatment and cardiac transplantation.

Infective endocarditis

Infective endocarditis is an illness caused by microbial infection of the cardiac valves or endocardium. The annual incidence is approximately 10 in 100,000 with 30-day mortality as high as 30%. It follows invasion of the bloodstream by microorganisms, most often from the mouth, gastrointestinal, genitourinary or respiratory tracts or skin. Platelets adhere to endothelial breaks and form vegetations, which are then colonized by circulating bacteria. Common sites of infection include bicuspid aortic valves and mitral valves, with prolapse and regurgitation.

Risk factors for infective endocarditis include abnormal or prosthetic heart valves (although 50% of cases occur with normal valves), structural heart defects, intravenous drug use, hypertrophic cardiomyopathy and immunocompromise.

Staphylococcus aureus spp is the commonest pathogen; others include *Streptococcus viridans*, Group D streptococci, *Streptococcus faecalis*, *Streptococcus intermedius* and *Staphylococcus epidermidis*, especially in intravenous drug users. *Pseudomonas aeruginosa*, organisms from the HACEK group (**H**aemophilus spp, **A**ggregatibacter actinomycetemcomitans, **C**ardiobacterium spp, **E**ikenella corrodens, **K**ingella kingae) and enterococci are some of the non-streptococci pathogenic causes.

Clinical features

The diagnosis should be suspected in a patient with fever and a new or changing heart murmur, unexplained positive blood cultures and unexplained new embolic events. Clinical features include:

- Infection: fever, malaise and lassitude, sweats, myalgia, arthralgia, weight loss, finger clubbing, anaemia.
- Heart disease: murmurs. In tricuspid endocarditis the patient may not have a murmur. Later in disease progression signs of tricuspid insufficiency or right-sided heart failure (raised venous pressure, pulsatile liver) can develop.
- Lung disease: embolic pneumonia, pleurisy or haemoptysis.
- Vascular phenomena: arterial emboli (most emboli are sterile but large fungal mycelia may embolize), intracranial haemorrhage, Janeway's lesions, conjunctival haemorrhages, septic pulmonary infarcts, mycotic aneurysm.

Table 28.16 Duke criteria for the diagnosis of infective endocarditis

Major criteria	• Blood cultures positive for endocarditis: typical organism in two separate blood cultures or persistently positive blood cultures • Endocardial involvement: positive echocardiogram (vegetation/oscillating intracardial mass, dehiscence of prosthetic valve, abscess, new valvular regurgitation)
Minor criteria	• Predisposition (e.g., mechanical valve, IVDU) • Fever (>38°C) • Vascular phenomena • Immunological phenomena • Positive blood culture that does not meet major criteria • Echocardiographic features consistent with the disease but not meeting major criteria

For a diagnosis of infective endocarditis, the patient must meet either two major criteria or one major with three minor criteria or five minor criteria. IVDU, Intravenous drug use.

- Immunological phenomena: examples include vasculitic skin lesions, glomerulonephritis, splinter haemorrhages, Roth spots in the retina and Osler nodes. They are classic signs of infective endocarditis but are often absent early in disease progression.

Table 28.16 lists the modified Duke criteria for diagnosis of infective endocarditis.

CLINICAL NOTES

INVESTIGATIONS IN INFECTIVE ENDOCARDITIS

- Blood cultures: numerous (at least three) sets from different sites at different times are needed and are a part of the diagnostic criteria.
- Full blood count and C-reactive protein: normochromic normocytic anaemia; raised inflammatory markers.
- Chest X-ray: in right-sided endocarditis multiple shadows resulting from embolic pneumonia and pulmonary infarction may be present.
- ECG: ischaemic changes due to coronary embolism or conduction defect due to the development of an aortic root abscess, look for a prolonged PR interval.
- Echocardiography: vegetations or paravalvular abscess formation. Negative transthoracic echocardiography findings do not exclude the diagnosis and transoesophageal echocardiography is preferred as it is more sensitive.

Management

Taking blood cultures should not delay treatment in an acutely unwell patient. Patients with endocarditis require a prolonged course of antibiotics, given intravenously in most cases. The exact regimen depends on the positive cultures plus local resistance patterns, which should be reflected in hospital-specific antibiotic guidelines. Empirical therapy should be started while culture results are awaited. Generally, cell-wall inhibitors (e.g., β-lactams or glycopeptides such as vancomycin) combined with an aminoglycoside (e.g., gentamicin) are a good first-line therapy. If fungal infection is suspected, antifungal agents should be added.

Surgical intervention may be needed for haemodynamic complications such as acute severe valvular regurgitation or valve obstruction by vegetations, for intractable heart failure, cardiac abscess formation and resistant infections.

CLINICAL NOTES

POSSIBLE CAUSES OF ENDOCARDITIS IN THE EVENT OF NEGATIVE CULTURES

- *Coxiella burnetii* (Q fever).
- Fungi (e.g., *Aspergillus*, *Histoplasma*).
- Partially treated bacterial endocarditis.
- Systemic lupus erythematous.
- Nonbacterial endocarditis associated with carcinoma.
- Atrial myxoma.

CLINICAL NOTES

THE ROLE OF ANTIBIOTIC PROPHYLAXIS IN INFECTIVE ENDOCARDITIS

NICE does not recommend routine antibiotic prophylaxis against infective endocarditis in at-risk patients undergoing dental, gastrointestinal or genitourinary, or upper and lower respiratory tract procedures.

At-risk patients include:

- Valve replacement
- Previous infective endocarditis
- Hypertrophic cardiomyopathy
- Acquired valvular heart disease with stenosis or regurgitation
- Structural congenital heart disease (excluding isolated ASD, fully repaired VSD and fully repaired patent ductus arteriosus)

Rheumatic fever

Acute rheumatic fever is a multisystem immune disease following infection with a group A β-haemolytic streptococcus. Antibodies generated against the bacteria bind to and damage the heart, nervous system, joints and skin. The multisystem involvement reflects the vasculitic nature of the underlying disease. It is rare in the developed world because of the use of antibiotics for pharyngeal infection and reduced virulence of the organism. It usually affects children aged 5 to 15 years but no age is immune. Risk factors include crowding and low socioeconomic status. The incubation period is 1 to 5 weeks after a throat infection.

The diagnosis of acute rheumatic fever is based on clinical findings organized by the Jones criteria. The presence of two major criteria or one major and two minor criteria, along with evidence of streptococcal infection, indicates a high probability of rheumatic fever (Table 28.17).

Major Jones criteria

Carditis (40%–50%)

There may be myocarditis (this can manifest itself with features of cardiac failure), endocarditis (the mitral valve is most commonly affected) or pericarditis. It is more evident in children, and may be asymptomatic or result in death in the acute stage. Carditis can lead to heart failure and chronic valvular heart disease. The initial mortality rate is low at 1%.

Polyarthralgia (80%)

This is the most common major criterion and usually presents as migratory joint pain affecting larger joints. The onset is sudden with signs of inflammation and limitation of movement. It responds well to antiinflammatory drugs and rarely leaves any residual deformity. Symptoms last for 3 to 6 weeks.

Chorea (Sydenham chorea) (10%)

Movements are choreoathetoid and involuntary, involving mainly the face and limbs, and may be unilateral. It is associated with emotional lability. There can be a latent period of 2 to 6 months. Symptoms last for approximately 6 months. It is commoner in girls. There may be no other signs of rheumatic fever.

Table 28.17 Revised Jones criteria for guidance in the diagnosis of rheumatic fever

Major	Minor
Polyarthritis	Fever (≥38.5°C)
Carditis	Polyarthralgia
Sydenham chorea	Previous rheumatic fever or rheumatic heart disease
Erythema marginatum	Raised levels of CRP and/or ESR
Subcutaneous nodules	ECG with prolonged PR interval

For a diagnosis of rheumatic fever, there must also be supporting evidence of preceding streptococcal infection.
CRP, C-reactive protein; ESR, erythrocyte sedimentation rate.

Erythema marginatum (5%)

This is a painless rash appearing as large, pink macules that spread quickly to give a serpiginous edge with a fading centre. The face is usually spared.

Subcutaneous nodules (rare)

These are round, firm and painless, ranging from 0.5 to 2 cm. They are mobile and occur mainly over bony prominences.

Management

Although antiinflammatory drugs (aspirin, NSAIDs, corticosteroids) relieve the pain and swelling of joints and can reduce the severity of cardiac involvement, evidence of their effectiveness in changing overall disease progression is lacking. Patients with evidence of an ongoing bacterial infection should be given antibiotics.

Atrial myxomata

These are rare, benign, primary tumours, usually in the left atrium, which are twice as common in women as men. They present with vague symptoms (e.g., fever, weight loss, general malaise, AF, left atrial obstruction or systemic emboli). Auscultation may reveal a diastolic 'tumour plop'. Erythrocyte sedimentation rate is characteristically raised. They are diagnosed by echocardiography, and treatment is by surgical excision.

CONGENITAL HEART DISEASE IN ADULTS

Congenital heart disease is any defect of the heart present at the time of birth. The disease may cause impairment of flow, contraction or electrical conduction. Broadly speaking, congenital heart disease affecting blood flow can be divided into acyanotic (left-to-right shunt, see Fig. 28.30) or cyanotic (right-to-left shunt).

Acyanotic conditions

Atrial septal defect

ASD accounts for 10% of congenital heart defects and is more common in women than in men. There are two types: ostium secundum ASD (the more common type) and ostium primum ASD. Ostium secundum ASD is confined to the fossa ovalis, and is a defect in the septum primum. Ostium primum ASD is a defect at the level of the tricuspid and mitral valves that lies at

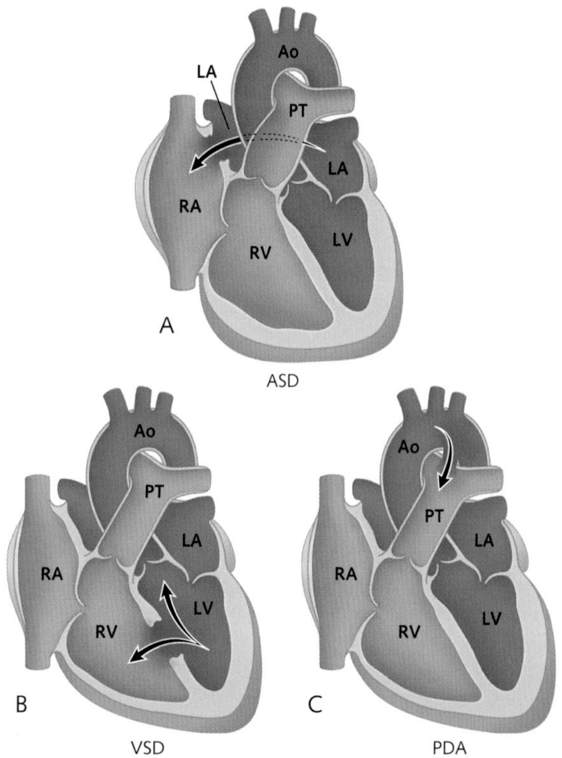

Fig. 28.30 Common congenital left-to-right shunts (*arrows* indicate the direction of blood flow). (A) Atrial septal defect (ASD). (B) Ventricular septal defect (VSD). (C) Patent ductus arteriosus (PDA). *Ao,* Aorta; *LA,* left atrium; *LV,* left ventricle; *PT,* pulmonary trunk; *RA,* right atrium; *RV,* right ventricle. (From Mitchell RN, et al. *Pocket Companion to Robbins and Cotran Pathologic Basis of Disease*, 10th ed. Elsevier; 2024.)

the inferior margin of the fossa ovalis. It belongs to the AV septal defect group.

The communication between the atria allows left-to-right atrial shunting. Atrial arrhythmias are common. In ostium primum ASD, there may be involvement of the mitral and tricuspid valves producing regurgitation.

Most patients are asymptomatic; a few have dyspnoea and weakness. The patient may have palpitations secondary to atrial arrhythmias, and right-sided heart strain may develop later in life. Auscultation reveals wide, fixed splitting of the second heart sound. The increased right-sided heart output gives rise to a pulmonary systolic flow murmur. A tricuspid diastolic flow murmur can be present with large defects. There may be a left parasternal heave of right ventricular hypertrophy.

Echocardiography reveals dilatation of the right-sided cardiac chambers. Cardiac catheterization demonstrates a step-up in oxygen saturation at the right atrial level due to the shunting of oxygenated blood from the left atrium to the right atrium.

Ventricular septal defect

VSD is the most common congenital heart lesion, accounting for approximately one-third of all malformations. Blood moves from the high-pressure left ventricle to the right ventricle. If the defect is large, pulmonary flow increases, leading to obliterative pulmonary vascular changes and an increase in pulmonary vascular resistance. The pulmonary arterial pressure may then equal the systemic pressure, reducing or reversing the shunt, and central cyanosis may develop (Eisenmenger syndrome).

A small defect (maladie de Roger) may cause no symptoms but there is a loud pansystolic murmur at the left sternal edge; it may close spontaneously. Larger VSDs produce breathlessness and fatigue. The apex beat is prominent as a result of left ventricular hypertrophy, and there may be a left parasternal heave if there is right ventricular hypertrophy with pulmonary hypertension. There is a thrill at the left sternal edge, as well as a pansystolic murmur in the same place. A mitral diastolic flow murmur implies a large shunt.

Echocardiography is diagnostic if the defect can be imaged. Cardiac catheterization will show a step-up in oxygen saturation at the right ventricular level due to the shunting of oxygenated blood from the left ventricle to the right ventricle. Left ventricular angiography produces opacification of the right ventricle through the defect.

Moderate and large defects should be closed surgically to prevent pulmonary hypertension and Eisenmenger syndrome.

Patent ductus arteriosus

PDA accounts for approximately 10% of congenital heart defects and is more common in women. The ductus arteriosus connects the pulmonary artery to the descending aorta but should close off at birth. Because the aortic pressure is higher than the pulmonary artery pressure throughout the cardiac cycle, the PDA produces continuous shunting from the aorta to the pulmonary artery, leading to an increased pulmonary venous return to the left side of the heart and an increased left ventricular volume load.

Patients with small shunts are usually asymptomatic. Large shunts lead to left ventricular failure with breathlessness. The pulse is collapsing. There may be left ventricular hypertrophy. There is a continuous machinery murmur with systolic accentuation loudest in the first or second left intercostal space. Patients are also more likely to develop lower respiratory tract infections.

Echocardiography shows dilatation of the left-sided cardiac chambers and abnormal flow across the ductus. Cardiac catheterization demonstrates a step-up in oxygen saturation at the pulmonary artery level.

Indometacin is effective only if given in utero or to preterm infants (stimulates duct closure by inhibiting prostaglandin synthesis). PDA closure is indicated for symptomatic patients or those with features of heart failure. This can be achieved with interventional radiology techniques or surgically.

Aortic coarctation

This accounts for 5% to 7% of congenital heart defects. It is more common in White people and men. It is associated with Turner syndrome, Marfan syndrome and berry aneurysms. There is a narrowing of the aorta at or just distal to the ductus arteriosus; the vast majority are distal to the origin of the left subclavian artery. The condition is a cause of secondary hypertension. It encourages the formation of a collateral arterial circulation involving the intercostal arteries. In 30% of patients, there is an associated bicuspid aortic valve.

In adults, the condition is often asymptomatic until long-standing hypertension becomes apparent. When present, symptoms include headache, left ventricular failure, stroke and endocarditis. On examination the femoral pulses are weak or absent and there is radiofemoral delay. The upper limbs may be hypertensive or have unequal BP, and the lower limbs have a low BP. There may be features of left ventricular hypertrophy. There is a mid-systolic or late-systolic murmur over the upper precordium or back due to turbulent flow through the coarctation. Collateral murmurs may be heard over the scapulae, and there may be an aortic systolic murmur of an associated bicuspid valve.

CXR shows tortuous and dilated collaterals that may erode the undersurface of the ribs to produce rib notching. There may be a double aortic knuckle due to stenosis and poststenotic dilatation. MRI and aortography confirm the diagnosis. Treatment is by surgical resection or balloon angioplasty.

Aortic and pulmonary stenosis

Clinical features and management of aortic stenosis have been covered previously in this chapter. The commonest congenital abnormality is a bicuspid valve (1%–2%) which results in chronic turbulent flow leading to calcification of the leaflets. Supravalvular aortic stenosis is associated with Williams syndrome.

Pulmonary stenosis is rare and often asymptomatic until severe. Patients can present with exertional dyspnoea, light-headedness and symptoms of right-sided heart strain. It is associated with Noonan syndrome and Alagille syndrome. In general, invasive intervention is recommended (valvotomy is very effective).

Cyanotic conditions

Tetralogy of Fallot

This represents 6% to 10% of cases of congenital heart disease. The four features composing the tetrad are:

- VSD
- Right ventricular outflow obstruction (pulmonary stenosis – infundibular or valvar)
- The aorta being positioned over the ventricular septum ('overriding aorta')
- Right ventricular hypertrophy

Because there is right ventricular outflow obstruction, the shunt through the VSD is from right to left (Fig. 28.31). This results in central cyanosis.

Children may present with deep cyanosis and syncope. Squatting helps to decrease the right-to-left shunt by increasing systemic resistance. Signs include cyanosis and finger clubbing. There is a parasternal heave and systolic murmur in the pulmonary area (second left intercostal space), P_2 is soft or absent, and there may be a growth retardation.

The heart is boot-shaped (coeur en sabot) and the pulmonary artery is small with oligaemic lung fields on a chest radiograph. Echocardiography can be diagnostic, but it may be necessary to proceed to cardiac catheterization studies to confirm the disorder.

Management is by total surgical correction. Palliative procedures as holding measures can be used (e.g., the modified Blalock–Taussig shunt, which produces an anastomosis between a subclavian artery and a pulmonary artery to increase pulmonary blood flow).

Transposition of the great arteries

TGA (Fig. 28.31) accounts for 5% of all congenital heart diseases. It is more common in males than females. The aorta arises from the right ventricle while the pulmonary vein from the left ventricle; this means that the systemic and pulmonary circulations instead of normal in-series arrangement, become parallel with deoxygenated venous blood pumped back into the body via the left ventricle and oxygenated pulmonary blood circulating back to the lungs. Different pathological variants exist, TGA without VSD, TGA with VSD and TGA with VSD and pulmonary stenosis. Clinical presentation depends on the anatomical type. If no VSD is present cyanosis is evident while in patients with a large VSD blood mixing means that cyanosis is minimal. Treatment is surgical.

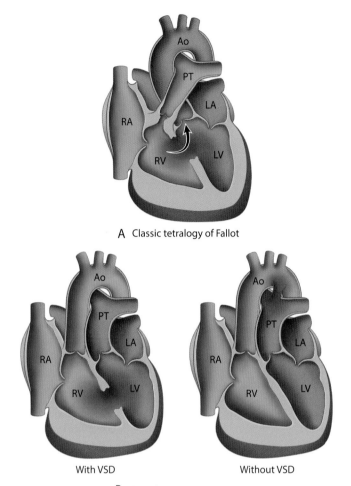

A Classic tetralogy of Fallot

With VSD   Without VSD

B Complete transposition

Fig. 28.31 Common congenital right-to-left shunts (cyanotic congenital heart disease). (A) Tetralogy of Fallot (*arrow* indicates direction of blood flow). (B) Transposition of the great arteries with and without VSD. *Ao*, Aorta; *LA*, left atrium; *LV*, left ventricle; *PT*, pulmonary trunk; *RA*, right atrium; *RV*, right ventricle; *VSD*, ventricular septal defect. (From Kumar V, et al. *Robbins & Kumar Basic Pathology*. 11th ed. Elsevier; 2023.)

Tricuspid atresia

Clinical features include cyanosis, right heart strain, heart failure and growth retardation. Neonates with significantly limited pulmonary blood flow can be managed with prostaglandins which prevent the closure of the ductus arteriosus allowing blood mixing. Definitive treatment is surgical.

Chapter Summary

- Cardiovascular disease is one of the biggest killers in the United Kingdom. Modifiable risk factors include hypertension, diabetes mellitus, obesity and smoking. It can present as stable angina or acute coronary syndrome. Both of those syndromes result from inadequate oxygenation of the cardiac muscle.
- Drug treatments for CVD include antiplatelet agents, nitrates, β-blockers, calcium channel blockers, potassium channel activators, angiotensin-converting enzyme (ACE) inhibitors and lipid-lowering drugs.
- Acute coronary syndrome is a medical emergency that includes ST elevation myocardial infarction, non-ST elevation myocardial infarction and unstable angina. It usually results from atherosclerotic plaque rupture. If STEMI is present, urgent percutaneous coronary intervention should be undertaken. Revascularization can be delayed in NSTEMI unless patients have an immediate or higher risk of death or future cardiovascular events.
- Atrial fibrillation is the most common sustained cardiac arrhythmia. Causes can include CVD, valvular disease, infection or electrolyte disturbances. Two approaches to treatment exist: rate control and rhythm control. Generally, rate control is recommended as the first-line option unless the patient has a reversible cause of the arrhythmia, heart failure, the AF is of new onset or rhythm control is deemed more suitable. Anticoagulation should be considered in all patients with AF.
- Heart failure is a clinical syndrome where the heart cannot meet the demands placed on it by the body. It can present as an acute problem or it can be of chronic nature. Acute heart failure is a medical emergency. ACE inhibitors and diuretics are the mainstay of treatment. β-Blockers, are used in chronic heart failure with preserved ejection fraction. In the context of heart failure with reduced ejection fraction optimal pharmacological treatments include ACE inhibitors or ARNI, β-blockers, mineralocorticoid and SGLT2 inhibitors. Nondrug treatments include implantable cardiac devices.
- Hypertension can be essential (no underlying cause identified) or secondary (to, e.g., kidney, vascular, endocrine or heart disease). Treatment includes a stepwise approach of introduction of drugs depending on the patient's age and ethnicity.
- Rheumatic fever is the most common cause of mitral stenosis. Aortic stenosis is usually the result of a calcified bicuspid valve.
- Pericarditis can lead to the development of cardiac tamponade. Cardiac tamponade is a medical emergency. Treatment is with pericardiocentesis.
- Hypertrophic obstructive cardiomyopathy is an autosomal dominant genetic disorder that leads to left ventricular hypertrophy and cardiac dysfunction. Patients are at risk of sudden cardiac death.
- *Staphylococcus aureus* is the commonest pathogen responsible for infective endocarditis. Modified Duke criteria are used for diagnosis.
- Rheumatic fever is a multisystem immune disease that follows infection with a group A β-haemolytic streptococcus.

UKMLA Conditions
Acute coronary syndromes
Aortic aneurysm
Aortic valve disease
Arrhythmia
Arterial thrombosis
Arterial ulcers
Cardiac arrest
Cardiac failure
Deep vein thrombosis
Essential or secondary hypertension
Infective endocarditis
Ischaemic heart disease

UKMLA Presentations
Breathlessness
Cardiorespiratory arrest
Chest pain
Cyanosis
Dizziness
Driving advice
Erectile dysfunction
Heart murmurs
Hypertension
Limb claudication
Low blood pressure
Palpitations

Continued

● Chapter Summary—cont'd

UKMLA Conditions
Mitral valve disease
Myocardial infarction
Myocarditis
Pericardial disease
Peripheral vascular disease
Pulmonary embolism
Pulmonary hypertension
Right heart valve disease
Vasovagal syncope

UKMLA Presentations
Peripheral oedema and ankle swelling

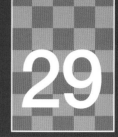
INTRODUCTION

In this chapter we review the clinical features, investigations and management of common respiratory conditions. The examination of the respiratory system is covered in Chapter 2 and important differentials for shortness of breath, cough and haemoptysis, alongside their examination findings are found in Chapters 5 and 6, respectively.

RESPIRATORY FAILURE

Respiratory failure is a dysfunction of gas exchange resulting in abnormalities of oxygenation or ventilation, leading to hypoxia (low blood oxygen levels) and/or hypercapnia (high blood carbon dioxide levels). Respiratory failure is present when the partial pressure of oxygen in arterial blood (PaO_2) is less than 8.0 kPa (in a patient breathing air at sea level). This can be divided into:

- **Type I (hypoxaemic) respiratory failure:** hypoxia combined with a normal or low partial pressure of CO_2 ($PaCO_2$). The primary cause is a ventilation–perfusion ($\dot{V}/\dot{Q}$) mismatch.
- **Type II (hypercapnic) respiratory failure:** hypoxia combined with a raised $PaCO_2$ (>6.0 kPa). The underlying cause is alveolar hypoventilation, with or without $\dot{V}/\dot{Q}$ mismatch (see also Clinical Notes: alveolar-arterial gradient).

The clinical features of respiratory failure can be thought of as those due to:

- *Hypoxaemia* (present in both type I and type II): dyspnoea, restlessness, central cyanosis and eventually impaired consciousness, or
- *Hypercapnia* (type II): headache, tachycardia with bounding pulse, tremor and clouding of consciousness.

An arterial blood gas (ABG) is essential to diagnose respiratory failure.

Investigations useful in respiratory failure include:

- Blood tests: full blood count (FBC) to look for anaemia, polycythaemia, leucocytosis; urea and electrolytes (U&Es); C-reactive protein (CRP); blood cultures if the patient is pyrexial.
- Imaging: chest X-ray (CXR); CT pulmonary angiogram (CTPA) if pulmonary embolism (PE) is suspected.
- Sputum microscopy, culture and sensitivities.
- Spirometry.

The course of the disease and its prognosis depends on the underlying disorder and the premorbid condition of the patient.

CLINICAL NOTES

ALVEOLAR–ARTERIAL GRADIENT

Alveolar–arterial (A–a gradient) is a measure used to determine the origin of hypoxemia (intrapulmonary or extrapulmonary). It is the difference between the alveolar (A) and arterial (a) oxygen concentration. It is calculated from the following formula:

$$A\text{–}a\ Gradient = [(FiO_2) \times (Atmospheric\ Pressure - H_2O\ Pressure) - (PaCO_2/0.8)] - PaO_2$$

An elevated A–a gradient indicates $\dot{V}/\dot{Q}$ mismatch, shunt or alveolar hypoventilation.

A depressed A–a gradient points towards hypoventilation or low inspired oxygen levels.

Type I respiratory failure (T1RF)

Causes
T1RF can occur as a result of:

- Low inspired oxygen concentration (FiO_2) (e.g., high altitude)
- $\dot{V}/\dot{Q}$ mismatch (e.g., PE, atelectasis)
- Shunting, for example, right-to-left shunt where mixing of oxygenated and nonoxygenated blood occurs (e.g., patent foramen ovale, atrial septal defects)
- Alveolar hypoventilation (e.g., neuromuscular disorders causing respiratory muscle weakness, chest wall deformities, interstitial lung disease (ILD))
- Altered gas diffusion (e.g., pneumonia, acute respiratory distress syndrome (ARDS), pulmonary fibrosis)

Management
In acute hypoxaemic respiratory failure, oxygen delivery to vital organs must be ensured. Hypoxia is life-threatening, and oxygen therapy is indicated to maintain saturations of more than 90% (PaO_2 >8 kPa). The British Thoracic Society (BTS) recommends target saturation of 94% to 98% for oxygen saturations

for most patients. Oxygen can be delivered via nasal cannula (up to 5 L/min), simple face masks (up to 10 L/min), nonrebreath masks (up to 15 L/min), venturi masks (specific FiO_2 per mask, 2–15 L) or assisted ventilation may be necessary (see Clinical Notes: assisted ventilation). Continuous positive airway pressure (CPAP) is particularly useful in T1RF.

Therapeutic objectives in T1RF include:

- Specific therapy of underlying causes (e.g., antimicrobial therapy for pneumonia, bronchodilators/steroids for asthma or chest drain insertion for pneumothorax).
- General supportive care: adequate hydration, nutrition and electrolyte balance.

CLINICAL NOTES

ASSISTED VENTILATION

'Assisted ventilation' describes the delivery of ventilatory support to assist or replace spontaneous respiration. Assisted ventilation is associated with airway and alveolar damage through mechanisms such as oxygen toxicity, volutrauma (overstretching), barotrauma (over pressure), biotrauma (shear forces) and cardiac overstimulation.

Modes of assisted ventilation include:

- High-flow nasal oxygen (HFNO): high-flow oxygen (heated and humidified) is delivered through nasal cannula, facilitating gas exchange. It can achieve an FiO_2 as high as 100% in a flow of up to 60 L/min. It generates positive end-expiratory pressure, impeding atelectasis and reduces the work of breathing. It is well tolerated by patients. Impaired respiratory drive is a contraindication to its use.
- Noninvasive ventilation (NIV): delivers oxygen without the use of an invasive artificial airway. NIV creates inspiratory and expiratory positive airway pressure leading to air moving via a pressure gradient. This cyclical mode of ventilation facilitates CO_2 clearance, airway opening and reduces the work of breathing. It is particularly useful in CO_2 retention or chronic obstructive pulmonary disease. High expiratory positive airway pressure reduces preload and therefore decreases stroke volume. 'BIPAP' (bi-level positive airway pressure – machine trade name) is a term often used to refer to NIV.
- Continuous positive airway pressure (CPAP): continuous positive pressure is delivered through all phases of ventilation, facilitating oxygenation. It promotes alveolar opening, increases the functional residual capacity and reduces left ventricular transmural pressure, increasing cardiac output. CPAP is particularly useful in obstructive sleep apnoea and congestive cardiac failure. Care should be taken in patients with low blood pressure as CPAP reduces venous return.

Invasive ventilation: support is administered with the use of an invasive artificial airway. This can be penetrating through the nose (nasotracheal), mouth (endotracheal) or skin (tracheostomy).

Type II respiratory failure (T2RF)

A rise in $PaCO_2$ should cause an increase in ventilation by central stimulation of the respiratory centres in the medulla, resulting in an increase in minute ventilation to lower $PaCO_2$. In T2RF, this mechanism fails, and there is effective alveolar hypoventilation. This can be due to several causes.

Causes

Type II respiratory failure can occur as a result of:

- Reduced breathing effort, including reduced central drive (e.g., sedation and brainstem disorders, obesity, drugs).
- Neuromuscular disease (e.g., Guillain–Barré syndrome, motor neurone disease, spinal cord lesions, poliomyelitis, myasthenia gravis and diaphragmatic palsy).
- Thoracic wall abnormalities (e.g., kyphoscoliosis).
- Increased airway resistance (e.g., asthma, chronic obstructive pulmonary disease (COPD), pneumonia and lung fibrosis).

Management

As in type I failure, ensuring adequate oxygenation is key. However, care must be taken when high oxygen concentrations are being delivered to patients with chronic T2RF, as they rely on their hypoxic drive for ventilation because of chronic CO_2 retention.

Oxygen therapy must be carefully controlled. Venturi masks are used to maintain oxygen saturations of 88% to 92% (target saturation for patients at risk of CO_2 retention). Oxygen concentration is titrated to achieve normoxaemia without acidosis (see BTS Guideline for oxygen use in adults in healthcare and emergency settings. May 2017). Assisted ventilation may be necessary (see Clinical Notes: assisted ventilation), NIV is particularly useful in T2RF.

Therapeutic objectives in T2RF include:

- Specific therapy of the underlying cause (e.g., antimicrobial and bronchodilator therapy for an infective exacerbation of COPD).
- General supportive care as for type I failure.

ASTHMA

Asthma is a disease of the airways characterized by an increased responsiveness of the tracheobronchial tree to many different stimuli, resulting in paroxysmal, reversible, airway obstruction. Asthma is episodic, with acute exacerbations interspersed by symptom-free periods. Most attacks are short (minutes to hours), with complete clinical recovery. In severe asthma, patients can experience some degree of airway obstruction daily, with accompanying symptoms.

Asthma is common, with a prevalence of approximately 12% of the population in the United Kingdom. The incidence is higher in children. In the United Kingdom, more than 1000 people die of acute asthma attacks every year.

Aetiology

Asthma is likely to be a combination of multiple environmental and genetic factors.

Often, those with asthma are atopic, with the production of IgE in response to an antigenic challenge. Atopic asthma can be associated with a personal or family history of allergy such as hayfever, urticaria and eczema. There may also be increased levels of IgE in the serum and a positive response to provocation tests (e.g., histamine or methacholine challenge).

'Intrinsic asthma' is a term used to describe patients with no personal or family history of allergy, negative skin test results and normal serum levels of IgE. Many develop typical symptoms following an upper respiratory tract infection.

Many patients do not fit into either category but fall into a group with a mixture of allergic and nonallergic features.

Pathophysiology

Many theories and mediators are proposed regarding the mechanisms for asthma. The role of IgE, various cytokines and chemokines, mast cells, histamine, eosinophils, leucotrienes, cell adhesion molecules and activated T lymphocytes – in particular the balance between Th1 and Th2 cells – provides much academic debate and has provided new therapeutic targets such as monoclonal antibodies against IgE.

The clinical features of asthma probably derive from chronic airway inflammation causing denuded airway epithelium, inflammatory cell infiltrate, mast cell activation and smooth muscle and mucous gland hypertrophy.

The two main pathophysiological events responsible for acute asthma exacerbations are bronchospasm (smooth muscle spasm leading to airway narrowing) and airway plugging secondary to excessive secretions. Vascular congestion and oedema formation are also involved.

A number of factors interact with normal airway responsiveness and provoke acute episodes, including:

- allergens (e.g., house dust mites and animal dander);
- drugs (e.g., β-blockers and nonsteroidal antiinflammatory drugs);
- environmental factors (e.g., climate conditions and air pollution);
- occupations (e.g., exposure to industrial chemicals, drugs, metals, dusts);
- infections (e.g., viral and bacterial);
- exercise;
- emotion;
- cigarette smoke.

Clinical features

The classic symptoms of asthma consist of shortness of breath, wheeze, chest tightness and cough. Nocturnal symptoms are very common due to diurnal variation. Symptoms may resolve spontaneously or may be relieved by treatment.

In its most typical form, asthma is an episodic disease and the symptoms coexist. At the onset of an attack, patients experience tightness in the chest, often with a nonproductive cough. Breathing becomes audibly harsh, speech is difficult, wheezing becomes prominent and expiration is prolonged as airflow is reduced. Patients are frequently tachypnoeic and tachycardic. If the attack is severe or prolonged, there may be a loss of breath sounds, and the wheeze becomes either very high-pitched or inaudible as airflow is severely compromised. Accessory muscles of respiration are used and pulsus paradoxus can develop.

Less typically, a patient with asthma may present with intermittent episodes of nonproductive cough or shortness of breath on exertion. Such patients often have normal physical examination findings but may wheeze after repeated forced exhalations or may show evidence of airway obstruction with spirometry.

Investigations

The diagnosis of asthma is established by demonstration of reversible expiratory airflow obstruction. The National Institute for Health and Care Excellence (NICE) recommends different investigations that can be used, including as standard:

- Fractional exhaled nitric oxide (FeNO) test, used to measure the level of airway inflammation – in adults positive if a result of 40 parts per billion (ppb) or more is obtained.
- Bronchodilator reversibility (BDR) test. In adults positive if improvement in the forced expiratory volume in 1 second (FEV$_1$) of 12% or more and increase in volume of 200 mL or more is observed following administration of a β$_2$-agonist.
- Spirometry: demonstrating an obstructive picture (FEV$_1$/FVC ratio <70%). Note, in asymptomatic patients, normal spirometry findings do not exclude asthma.

Other tests:

- Peak expiratory flow rate (PEFR) diurnal variation: positive if variability is greater than 20% on more than 3 days in a week for 2 weeks. Used if diagnosis is uncertain following above testing.
- Direct bronchial challenge test with histamine or methacholine – positive if provocative concentration of methacholine causing a 20% fall in FEV$_1$ (PC20) is 8 mg/mL or less. Use following above tests if diagnosis remains uncertain.

Once the diagnosis has been confirmed, measurement of PEFR at home, or FEV$_1$ in the clinic, can be used to monitor the course of the illness and the effectiveness of therapy. Eosinophilia and high serum IgE levels may be supportive but are not specific for asthma. Very high serum IgE levels or eosinophilia is not typical for asthma and may indicate asthma plus another diagnosis (e.g., allergic bronchopulmonary aspergillosis (ABPA)).

CLINICAL NOTES

DIFFERENTIAL DIAGNOSIS OF ASTHMA

- Chronic obstructive pulmonary disease
- Upper airway obstruction: tumour, vocal cord dysfunction and laryngeal oedema
- Endobronchial disease: foreign body aspiration, neoplasm, bronchial stenosis
- Left ventricular failure
- Carcinoid tumours
- Recurrent pulmonary emboli
- Eosinophilic pneumonia
- Systemic vasculitis with pulmonary involvement

Management

Chronic asthma requires long-term management (see BTS/Scottish Intercollegiate Guidelines Network (SIGN) asthma guideline, July 2019; NICE, 2017. Asthma: diagnosis, monitoring and chronic asthma management). A patient-centred model of care, which should characterize supporting all patients with a chronic illness, should be applied (i.e., patient education and empowerment, pharmacological therapy and a multidisciplinary approach in hospital and the community).

The therapeutic targets of medications used for asthma include:

- Drugs that inhibit smooth muscle contraction (e.g., β$_2$-agonists, anticholinergics and methylxanthines such as theophylline)
- Drugs that prevent or reverse airway inflammation (e.g., corticosteroids)
- Drugs that modify the action of leucotrienes (e.g., leucotriene antagonists)

Emergency management

Emergency treatment of acute asthma is one of the most common emergencies seen in medical practice. Senior help should be involved early. The features, approach to assessment and treatment of these patients are summarized in Table 29.1.

COMMON PITFALLS

- Raised respiratory rate in a patient who appears otherwise well may be the only sign of a severe attack.
- Silent chest with no evidence of wheeze in a patient with asthma attack signifies poor air entry and is a very poor prognostic sign.
- Patients with increased work of breathing will tire after a period. Reduced respiratory rate (exhaustion) and/or altered state of consciousness (CO$_2$ retention) is a sign of deterioration.

HINTS AND TIPS

Remember to ask patients their best PEFR readings – severity of attacks is graded using this.

Long-term management

The aim of management is control of the disease. Patient education, enabling self-management, is essential and involves

Table 29.1 Checklist for the emergency assessment and treatment of acute asthma

Tasks to consider	Comment
Assessment	Clinical features indicating acute severe asthma (any one of): • inability to complete sentences in one breath • respiratory rate ≥25/min • heart rate ≥110 bpm • peak flow rate 33%–50% best or predicted Features indicating life-threatening attack (if any present): • peak expiratory flow rate <33% best or predicted • oxygen saturation <92% • PaO_2 <8 kPa • $PaCO_2$ normal • cyanosis • poor respiratory effort • silent chest • altered conscious level • exhaustion • arrhythmia • hypotension
Immediate management (in hospital)	Oxygen: aim for saturations of 94%–98% Oxygen-driven nebulizers of: • salbutamol (5 mg): back to back • ipratropium bromide (500 μg) if severe attack Corticosteroids (hydrocortisone 100 mg IV or prednisolone 40–50 mg PO Magnesium sulphate IV (bronchodilatory effect) (1.2–2 g over 20 min) Early senior clinical review and ITU referral Intravenous bronchodilators (aminophylline or salbutamol) may be considered if no improvement
Criteria for hospital admission	• Any life-threatening attack • All severe attacks that do not respond to initial treatment • Previous near-fatal asthma If recovered and peak expiratory flow rate >75% best 1 hour after treatment, consider discharge from the accident and emergency department. Low threshold for admission in afternoon/evening attack or known nocturnal symptoms.
Referral to intensive care	• Persisting or worsening hypoxia • Worsening peak flow despite treatment • Exhaustion or poor respiratory effort • Hypercapnia or acidosis on ABG measurements • Coma or respiratory arrest
Further investigations	Consider: • CXR: if other disease is considered (pneumothorax, infection) • Regular ABG measurements • Bloods (FBC, U&Es) • ECG
Duration of hospital stay	Until symptoms and lung function are stable – on discharge medication for 12–24 hours Peak expiratory flow rate >75% best or predicted Peak expiratory flow rate diurnal variation <25%
Drugs on discharge	Oral steroids (minimum 5 days) Inhaled steroid therapy Inhaled short-acting β_2-agonist Other medications as per stepwise plan
Treatment changes on discharge	GP review within 48 hours of discharge Clinic follow-up arranged within 4 weeks Inhaler technique reviewed Appropriate lifestyle advice given Patient action plan to promote self-management Drug level monitoring if needed

ABG, *Arterial blood gas;* CXR, *chest X-ray;* ECG, *electrocardiogram;* FBC, *full blood count;* $PaCO_2$, *partial pressure of carbon dioxide;* PO_2, *partial pressure of oxygen;* U&Es, *urea and electrolytes.*

identifying triggers and avoiding precipitants (e.g., smoking), monitoring the severity of the illness (PEFR diaries) and adherence to medication. Regular multidisciplinary reviews are important.

A stepwise approach to management of asthma is recommended. The BTS/SIGN guidelines are summarized in Table 29.2. Treatment is stepped up when symptoms are not controlled and should be reduced to the lowest feasible level when control is achieved. Ensure adherence and inhaler technique, and consider the use of spacer devices at each step. If control remains poor despite steps 1 to 3, referral to specialist care is warranted to consider other treatments (e.g., long-acting muscarinic antagonists, theophyllines or monoclonal antibodies). A 'rescue' course of prednisolone can be given at any time and with any step to cover an exacerbation.

In patients aged 6 years or older with poorly controlled (requiring at least four courses of oral corticosteroids in the previous year) severe persistent confirmed allergic IgE-mediated disease, the anti-IgE monoclonal antibody omalizumab may be used, as recommended by NICE.

HINTS AND TIPS

If asthma control is poor, do not forget to assess inhaler technique.

Drug therapy should be kept as simple as possible. Many patients find the division of drugs into 'preventers' and 'relievers' useful to understand their disease and its treatment.

COMMUNICATION

Asthma control can be greatly improved with a clear self-management plan enabling the patient to lead in the symptom control. Asthma nurse specialists and physiotherapists can be crucial in promoting independence.

All patients with asthma should have a personalized asthma action plan.

COMMUNICATION

The Royal College of Physicians devised three simple questions that aid in determining asthma control:

- Have you had difficulty sleeping because of your asthma symptoms (including cough)?
- Have you had your usual asthma symptoms during the day (e.g., cough, wheeze, chest tightness or breathlessness)?
- Has your asthma interfered with your usual activities (e.g., housework, work, school)?

Table 29.2 Stepped care plan for the management of chronic asthma (BTS/SIGN 2019)

Step	Measures
All: Intermittent reliever therapy	Inhaled short-acting β_2-agonist as required
1. Regular preventer therapy	Start low-dose inhaled steroids (ICS) regularly (e.g., beclomethasone, budesonide or fluticasone)
2. Initial add-on therapy	Add long-acting β_2-agonist (LABA) regularly[a]
3. Additional controller therapies	Increase dose of ICS to medium dose **OR** add leucotriene receptor antagonist (LTRA)[a] Note – if no response to LABA consider stopping
4. Specialist therapies	Refer to specialist care

[a]Note: NICE guidance (April 2022) recommends step 2: add LTRA followed by step 3: add LABA.

CHRONIC OBSTRUCTIVE PULMONARY DISEASE

The term 'COPD' includes both chronic bronchitis and emphysema, and is caused by chronic inflammation. It is defined by expiratory airflow limitation with an FEV_1 to forced vital capacity ratio of less than 0.7 and limited reversibility with bronchodilators.

Chronic bronchitis is defined as excessive mucus production sufficient to cause cough with sputum for at least 3 months of the year for more than two consecutive years, in the absence of another condition known to cause sputum production. Emphysema is permanent, abnormal distension of the air spaces distal to the terminal bronchioles with destruction of alveolar walls.

Aetiology

Cigarette smoking

Cigarette smoking is the most commonly identified factor in COPD, thought to be causative in 90% of cases. Prolonged cigarette smoking impairs ciliary movement, inhibits function of alveolar macrophages (dust cells) and leads to hypertrophy and hyperplasia of mucus-secreting glands. An accurate smoking history should be taken and expressed as a pack year history (20 cigarettes per day for 1 year equates to 1 pack year).

Alpha-1 (α1) antitrypsin deficiency

α_1-Antitrypsin is a protease inhibitor, encoded by a gene on chromosome 14, that protects cells against protease such as neutrophil elastases. Patients homozygous (1 in 625 to 1 in 2000) for a deficiency of α_1-antitrypsin (genotype ZZ) have a greatly increased incidence of early-onset emphysema. The defect is in α_1-antitrypsin release from the liver, where the protein is synthesized. Patients with the ZZ genotype have blood levels 10% of those with the normal MM genotype. As well as being at increased risk of developing emphysema, patients with the ZZ genotype are also at risk of chronic liver disease.

Occupation

Occupational exposure to a variety of dusts and fumes (e.g., gold and coal mining) may contribute to the development of COPD, particularly in nonsmokers, and results in a higher prevalence of chronic bronchitis among employees.

Pathophysiology

The hallmark of chronic bronchitis is hypertrophy of the mucus-producing glands found in the submucosa of large cartilaginous airways. Postmortem lungs show goblet cell hyperplasia, mucosal and submucosal inflammatory cells, oedema, peribronchial fibrosis, intraluminal mucous plugs and increased smooth muscle in small airways. Inflammation in chronic bronchitis occurs at the alveolar epithelium, and differs from the predominantly eosinophilic inflammation of asthma by the predominance of T lymphocytes and neutrophils.

Emphysema is classified according to the pattern of involvement of the gas-exchanging units (acini) of the lung distal to the terminal bronchiole. In centriacinar emphysema the distension and destruction are mainly limited to the respiratory bronchioles (more prominent in the upper lobes), with relatively less change peripherally in the acinus; these are the changes found in smokers. Panacinar emphysema involves both the central and the peripheral portions of the acinus; these changes are those seen in α_1-antitrypsin deficiency and occur more commonly in the lower lobes.

The chronic airflow limitation is a consequence of small airway disease. There is narrowing and blockage of small airways by an inflammatory bronchiolitis, alongside airways collapse in expiration due to the loss of elastic recoil and radial traction to balance the positive transmural pressure. This limits airflow and results in the air trapping and hyperinflation seen on CXR and lung function tests.

Clinical features

The most common feature of COPD is breathlessness – initially during activity but progressively at rest. Other symptoms include cough, sputum production (particularly in chronic bronchitis), wheeze, prolonged expiratory phase and fatigue. Patients with severe COPD may develop chronic respiratory failure (T2RF). Most patients have features of both chronic bronchitis and emphysema.

An acute exacerbation of COPD is a common cause for hospital admission, and is defined as a sudden worsening of symptoms (increased cough, sputum production and dyspnoea). This can be caused by a bacterial or viral infection (infective exacerbation (IECOPD)) or other trigger (noninfective exacerbation (NIECOPD)).

Patients may present in respiratory distress: increased respiratory rate, use of accessory muscles of respiration, pursed lip breathing and drowsiness.

Investigations

Diagnosis is established on the basis of history, examination and demonstrating airflow obstruction with no or limited reversibility. Spirometry is the gold standard. A CXR may show hyperexpansion and is used to rule out alternative diagnoses. An FBC should be routinely performed to identify anaemia or polycythaemia. The body mass index needs to be calculated for all patients. There may be an overlap between asthma and COPD, and it may be difficult to differentiate between them. Table 29.3 lists the characteristic features of COPD and asthma.

Patients who present with an acute exacerbation of symptoms require a CXR, serial ABG measurements, blood tests (FBC, U&E, CRP) and an ECG. If an IECOPD is suspected, blood cultures should be sent to the laboratory if patients are pyrexial. Sputum cultures, legionella and pneumococcal urinary antigen testing and a respiratory virus screen should be considered.

Management

Management of patients with COPD is based on an accurate diagnosis, assessment of the severity of symptoms and degree of airflow obstruction, smoking status, the extent of disability and frailty, frequency of exacerbations and hospital admissions and ensuring optimal medical therapies are in place.

Severity is based on FEV_1, as measured by spirometry, which is compared with the predicted value (based on age, sex, height) and expressed as a percentage (FEV_1 % predicted):

- Stage 1 (mild): ≥80% with symptoms present
- Stage 2 (moderate): 50%–79%

Table 29.3 Clinical features to help differentiate chronic obstructive pulmonary disease and asthma

Features	COPD	Asthma
Smoker or ex-smoker	Nearly all	Possibly
Chronic productive cough	Common	Uncommon
Symptoms at age <35 years	Rare	Often
Dyspnoea	Persistent and progressive	Variable
Nocturnal waking with cough or breathlessness	Uncommon	Common
Significant diurnal or day-to-day variability of symptoms	Uncommon	Common

COPD, Chronic obstructive pulmonary disease.

- Stage 3 (severe): 30%–49%
- Stage 4 (very severe): <30%

Care should be via a multidisciplinary team approach and include:

- Smoking cessation: the single most important intervention to modify the natural course of the disease. It will not repair damaged lung tissue, but the rate of decline in FEV_1 with time will revert to that of a nonsmoker. Help from smoking cessation specialists and pharmacological assistance (nicotine replacement, varenicline or bupropion) may increase effectiveness.
- Patient education with a personalized self-management plan.
- Treatment of comorbidities (remember to consider bone health as increased risk of osteoporosis with high steroid use).
- Pneumococcal and influenza vaccination.
- Optimizing pharmacological therapies (see later).
- Pulmonary rehabilitation (a multidisciplinary programme of graded exercise, nutritional advice, psychological support and patient education; this relieves symptoms and reduces exacerbations and can increase exercise ability).
- Treatment of acute exacerbations.
- Management of cor pulmonale (right-sided heart failure secondary to pulmonary dysfunction), if present.
- Home oxygen therapy and/or home noninvasive ventilation (NIV) in persistent hypercapnic respiratory failure nonresponsive to medical treatment.
- Consideration of advanced care planning in end-stage COPD (see Communication box).

Short-term management

General principles of treatment of exacerbations of COPD include:

- Oxygen therapy (see clinical notes: oxygen use in COPD in the acute setting)
- High-dose β_2-agonists and anticholinergics
- Antibiotics if infection is suspected
- Systemic steroids (if oral therapy is indicated, 30 mg prednisolone for 7–14 days)
- Chest physiotherapy
- Theophylline if appropriate
- Assisted ventilation

HINTS AND TIPS

In acidotic or hypercapnic patients, air, not oxygen, should be used to drive nebulizers.

Long-term management

Inhaled therapies

These Include:

- Short-acting β_2-agonists (SABA, e.g., salbutamol and terbutaline)
- Long-acting β_2-agonists (LABA, e.g., salmeterol and formoterol)
- Anticholinergics (short acting: SAMA, e.g., ipratropium bromide, or long acting: LAMA, e.g., tiotropium)
- Corticosteroids (ICS, e.g., fluticasone and budesonide)
- Phosphodiesterase inhibitors (e.g., theophyllines)

Treatment is via a step-wise approach and up-titrated if there are ongoing exacerbations or symptoms causing limitations. Drugs can be delivered through inhalers, spacer devices or nebulizers. Initial management is with a SABA or SAMA as required, then uptitrated as follows:

- Step 1 if no features of asthma or steroid responsiveness: LABA+LAMA
- Step 1 if features of asthma or steroid responsiveness: LABA+ICS
- Step 2: LABA+LAMA+ICS

When titrating therapy, symptomatic relief, quality of life, patient preference, side-effect profile and cost should be considered.

Other therapies

- Oral steroids are used in exacerbations of COPD, and some patients take them long-term, but this is not recommended.
- Oral theophylline may be considered following SABA and LABA use, or in those who cannot use inhaled therapies.
- Oral mucolitics (e.g., carbocysteine): considered in patients with chronic productive cough.
- Oral phosphodiesterase-4 inhibitors (roflumilast): by respiratory specialist if persistent symptoms/exacerbations.
- Long-term oxygen therapy (LTOT) is indicated in:
  - Stable, nonsmokers, with PaO_2 <7.3 kPa.
  - Stable, nonsmokers, with PaO_2 7.3 to 8.0 kPa and one of the following: pulmonary hypertension, peripheral oedema, nocturnal hypoxaemia or secondary polycythaemia.
- Prophylactic antibiotics: by respiratory specialist if >3 exacerbations require steroids with at least one hospital admission in 1 year. Treatment with azithromycin 500 mg 3 times per week.
- Bullectomy or lung volume reduction surgery: some patients may be suitable to relieve symptoms.
- Lung transplantation: In end-stage disease, is an option for some, often younger, patients.

BRONCHIECTASIS

Bronchiectasis is abnormal and permanent dilatation and thickening of the bronchioles secondary to chronic inflammation leading to irreversible damage to the bronchial wall. It is associated with bacterial colonization. It can be focal, involving airways supplying a region of the lung, or diffuse, involving airways in a more widespread manner.

Bronchiectasis is commonly caused by severe lower respiratory tract infections. Adenovirus and influenza virus are the main viral causes; infections with necrotizing organisms (e.g., *Mycobacterium tuberculosis* (TB) or anaerobes) remain important. It can also be congenital, associated with conditions such as ABPA or those causing immunodeficiency or poor mucociliary clearance (e.g., cystic fibrosis, α_1-antitrypsin deficiency or Kartagener syndrome (primary ciliary dyskinesia)).

Clinical features

Patients typically present with persistent or recurrent cough and purulent sputum production. Intermittent haemoptysis occurs in more than half of cases and can cause massive bleeding. Physical examination of the chest may reveal any combination of coarse crepitations and wheeze, reflecting the damaged airways containing significant secretions. Clubbing may be present.

Investigations

Those with suspected bronchiectasis should be referred to a respiratory specialist for diagnosis. High-resolution CT (HRCT) is the gold standard investigation and confirms the diagnosis. Initial investigations prior to referral may include:

- CXR : may show 'tramline shadows' due to bronchial wall thickening.
- Spirometry: to assess lung function and reversibility
- Sputum culture: to guide antibiotic therapy.

Testing for underlying causes (e.g., immunodeficiency, cystic fibrosis) should be considered.

Management

Sustained lung damage is irreversible and therefore therapy is aimed at halting or slowing down the progression of the disease. The underlying cause should be managed with appropriate treatment (e.g., antituberculous drugs for TB or steroids for ABPA). Regular airway clearance physiotherapy is recommended. Antibiotics should be used according to organism sensitivities. Lung resection surgery is occasionally effective for localized bronchiectasis.

PNEUMONIA

Pneumonia is an infection of the pulmonary parenchyma (i.e., the functional lung tissue) causing chest signs and symptoms (cough, shortness of breath, wheeze, sputum, fever, chest pain/discomfort). A CXR demonstrating consolidation can confirm the diagnosis. It is a common condition with high mortality rates. Many bacterial species, viruses, fungi and parasites can cause pneumonia. Empirical antimicrobial treatment is often commenced before the causative micro-organism is identified, after which therapy is adjusted accordingly.

COMMUNICATION

It is important to communicate to patients that their symptoms should abate once treatment has been started; however, it may take time for them to get back to their baseline. NICE recommends providing the following information:

- 1 week: fever should have resolved.
- 4 weeks: chest pain and sputum production should have substantially reduced.
- 6 weeks: cough and breathlessness should have substantially reduced.
- 3 months: most symptoms should have resolved but fatigue may still be present.
- 6 months: most people will feel back to normal.

Aetiology

Community-acquired pneumonia (CAP)

A CAP develops out of hospital or within 48 hours of admission. Causes include *Streptococcus pneumonia* (pneumococcus; most common), *Haemophilus influenzae* and *Staphylococcus aureus*. Twenty percent of infections in adults are thought to be of viral origin. In preexisting lung disease (e.g., COPD/bronchiectasis), organisms such as *Pseudomonas aeruginosa* and *Moraxella catarrhalis* are more common. Severity and management of a CAP is guided by the CURB-65 score (see Clinical Notes: CURB-65 score).

Atypical pneumonia

This is caused by organisms such as *Mycoplasma*, *Legionella* and *Chlamydia* species. They can be acquired in the community or in institutions. Detailed travel history, occupational and social history are important in identifying risk factors.

Hospital-acquired pneumonia (nosocomial - HAP)

A HAP is a new-onset pneumonia that develops 48 hours or more after admission to hospital. It can be caused by all of the aforementioned agents, but Gram-negative organisms such as *Pseudomonas* and *Klebsiella* are responsible for most cases.

Aspiration pneumonia

Aspiration pneumonia occurs as a result of aspiration of foreign material, usually oral or gastrointestinal contents, into the airway. This is most commonly because of the inability to protect the airway such as after a stroke or with a decreased consciousness level. Anaerobic organisms may be implicated.

Opportunistic pneumonia

Opportunistic pneumonia occurs in predisposed individuals. Patients with cystic fibrosis are at increased risk of *Pseudomonas* pneumonia because of changes in the composition of airway surface mucus. Immunocompromised patients (e.g., HIV positive, organ transplant patients) are at increased risk of fungal (e.g., *Aspergillus*), *Pneumocystis jiroveci* (formerly *Pneumocystis carinii*) or viral (e.g., CMV, herpes simplex virus) pneumonia. Ventilated patients are at increased risk of ventilator-associated pneumonia, commonly caused by *Pseudomonas* or *Klebsiella*.

Clinical features

Typical

Typical pneumonia is characterized by fever, chills, tachypnoea, dyspnoea, cough productive of purulent sputum and, in some cases, pleuritic chest pain. The causative pathogens are usually *S. pneumonia*, *S. aureus*, *M. catarrhalis* and *H. influenzae*.

Atypical

It was traditionally stated that 'atypical' pneumonia has a more gradual onset, a dry cough and extrapulmonary symptoms (headache, muscle aching, fatigue, sore throat, nausea, vomiting and diarrhoea). The term 'atypical pneumonia' remains in use but it is the organisms that are 'atypical' and not the symptoms. Causative pathogens include *Mycoplasma pneumonia*, *Legionella pneumophila*, *Chlamydophila* species and *Coxiella burnetii* (causing Q fever). Viruses, fungi and protozoa can also be implicated.

Investigations

Bedside

- Blood tests: FBC: neutrophilia may be present, U&Es: raised urea level is indicative of dehydration and is a part of the CURB65 score (see Clinical Notes box), CRP: level may be raised and can help in assessing response to treatment.
- ABG: T1RF may be present.
- Blood cultures in pyrexic patients, before commencement of antibiotic therapy may help in determining the cause.
- Sputum sample for microbiology, culture and sensitivities.
- If clinically indicated, pneumococcal and *Legionella* urinary antigens; respiratory virus and COVID-19 screen.

Imaging

- CXR: diffuse or lobar pulmonary infiltrates may be seen. Air bronchograms are characteristic of consolidation. Pleural effusions, pulmonary cavitation or hilar lymphadenopathy may be present. Cavitating lesions may be caused by TB, oral anaerobic bacteria, enteric gram-negative bacilli, *S. aureus*, *Pseudomonas*, *Legionella*, *Aspergillus* spp. and fungi.
- CT: not commonly used as a first-line imaging modality. However, if the CXR is suggestive of a space-occupying lesion, a CT scan would be indicated.

Other tests

- Pleural tap: if pleural effusion present. May be aspirated +/- drained if empyema or parapneumonic effusions (see later: pleural effusion). The fluid should be sent for microscopy, culture and sensitivity testing. If a sinister cause is suspected, a sample should be sent for cytology.
- Bronchoscopy: in pneumonia this is mainly used to collect samples that could aid in identifying the causative pathogen, particularly if the patient is nonproductive of sputum. This can be achieved by either bronchoalveolar lavage or transbronchial biopsy at the site of the pulmonary consolidation.

Management

Pneumonia is a leading cause of sepsis (see Clinical Notes: sepsis). The mainstay of treatment for pneumonia is antibiotics. It is important to differentiate the underlying cause of the pneumonia (i.e., CAP, HAP or aspiration pneumonia) as this will help guide antibiotic choice due to underlying organisms. Often for a CAP, atypical infections are covered with addition of a macrolide (e.g., clarithromycin) or a tetracycline (e.g., doxycycline) alongside a penicillin-based antibiotic (or alternative regimen if penicillin allergy). For aspiration pneumonia, often anaerobic causative organisms need to be covered (i.e., addition of metronidazole). However, check hospital-specific guidelines as pathogen prevalence and local antibiotic sensitivities differ. Hypoxia should be treated with oxygen, dehydration treated with fluids and pleuritic pain treated with analgesia (see Clinical Notes: pleuritic chest pain). Saline nebulizers and chest physiotherapy are also of benefit to aid sputum clearance.

CLINICAL NOTES

PLEURITIC CHEST PAIN

Appropriate management of pleuritic chest pain is extremely important. Pain will hinder recovery by reducing mobility and cough effectiveness. This will lead to inadequate sputum clearance and can worsen the course of the disease. Mild pleuritic chest pain can be treated with paracetamol and nonsteroidal antiinflammatory drugs (unless contraindicated). Moderate and severe pain may require opiates.

CLINICAL NOTES

SEPSIS

Sepsis is a syndrome caused by the body's abnormal response to infection, associated with organ dysfunction. It is a life-threatening condition with very high morbidity and mortality rates. As such, early recognition and management are key (see Clinical Notes: sepsis six).

CLINICAL NOTES

SEPSIS SIX

Sepsis six is a care bundle used for early management of sepsis that was developed to improve patient outcomes. It consists of six steps which should be delivered within 1 hour of diagnosis:

- oxygen
- blood cultures
- serum lactate measurement
- empirical intravenous antibiotics
- intravenous fluids
- urine output measurement

PULMONARY EMBOLISM (PE)

PEs are a common, potentially fatal and frequently missed diagnosis. It results from obstruction of a pulmonary artery, causing hypoxia and circulatory collapse. Venous thrombosis is the most common cause, whereas fat (after long bone fracture/orthopaedic surgery), air (e.g., after central venous catheter insertion) or amniotic fluid emboli are less frequent.

Risk factors include immobility (e.g., long-haul travel, during illness), surgery, malignancy, infections such as COVID-19 (see Chapter 38), obesity, pregnancy, contraceptive pill use and thrombophilic conditions (e.g., factor V Leiden).

A PE may be classed as 'provoked' when associated with a risk factor within the past 3 months or 'unprovoked' if not.

Clinical features

Dyspnoea is the most frequent symptom with tachypnoea and unexplained tachycardia the most frequent signs in PEs. Dyspnoea, syncope, hypotension or cyanosis indicates a massive PE, whereas pleuritic chest pain, cough or haemoptysis often suggests a small embolism located near the pleura. On examination, young or previously healthy individuals may simply appear anxious but otherwise well, even with a large PE.

NICE recommends assessment of the clinical probability of a PE by the use of the two-level Wells score (Table 29.4). A score of more than 4 points means PE is likely and a CTPA should be undertaken. A score of 4 points or less means PE is unlikely and a D-dimer should be undertaken. If the D-dimer is positive then CTPA should be requested, if negative alternative diagnoses should be considered.

HINTS AND TIPS

If haemodynamically stable (no tachycardia, hypotension, shock, collapse or pallor) and nonpregnant/within 6 weeks of childbirth, interim anticoagulation (see Management) may be considered whilst awaiting CTPA. In practice, this may be on an urgent outpatient basis (e.g., via same-day emergency care services).

Table 29.4 Well score to assess the probability of pulmonary embolism

	Score
Clinical features of DVT	3.0
Alternative diagnosis is less likely than PE	3.0
Tachycardia (HR >100 bpm)	1.5
Immobilization (>3 days)/surgery in previous 4 weeks	1.5
History of DVT or PE	1.5
Haemoptysis	1.0
Malignancy (either treated within 6 months or palliative)	1.0

A score of 4 points or less means PE is unlikely; a score of more than 4 points means PE is likely.
DVT, Deep vein thrombosis; PE, pulmonary embolism.

Investigations

- ABG: often normal, but can show hypoxaemia, low $PaCO_2$ (secondary to hyperventilation) or acidosis.
- D-dimer: its main value is as a negative result to exclude thromboemboli in low-risk patients.
- ECG: often normal but sinus tachycardia is the most common finding; right bundle branch block and right ventricular strain are indicative. The $S_1Q_3T_3$ pattern (deep S wave in I, Q waves in III and inverted T waves in III) is 'textbook' but uncommon.
- CXR: usually normal but may show atelectasis or a small wedge shadow (Hampton hump).
- CTPA: the gold standard for diagnosing PE. It allows visualization of the pulmonary vasculature.
- $\dot{V}/\dot{Q}$ scanning (isotope lung scanning): looking for a mismatch defect. This method requires a normal CXR.
- Lower limb venous ultrasound scan: to confirm deep vein thrombosis (DVT).
- Echocardiography may show evidence of acute right ventricular dysfunction, especially in significant PEs causing haemodynamic instability.

Management

Follow the ABCDE approach in initial management. NICE guidelines recommend the following treatment:

- Haemodynamically unstable patients with a PE should be considered for thrombolytic therapy or embolectomy. In the event of a cardiac arrest, if a decision to treat the patient with thrombolysis is made, it is recommended that CPR be continued for 60 to 90 minutes after administration of the drug or until the return of spontaneous circulation.

- Patients with confirmed DVT or PE should receive suitable anticoagulation. Apixaban or rivaroxaban is recommended first line. Low-molecular-weight heparin (LMWH), dabigatran, edoxaban or vitamin K antagonists (warfarin) are alternatives. Choice on anticoagulation should be based on contraindications, comorbidities and patient choice.
- Anticoagulation should be continued for a minimum of 3 months. NICE recommends considering stopping anticoagulation at 3 months (3–6 months in active cancer) in a provoked PE, where the provoking factors have been resolved. In an unprovoked PE, anticoagulation beyond 3 months should be considered, with discussion on risk/benefits with the individual.
- In renal failure (creatinine clearance <15 mL/min/stage V CKD) only LMWH, unfractionated heparin (UFH) or warfarin is licenced.
- Inferior vena cava filters (temporary or permanent) are implantable devices recommended for use in patients with contraindications to anticoagulation or those with recurrent thromboembolisms despite adequate drug therapy.
- In unprovoked PE, investigation of underlying causes needs to be undertaken (e.g., thrombophilia testing (see Chapter 37), review for clinical symptoms/signs of malignancy).

HINTS AND TIPS

Patients who have recurrent thromboembolic events, or who have had a thromboembolic event with a strong family history, should be screened for recognized hypercoagulable states. Lifelong anticoagulation may be necessary.

LUNG CANCER

The World Health Organization reports that lung cancer was the most common cause of cancer death worldwide in 2020. In the United Kingdom, more than 48,000 new cases are diagnosed every year. The 10-year survival rate is as low as 10%, and the 5-year survival rate is 16%. The term 'lung cancer' is usually reserved for primary tumours arising from the respiratory epithelium (bronchi, bronchioles and alveoli) rather than metastases from distant malignancies. However, lung metastases are common with sites of origin including the gastrointestinal tract, kidney, ovary, bone, breast and prostate.

Lung cancer types can be divided into two main groups (approximately 90%):

- Small cell lung cancer (SCLC, 15%–20%): arises from central airways, it grows rapidly and spreads early.
- non-small cell lung cancer (NSCLC, 80%–85%)
  - Adenocarcinoma (including bronchioloalveolar cell carcinoma): usually located peripherally, more common in nonsmokers. Arises from epithelial mucous cells.
  - Squamous cell carcinoma: most common type of lung cancer, from the large airways, usually located centrally, it grows slowly and spreads late.
  - Large cell (anaplastic) carcinoma: heterogeneous group of undifferentiated tumours.

The remainder (approximately 10%) include undifferentiated carcinomas, carcinoids and rarer tumour types (e.g., mesothelioma arising from the pleura following asbestos exposure or bronchoalveolar cell lung cancer). All cell types have different natural histories and responses to therapy, and therefore a correct histological diagnosis is essential to appropriate management.

Aetiology

In the United Kingdom, 72% of lung cancers are attributable to smoking (71% active smoking, 1% second-hand smoke). Cigarette smoke contains numerous well-documented carcinogens. The risk of developing lung cancer rises with the number of smoking pack years (Table 29.5). Smoking cessation improves patient outcomes and reduces the risk of developing lung cancer.

Other risks are much less common and include increasing age, radon exposure, asbestos exposure and previous or current lung disease. Mutations in the epidermal growth factor receptor tyrosine kinase (EGFR-TK) are of importance in NSCLC.

Pathology

Like other carcinomas, lung cancer is not caused by a single insult but follows the pattern of cellular dysplasia progressing to carcinoma and spread as the burden of genetic damage accumulates and key oncogenes are mutated.

Clinical features

Unexplained or persistent (duration of more than 3 weeks) cough, dyspnoea, voice hoarseness, lymphadenopathy (cervical or supraclavicular) and stridor, as well as unexplained haemoptysis in people aged 40 years or older and signs of superior vena cava obstruction (SVCO; face or neck swelling with raised jugular venous pressure) should raise the suspicion of lung cancer and warrant urgent CXR referral. Clubbing and tar staining of the fingers may be present. As with any type of malignancy, patients can exhibit systemic symptoms such as anorexia, cachexia, fatigue, malaise and unintentional weight loss.

Table 29.5 The risk of death from lung cancer related to the number of cigarettes smoked

Pattern of smoking	Deaths per 100,000 people	Relative risk
Never smoked	14	1
Ex-smoker	58	4
Current smoker		
1–14 cigarettes/day	105	7.5
15–24 cigarettes/day	208	15
>25 cigarettes/day	355	25

Local invasion of the tumour, depending on the structures involved, may lead to the following symptoms:

- Endobronchial growth: this may result in cough, haemoptysis, wheeze, stridor, dyspnoea and postobstructive pneumonitis (fever and productive cough).
- Invasion of the chest wall: this could cause pain (pleural or chest wall involvement), cough, dyspnoea and symptoms of lung abscess due to tumour cavitation.
- Transbronchial spread: (especially bronchioloalveolar carcinoma) produces growth along multiple alveolar surfaces with resultant impairment of oxygen transfer, dyspnoea, hypoxia and the production of copious sputum.
- Invasion of other thoracic structures: this may lead to airway obstruction, oesophageal compression with dysphagia, recurrent laryngeal nerve paralysis with hoarseness, phrenic nerve paralysis with elevation of the hemidiaphragm, dyspnoea and sympathetic nerve paralysis with Horner syndrome (ptosis, miosis, enophthalmos and ipsilateral facial loss of sweating).
- Pancoast tumour: grows in the apex of the lung extends locally with involvement of the eighth cervical and first and second thoracic nerves of the brachial plexus. There is shoulder pain, which characteristically radiates in the ulnar distribution of the arm, often with destruction of the first and second ribs seen on CXR.
- Other problems of regional spread include: superior vena cava syndrome from vascular obstruction, pericardial and cardiac extension with resultant effusion or tamponade, lymphatic obstruction with resultant pleural effusion and lymphangitic spread through the lungs with hypoxaemia and dyspnoea.

Paraneoplastic syndromes

Lung cancer can also present as a paraneoplastic syndrome. Lung cancer patients may have signs and symptoms that result from extra-pulmonary organ dysfunction unrelated to space-occupying metastases. Most commonly they are due to tumour secretory products. Important paraneoplastic syndromes associated with lung cancer are listed in Table 29.6. Resection of the primary tumour may result in resolution of symptoms.

Table 29.6 Important paraneoplastic syndromes associated with lung cancer

Organ/system	Syndrome	Lung cancer histological type
Endocrine and metabolic	Cushing syndrome	Small cell
	SIADH	Small cell
	Hypercalcaemia	Squamous cell
	Gynaecomastia	Large cell
Connective tissue and bone	Clubbing and HPOA	Squamous cell, adenocarcinoma and large cell
Neuromuscular	Peripheral neuropathy	Small cell
	Subacute cerebellar degeneration	Small cell
	Eaton–Lambert myasthenic syndrome (myasthenia)	Small cell
	Dermatomyositis	All
Haematological	Anaemia	All
	DIC	All
	Eosinophilia	All
	Thrombocytosis	All
Cardiovascular	Thrombophlebitis	Adenocarcinoma
	Nonbacterial thrombotic endocarditis	Adenocarcinoma

DIC, *Disseminated intravascular coagulation;* HPOA, *hypertrophic pulmonary osteoarthropathy;* SIADH, *syndrome of inappropriate antidiuretic hormone secretion.*

Investigations

- CXR: abnormal in most cases. Common findings include hilar masses (squamous and small cell), peripheral masses (adenocarcinoma), atelectasis, infiltrates, cavitation (squamous cell) and pleural effusions. Compare the CXR with old CXRs if possible.
- CT: contrast-enhanced chest CT (including lower neck) for diagnosis alongside CT abdomen/pelvis (for staging purposes). The disease is staged on the basis of the Tumour Node Metastasis (TMN) classification, which directs treatment decisions and prognosis.
- Positron emission tomography – CT: all patients with potential for curative treatment.
- MRI: not routinely recommended for staging purposes unless superior sulcus tumour is present.

- Head imaging: consider head CT and MRI (if CT findings are normal) in patients with suspected intracranial disease.
- Options for diagnostic pathology include biopsy of either the mass or the lymph nodes. NICE recommends image-guide biopsy of the lesion or nodes in peripheral lung lesions; flexible bronchoscopy in those with central lesions; and endobronchial ultrasound-guided transbronchial needle aspiration (EBUS-TBNA) and/or endoscopic ultrasound-guided fine-needle aspiration (EUS-FNA) for assessment of intra thoracic lymph nodes. Surgical staging is also possible if EBUS-TBNA/EUS-FNA is negative.
- Sputum cytology: patients with centrally located lesions in whom other tests are contraindicated.
- EGFR-TK genetic testing in locally advanced or metastatic NSCLC.

Management

Smoking cessation is crucial but should not delay treatment. Histological classification and staging of the tumour will guide treatment.

Small cell lung cancer
- In those diagnosed with SCLC, urgent oncological review is recommended.
- SCLCs have often already spread at the time of presentation. In those who present with early disease (T1a–2a, N0, M0) surgery may be considered. In those with limited-stage disease (T1–4, N0–3, M0), upfront chemotherapy is offered. Concurrent radiotherapy may also be offered as appropriate.
- In advanced disease, chemotherapy (+/– immunotherapy) may be offered.

Non-small cell lung cancer
- In those with curative intent:
  - Cardiovascular and lung functions require assessment.
  - Surgery should be offered first line (lobectomy most commonly).
  - Radiotherapy treatment if surgery is contra-indicated or declined, this may be given with chemotherapy alongside in stage 2 or 3 disease.
  - Adjuvant chemotherapy (post surgery/radiotherapy) may also be given depending on staging.
- In noncurative disease:
  - Treatment is directed by presence of any targetable mutations, PDL-1 (programmed death-ligand 1) status and cell origin (squamous or nonsquamous). It may include chemotherapy, immunotherapy or targeted treatment, either alone or in combination.

Management of symptoms plays a crucial role. Breathlessness may respond to opiates or sublingual lorazepam.

Radiotherapy may also be used to relieve symptoms (endobronchial obstructive, bone pain secondary to metastases or SVCO). Patients with endobronchial obstruction may undergo palliative debulking or stenting. Symptomatic malignant pleural effusions can be aspirated or drained, with consideration of talc pleurodesis to reduce recurrence or a permanent drain (indwelling pleural catheter (IPC)) to allow recurrent drainage. Brain metastasis may require steroids and antiseizure medications, and radiotherapy may be considered.

COMMUNICATION

Patients are rarely surprised when the final diagnosis of lung cancer is explained to them. Ask open questions and seek their opinion as to what might be wrong with them; this can enable cancer to be discussed more easily as they have used the word first.

TUBERCULOSIS

TB is a chronic granulomatous disease caused by a cell-mediated immune response to bacteria belonging to the *M. tuberculosis* complex. It is an airborne disease that usually affects the lungs, although extrapulmonary involvement can occur. If properly treated, TB caused by drug-susceptible strains is curable in virtually all cases.

Of the pathogenic species belonging to the *M. tuberculosis* complex, the most frequent and important agent of human disease is *M. tuberculosis*. Closely related organisms that can also infect humans include *Mycobacterium bovis* (the bovine tubercle bacillus, once an important cause of TB transmitted by unpasteurized milk) and *Mycobacterium africanum*.

M. tuberculosis is a rod-shaped, non-spore-forming, aerobic bacterium. Although strictly gram-positive, it may not stain readily, and is often neutral on Gram staining. However, once stained, the bacilli cannot be decolorized by acid, a characteristic justifying their classification as acid-fast bacilli (AFB).

In most developed countries the incidence of TB fell until the 1980s. It then reached a plateau, and began to increase again in the United Kingdom until 2012. This was due to an increase in susceptible groups, including the elderly, immigrants, people from ethnic minorities, those with alcohol dependence, the homeless and the immunocompromised (both iatrogenic and pathological; HIV is the most important group of the latter, as those with HIV are 16-fold more likely to develop active TB). Worldwide, TB remains a leading cause of death. Multidrug-resistant strains of TB continue to be a global problem.

Pathogenesis

TB is usually classified as pulmonary or extrapulmonary. Before HIV infection, 80% of all cases of TB were limited to the lungs; now two-thirds of HIV-infected patients with TB have both pulmonary and extrapulmonary disease, or even extrapulmonary disease on its own.

Pulmonary tuberculosis

Pulmonary TB can be classified as primary or secondary.

Primary pulmonary TB results from an initial infection with tubercle bacilli. Alveolar macrophages take up the inhaled pathogens for transit to hilar lymphoid tissue, facilitating the host's immune response and control of the infection. Occasionally, dissemination occurs and bacteria are spread to various parts of the body via blood or lymphatic fluid, where granulomas containing the organisms are formed. In most cases, host immunity mechanisms lead to spontaneous healing of these lesions and elimination of the bacteria. In some cases, pathogens persist in a dormant state (termed latent TB – see later). A ghon focus is a calcified caseating granuloma that indicates past primary infection.

Patients with impaired immunity who develop primary pulmonary TB may progress rapidly to clinical illness. This may result from spread of infection by:

- Pleural effusion: may lead to tuberculous empyema.
- Necrosis and acute cavitation of the primary lesion: known as 'progressive primary TB'.
- Bloodstream dissemination: resulting in miliary TB with a possible tuberculous meningitis.

Reactivation of dormant bacteria leads to secondary TB. This is usually a result of debility or immunocompromise and tends to localize to the apical and posterior segments of the upper lobes. CXR changes can range from small infiltrates to extensive cavitation. Widespread involvement of the lung with coalescing lesions produces tuberculous pneumonia.

The pathogenicity of *M. tuberculosis* varies, with one-third of untreated patients dying of severe pulmonary TB within weeks or months, whereas the rest undergo spontaneous remission or proceed along a chronic course often involving lung fibrosis.

Extrapulmonary tuberculosis

This most commonly involves lymph nodes, the pleura, genitourinary tract, bones and joints, meninges, liver, gut and peritoneum.

Clinical features

TB is a disease of insidious onset, with primary infection usually being asymptomatic. Clinical features of secondary TB are nonspecific and differ depending on the organs affected.

Systemic
- B-symptoms: night sweats, fevers and weight loss.
- Fatigue.
- Anorexia.
- Clubbing.

Pulmonary
- Cough: chronic and productive.
- Chest pain.
- Dyspnoea.
- Haemoptysis.
- Crepitations: involved areas.
- Wheeze: partial bronchial obstruction.

Extrapulmonary

This is dependent on the organ system affected. Common manifestations include:

- The central nervous system (CNS): TB meningitis, tuberculomas: meningism, photophobia, reduced conscious level, focal neurological signs.
- Lymphadenopathy.
- Abscesses.
- Genitourinary: dysuria, frequency, epididymitis, salpingitis.
- Musculoskeletal: Pott disease – vertebral TB.
- Cardiovascular: pericardial TB.

Investigations

A high index of suspicion for TB, especially in at-risk groups, is necessary. TB should be included in the differential diagnosis in patients with febrile illnesses, cervical lymphadenopathy or focal infiltrates on CXR. The diagnosis is based on the finding of AFB by microscopy of a diagnostic specimen such as sputum or tissue (e.g., lymph node biopsy) using either auramine staining and fluorescence microscopy or the more traditional light microscopy of specimens using the Ziehl–Neelsen stain.

Pulmonary TB
- CXR: may show the typical picture of upper lobe infiltrates, with or without cavitation.
- Sputum samples: three sputum samples (including one early morning, where able) in patients with suspected pulmonary TB for AFB smear and mycobacterial culture and sensitivity

testing. Most species of mycobacterium, including *M. tuberculosis*, are slow growing, so 4 to 8 weeks may be required before growth is detected and antibiotic sensitivity can be assessed. Newer molecular biological techniques, such as the rapid diagnostic nucleic acid amplification test, can confirm the presence of *M. tuberculosis* more quickly and give drug sensitivities.
- If unable to provide sputum samples, other tests such as bronchoscopy with bronchoalveolar lavage or transbronchial biopsy (especially with miliary TB).

CLINICAL NOTES

'Smear-positive' patients (confirmed AFB on sputum smear) should be considered infectious and should be isolated.

HINTS AND TIPS

If patients cannot produce a sputum sample, consider saline nebulizers to help them expectorate.

Extrapulmonary TB

When extrapulmonary TB is suspected, specimens of involved sites may include:

- Cerebrospinal fluid: tuberculous meningitis.
- Lymph node biopsy.
- Pleural fluid and pleural biopsy samples: pleural disease.
- Bone marrow: miliary TB.
- Liver biopsy: miliary TB.
- Early morning urine: renal TB.

In all cases specimens are sent for AFB microscopy, stain and culture.

Positive tuberculin testing indicates exposure to mycobacteria or vaccination and not active disease and is best used in contact tracing and public health screening. The Mantoux test is commonly used (previously heaf test was used). This involves an intradermal injection of purified protein derivative and then observation of the response. The Mantoux test results may be falsely positive in BCG (bacillus Calmette–Guérin)-vaccinated individuals (see Clinical Notes: TB vaccination). In those patients, because of the questionable reliability of the Mantoux test, interferon-gamma testing (interferon-gamma release assay, IGRA) is recommended as a first-line test.

False negatives are possible in active TB, especially in miliary TB or if the patient is immunosuppressed, for example, HIV infection.

Latent TB should be considered and screened for in those who are immunocompromised or close contacts of those with confirmed pulmonary TB. In the United Kingdom, screening is also undertaken in new entrants to the United Kingdom from high TB prevalent countries and NHS employees who are working with patients or clinical specimens. If screening is positive – the individual should be assessed for active TB (symptoms and CXR). If there is no sign of active TB, latent TB should be referred to the local TB multi-disciplinary team to consider treatment.

> ### CLINICAL NOTES
>
> Prior to initiation of biologic agents (e.g., anti-TNF-alpha agents such as infliximab) active and latent TB should be screened for and monitoring for symptoms is required during and after treatment. Screening involves history (including risk factor assessment) and examination, followed by chest X-ray and IGRA testing.

Management

TB is a notifiable disease in the United Kingdom. Public health authorities should be informed for contact tracing. Patients should be referred to a specialist TB physician if available. NICE recommends treatment as follows:

- Active TB without CNS involvement:
  - Initial phase: rifampicin, isoniazid, pyrazinamide and ethambutol for 2 months.
  - Continuation phase: rifampicin and isoniazid for another 4 months.
- Active TB with CNS involvement:
  - Initial phase: rifampicin, isoniazid, pyrazinamide and ethambutol for 2 months.
  - Continuation phase: rifampicin and isoniazid for another 10 months.
  - High-dose dexamethasone or prednisolone, weaned down over a period of 4 to 8 weeks.
- In single drug-resistant TB, the remaining three drugs are given for treatment in the initial phase, but the continuation phase may be longer depending on the resistant drug.
- Multidrug resistant TB: requires prolonged treatment of often 18 to 24 months with multiple drugs (often six or more) and surgical intervention may be considered.
- Latent TB: in those aged 35 to 65 years treatment is usually recommended. Outside of this age group risk of hepatotoxicity with anti-TB agents must be considered alongside the risk of progression to active TB and

advantages/disadvantages of treatment are discussed with the patient. This is usually a combination of rifampicin and isoniazid for 3 months, or isoniazid alone for 6 months.

> ### PATIENT SAFETY
>
> Adherence to treatment is a serious issue in tuberculosis. Successful drug therapy relies on compliance with treatment. Supervised therapy in at-risk groups (e.g., the homeless population) may improve outcomes. Directly observed therapy, short course in which medications are taken three times per week under supervision can also be helpful.

> ### CLINICAL NOTES
>
> #### ANTITUBERCULOSIS MEDICATION – SIDE EFFECTS
>
> - Isoniazid: liver toxicity, peripheral neuropathy. Pyridoxine therapy is usually started alongside to minimize the neurological side effects.
> - Rifampicin: stains body secretions and urine pink/orange, liver toxicity, hepatic enzyme inducer, thrombocytopenia.
> - Pyrazinamide: liver toxicity, high uric acid levels, gout, arthralgia.
> - Ethambutol: visual disturbances such as altered visual acuity, visual field defects, optic neuritis leading to colour blindness.
>
> Check liver function test results and urea and electrolyte levels before commencement of treatment. Visual acuity should be tested before ethambutol use.

> ### CLINICAL NOTES
>
> #### TB VACCINATION
>
> Bacillus Calmette–Guérin (BCG) was derived from an attenuated strain of M. bovis and was first administered to humans in 1921. Many BCG vaccines are now available worldwide; all are derived from the original strain, but the vaccines differ in efficacy. The vaccine is safe and rarely causes serious complications. It should not be given to HIV-positive patients.

BCG vaccination induces purified protein derivative (PPD) reactivity, but the magnitude of PPD skin test reactions after vaccination does not predict the degree of protection afforded. The UK Department of Health and Social Care recommends vaccination of all infants and children younger than 16 years at high risk of TB. Routine BCG vaccination is no longer offered to all PPD-negative children at the age of 12 years.

PNEUMOTHORAX

A pneumothorax is the presence of air in the pleural space (i.e., between the visceral pleura covering the lung and the parietal pleura covering the inside of the chest wall) leading to lung collapse. Risk factors for pneumothorax include smoking, increased height, male sex, increasing age, Marfan syndrome and underlying lung disease. The following distinctions are made between the different types of pneumothorax:

- Spontaneous pneumothorax: occurs without trauma to the thorax.
- Primary spontaneous pneumothorax: occurs in the absence of lung disease, usually due to the rupture of an apical pleural bleb that lies within or immediately under the visceral pleura. Approximately 25% of patients will have a recurrence.
- Secondary spontaneous pneumothorax: occurs in the presence of preexisting lung disease (e.g., COPD).
- Traumatic pneumothorax: penetrating or nonpenetrating chest injuries.
- Tension pneumothorax: the pressure in the pleural space is positive throughout the respiratory cycle, leading to increasing pressure and mass effect on the mediastinum.
- Iatrogenic pneumothorax: occurs following medical treatment (e.g., central venous catheter insertion, mechanical ventilation, thoracic needle aspiration).
- Catamenial pneumothorax: secondary to thoracic endometriosis; occurs during menstruation.

Clinical features

Clinical features of pneumothorax include:

- pleuritic chest pain on the affected side
- shortness of breath
- tachycardia
- decreased chest expansion, hyperresonance on percussion and diminished breath sounds

A CXR will confirm the diagnosis by demonstrating a line of visceral pleura with absent lung markings beyond the line.

Pneumothoraces classified as large or small, on the basis of the presence of a visible rim of air less than 2 cm or more than 2 cm between the lung and chest wall at the level of the hilum on a plain CXR.

In a large tension pneumothorax a patient may be in extremis (hypotension, tachycardia, extreme dyspnoea) which is a medical emergency (see Clinical Notes: tension pneumothorax) and is treated on clinical diagnosis.

Management

Management of a pneumothorax is via aspiration or a chest drain. The treatment algorithm for primary and secondary pneumothoraces is shown in Fig. 29.1. Small-diameter Seldinger chest drains are preferred for nontraumatic pneumothorax. Pleurodesis or surgery, by thoracoscopy or thoracotomy, may be indicated or considered to prevent recurrence. Emergency management of a tension pneumothorax is via emergency thoracocentesis. (see Clinical Notes 'Tension Pneumothorax').

CLINICAL NOTES

TENSION PNEUMOTHORAX

A tension pneumothorax is a medical emergency. It is a well-recognized cause of cardiac arrest. Patients are acutely short of breath, tachypnoeic and tachycardic. Breath sounds are absent on the affected side, and the trachea is deviated away from the side of the lesion. Treatment includes oxygen and emergency thoracocentesis (into the second intercostal space in the midclavicular line, on the side of the pneumothorax usually just above the rib margin to avoid the neurovascular bundle).

PLEURAL EFFUSION

A pleural effusion is an accumulation of excess fluid in the pleural space. This can be caused by pulmonary, pleural or extrapulmonary disease. The fluid is often described as being an exudate or transudate, depending on its composition. The Light criteria are classically used to distinguish between the two (see later).

If the fluid is blood, this is called a 'haemothorax', if it is puss, it is called 'empyema' and if it is chyle, it is called 'chylothorax'.

Exudative effusions are due to increased capillary permeability with or without diminished fluid resorption; they are most commonly unilateral and caused by:

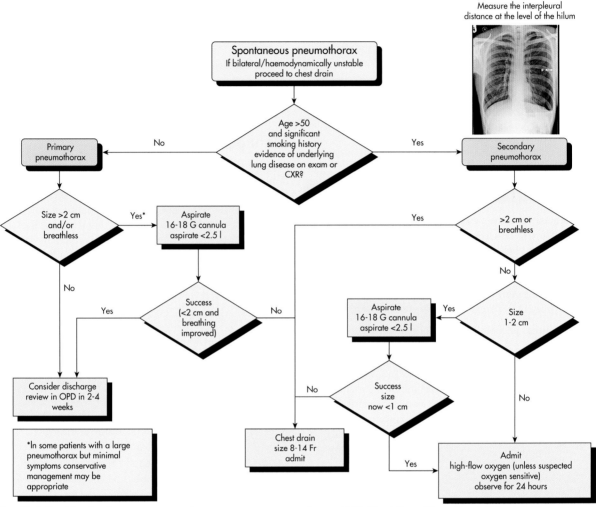

Fig. 29.1 Algorithm for the management of a spontaneous pneumothorax. *CXR*, Chest X-ray (From Macduff A, et al. *Management of spontaneous pneumothorax: British Thoracic Society pleural disease guideline. Thorax* 65:ii18-ii31; 2010.)

- infection (parapneumonic effusion: 'simple' if pH >7.2 and 'complicated' if pH <7.2; empyema if frank pus on aspiration)
- malignancy
- pulmonary emboli
- connective tissue disease (e.g., rheumatoid arthritis)
- pancreatitis

Transudative effusions tend to be bilateral and are due to decreased oncotic pressure or elevated hydrostatic pressure across the pleural membranes, as in:

- heart failure
- cirrhotic liver disease
- hypoalbuminaemia (e.g., liver disease, nephrotic syndrome)

- constrictive pericarditis
- hypothyroidism
- Meigs syndrome – in conjunction with a benign ovarian tumour (commonly a fibroma)

Clinical features

The accumulation of fluid within the pleural space is generally asymptomatic until it is large enough to cause respiratory compromise. Symptoms include breathlessness, particularly on exertion, and sometimes chest pain or cough. The examination findings include decreased breath sounds, stony dull percussion note and decreased expansion on the affected side. History taking should cover:

- Evidence of cardiac failure and ischaemic heart disease.
- Evidence of recent pneumonia: empyema and a reactive effusion may develop, especially if symptoms of infection persist.
- Evidence of malignancy: lung primary, metastatic disease and mesothelioma (asbestos exposure).

Investigations

- CXR: confirms the presence of an effusion and whether it is bilateral or unilateral. However, effusions smaller than 200 mL will not usually show up on a CXR. It may also show underlying malignancy, pleural plaques/thickening or heart failure. A repeat CXR should be performed after aspiration or chest drain insertion.
- Ultrasound scanning can visualize even small pleural effusions. Direct ultrasound vision is recommended for chest drain insertion.
- CT scanning may be required to further evaluate the underlying cause.

A sample of the effusion should be obtained by pleural aspiration. Its gross appearance should be noted and then sent for the following tests:

- pH: pH less than 7.2 in conjunction with pneumonia implies an infected pleural space.
- Protein and lactate dehydrogenase (LDH): this should be done with paired serum samples. Traditionally, effusions are divided into:
  - Exudative: protein level greater than 30 g/dL.
  - Transudative: protein level less than 30 g/dL. If the serum protein level is low, then this is a less useful cut-off and the Light criteria are more sensitive and specific. These state that if one of the following is true, then the fluid is exudative:
    - pleural fluid protein/serum protein ratio greater than 0.5;
    - pleural fluid LDH/serum LDH ratio greater than 0.6;
    - pleural fluid LDH level more than two-thirds of the upper serum LDH reference level.
  - Gram stain, culture and sensitivities: for bacterial infection. If there is suspicion of TB, then stain and culture for *Mycobacterium* spp. should be requested.
  - Cytology: for malignancy and differential cell count.

Further investigations may include pleural biopsy, thoracoscopy and bronchoscopy which are likely to need specialist involvement.

Management

The underlying diagnosis should be sought and then treated. Many effusions will resolve with this alone, particularly if they are due to cardiac failure. If the history and fluid analysis suggest pleural infection (see 'Red Flag'), then it should be drained in addition to antibiotic therapy. Drainage is usually achieved by insertion of a chest drain. If malignancy is confirmed and the effusion is causing symptoms, then drainage and pleurodesis with a sclerosing agent such as talc should obliterate the pleural space, preventing reaccumulation. For recurrent pleural effusions, an IPC may be considered to allow fluid to be drained in the community to relieve symptoms.

CLINICAL NOTES

Chest drains are inserted under ultrasound guidance using the Seldinger technique. The drain is inserted in the safe triangle (formed anteriorly by the lateral border of the pectoralis major, inferiorly by the fifth intercostal space and laterally by the anterior border of the latissimus dorsi). Post procedure the patient will require a CXR to check position of the drain and to review for a pneumothorax. Fluid should be drained at a rate no faster than 2 L in 24 hours.

RED FLAG

Pleural infections (empyema and complicated parapneumonic effusions) are associated with a high mortality rate. A pleural drain is indicated in a pleural infection when frank pus is aspirated, pleural fluid pH <7.2 or organisms are cultured from pleural aspirate.

INTERSTITIAL LUNG DISEASE

ILD is an umbrella term for a heterogeneous group of disorders that affect the lung parenchyma. Prolonged damage to the cells leads to cellular proliferation and scarring with chronic loss of lung function (pulmonary fibrosis). Pulmonary fibrosis for which no obvious cause can be identified is termed 'idiopathic pulmonary fibrosis' (IPF).

Aetiology

ILD can be classified into conditions with and without a known cause.

Known cause:

- Environmental agents: asbestosis, silicosis, pneumoconiosis;

- Drugs: sulfasalazine, gold, amiodarone, methotrexate, oxygen, nitrofurantoin.
- Systemic disease: connective tissue disorders (systemic lupus erythematosus, rheumatoid arthritis, systemic sclerosis), neoplasia, vasculitides (granulomatosis with polyangiitis (previously known as 'Wegener granulomatosis')), eosinophilic granulomatosis with polyangiitis (previously Churg–Strauss syndrome), microscopic polyangiitis), sarcoidosis, inflammatory bowel disease.

Unknown cause:

- IPF
- usual interstitial pneumonia
- cryptogenic organizing pneumonia

Clinical features

Most patients present with a nonproductive cough, slowly progressive dyspnoea, fatigue, weight loss and occasionally haemoptysis. CXR may show reticulonodular shadowing and loss of lung volume. Careful history taking including occupational and environmental risks, travel, medications, past illness, smoking and family history is important to find a cause. Examination may show cyanosis, finger clubbing and bilateral fine-end inspiratory crackles. As the disease progresses, cor pulmonale may develop.

Investigations

- Bloods: FBC, erythrocyte sedimentation rate, U&Es, calcium, liver function tests, serum angiotensin-converting enzyme (ACE) and autoantibodies to look for a cause.
- CXR: is often the first modality of imaging. In sarcoidosis the stages of the disease are classified according to the appearance on CXR (Table 29.7).
- HRCT: provides more detailed diagnostic and prognostic information. 'Ground glass' changes on HRCT usually indicate mild ILD, whereas 'honeycomb' changes signify marked fibrosis and poor prognosis.
- Other tests include: pulmonary function tests (usually restrictive pattern), bronchoalveolar lavage or lung biopsy. Lung biopsy should be considered to differentiate between the various subtypes of interstitial pneumonia. Only usual interstitial pneumonia can be accurately diagnosed by HRCT.

Management

Therapy depends on the origin and the underlying cause of the disease. For instance, if ILD is thought to be a result of a certain drug, use of that medication should be discontinued. In

Table 29.7 Chest X-ray stages of sarcoidosis

Stage 1	Bihilar lymphadenopathy
Stage 2	Bihilar lymphadenopathy and pulmonary infiltrates (reticulonodular shadowing)
Stage 3	Bilateral pulmonary infiltrates
Stage 4	Fibrocystic sarcoidosis typically with upward hilar retraction, cystic and bullous changes

connective tissue disease-related ILD, immunosuppression is indicated. Management of complications is as they develop. In end-stage disease, referral for transplantation may be indicated.

Idiopathic pulmonary fibrosis

IPF is a progressive disorder of unknown origin. It is associated with high morbidity and mortality (median survival from the time of diagnosis is 3 years). It is the most common of the ILDs.

There is currently no curative therapy for IPF, and treatment is supportive. This includes pulmonary rehab, thalidomide (for persistent cough, unlicensed use), orally administered N-acetylcysteine (unlicensed use) and, in selected patients, immunosuppression. Patients with forced vital capacity between 50% and 80% can be considered for treatment with pirfenidone or nintedanib (immunosuppressants with antifibrotic actions). Nintedanib is a tyrosine kinase inhibitor.

Sarcoidosis

Sarcoidosis is a multisystem chronic inflammatory disorder of unknown origin. The most commonly affected sites include the lungs, skin and eyes. Pathophysiology involves formation of noncaseating granulomas. Almost half of individuals with sarcoidosis are asymptomatic, and the disease is an incidental discovery. Symptoms can be nonspecific and include fever, fatigue, malaise and weight loss. Pulmonary disease can present with dyspnoea and a nonproductive cough. Heerfordt syndrome is a manifestation of sarcoidosis and includes uveitis, facial nerve palsy and parotid gland swelling. Löfgren syndrome is a triad of fever, bilateral hilar lymphadenopathy with arthralgia and erythema nodosum. Serum ACE levels are elevated in most patients with sarcoidosis, but sensitivity and specificity are limited. Often treatment is not required, and careful discussion on benefit of treatments should be discussed with the patient. Management includes systemically acting corticosteroids as initial treatment and may be continued as maintenance. Antimetabolites (e.g., methotrexate) or biological agents (e.g., antitumour necrosis factor inhibitors – infliximab) can be used as second- and third-line agents, respectively.

Occupational lung disease

Many acute and chronic lung diseases are directly related to occupational exposure to inorganic and organic dusts. A number of different clinical syndromes may result, and these are listed in Table 29.8. They are important as they are largely preventable through increased awareness and improved workplace conditions.

Aspergillus and the lung

Aspergillus is a genus of fungi consisting of several hundred species. Organisms belonging to this group are mainly found in soil and other organic materials. *Aspergillus fumigatus* and *Aspergillus niger* are pathogens most commonly implicated in human disease. Normally, *Aspergillus* spp.-associated disorders occur in patients with a compromised immune system.

Pulmonary aspergillosis is a respiratory disease caused by *Aspergillus* spp. Many clinical syndromes have been described:

- Allergic bronchopulmonary aspergillosis (ABPA): a combined type I and type III hypersensitivity disorder. It occurs in patients with asthma, cystic fibrosis and bronchiectasis. It is characterized by bronchospasm, peripheral blood eosinophilia, *Aspergillus* precipitins and raised IgE levels with pulmonary infiltrates. It can lead to bronchiectasis. Treatment is with corticosteroids and antifungals.
- Severe asthma with fungal sensitization (SAFS): *A. fumigatus* and *Candida albicans* are the most common offenders. Treatment is as for asthma with antifungals.
- Aspergilloma: presence of a cluster of mould in a body cavity secondary to *Aspergillus* spp. colonization. Surgical resection remains the most effective treatment.
- Invasive aspergillosis: disseminated infection in immunocompromised patients. Treatment is with antifungal therapy.
- Chronic necrotizing pulmonary aspergillosis.
- *Aspergillus clavatus* causes a type of extrinsic allergic alveolitis (EAA) also referred to as 'malt worker's lung'. Treatment is with oral steroids; if it is left untreated, pulmonary fibrosis may develop.

HYPOVENTILATION SYNDROMES AND SLEEP-RELATED RESPIRATORY DISORDERS

Apnoea is defined as an intermittent cessation of respiratory airflow (>10 seconds), which often occurs during sleep.

Table 29.8 Common occupational lung diseases

Disease	Causes	Lung injury
Chronic fibrotic lung disease	Coal workers' pneumoconiosis Silicosis Asbestosis	Diffuse nodular infiltrates on chest X-ray
Hypersensitivity pneumonitis	Mouldy hay (farmer's lung) Avian proteins (bird fancier's lung)	Restrictive pulmonary dysfunction
Obstructive airway disorders	Grain dust Wood dust Tobacco Pollen Synthetic dyes Formaldehyde	Occupational asthma
Toxic lung injury	Irritant gases	Pulmonary oedema Bronchiolitis obliterans
Lung cancer	Asbestos	Mesothelioma
	Arsenic Chromium Hydrocarbons	All lung cancer types
Pleural diseases	Asbestos Talc	May cause benign effusions and plaques

Hypopnoea is a reduction in breathing (>10 seconds). The most common cause of sleep-disordered breathing is obstructive sleep apnoea (OSA); other hypoventilatory disorders are much less common.

Sleep apnoea is divided into three types:

- Central sleep apnoea: apnoea with a patent upper airway. The cause is central in origin and usually involves dysregulation in the functioning of the respiratory centres in the brainstem.
- OSA: apnoea despite continuing respiratory effort because of complete or partial upper airway occlusion.
- Mixed apnoea.

Obstructive sleep apnoea/hypopnoea syndrome (OSAHS)

This is OSA resulting in irregular night-time ventilation and excessive daytime sleepiness. The symptoms include snoring, poor concentration, unrefreshing restless sleep, daytime somnolence, morning headaches and reduced cognitive function. Risk factors include obesity, increasing age, male sex, neck circumference, sedative drugs and alcohol.

Obesity hypoventilation syndrome (OHS)

This is OSA characterized by hypoventilation associated with obesity and daytime hypercapnia and is also known as 'Pickwickian syndrome'. Night-time hypoventilation is more profound here than OSA alone. This may cause poor night-time sleep and, in chronic untreated cases, lead to congestive cardiac failure and cor pulmonale.

Management

The Epworth sleepiness scale is used in preliminary assessment of OSA syndromes and respiratory polygraphy, polysomnography or sleep studies may be arranged for diagnosis.

Management of OSA includes weight reduction, avoidance of alcohol at night, smoking cessation, intraoral devices (e.g., mandibular advancement device) and avoidance of sleeping supine. Sleep hygiene advice should be given. CPAP remains the gold standard treatment to splint open the upper airway during sleep. Rarely surgical intervention (tonsillectomy, oropharyngeal surgery) may be recommended.

RED FLAG

Remember those with excessive sleepiness in OSA syndromes may fall asleep during daytime activities. The driver and vehicle licensing agency (DVLA – UK) has strict guidance on when they must be notified. This includes those who have 3 months of excessive sleepiness with suspected or confirmed mild OSA and those diagnosed with moderate/severe OSA with excessive sleepiness.

Congenital central hypoventilation syndrome (CCHS)

CCHS (previously Ondine's curse), is a fatal respiratory condition if left untreated. It can be congenital or as a result of a significant neurological injury. The condition is characterized by episodes of central apnoea secondary to autonomic failure at the level of the brainstem. It is a rare condition that may be associated with Hirschsprung disease and neuroblastoma. Treatment used to involve tracheostomy and lifelong mechanical ventilation. More recently biphasic cuirass ventilation and phrenic nerve pacing have been successfully used to manage the condition.

ACUTE RESPIRATORY DISTRESS SYNDROME

ARDS is a life-threatening condition characterized by severe respiratory failure secondary to noncardiogenic pulmonary oedema on a background of acute alveolar injury. The pathogenesis is complex, but involves capillary leak, marked lung inflammatory response, surfactant dysfunction, coagulopathy and atelectasis.

ARDS is defined by:

- Acute onset lung injury (within 1 week of exposure to a well-recognized risk factor)
- New bilateral infiltrates on CXR (Fig. 29.2)

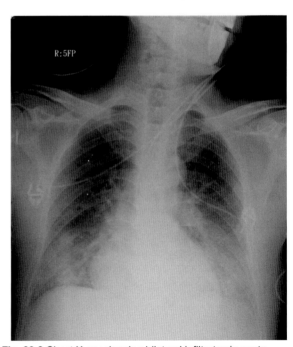

Fig. 29.2 Chest X-ray showing bilateral infiltrates in acute respiratory distress syndrome. (Reprinted from Su Y-J, Kung C-T, Lee C-H, et al. An industrial worker hospitalized with paralysis after an aerosolized chemical exposure. *American Journal of Kidney Diseases* 2010; 56:A38–A41, with permission from Elsevier.)

- Noncardiogenic origin of pulmonary oedema
- Refractory hypoxaemia: PaO_2/FiO_2 of 39.9 kPa or less

ARDS can develop as a result of sepsis, pneumonia, trauma, severe burns, pancreatitis, disseminated intravascular coagulopathy (DIC), blood transfusions, drug reactions and near drowning. Hypoxaemia results from noncardiogenic pulmonary oedema. Prognosis in ARDS is poor. Mortality of severe ARDS is close to 50%. Most survivors have residual impairment of lung function.

> **CLINICAL NOTES**
>
> Sepsis is the most common cause of ARDS. Remember that the source may be from sites other than the lungs – a patient presenting with sepsis secondary to an *Escherichia coli* urinary tract infection may develop ARDS.

Management

ARDS should be managed in an intensive care unit. The mainstay of therapy is the use of lung protective strategies and treatment of the underlying cause. Most patients require mechanical ventilation.

- Lung protective measures: low tidal volume ventilation at lower pressures, negative fluid balance.
- Permissive hypercapnia.
- Lung recruitment manoeuvres (e.g., proning, high-frequency oscillatory ventilation, corticosteroids), higher positive end-expiratory pressure.
- Extracorporeal membrane oxygenation (ECMO).
- Cardiovascular support: ARDS is often associated with multiorgan distress or failure. Invasive haemodynamic monitoring such as with arterial and central venous lines is used to monitor fluid balance, blood pressure and cardiac output (PiCCO line). If blood pressure remains low despite adequate fluid resuscitation, inotropes such as noradrenaline may be indicated.

COVID-19 PNEUMONITIS

COVID-19 (coronavirus disease-2019) is caused by SARS-CoV-2 (severe acute respiratory syndrome-CoV-2), which initially presented in December 2019 in Wuhan, China, leading the WHO to declare a pandemic in March 2020. It can be asymptomatic, or present with a wide range of symptoms, commonly fever, anosmia, cough and shortness of breath. The disease process can range from mild to life-threatening. Respiratory symptoms are driven by a viral pneumonitis, often with a severe hypoxaemia disproportionate to symptoms, which may progress to an ARDS-type picture.

Typical CXR findings are bilateral, patchy, peripheral ground-glass opacities. CT scanning may similarly demonstrate ground-glass opacities (with or without septal thickening), consolidation and evidence of fibrosis (e.g., traction bronchiectasis).

Management of acute hypoxaemic respiratory failure in COVID-19 pneumonitis includes:

- Oxygen: to maintain target saturation of ≥92%. It is recommended to use venturi masks to deliver a set oxygen concentration.
- Awake proning: asking patients who are able, to lie on their front (prone) has shown benefit (in reducing need for intubation) for those in hospital who are not intubated and have higher oxygen needs (FiO_2 >40%).
- NIV: Studies such as the RECOVERY-RS trial sought to compare CPAP, high-flow nasal oxygen (HFNO) and standard oxygen delivery in the management of those with COVID-19 in acute respiratory failure. NICE guidelines suggest the following:
  - CPAP; consider CPAP when
    - hypoxaemia persists despite supplemental oxygen with FiO_2 ≥40%, and either;
    - escalation to invasive ventilation is not immediately needed, or it has been agreed that escalated beyond CPAP is not appropriate.
  - HFNO: evidence does not show benefit over standard oxygen therapy in individuals where escalation to invasive ventilation is appropriate. Consider using HFNO when:
    - CPAP is not tolerated but humidified oxygen at high flow rates is needed;
    - oxygen saturations are not maintained despite maximum standard oxygen delivery, CPAP is not suitable;
      - they do not need immediate invasive ventilation;
      - escalation to invasive ventilation is not suitable;
      - they are weaning, or require a break, from CPAP.
- Invasive ventilation: the timing of intubation can be challenging in COVID-19 and early consideration of suitability for treatment escalation should be made (see Clinical Notes: TEPs). General principles are similar to ARDS management, however aiming for neutral fluid balance. Many of those requiring respiratory support may also require multiorgan support including cardiovascular support and renal replacement therapy.

On recovery and subsequent discharge, those with COVID-19 with CXR changes will require further follow-up. In mild-moderate cases (in general, community or ward-based management) a CXR is recommended at 12 weeks post discharge. In severe cases (in general HDU or ICU-based management), a review including a post-COVID-19 holistic assessment at 4 to 6 weeks post discharge and a CXR with face-to-face assessment at 12 weeks post discharge is recommended. In those whose CXR at 12 weeks does not return to normal, further assessments including pulmonary function testing or CT imaging may be considered.

For further information on COVID-19 including epidemiology, pathophysiology, long COVID, severity classification and management including therapeutics, see Chapter 38.

CLINICAL NOTES

TEPs

Treatment escalation plan (TEP) forms are increasingly used across hospital trusts to aid discussion and documentation of appropriate ceilings of care for an individual in discussion with patients and families. This generally is divided into full escalation (level 3 care – ICU support), high-care support (level 2) and ward-based (level 1 or level 0) ceilings of care. These are separate to DNACPR (do not attempt cardiopulmonary resuscitation) forms and advanced care directives, which should also be considered when reviewing TEPs.

CYSTIC FIBROSIS

Cystic fibrosis is a multisystem autosomal recessive disorder that results from mutations in the cystic fibrosis transmembrane conductance regulator (*CFTR*) gene located on chromosome 7. Its function involves regulation of chloride and water movement across the cell membrane. Close to 2000 mutations have been identified but the ΔF508 mutation is most common accounting for approximately 70% of cases worldwide. Cystic fibrosis occurs in 1 in 2500 live births; 1 person in 25 is a carrier.

Clinical features

Cystic fibrosis is characterized by:

- Chronic airway infection and inflammation leading to bronchiectasis and progressive airway obstruction
- Exocrine and endocrine pancreatic insufficiency
- Intestinal and hepatic dysfunction
- Abnormal sweat gland function
- Urogenital dysfunction (obstructive azoospermia in males)

The signs and symptoms typically occur in childhood, but cystic fibrosis is diagnosed in up to 5% of patients in adulthood.

Because of neonatal screening programmes for cystic fibrosis (at day 6 of life), clinical presentation of cystic fibrosis has become less frequent. Respiratory problems, such as recurrent infections or sputum overproduction, are the most common initial concerns in newly presenting patients.

The diagnosis of cystic fibrosis rests on a combination of clinical criteria, analysis of sweat chloride (the 'sweat test') and genotyping. Faecal elastase testing is a useful screening and monitoring test for exocrine pancreatic function impairment.

Management

A multidisciplinary approach leads to better patient outcomes. Improvements in supportive therapy mean that the median survival is now 40 years. Management strategies are aimed at preventing and treating respiratory problems. They include airway clearance techniques and mucoactive agents (first-line dornase alfa – a recombinant human deoxyribonuclease) to promote clearance of secretions. Control of pulmonary infection with regular sputum samples and prophylactic antibiotics alongside adequate nutrition (pancreatic enzyme and fat-soluble vitamin supplements) is required. Pneumococcus and influenza vaccinations are recommended. Patients should be monitored for diabetes, liver disease and intestinal obstruction. As irreversible complications arise, heart–lung transplantation may be an option for some. Gene therapy for cystic fibrosis remains an ongoing area of interest in clinical trials.

CLINICAL NOTES

PATHOGENS COLONIZING LUNGS OF PATIENTS WITH CF

The pathogens that most commonly colonize the lungs of patients with cystic fibrosis are *Staphylococcus aureus*, *Pseudomonas aeruginosa*, *Escherichia coli*, *Klebsiella pneumonia* and *Burkholderia cepacia*.

COMMUNICATION

The transition from paediatric to adult care is difficult for both patients and their parents. Patients need to build relationships with a new medical team at a time when they are becoming independent adults. This may be hard for parents, who have often spent most of their time caring for their child. Support should be offered to both parties to help facilitate this transition.

Chapter Summary

- Respiratory failure is a medical emergency. Type I is associated with hypoxia with normal CO_2 levels, type II is hypoxia with hypercapnia.
- Severe or life-threatening asthma is a medical emergency. Initial management includes oxygen, steroids and salbutamol and ipratropium bromide nebulizers.
- COPD is a disease commonly associated with smoking. It tends to present with chronic dyspnoea and productive of sputum cough. Emergency management is similar to that of asthma; however, controlled oxygen delivery via venturi mask, with oxygen saturation targets of 88% to 92% are preferred.
- The most common pathogens responsible for community-acquired pneumonia are pneumococcus, *Haemophilus influenzae* and *Staphylococcus aureus;* atypical pneumonia is most commonly caused by *Mycoplasma*, *Legionella* and *Chlamydia* species; hospital-acquired pneumonia is most commonly caused by gram-negative species such as *Pseudomonas* and *Klebsiella.* If aspiration pneumonia is suspected, antibiotic treatment should include anaerobic organism cover.
- CURB65 is a useful tool that helps to assess the risk of death in patients presenting with a community-acquired pneumonia.
- Venous thrombosis is the most common cause of pulmonary embolism. A CTPA is the gold standard for diagnosis. Haemodynamically unstable patients with pulmonary embolism should be considered for thrombolysis.
- Lung cancer is the most common cause of cancer death worldwide. Adenocarcinoma is more common in nonsmokers, and is usually located in the peripheries of the lung; squamous cell carcinoma tends to affect the large airway; small cell carcinoma is the most aggressive type of lung cancer, and grows fast and spreads early.
- Tuberculosis (TB) is a chronic granulomatous disease that can affect various organs in the body. Treatment of pulmonary tuberculosis is with 6-month therapy with four different drugs for the first 2 months and two drugs for the remaining 4 months. If central nervous system involvement then TB treatment is continued for 12 months.
- Tension pneumothorax is a medical emergency and should be managed with an A–E approach and immediate decompression. This is achieved by thoracocentesis with a large-bore cannula into the second intercostal space in the midclavicular line.
- Pleural effusions can be exudative or transudative. Exudative effusions are most commonly unilateral and a result of infection or malignancy. Transudative effusions tend to be bilateral and a result of heart failure, hypoalbuminemia or liver disease.
- Idiopathic pulmonary fibrosis is the most common of the interstitial lung diseases. It is a progressive disease of unknown cause. Treatment is supportive.
- Acute respiratory distress syndrome is a life-threatening complication of an acute lung insult. The most common causes include sepsis, pancreatitis and trauma. It is managed in an intensive care setting.
- COVID-19 infections can cause a range of symptoms, which can range from mild to life-threatening. Respiratory symptoms are driven by a viral pneumonitis, often with a severe hypoxaemia disproportionate to symptoms, which may progress to an ARDS-type picture, requiring ventilatory support.
- Cystic fibrosis is an autosomal recessive disorder that affects the *CFTR* gene. The most common mutation is ΔF508. This leads to abnormalities in electrolyte transport across epithelial cell membranes in predominantly the lung, pancreas, gastrointestinal tract, genitourinary tract and skin.

Continued

Chapter Summary—Cont'd

UKMLA Conditions
Asbestos-related lung disease
Asthma
Asthma COPD overlap syndrome
Breathlessness
Bronchiectasis
Cardiac arrest
Chronic obstructive pulmonary disease
Cough
COVID-19
Cystic fibrosis
Deep vein thrombosis
Fibrotic lung disease
Hospital-acquired infections
Lower respiratory tract infection
Lung cancer
Lymphadenopathy
Metastatic disease
Obesity
Obstructive sleep apnoea
Occupational lung disease
Pneumonia
Pneumothorax
Pulmonary embolism
Pulmonary hypertension
Respiratory failure
Sarcoidosis
Squamous cell carcinoma
Tuberculosis
Upper respiratory tract infection
Vaccination
Wheeze

UKMLA Presentations
Anosmia
Breathlessness
Cardiorespiratory arrest
Chest pain
Cough
Cyanosis
Fever
Haemoptysis
Hoarseness and voice change
Pain on inspiration
Pleural effusion
Snoring
Wheeze

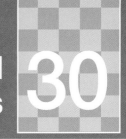
UPPER GASTROINTESTINAL TRACT

Oesophageal disorders

Gastro-oesophageal reflux disease

The lower oesophageal sphincter (LOS) normally prevents significant acid reflux into the oesophagus. Other antireflux mechanisms include the intraabdominal section of the oesophagus, the diaphragmatic crura and the folds of gastric mucosa. These mechanisms fail in gastro-oesophageal reflux disease (GORD).

Clinical features

These are described in Chapter 10. It is important to note that the presentation may be difficult to distinguish from that of angina (including nonspecific ECG changes), and that atypical symptoms such as nocturnal asthma or laryngeal discomfort may occur. Severe oesophagitis may be associated with occult and/or overt gastrointestinal (GI) bleeding and iron-deficiency anaemia.

Investigations

These are outlined in Chapter 10.

Endoscopy is indicated in those older than 55 years, and in those with symptoms lasting more than 4 weeks, dysphagia, abdominal mass, weight loss and persistent symptoms despite testing for *Helicobacter pylori* (*H. pylori*) and treatment (lifestyle changes and antacids). Antacid treatment can mask serious disease and, if possible, it should be stopped at least 2 weeks before endoscopy.

CLINICAL NOTES

NATIONAL INSTITUTE FOR HEALTH AND CARE EXCELLENCE (NICE) GUIDANCE ON THE MANAGEMENT OF PROVEN GORD

- Lifestyle modifications in GORD
  - Avoid identified or precipitating dietary factors.
  - Eat smaller meals.
  - Raise the head of the bed.
  - Do not eat 3 to 4 hours before going to bed.
  - Encourage weight loss, if applicable.
  - Smoking cessation.
  - Reduce stress levels.

- Avoid drugs that reduce lower oesophageal sphincter pressure (theophylline, nitrates, calcium channel blockers, β-blockers, α-blockers, benzodiazepines, tricyclic antidepressants, anticholinergics and caffeine).
- Full-dose proton pump inhibitor (PPI) therapy for 1 month.
- Clinical judgement should be used to offer a *H. pylori* 'test-and-treat' approach versus full-dose PPI for 4 weeks. Leave a 2-week washout period after PPI before testing for *H. pylori* with a breath test or a stool antigen test.

Management

See Clinical Notes: management of GORD.

First-line treatment involves lifestyle modification advice and full-dose proton pump inhibitor (PPI) therapy (e.g., omeprazole) for 4 weeks. In patients with a poor response to these measures, consider a further 4 weeks of PPI therapy. An increase in dosage or an alternative PPI can also be considered. A histamine (H$_2$)-receptor antagonist, such as famotidine, may be useful in patients with nocturnal symptoms. Additional agents include antacids (e.g., alginate preparations, such as Gaviscon, that form a 'foam raft').

Offer people who test positive for *H. pylori* a 7-day, twice-daily course of treatment with a PPI and amoxicillin with either clarithromycin or metronidazole (taking into account previous exposure to either of these). If penicillin is allergic, offer a PPI, bismuth, metronidazole and tetracycline.

Treatment is aimed at symptomatic relief. Surgery is rarely indicated, and only if symptoms are severe despite maximum medical management and there is pH monitoring evidence of active acid reflux during symptomatic episodes. A full-dose PPI long-term as maintenance treatment can be offered if symptoms of severe oesophagitis are controlled.

Complications

Benign oesophageal stricture—This usually occurs in patients older than 60 years and causes intermittent dysphagia. The stricture is usually dilated endoscopically, and surgery is rarely required. Acid secretion is controlled pharmacologically.

Hiatus hernia—This is the herniation of part of the stomach, commonly the proximal part, into the chest cavity. Hiatus hernias are generally asymptomatic but may be associated with acid reflux causing dyspeptic symptoms (see later and Chapter 10). Since hiatus hernias are associated with increased body mass index (BMI), weight loss is usually advisable. A hiatus hernia rarely requires treatment other than symptomatic management for acid reflux (see earlier). Occasionally surgery is indicated, which involves wrapping the fundus of the stomach around the LOS (Nissen fundoplication).

There are two types of hiatus hernia:

Sliding hiatus hernia—The gastro-oesophageal junction 'slides' through the oesophageal hiatus into the thorax. This type accounts for 80% of hiatus hernias.

Rolling (or paraoesophageal) hiatus hernia—The LOS remains below the diaphragm but part of the stomach rolls up into the chest next to the oesophagus (20% of cases). Occasionally this results in gastric volvulus, resulting in severe pain and requiring surgery.

Barrett oesophagus

This is intestinal metaplasia from squamous to columnar epithelium following long-standing acid reflux and, although visible macroscopically, it is confirmed histologically following endoscopic biopsy. It is significant as it is premalignant for oesophageal adenocarcinoma (see later).

Eosinophilic oesophagitis

This is a hypersensitive inflammatory condition of the oesophagus. The condition more commonly affects children and young adults, and presents with symptoms of dyspepsia, dysphagia and food impaction. The diagnosis is based on the histological appearance of endoscopic biopsy samples. Treatment involves allergy testing and allergen avoidance. Swallowed liquid cortisone may help. Recent evidence suggests a role for PPIs in symptom control and potential remission of the underlying disorder. Severe strictures may require endoscopic balloon dilatation. GORD also leads to eosinophil infiltrate, so it can be difficult to distinguish.

Oesophageal motility disorders

These can give rise to dyspepsia (see Chapter 10), pain, dysphagia, odynophagia and regurgitation. Causes include old age, diabetes mellitus, neurological disorders affecting the brainstem, systemic sclerosis, achalasia (see later) and diffuse oesophageal spasm. The diagnosis can be suggested by chest X-ray (CXR) or barium swallow appearances, but oesophageal manometry is the definitive investigation. Treatment options are dependent on cause, and include antispasmodic drugs, botulinum toxin injection, balloon dilatation and surgery.

Achalasia

Achalasia is failure of relaxation at the distal end of the oesophagus due to an underlying neuromuscular problem, commonly the ganglionic cells in the myenteric plexus. Because there is a functional obstruction distally, it causes progressive dilatation, tortuosity, incoordination of peristalsis and often hypertrophy of the proximal oesophagus, which can lead to large volumes of food and saliva accumulating in the dilated oesophagus.

The condition affects males and females equally, and has a peak incidence in the third and fourth decades of life. Diagnosis is on barium swallow (or a water contrast swallow if there is risk of aspiration), which usually precedes endoscopy and manometry. The condition is incurable, but management with botulinum toxin or endoscopic balloon dilatation can provide symptomatic relief. Occasionally surgery (Heller cardiomyotomy) can be performed to permanently dilate the lower 3 to 4 cm of the oesophagus. This procedure, however, may lead to reflux oesophagitis.

Oesophageal cancer

The incidence in the United Kingdom is 15 in 100,000, and is expected to fall by 3% by 2035, but is higher in China and parts of Africa. It is commoner in men, heavy drinkers and smokers. Predisposing factors include Plummer–Vinson syndrome, achalasia, coeliac disease and tylosis (hyperkeratosis of the palms and soles).

In general, squamous cell carcinomas occur in the upper and mid-oesophagus. Adenocarcinoma typically arises in columnar epithelium of the lower oesophagus. Worldwide, squamous cell carcinoma predominates. Barrett oesophagus increases the risk of adenocarcinoma by 40-fold.

Clinical features

The incidence peaks in the seventh decade. General features of malignancy occur, including weight loss, anorexia and lassitude. Local features include dysphagia (initially to solids progressing to liquids), retrosternal pain and odynophagia. Direct invasion of surrounding structures and regional lymph node involvement are common. Metastases to other organs and distant lymph nodes may occur.

Investigations

Endoscopy with biopsy, and barium swallow are the main diagnostic investigations. CT and/or MRI scanning, liver ultrasound scanning and bronchoscopy are commonly performed as part of the staging process. Occasionally a staging laparoscopy is performed if there is a significant infradiaphragmatic component, in people with potentially curable malignancy.

Management

Surgery may be considered, depending on the tumour stage/grade and the fitness of the patient, but it carries high morbidity and mortality. Open or minimally invasive approaches can be employed, alongside lymph node resection. Radiotherapy and chemotherapy may play a role, either as a neoadjuvant or adjuvant treatment. Often palliation is the only option, and this may include endoscopic dilatation, stent placement, laser photocoagulation and/or radiotherapy with the aim of maintaining patency of the oesophageal lumen. The overall survival rate in advanced disease is poor, at around 4% at 5 years.

Gastroduodenal disorders

Gastroduodenitis and peptic ulcer disease

Acute gastritis and ulceration can result from nonsteroidal antiinflammatory drug (NSAID) use, steroids, alcohol, smoking or severe stress or burns (Curling ulcer). Chronic gastritis complicates *H. pylori* infection, autoimmune gastritis (e.g., pernicious anaemia) and long-term NSAID use. Most chronic gastritis is asymptomatic, but it may be a risk factor for malignant change.

Peptic ulcer disease most commonly occurs in the duodenum, followed by the stomach, oesophagus and jejunum in Zollinger–Ellison syndrome (see Gastrinoma section) or after a gastroenterostomy. It may occur in a Meckel diverticulum with ectopic gastric mucosa. Its prevalence is 15% to 20%, and incidence increases with age. It is commoner in men.

H. pylori infection is associated with 95% of duodenal ulcers and 80% of gastric ulcers. NSAIDs are the second biggest cause, and it is important, when you are taking a history, to specifically ask about the use of over-the-counter medication. Gastric ulceration is a mode of presentation of gastric cancer.

The three main complications secondary to peptic ulceration are bleeding, perforation and pyloric stenosis (occurs because of oedema surrounding the ulcer or from scar formation on ulcer healing). Perforation is more common in duodenal ulcers than in gastric ulcers.

Clinical features

Dyspepsia is the commonest mode of presentation (see Chapter 10). Duodenal ulcers classically present with pain typically before meals or at night, which is relieved by eating. Gastric ulcers may present with pain related to meals, that is relieved by antacids. Anorexia, vomiting and weight loss should lead to the suspicion of gastric carcinoma.

Examination findings are often normal, or reveal epigastric tenderness. A mass suggests carcinoma, and a succussion splash may suggest pyloric obstruction.

Investigations

These are described in Chapter 10. Endoscopy is the investigation of choice. All gastric ulcers should be biopsied to exclude malignancy, but duodenal ulcers are nearly always benign; biopsy specimens should be taken for *H. pylori* at endoscopy. Acid secretion status may be assessed if Zollinger–Ellison syndrome is suspected by measurement of fasting gastrin level.

Management

The patient should be advised to modify exacerbating factors such as smoking, diet, alcohol consumption and stress. Use of NSAIDs should be stopped, and alternative analgesia, such as paracetamol or opioids, should be offered.

Drug therapy

PPIs, antacids and H_2-antagonists all help with symptomatic relief. See NICE guidelines for details on treatment.

Other therapy

PPIs should be prescribed and *H. pylori* testing performed. If the result is positive, PPI therapy should be continued for 2 months, and then *H. pylori* eradication should be undertaken. Testing for *H. pylori* should be repeated 4 to 8 weeks after completion of eradication therapy if the patient was known to have gastric ulcers or if symptoms persist. If the result is positive, expert advice should be sought. Treatment failure may indicate poor adherence or antibiotic resistance; if the result is negative, clinical reevaluation and investigation is required.

All gastric ulcers should be followed up with endoscopy/biopsy until they have completely healed because of the risk of an underlying malignancy.

Surgery is usually considered when medical treatment has failed, or for complications that include persistent haemorrhage, perforation or pyloric stenosis. Surgical procedures include partial gastrectomy or highly selective vagotomy and pyloroplasty (rarely performed now). Haemorrhage may be controlled endoscopically by injection of adrenaline or diathermy, laser photocoagulation or heat probe and application of endoscopically placed clips. Perforations are usually oversewn with an omental plug.

Upper gastrointestinal tract haemorrhage

HINTS AND TIPS

A carefully taken history may help with the diagnosis in haematemesis. In Mallory–Weiss syndrome, oesophageal tears are associated with violent retching or vomiting, and the initial vomitus is usually free of blood.

Upper GI tract bleeding is a medical emergency when acute, and carries a 10% mortality rate. It commonly presents with melaena and/or haematemesis. Peptic ulcers and oesophageal varices are the most common causes. The approach to taking an appropriate history, examination and developing a complete differential diagnosis is discussed in Chapter 11.

Management

Immediate treatment—As with any medical emergency, start with the ABCDE approach (see Chapter 2). It is essential to establish whether the patient is haemodynamically compromised.

- Ensure the airway is protected and administer high-flow oxygen if hypoxia is present.
- Establish intravenous access with two large-bore cannulas (>16 gauge); send blood for sampling and cross-match.
- Intravenous fluids should be given while you are awaiting cross-matched blood. If bleeding is profuse, use O-negative blood and follow the local massive blood loss protocol (see Chapter 2).
- Clotting should be corrected with platelets, fresh frozen plasma and, in patients taking warfarin, prothrombin complex concentrate (e.g., Octaplex, Beriplex) and vitamin K.
- Fluid resuscitation should be titrated to the patient's haemodynamic status: low blood pressure (systolic blood pressure <80 mmHg), tachycardia and low urine output (<30 mL/kg per hour) all indicate severe hypovolaemia.

Risk should be assessed for all patients with an acute upper GI tract bleed. The Blatchford scoring system is used initially, followed by the full Rockall score once endoscopy has been performed (Tables 11.2 and 11.3). Immediate endoscopy is offered to unstable patients; all other patients should undergo the investigation within 24 hours of admission.

In stable patients who are not actively bleeding and not anaemic, conservative management is indicated. This includes bed rest, nil by mouth and close monitoring of the pulse, blood pressure, respiratory rate and fluid balance.

Endoscopy is both diagnostic and therapeutic. It will reveal the cause of bleeding in more than 80% of cases. If there is active bleeding, adrenaline can be injected, or bleeding vessels can be coagulated with a heat probe or with laser therapy or ligated with a mechanical method (e.g., clips, bands). PPIs are given to patients with bleeding ulcers but are not recommended before endoscopy in suspected non-variceal bleeds.

In variceal bleeding, vasoconstrictor therapy with terlipressin is used at presentation to reduce splanchnic blood flow and therefore portal pressure. Prophylactic antibiotic treatment is also offered in these cases.

Interventional radiology or surgery is indicated if it is not possible to control persistent or recurrent bleeding with medical management. In variceal bleeding, a Sengstaken–Blakemore tube can be passed through the oesophagus, with balloons to compress varices at the oesophagogastric junction. In oesophageal varices, transjugular intrahepatic portosystemic shunt lowers portal pressure by creating a shunt to the systemic circulation.

Mortality associated with first-time presentation of variceal bleeding is as high as 20%. The 2-year recurrence risk is approximately 80%. Adverse prognostic factors include jaundice, ascites, hypoalbuminaemia and encephalopathy (i.e., other features of decompensated liver failure).

Gastric cancer

The incidence of gastric carcinoma is around 10 in 100,000, and it is more common in men and the elderly. *H. pylori* is associated with 32% of stomach cancers in the United Kingdom. Suggested dietary links include alcohol, processed meat and nitrates, which are converted to nitrosamines by bacteria. It occurs more often in Japan because of the higher fish intake resulting in a high level of nitrosamines. It is commoner in those who are overweight, in smokers and in patients with blood group A.

Other predisposing conditions include pernicious anaemia, chronic gastritis with atrophy, areas of intestinal metaplasia and partial gastrectomy.

Most cancers are adenocarcinomas and affect mainly the pylorus and antrum. They are polypoid or ulcerating lesions with rolled edges. Less common are leather-bottle-type adenocarcinomas (linitis plastica).

Clinical features

General features of malignancy may be present (weight loss, anorexia, etc.). Local features may include dyspeptic symptoms (see Chapter 10), nausea and vomiting, dysphagia, GI bleeding or iron-deficiency anaemia and a palpable epigastric mass or tenderness. A Virchow node (enlarged lymph node in the left supraclavicular fossa) indicates metastatic disease. The most common sites for spread are liver, bones, brain and lung. Transcoelomic spread may occur (e.g., to ovaries – Krukenberg tumour). Paraneoplastic features include dermatomyositis and acanthosis nigricans but these are rare.

Diagnosis is made on gastroscopy with multiple biopsies for histology. Endoscopic ultrasound and CT/MRI scanning are used for staging. Occasionally, a diagnostic laparoscopy is indicated to assess spread from locally advanced tumours.

Management

Surgery is the only curative option. Depending on the position and extent of the tumour, the patient may have a partial or a total gastrectomy. Endoscopic mucosal resection is offered for early-stage cancers. The 5-year survival rate in advanced disease is 5%. The 5-year survival rate with gastrectomy is around 20%. Palliation may involve the use of chemotherapy, radiotherapy and surgery. Targeted therapy with trastuzumab (Herceptin), a monoclonal antibody that inhibits human epidermal growth factor receptor 2 (HER2), increases survival rates in advanced, HER2-positive gastric cancers.

Gastrointestinal stromal tumour

A GI stromal tumour (GIST) is a mesenchymal tumour of the GI tract that is commonly benign (70%–80%) but may be malignant.

The tumours are mostly solitary and can occur anywhere in the GI tract. Malignant spread tends to be intraabdominal and to the liver; very rarely the tumour metastases to lungs or bone. The clinical features are dependent on tumour size and location, but often include nausea, pain and occult bleeding. GIST is unusual in people younger than 50 years and is associated with neurofibromatosis type I. Treatment is surgical: local excision with or without targeted therapy with the tyrosine kinase inhibitors imatinib and sunitinib. The 2-year survival rate with advanced disease is now 80% because of advances in monoclonal technologies.

Small bowel disorders

Malabsorption

The clinical features of malabsorption were outlined in Chapter 13 and include anorexia, weight loss and lethargy, abdominal distension and increased borborygmi, steatorrhoea, wasting, clubbing, petechiae (secondary to vitamin K deficiency), anaemia (iron-, vitamin B_{12}- and folate-deficiency anaemia), paraesthesia, bone pain and tetany (secondary to hypocalcaemia), oedema, leuconychia and ascites (secondary to hypoproteinaemia) and peripheral neuropathy (secondary to vitamin B deficiency). There may also be signs of the underlying disease (e.g., jaundice or lymphadenopathy with lymphomas). Causes of malabsorption are outlined in Table 30.1.

Coeliac disease

Coeliac disease is a T-cell-mediated autoimmune gluten-sensitive enteropathy. Present in gluten-containing food, proteins called prolamins, including α-gliadin, trigger T-cell-mediated damage to the duodenal and jejunal mucosa, leading to villous atrophy and malabsorption. Gluten is a component of wheat, barley and rye.

The UK prevalence of coeliac disease is around 1 in 100 people. It is commoner in females and can occur at any age. It is a multigenetic disorder, associated with HLA-DQ protein, with DQ2 and DQ8 isoforms of HLA-DQ present in more than 95% of cases. Immunogenic mechanisms and environmental factors (e.g., viral infections) may also play a role.

Clinical features—Symptoms may be nonspecific (e.g., lethargy and malaise). Classically, there is a history of diarrhoea or steatorrhoea, with abdominal discomfort, and sometimes weight loss. Other features include mouth ulcers, anaemia (folate or iron deficiency; vitamin B_{12} deficiency is rare as the stomach and terminal ileum are not involved) and less commonly failure to thrive (children), osteomalacia, tetany, neuropathies, myopathies and hyposplenism.

Patients with coeliac disease are at increased risk of developing other autoimmune disease (e.g., thyroid disease and insulin-dependent diabetes) and small bowel lymphomas and adenocarcinomas. Dermatitis herpetiformis, which is a chronic subepidermal blistering skin disorder, is the classic skin manifestation of coeliac disease.

Investigations—The 2015 NICE guidelines recommend serological testing in patients presenting with any of the following: persistent unexplained abdominal or GI symptoms, faltering growth, prolonged fatigue, unexpected weight loss, severe or persistent mouth ulcers, unexplained iron, vitamin B_{12} or folate deficiency, autoimmune disease (including type 1 diabetes) and irritable bowel syndrome (IBS) (in adults).

First-line testing includes testing for total immunoglobulin A (IgA) and IgA tissue transglutaminase (tTG). If IgA tTG test results are weakly positive, IgA endomysial antibody (EMA) testing is performed. If IgA is deficient (total IgA 0.07 g/L or less), testing for immunoglobulin G (IgG) EMA, IgG deamidated gliadin peptide or IgG tTG should be considered. Duodenal biopsy showing villous atrophy with chronic inflammation in the lamina propria is needed for diagnosis. Testing is only accurate in patients who do not have a gluten-free diet.

Table 30.1 Causes of malabsorption

Cause	Examples
Biliary insufficiency	Primary biliary cirrhosis, biliary obstruction, cholestyramine, ileal resection (impaired enterohepatic circulation)
Pancreatic insufficiency	Chronic pancreatitis, pancreatic carcinoma, cystic fibrosis, Zollinger–Ellison syndrome (pancreatic enzymes inactive at low pH because of gastric acid hypersecretion)
Abnormalities of the small bowel mucosa	Coeliac disease, Whipple disease, tropical sprue, radiation enteritis, small bowel resection, brush border enzyme deficiency (e.g., lactase deficiency), drugs (e.g., metformin), amyloid, hypogammaglobulinaemia (also predisposes to infection), intestinal lymphangiectasia, lymphoma, abetalipoproteinaemia, ischaemia
Bacterial overgrowth	Especially in diverticula and postoperative blind loops. Also in dilated areas of small bowel in systemic sclerosis
Infection	Giardiasis, diphyllobothriasis, strongyloidiasis, tuberculosis
Intestinal hurry	Postgastrectomy dumping, after vagotomy, gastrojejunostomy, short bowel syndrome (multiple resections, e.g., Crohn disease)

Management—Treatment is a lifelong gluten-free diet and deficient nutrient replacement (e.g., vitamin D). Patient advice and education are key. Patients should be reviewed annually. Refractory disease is rare when the diet is truly gluten-free, but steroids and azathioprine can be considered.

Pancreatic insufficiency (see later)

Bacterial overgrowth—Although bacterial overgrowth may occur spontaneously, especially in the elderly, it is normally associated with a structural abnormality of the small intestine (e.g., in diverticula or postoperative blind loops of bowel). Aspiration of jejunal contents reveals *Escherichia coli* or *Bacteroides* spp. In concentrations greater than 10^5/mL as part of a mixed flora. The bacteria can deconjugate bile salts, which can be detected in aspirates; this deficiency of conjugated bile salts leads to steatorrhoea. The bacteria also metabolize vitamin B_{12}, leading to deficiency. Management involves correction of the underlying disorder and vitamin replacement. If this is not possible, broad-spectrum antibiotic therapy, including anaerobic cover with metronidazole, should be initiated.

Tropical sprue

This is a severe malabsorption disease, usually accompanied by diarrhoea and malnutrition. It occurs in most tropical or subtropical regions. The cause is unknown but is thought to be of infective origin. Jejunal histology shows partial villous atrophy and inflammation. The mainstay of treatment involves fluid, electrolyte and nutritional replacement (folic acid, vitamin B_{12}). Occasionally antibiotic treatment with tetracycline is needed.

Whipple disease

This is a rare cause of malabsorption, usually affecting men older than 50 years. Symptoms include steatorrhoea, fever, chronic cough, weight loss, arthralgia, lymphadenopathy and sometimes involvement of the heart, lung and brain. Histologically, cells of the lamina propria are replaced by macrophages that contain periodic acid–Schiff-positive glycoprotein granules. The organism responsible is *Tropheryma whippelii*. Treatment is with antibiotics long-term (1–2 years).

Neuroendocrine tumours of the bowel

These tumours are rare.

Carcinoid tumours often occur in the small bowel, and the other tumours discussed later arise in the pancreas. They arise from amine precursor uptake and decarboxylation (APUD) cells, which secrete a number of hormones (e.g., gastrin, glucagon and vasoactive intestinal peptide (VIP)). Pancreatic endocrine tumours may occur with other endocrine tumours as part of multiple endocrine neoplasia syndromes (see Chapter 33).

Carcinoid tumours

These are slow-growing tumours that originate from the enterochromaffin cell (neural crest) of the intestine. They may appear in the appendix (45%), terminal ileum (30%), rectum (15%) or other site in the GI tract, ovaries, testis or the lung. They have malignant potential; 80% of large tumours will metastasise. Presentations include appendicitis, intussusception and obstruction. Carcinoid syndrome is associated with 30% of intestinal neuroendocrine tumours.

Carcinoid syndrome

This is a paraneoplastic syndrome that occurs as a result of the release of pharmacologically active mediators (e.g., 5-hydroxytryptamine (5-HT), prostaglandins and kinins) from carcinoid tumours into the systemic circulation. It occurs in approximately 5% of cases, and only when there is hepatic involvement, allowing products to avoid first-pass metabolism in the liver and reach the systemic circulation. Clinical features include flushing (which may be prolonged and lead to telangiectasia), abdominal pain, diarrhoea, bronchospasm and oedema (associated with pulmonary stenosis or tricuspid regurgitation).

Diagnosis is by measurement of 5-hydroxyindoleacetic acid (5HIAA, a 5HT metabolite) in 24-hour urine collection. Plasma chromogranin A levels correlate directly with tumour burden. Localization of the tumour is with the use of indium-111 octreotide scintigraphy or PET scans. Occasionally, abdominal CT scan or laparoscopy/laparotomy is needed.

Management includes avoidance of flushing precipitants (e.g., alcohol, coffee). Surgery (with or without chemotherapy) is best for localized tumours, and may be curative. Octreotide alleviates flushing and diarrhoea. Other useful drugs include cyproheptadine (an antihistamine with 5-HT and calcium channel-blocking properties) and methysergide (which also blocks 5-HT). Targeted radiotherapy (e.g., ^{131}I-metaiodobenzylguanidine or peptide receptor radionuclide therapy) is highly effective. Other procedures include enucleation of liver metastases, hepatic artery ligation, embolization and 5-fluorouracil injection.

Median survival is variable, and can range from 3 years in metastatic disease to 15 years in some individuals.

Gastrinoma

This is usually due to a gastrin-secreting pancreatic adenoma, which stimulates excessive acid production, leading to multiple recurrent ulcers in the stomach and duodenum. Approximately half are malignant and 10% are multiple. They cause a clinical syndrome called Zollinger–Ellison syndrome. Patients commonly have diarrhoea (due to upper intestinal tract low pH) and steatorrhoea (due to low pH-driven diminished lipase activity). The diagnosis is made from a raised fasting serum gastrin level; the gastric acid output is also raised. Treatment is by removal of the primary tumour (provided there is no evidence of metastases) and use of omeprazole or octreotide.

Insulinomas

These are tumours of the beta cells of the pancreas; 5% are malignant and 5% are multiple. The patient presents with recurrent or fasting hypoglycaemia, which may manifest itself in bizarre behaviour, epilepsy, dementia or confusion. Treatment is by surgical excision of the tumour. If surgery is not feasible, diazoxide or octreotide is useful. Fasting hypoglycaemia is discussed in Chapter 33.

VIPomas

These tumours release VIP, which produces intestinal secretions leading to watery diarrhoea, hypokalaemia and sometimes achlorhydria. Diagnosis is by high serum levels of VIP. The tumour should be resected if possible. Octreotide is useful for controlling symptoms.

Glucagonomas

These are tumours of the alpha cells of the pancreas, which release glucagon. Symptoms include diabetes, diarrhoea, a necrolytic migratory erythematous rash, weight loss, anaemia and glossitis.

LOWER GASTROINTESTINAL TRACT

Colorectal disorders

Colorectal neoplasia

Benign disease

Colonic polyps are common and are often found incidentally during investigation of coincidental gastro-intestinal symptoms such as pain, altered bowel habit or bleeding haemorrhoids. They may be benign or neoplastic (commoner), and may be sessile or pedunculated; they can range from a few millimetres to 10 cm in diameter, and may be solitary or multiple.

Adenomatous polyps (neoplastic) are usually asymptomatic but may bleed and lead to iron-deficiency anaemia. Sessile villous adenomas of the rectum may present with profuse diarrhoea and hypokalaemia. Most colonic carcinomas originate from adenomas. Once a polyp is found, it should be removed endoscopically. NICE recommends colonoscopic surveillance only if the polyps have high-risk features, with repeat colonoscopy at 3 years. If there is no high-risk feature then the patient should just follow routine bowel screening.

Familial adenomatous polyposis is a genetic disorder that can have different inheritance patterns. In most severe cases, where the adenomatous polyposis coli gene (*APC*) is mutated, it is autosomal dominant. Patients have multiple polyps throughout the GI tract, with the lifetime risk of malignant transformation reaching 100%. In high-risk patients, colectomy with ileorectal anastomosis may be performed, with continued surveillance of the rectal stump.

Peutz–Jeghers syndrome is an autosomal dominant disease that consists of mucocutaneous pigmentation and hamartomatous polyps (nonneoplastic) anywhere along the GI tract, most commonly in the small bowel.

Colorectal cancer

Colorectal carcinoma is the fourth most common cancer in the United Kingdom, with more than 40,000 new cases registered every year. The incidence increases with age. Risk factors include high red and processed meat intake, alcohol consumption, smoking, low-fibre diet, high BMI, family history (especially significant if affected before 60 years of age), inflammatory bowel disease (IBD) and polyposis syndromes. The vast majority of neoplasms are adenocarcinomas. The colon is the more common site of disease and accounts for two-thirds of colorectal cancers. Two-thirds of tumours occur with ulceration and spread by direct infiltration, invading the lymph nodes and blood vessels, leading to metastases.

Hereditary nonpolyposis colon cancer (also known as 'Lynch syndrome') is a dominantly inherited mutation of a DNA mismatch repair gene. Affected family members develop right-sided cancers at an early age. Colonoscopic surveillance every 2 years from the age of 25 years is usually recommended. Daily aspirin, to be taken more than 2 years, is considered to reduce risk.

Clinical features—General features of malignancy include weight loss, anorexia and lethargy. Other features depend on the site of the tumour. Left-sided tumours present with abdominal pain, altered bowel habit, bowel obstruction and rectal bleeding. Right-sided tumours can become large and remain asymptomatic (as the stool has a liquid consistency here). They may present with iron-deficiency anaemia. Any persistent change in bowel habit or rectal bleeding must be investigated.

Examination should always include a digital rectal examination. The tumour may be detected as an abdominal mass, and hepatomegaly may be felt with liver metastases. Liver metastases are present in around 20% to 25% of cases at diagnosis.

Investigations

Screening—Faecal occult blood testing is a part of the NHS Bowel Cancer Screening Programme. It is available to those aged 60 to 74, and is offered every 2 years. The program is currently being expanded to include all adults between 50 and 74. These home tests potentially detect faecal blood, which may be an early sign of colorectal cancer. Colonoscopy is offered to those with an abnormal result. The faecal occult blood test has a sensitivity of about 60% and a positive predictive value of 5% to 10%.

Bedside
- Full blood count (FBC) for microcytic anaemia (blood loss).
- Urea and electrolytes (U&Es) to detect electrolyte abnormalities common with diarrhoea.
- Liver function tests (LFTs) to monitor liver function.
- Tumour markers (carcinoembryonic antigen (CEA)) to monitor response to treatment (has a negative prognostic significance).

Other
- CT (contrast CT of chest, abdomen and pelvis for staging).
- MRI (for staging in patients with rectal disease).
- CT colonography.
- Colonoscopy and biopsy (the gold standard).
- Flexible sigmoidoscopy then barium enema (in patients unfit for colonoscopy: the detection rate is around 60%).

Staging
- Contrast-enhanced CT of chest, abdomen and pelvis for all colorectal cancers – modified Duke classification (Table 30.2).
- Additional MRI for patients with rectal cancer to assess surgical margins and lymph nodes.
- Endorectal ultrasound examination for rectal cancers.

Management and prognosis

NICE guidelines on the management of colorectal cancer were last updated in December 2021. All new cases are discussed at a multidisciplinary team meeting. More than 90% of primary tumours can be resected surgically. Neoadjuvant radiotherapy and chemotherapy may be used preoperatively to shrink the mass or to relieve symptoms and/or improve survival in patients with advanced disease. The prognosis is summarized in Table 30.2.

HINTS AND TIPS

Adjuvant chemotherapy is given after surgery to reduce the statistical chance of relapse due to occult disease. Neoadjuvant chemotherapy is given before surgery, often to shrink or downstage the tumour.

Diverticular disease

A diverticulum is an outpouching of the wall of the gut (mucosa herniates through the muscle layer). Diverticula can present anywhere in the gut but are most common in the colon, especially the sigmoid colon and descending colon. They occur because of high intracolonic pressure with weakness of the colonic wall. Diverticulosis is the presence of asymptomatic diverticula, and diverticulitis is inflammation within a diverticulum. The incidence increases with age, and affects up to 50% of the population older than 50 years, although most people are asymptomatic. It is more common in women than in men.

Clinical features

There may be nonspecific colicky left-sided abdominal pain (that may be relieved by defecation), tenderness, nausea and flatulence. There may be a change in bowel habit with constipation or diarrhoea. Pyrexia and more severe pain are present with diverticulitis. Diverticula may perforate and lead to localized or generalized peritonitis or fistula formation (e.g., vesicocolic leading to pneumaturia and recurrent urinary tract infections, rectovaginal or intestinal fistulas). Rectal bleeding may occur, and is usually sudden and painless. Subacute obstruction may occur because of stricture formation.

Investigations

In the acute setting an FBC, U&E measurement, LFTs, amylase measurements and arterial blood gas tests are all indicated, as these patients tend to present with an acute abdomen. If the patient is pyrexial, blood cultures should be sent to the laboratory. Plain abdominal X-ray and erect CXR should be performed (to rule out obstruction and/or perforation), but a CT scan is the imaging modality of choice. If there is rectal bleeding, proctoscopy may be indicated. Colonoscopy is contraindicated in the acute setting as it may cause colonic perforation, but should be performed once the acute episode has resolved.

Management

In acute diverticulitis, treatment includes analgesia (avoid NSAIDs), adequate hydration and broad-spectrum antibiotics (to cover anaerobic and gram-negative bacteria). Profuse rectal bleeding may require blood transfusion. Between 15% and 30%

Table 30.2 Modified Duke classification of colorectal carcinoma

Tumour stage	Definition	Percentage of cases	Five-year cancer-related survival (%)
A	Confined to bowel wall	10	90
B	Beyond bowel wall/no metastases	35	70
C	Involves lymph nodes	30	30
D	Distant metastases/residual disease after surgery	25	<5

of patients will need surgery. Abscesses may need to be drained, and peritonitis following perforation or obstruction may necessitate resection with or without colostomy. Treatment of fistulas is surgical.

For diverticulosis, a high-fibre diet is recommended, and soluble fibre supplements and bulk-forming agents can be prescribed. Antispasmodics may provide symptomatic relief when colic is a problem but are not routinely recommended. Drugs that slow intestinal motility (e.g., codeine and loperamide) could exacerbate symptoms and are contraindicated.

Clostridium difficile and pseudomembranous colitis

Clostridium difficile is an anaerobic, gram-positive bacterium that can cause anything from mild diarrhoea to severe inflammation and perforation of the colon in pseudomembranous colitis (PMC). Colonization by *C. difficile* is encouraged by broad-spectrum antibiotic therapy, which eliminates other normal gut bacteria. All antibiotics but in particular cephalosporins, β-lactam inhibitors, clindamycin, macrolides and fluoroquinolones have been implicated in the infection. Other medications such a PPIs can also predispose to developing the condition.

There should be a suspicion of *C. difficile* infection in any inpatient who develops diarrhoea after a period of antibiotic therapy. It is usually of acute onset but may run a chronic course. Diarrhoea may be associated with fever and abdominal cramps. As with all causes of colitis, if severe, toxic dilatation of the colon can occur. Spread is through the faecal–oral route, and handwashing with water and soap is of paramount importance for infection control.

Diagnosis is by demonstration of *C. difficile* toxin in faeces. The most commonly used test is the stool cytotoxin test. Sigmoidoscopy in patients with PMC reveals an erythematous, ulcerated mucosa, which is covered by a membrane.

Management involves stopping use of the antibiotics and patient isolation. Orally administered metronidazole or vancomycin are used as specific treatments. Careful attention should be paid to fluid and electrolyte balance.

Lower gastrointestinal tract bleeding

The differential diagnosis of lower GI tract bleeding is shown in Table 30.3.

Lower GI tract bleeding may be occult and chronic, presenting with iron-deficiency anaemia and general lethargy and fatigue. Fresh bright red bleeding most commonly originates in the lower GI tract, whereas blood mixed in with stool is usually from higher in the tract. Most common causes of low GI tract bleeding are benign.

Acutely unwell patients need to be resuscitated first with use of the ABCDE approach. Once the patient is stable, investigations to

Table 30.3 Differential diagnosis of lower gastrointestinal tract bleeding

Anal fissure
Haemorrhoids
Inflammatory bowel disease
Infective colitis
Gastrointestinal carcinoma: sigmoid, caecum, rectum
Ischaemic colitis
Diverticulitis
Intestinal polyps
Vascular abnormalities: angiodysplasia, arteriovenous malformations
Meckel diverticulum
Peutz–Jeghers syndrome
Osler–Weber–Rendu disease
Endometriosis

determine the cause of bleeding are performed. Flexible sigmoidoscopy and/or colonoscopy and CT colonography are aimed at investigating the patient for colorectal cancer. CT angiography should be considered if vascular abnormalities are suspected. Stool samples are sent to exclude an infectious cause. More specialized tests such as capsule endoscopy can be performed if the initial investigations were inconclusive and small bowel disease is suspected.

Ischaemic colitis

Acute ischaemia of the bowel may occur and is often embolic (e.g., due to atrial fibrillation). This is a surgical emergency. It is suggested by disproportionate abdominal pain, haemodynamic shock and a relative absence of clinical signs with a metabolic acidosis with high lactate level, and a history of ischaemic heart disease.

Chronic intestinal ischaemia usually relates to low flow in the inferior mesenteric artery and therefore affects the descending colon. Severe postprandial pain occurs ('gut claudication') with rectal bleeding and diarrhoea. There is often pyrexia, tachycardia and leucocytosis. It usually settles with conservative management. Diagnosis is difficult, but revascularization may be attempted following angiography. Occasionally gangrene of the affected gut segment occurs, warranting surgical resection. Mortality is high.

Microscopic colitis

This is defined by the triad of chronic watery diarrhoea, normal colonoscopy findings and histopathological evidence of increased inflammatory cells within colonic biopsy specimens. The condition is associated with other autoimmune conditions such as Sjögren syndrome and coeliac disease, and commonly affects middle-aged women. Treatment is symptomatic with antidiarrhoeal drugs or occasionally budesonide.

Irritable bowel syndrome

Clinical features

Irritable bowel syndrome (IBS) is a functional bowel disease characterized by **A**bdominal pain or discomfort, **B**loating and/ or **C**hange in bowel habit. The diagnosis is symptom based, and at least one of those cardinal symptoms must be present for a minimum of 6 months. Cramping and alternating periods of diarrhoea and constipation are often present but predominance of either diarrhoea or constipation also occurs. Some people have a sense of incomplete evacuation or 'rectal dissatisfaction'. Passage of mucus may occur. Symptoms may be precipitated by certain foods, drugs (e.g., antibiotics) or stress. Other features such as tiredness, nausea, backache and bladder symptoms are common. Rectal bleeding is not a feature and prominent nocturnal symptoms point away from the diagnosis.

Investigations

The term 'diagnosis of exclusion' is not encouraged now as it belittles symptoms. However, it is important not to miss more serious disease (e.g., IBD or malignancy). Investigations include FBC, erythrocyte sedimentation rate (ESR), C-reactive protein (CRP) level, antibody testing for coeliac disease, faecal calprotectin level (if IBD is suspected) and cancer antigen 125 (CA125) level (if ovarian cancer is suspected). CT or colonoscopy should be considered in older patients or in patients in whom colonic carcinoma is suspected.

Management

The NICE guidelines on IBS were updated in April 2017. Patient education is important. Lifestyle advice should be given. Soluble fibre, such as ispaghula husk (psyllium), can be used to increase the amount of dietary fibre, whereas consumption of insoluble fibre (such as bran) and aggravating foods, caffeine, alcohol and fizzy drinks should be discouraged. In some patients there may be important psychological aggravating factors that respond to reassurance or cognitive behavioural therapy. Antimotility drugs such as loperamide may relieve diarrhoea, whereas laxatives help with constipation. Antispasmodics (e.g., mebeverine) may relieve pain. Tricyclic antidepressants should be considered if there is no improvement. Some patients derive benefit from a fermentable oligosaccharide, disaccharide, monosaccharide and polyol (FODMAP) diet in collaboration with a dietitian.

NONULCER DYSPEPSIA

'Nonulcer dyspepsia' encompasses a heterogeneous group of patients with dyspeptic symptoms (see Chapter 10) and no macroscopic mucosal abnormality.

The cause of their symptoms is unclear but is likely to be multifactorial and include acid, dysmotility, *H. pylori* infection and depression. Satisfactory management is often difficult for the patient and clinician to achieve. Lifestyle advice is given regarding smoking, alcohol consumption, obesity, etc. Use of culprit drugs, such as NSAIDs, should be stopped if possible. Antisecretory therapy is used and is titrated to the lowest-cost preparation that achieves symptom control. Those who are *H. pylori*-positive should undergo eradication therapy.

> **HINTS AND TIPS**
>
> In irritable bowel syndrome it is important to gain the patient's confidence. Investigations should be sufficient to exclude other important diagnoses. The diagnosis should then be made with appropriate explanation and advice, otherwise patients may move from doctor to doctor seeking further investigation.

Inflammatory bowel disease

> **HINTS AND TIPS**
>
> Extraintestinal manifestations of inflammatory bowel disease include **a**phthous ulcers, **p**yoderma gangrenosum, **i**ritis, **e**rythema nodosum, **s**clerosing cholangitis, **a**rthritis and **c**lubbing. A helpful mnemonic to remember these is A PIE SAC.

General overview

Ulcerative colitis and Crohn disease are collectively termed 'inflammatory bowel disease' (IBD). The two conditions differ in their natural history and response to treatment, but both follow a relapsing and remitting course (Table 30.4).

The primary cause of IBD is unknown, although 10% of patients have a first-degree relative with the disease, suggesting a combination of environmental and genetic factors. It may result from a genetically determined, inappropriately severe and/or prolonged inflammatory response to a dietary or microbial product. Abnormalities of colonic epithelial cell metabolism have also been reported in ulcerative colitis, and there are associations with long-term use of NSAIDs and antibiotics, although the significance is uncertain. Stress tends to exacerbate symptoms rather than cause the disease.

Table 30.4 Features of Crohn disease and ulcerative colitis

Feature	Crohn disease	Ulcerative colitis
Pathology	Transmural inflammation	Only mucosa and submucosa inflamed
	Fissuring ulcers: cobblestone mucosa	Mucosal ulcers: pseudopolyps
	Noncaseating granulomata	Crypt abscesses
	Can involve whole GI tract. Skip lesions	Continuous involvement proximally from rectum to affect variable length of colon
Clinical	Diarrhoea with or without rectal bleeding	Diarrhoea: often with blood and mucus
	Abdominal pain and fever prominent	Abdominal pain less prominent. Fever may be present
	Anal/perianal and oral lesions	
	Narrowing causing obstructive symptoms	
Associations	Increased incidence in smokers	Decreased incidence in smokers
	Cholelithiasis Renal calculi	Increased primary biliary cirrhosis, sclerosing cholangitis, chronic active hepatitis
	Extraintestinal manifestations of IBD (see later)	Other extraintestinal manifestations of IBD are less common than in Crohn disease
Complications	Fistulas (enteroenteral, enterovaginal, enterovesical, perianal)	No fistulas
	Strictures causing bowel obstruction	Toxic megacolon (in acute colitis)
	Carcinoma (related to colitis)	Carcinoma
	Iron-deficiency anaemia	
	Abscess formation	
	Vitamin B_{12} deficiency (terminal ileum commonly involved)	Iron-deficiency anaemia

GI, Gastrointestinal; IBD, inflammatory bowel disease.

There may be a history of atopy, autoimmune disease and the presence of circulating immune complexes and antibodies to colonocytes and neutrophils in ulcerative colitis. The presence of perinuclear antineutrophil cytoplasmic antibodies (p-ANCA) indicates ulcerative colitis, whereas the presence of anti-*saccharomyces cerevisiae* antibody (ASCA) indicates Crohn disease.

Ulcerative colitis

This is an idiopathic chronic relapsing inflammatory disease that always involves the rectum and extends proximally in continuity to affect a variable length of the colon. Although the small bowel is spared, there may be some 'backwash ileitis' secondary to ileocaecal valve incompetence. It is commoner in the Western world, with an incidence of about 10 to 20 in 100,000 per year. It is most commonly diagnosed at the age of 15 to 25 years, with a smaller peak at 55 to 65 years. There is no major sex difference. Patients with ulcerative colitis have no change in the overall standardized mortality ratio compared with the general population, although subgroups, such as those with extensive acute colitis, have higher mortality. The lifetime risk of developing colorectal cancer in people with ulcerative colitis is increased about twofold. The cumulative incidence is around 18% at 30 years.

Clinical features—The severity of diarrhoea and systemic upset depends on the extent of the disease and depth of mucosal ulceration.

Active subtotal or total ulcerative colitis causes frequent bloody diarrhoea, often with fever, malaise, anorexia, weight loss, abdominal pain, tenesmus, anaemia and tachycardia. With proctitis, the characteristic symptoms are rectal bleeding and mucus discharge, but the stool is well formed and general health is maintained. The patient is usually symptom-free between relapses.

Patients may present with complications. These can be local or extraintestinal. Local complications include:

- toxic megacolon
- perforation
- massive haemorrhage (rare)

Extraintestinal complications include:

- erythema nodosum, pyoderma gangrenosum, vasculitis (skin)
- anterior uveitis, episcleritis, conjunctivitis (eyes)
- large joint arthropathy, sacroiliitis, ankylosing spondylitis (joints)

- pericholangitis, sclerosing cholangitis, cirrhosis, autoimmune hepatitis, cholangiocarcinoma (liver)
- arterial and venous thrombosis (vasculature)

Investigations—Sigmoidoscopy and rectal biopsy show inflamed mucosa. If the disease is active, there may be pus and blood, visible ulceration and contact bleeding. Colonoscopy will show the extent of the disease. Ulcers and pseudopolyps may be seen. Other types of colitis should be excluded, and stool microscopy and culture are needed to exclude infection. Blood tests may show anaemia and raised levels of inflammatory markers (white cell count (WCC), ESR, CRP).

Histology shows inflammatory cells infiltrating the lamina propria with crypt abscesses. There is little involvement of the muscularis mucosae, and there is a reduction in the number of goblet cells.

In the patient with acute colitis, abdominal X-ray should be performed to look for colonic dilatation and evidence of mucosal oedema. An erect CXR is often performed in the acute setting to exclude perforation (60%–80% sensitive).

Management—A multidisciplinary approach is preferred with gastroenterologists, nursing staff and stoma therapists in collaboration with primary healthcare teams. Liaison with the colorectal surgical team at an early point is encouraged. Specific nutritional, haematinic and electrolyte deficiencies may require correction. Use of NSAIDs should be avoided, and opiates should be used only on specialist advice.

Patient mortality with acute colitis increases significantly in the case of perforation. In order to minimize the risk of complications, management is directed at stratifying patients in terms of severity, treating them accordingly to induce remission and carefully selecting those requiring emergency colectomy (Table 30.5).

Drug therapy—The mainstay of therapy in the acute phase is steroids (with bone protection) with the addition of a 5-aminosalicylic acid such as mesalazine. Patients should be weaned off steroids after the acute episode. Steroids are not used as a maintenance agent. Tacrolimus can be added in cases of inadequate response to steroid treatment. Ciclosporin is used as a salvage therapy in persistent disease; however, it is associated with high toxicity levels and severe side effects.

Mesalazine is used to maintain remission in mild to moderate disease. Thiopurines such as azathioprine or mercaptopurine are used if aminosalicylates alone are not effective or if the patient has two or more exacerbations per year requiring steroid treatment or after a single severe episode. It may take up to 4 months to effect a noticeable clinical benefit with azathioprine. Serious adverse effects include bone marrow suppression (resulting in, e.g., neutropenia) and cholestatic jaundice, necessitating blood checks fortnightly for 1 month, then monthly for 2 months, then 2 to 3 monthly. Thiopurine methyltransferase (TPMT) activity should be measured before commencement of treatment with thiopurines. TPMT is an enzyme that metabolizes these drugs, and its activity differs greatly amongst the population.

Anti-tumour necrosis factor-α (TNF-α) monoclonal antibodies such as infliximab, adalimumab and golimumab are effective agents used in moderate to severe disease refractory to conventional therapy.

If patients are systemically unwell (tachycardia, hypotension, fever, dehydration, tender abdomen) and have more than eight bowel movements per day, they should be admitted to hospital:

- Nil by mouth, intravenous fluids, close monitoring of observations, stool record.
- Intravenously administered hydrocortisone in divided doses throughout the day.
- Antibiotics for any accompanying infection (usually gram-negative).
- If improved at 5 days, commence oral steroid therapy.
- If failing to respond, some advocate the careful use of ciclosporin or infliximab to induce remission.
- Indications for emergency colectomy: continuing deterioration despite medical therapy; toxic dilatation of the colon; perforation.

Surgical intervention—Surgery is curative for colonic disease, although not for extraintestinal complications. Options include proctocolectomy with ileoanal pouch, permanent ileostomy or rarely subtotal colectomy with ileorectal anastomosis. Surgery may be considered electively for chronic intractable ulcerative colitis, colonic carcinoma, persistent mucosal dysplasia or growth retardation in children. The emergency indications are summarized in the last point of the preceding list. Many cases can now be done laparoscopically.

Prognosis and monitoring—Approximately 70% of untreated patients relapse annually, and up to 30% eventually require surgery, although the overall mortality is close to that of the general population. The main risks to life are severe attacks of the disease and colonic cancer. NICE recommends that patients with the disease extending beyond the rectum should be offered colonoscopic surveillance at 10 years. Additionally, the person-specific risk of neoplastic metaplasia should be calculated. Low-risk patients should be offered colonoscopy at 5 years, intermediate-risk patients should be offered colonoscopy at 3 years and high-risk patients should be offered colonoscopy at 1 year.

Crohn disease

Crohn disease can affect any part of the GI tract from the mouth to the anus. The involvement is not confluent ('skip lesions')

Table 30.5 Truelove and Witts classification for severity of ulcerative colitis

Activity	Mild	Moderate	Severe
No. of bloody stools/day	<4	4–6	>6
Temperature (°C)	Normal	37–37.8	>37.8
Heart rate (bpm)	Normal	Intermediate	>90
Hb (g/dL)	>11	10.5–11	<10.5
ESR (mm/h)	<20	20–30	>30

ESR, *Erythrocyte sedimentation rate;* Hb, *haemoglobin.*

(Table 30.4). It most frequently affects the ileocaecum or colon or ileum alone. The prevalence is approximately 50 to 100 in 100,000. Patients with Crohn disease have increased overall mortality compared with the general population. Peak onset is at the age of 15 to 30 years. The risk of colorectal cancer is comparable to that of people with ulcerative colitis.

Clinical presentation—The patient has diarrhoea and abdominal pain. There may be a fever, anaemia and weight loss. Associated complications are as with ulcerative colitis, and also clubbing, renal stones, amyloidosis and granulomata around body organs.

The presentation depends on the site of the disease and on the tendency to perforate or fistulate rather than to fibrose and stricture, which is probably determined by genetic factors. Terminal ileal disease presents with right iliac fossa pain, often with an associated mass. This may present acutely, mimicking appendicitis, or chronically, mimicking IBS. Strictures lead to GI obstruction.

Colonic Crohn disease is distinguishable from ulcerative colitis by the presence of skip lesions (multiple lesions with normal bowel in between), rectal sparing, perianal skin tags or fistulas with or without granulomata on biopsy, although the distinction is unclear in up to 10% of patients.

Investigations—Diagnosis is made by endoscopy and biopsy of lesions. Histology demonstrates transmural inflammation with an inflammatory cell infiltrate and noncaseating granulomata (in 30%). CT (or MRI) of the small and large bowel shows skip lesions, a coarse cobblestone appearance of the mucosa and, later, fibrosis producing narrowing of the intestine with proximal dilatation. MRI is particularly useful for evaluation of fistulas and abscesses, and should be used as the first-line imaging investigation in pelvic disease. Blood tests may show anaemia (potentially due to terminal ileum involvement and a resulting inability to absorb vitamin B_{12}). Serum CRP level can be elevated in active disease and is a useful marker of response to treatment. ESR has a similar role. Stool samples should be sent for microscopy and culture to exclude infection. Faecal calprotectin level reflects the degree of intestinal inflammation.

Management—In most cases of active Crohn disease, there are three therapeutic alternatives: drugs, diet and surgery. These options should be discussed with the patient.

Drug and diet therapy—Some patients manage with symptomatic therapy alone (e.g., loperamide or codeine phosphate) provided there is no evidence of obstruction or active colitis. Cholestyramine (an ion-exchange resin) is useful for diarrhoea due to terminal ileal disease or previous resection as it prevents conjugated bile acids from entering the colon. However, it should not be given at the same time as other medications as it impairs their absorption. Haematinics may require replacement, although anaemia often abates as disease activity falls.

Acute attacks are often treated with corticosteroids, but as with ulcerative colitis, these have no effect on reducing the rate of relapse. Their inappropriate use must be avoided because of their side-effect profile. Budesonide is a corticosteroid analogue with rapid hepatic conversion, and therefore reduced systemic side effects. It is less effective and should be used only if conventional steroids are contraindicated. Azathioprine therapy is often started during the acute attack and used as maintenance treatment. Methotrexate should be considered if thiopurines cannot be used. Infliximab and adalimumab are recommended for use in severe cases resistant to other drugs. Vedolizumab (anti-$\alpha_4\beta_7$ integrin monoclonal antibody) should be used only when anti-TNF-α agents fail.

Patients with colonic involvement may benefit from a 5-aminosalicylic acid compound. Antibiotics also have a role. Metronidazole is effective in colonic and perianal disease and in prevention of recurrence following bowel resection. If it is used for longer than 3 months, there is a risk of peripheral neuropathy. Other antibiotics are also used.

Elemental or polymeric diets are useful for inducing remission in small bowel disease but are expensive and unpalatable, so adherence is often poor.

Some patients can be maintained in remission without drug therapy – the importance to patients with Crohn disease of stopping smoking must be emphasized.

Surgical intervention—Surgery should be avoided if possible. It is indicated for:

- Patients in whom the disease is limited to distal portion of the ileum.
- Failure of medical therapy with acute or chronic illness causing ill health.
- Complications: abscess, obstruction, perforation, toxic dilatation, fistulas not responding to conservative treatment with antibiotics.
- Failure to grow (children).

Small bowel strictures can be widened (stricturoplasty), whereas those elsewhere need resection. Postoperative fistulas used to be a common complication but are now rare, partly because of the use of perioperative antibiotics, particularly metronidazole. After surgical resection, approximately half of patients remain symptom-free for 5 years and half require further surgery within 10 years.

Prognosis—Around 10% to 20% of patients remain asymptomatic for 20 years after the first or second episode of symptomatic disease. Around 50% of patients need at least one surgical resection within their lifetime, particularly if the small and large bowel are involved. The principles for colorectal cancer screening are the same as for ulcerative colitis.

HEPATOBILIARY SYSTEM

Gallbladder disorders

Gallstones and biliary colic

Gallstone-related disease is a common diagnosis in those admitted to hospital with abdominal pain. Risk factors include increasing age, obesity and weight-cycling, smoking, diabetes, female sex and oral contraceptive or hormone replacement therapy use.

Bile contains cholesterol, bile pigments and phospholipids; the relative concentrations of these determine the kind of stone that is formed. Pigment stones (10%) are small and radiolucent, and they are occasionally associated with haemolytic anaemia due to increased formation of bile pigment from haemoglobin. Cholesterol stones (10%) are large, often solitary and radiolucent. Mixed stones (80%) contain calcium salts, pigment and cholesterol. Only 15% to 20% of gallstones are radio-opaque, whereas approximately 90% of renal stones are radio-opaque.

Clinical features

Approximately 10% to 25% of the UK population have gallstones, 80% of which are asymptomatic. The commonest complications are biliary colic, acute cholecystitis and obstructive jaundice. Other presentations are uncommon or rare, and include cholangitis (infection of the bile ducts causing right upper quadrant pain, jaundice and fever with rigors – Charcot triad), chronic cholecystitis (chronic inflammation secondary to repeated episodes or acute cholecystitis), pancreatitis, empyema and gallstone ileus, where the gallstone perforates the gallbladder, ulcerates into the duodenum and passes on to obstruct the terminal ileum.

Biliary colic is the most common presentation, classically with pain in the upper abdomen or right upper quadrant. Typically, the pain lasts for more than 30 minutes, but less than 8 hours, is colicky in nature, and is often severe and may be associated with nausea and vomiting, but not associated with fever or abdominal tenderness.

Investigations

- LFTs may show a cholestatic picture if a gallstone is impacted in the common bile duct (CBD) (see Chapter 14).
- Ultrasound examination is useful in diagnosing gallstones, cholecystitis and stones in the bile duct.
- Magnetic resonance cholangiopancreatography (MRCP) should be used if ultrasound examination has not demonstrated CBD stones but the bile duct is dilated and/or LFT results are abnormal. Endoscopic ultrasound examination may be useful if MRI is not possible.
- Haemolysis screen: if pigment stones are suspected or found operatively.

Management

> **HINTS AND TIPS**
>
> Most asymptomatic gallstones do not need treatment. Asymptomatic CBD stones, however, should be treated in the same way as symptomatic CBD stones, as stones in the biliary tree can cause obstructive jaundice, cholangitis and pancreatitis.

In symptomatic gallstones, treatment is often by cholecystectomy (ideally laparoscopic), which may be performed immediately or after a delay. Care should be taken in patients with nonspecific upper abdominal symptoms to confirm that gallstones found on investigation are the true cause of symptoms. In biliary colic, cholecystectomy is usually reserved for recurrent episodes.

Patients with symptomatic CBD stones associated with cholangitis require resuscitation and intravenous antibiotics. In the presence of duct dilatation, endoscopic retrograde cholangiopancreatography (ERCP) with sphincterotomy is usually performed, allowing the removal of stones. A stent may be placed if stones cannot be retrieved. Other options include an 'on-table' cholangiogram during open or laparoscopic surgery to assess the presence of stones in the CBD.

Acute cholecystitis

Clinical features

Acute cholecystitis is most common in overweight, middle-aged women but may occur at any age. Risk factors include gallstones or biliary sludge (95% of patients), female sex, increasing age, obesity or rapid weight loss and pregnancy. It typically follows the impaction of a stone in the cystic duct or Hartmann pouch (at the junction of the gallbladder neck and the cystic duct). If the stone moves to the CBD, jaundice may occur. The signs and symptoms are like those of biliary colic, but in addition there is fever and tenderness in the epigastrium or right upper quadrant, and there may be rigors, vomiting, local peritonism or a gallbladder mass. Murphy sign may be positive; this is increased pain on inspiration when the tips of the fingers are placed under the costal margin in the right upper quadrant, due to an inflamed gallbladder impinging on the examiner's fingers. The test is only considered positive when the same manoeuvre performed in the left upper quadrant does not elicit pain.

> **CLINICAL NOTES**
>
> The differential diagnosis of acute cholecystitis includes:
>
> - Biliary colic
> - Cholangitis
> - Appendicitis in an anatomical variant of an appendix located higher than normal within the abdominal cavity
> - Perforated peptic ulcer
> - Pancreatitis
> - Right basal pneumonia
> - Myocardial infarction

Investigations

WCC is elevated and the levels of inflammatory markers are raised (unlike in biliary colic). A CXR, an ECG and serum amylase and troponin measurements should be taken to help exclude differential diagnoses. Ultrasound scan will commonly show a thickened gallbladder wall and stones with or without CBD dilatation.

Management

Management is usually conservative initially, unless complications ensue (e.g., perforation of the gallbladder). The patient should be asked to fast and should be given intravenous fluids, offered effective analgesia and prescribed antibiotics (e.g., amoxicillin and metronidazole intravenously) followed by oral co-amoxiclav; gentamicin should also be given intravenously if the patient is showing signs of sepsis. Laparoscopic cholecystectomy is the treatment of choice, and the current trend is to perform this acutely, within 1 week of diagnosis, to prevent recurrent episodes. Occasionally the inflammation is allowed to settle and a cholecystectomy is performed after 2 to 3 months. Open cholecystectomy is performed in the case of perforation.

Chronic cholecystitis

Recurrent episodes of cholecystitis are usually associated with gallstones, and can lead to intermittent colic and chronic inflammation. It may be asymptomatic, present as a more severe case of acute cholecystitis or present as 'flatulent dyspepsia': abdominal discomfort, bloating, nausea, flatulence and intolerance of fats. Right upper quadrant USS is the diagnostic investigation of choice; hyperenhancement of the gallbladder wall is the most common sign seen. The preferred treatment of choice is elective laparoscopic cholecystectomy. Patients who are not a good candidate for surgery can be managed expectantly, and are advised to stick to a low-fat diet to help reduce the frequency of symptoms.

Biliary tract cancer

Cholangiocarcinoma

This is a carcinoma arising in any part of the biliary tree, but most cholangiocarcinomas are extrahepatic. More than 90% of cholangiocarcinomas are ductal adenocarcinomas, and the remainder are squamous cell tumours. Patients usually present with obstructive jaundice or systemic symptoms. Risk factors include increasing age, primary sclerosing cholangitis and chronic intraductal gallstones.

Surgery is the only curative option, but less than one-third are resectable at diagnosis. Prognosis is poor (10%–40% at 5 years, average survival of 10–12 months from diagnosis). ERCP and stenting are used for palliation of jaundice, and chemotherapy is used for locally advanced or metastatic unresectable cholangiocarcinoma.

Gallbladder cancer

This is a rare cancer, and 85% of cases are adenocarcinoma. It is more common in women, smokers and those with a family history; the risk increases with age, particularly after 70 years. The tumour typically arises in the fundus, and is often discovered incidentally during cholecystectomy. Curative treatment requires surgery, the extent depending on the staging. Prognosis is very poor (10% 5-year survival rate) as most cases are diagnosed late.

Cancer of the ampulla of Vater

This tumour arises in the distal 1 cm of the CBD. Patients present with anorexia, nausea, vomiting, jaundice, pruritus or weight loss. Patients may present relatively early (compared with pancreatic cancer) because of the tumour location causing biliary obstruction. A curative Whipple procedure is preferred for early cancer (proximal pancreaticoduodenectomy with antrectomy). This is best done at a centre with specific expertise and experience in the procedure. Stenting may be used for palliation. The overall survival rate at 5 years is 20%.

Pancreatic disorders

Acute pancreatitis

Acute pancreatitis is an acute inflammatory condition of the pancreas causing local and systemic reactions. The incidence is approximately 3 cases per 10,000 population in the United Kingdom. Around 75% of cases are secondary to either gallstones or alcohol consumption, and a careful alcohol history and symptoms/signs of gallstone disease should be sought. Other causes include ERCP, surgery or trauma, toxins and drugs, hyperglyceridaemia and autoimmune disease.

HINTS AND TIPS

The causes of pancreatitis can be recalled from the mnemonic GET SMASHED:

- Gallstones
- Ethanol
- Trauma
- Steroids
- Mumps
- Autoimmune diseases
- Scorpion stings
- Hypertriglyceridaemia
- ERCP
- Drugs (e.g., azathioprine or thiazide diuretics)

Clinical features

Pancreatitis typically causes acute onset severe epigastric abdominal pain radiating to the back. Nausea and vomiting are common. Patients are dehydrated and quite unwell when they present, and must be assessed for signs of shock. Jaundice may be present. On examination, there may be abdominal tenderness with guarding and rebound tenderness. Tachycardia, fever, hypotension and sweating may be present. Bruising around the umbilicus (Cullen sign) or in the flanks (Grey Turner sign) are classic signs in pancreatitis.

Pancreatitis can lead to serious complications such as acute respiratory distress syndrome (ARDS), sepsis or disseminated intravascular coagulation.

Investigations

Bedside

- Serum amylase: level often markedly raised (more than three times the normal level). However, a normal amylase level does not exclude pancreatitis (this is especially true in acute attacks on a background of previous episodes when pancreatic tissue mass may be reduced). Amylase level is also raised with cholecystitis, perforated viscus (e.g., a duodenal ulcer) and even in ectopic pregnancy, but usually to a lesser extent. Serum lipase is more sensitive and specific, but the test is not always available.
- Serum calcium, magnesium and phosphate: levels may be low and replacement may be needed.
- FBC: WCC is usually raised.
- U&Es: raised urea level is an indicator of severity.
- LFTs: may show an obstructive picture.
- Fasting serum glucose: level often raised in pancreatitis.
- Arterial blood gases: metabolic acidosis. Po_2 is also measured, and this is important in prognosis.
- ECG: to exclude myocardial infarction.

Imaging

- Abdominal X-ray: gallstones, pancreatic calcification indicating previous inflammation, an absent psoas shadow due to retroperitoneal fluid and a distended loop of jejunum ('sentinel loop').
- Erect CXR: widened mediastinum in aortic dissection; gas under the diaphragm in perforated peptic ulcer. In severe cases, pleural effusion or ARDS.
- Abdominal ultrasound or endoscopic ultrasound examination: allows visualization of gallstones and duct dilatation.
- Abdominal CT scan: within 48 hours for severe pancreatitis, within 7 days for those failing to improve (suspected pancreatic necrosis), delayed for detection of pseudocyst.
- MRCP may be indicated to detect occult microlithiasis, neoplasms, chronic pancreatitis or anatomical abnormalities, or if the person is not improving clinically as expected.

Table 30.6 Modified Glasgow severity scoring in acute pancreatitis

Mnemonic	
Po_2	Arterial Po_2 <8 kPa
Age	Age >55 years
Neutrophils	WCC >15 × 10^6/L
Calcium	Corrected calcium concentration <2.0 mmol/L
Renal	Urea concentration >16 mmol/L
Enzymes	Enzyme concentrations: LDH >600 U/L; AST >125 mmol/L
Albumin	Albumin concentration <32 g/L
Sugar	Fasting glucose concentration >10 mmol/L

Each element scores 1 point: 0 or 1, mild pancreatitis; 2, moderate pancreatitis; 3 or more, severe pancreatitis.
AST, Aspartate aminotransferase; LDH, lactate dehydrogenase; Po_2, partial pressure of arterial oxygen; WCC, white cell count.

Multiple prognostic scoring systems have been validated to determine severity, guide management and predict mortality; the Modified Glasgow Acute Pancreatitis Severity Score (Imrie score) is the most commonly used (Table 30.6). An alternative prognostic scoring system is the Acute Physiology and Chronic Health Evaluation II (APACHE-II) score, which also considers chronic health problems. Any patient with severe pancreatitis should be discussed with staff from the intensive care unit/high-dependency unit as multiple organ dysfunction syndrome can evolve quickly.

Mortality is 5% in mild disease and around 30% in severe disease. Recurrence is uncommon in patients who recover. Death may be from shock, renal failure, sepsis or respiratory failure. Other complications include hypocalcaemia due to the formation of calcium soaps, transient hyperglycaemia, pancreatic abscess requiring drainage and pseudocyst (fluid in the lesser sac presenting as a palpable mass), persistently raised serum amylase levels or LFT values and fever. Patients should be investigated to exclude gallstones, and alcohol should be avoided.

Management

Patients with pancreatitis are usually managed conservatively. Aggressive rehydration, analgesia and electrolyte replacement are important. Careful fluid and electrolyte balance monitoring should be emphasized. In patients who are unable to tolerate oral intake a nasogastric tube should be inserted for nutritional support, with return to enteral feeding as early as possible. Treatment with antibiotics is commenced if an infective cause is suspected or there is evidence of infected pancreatic necrosis and/or associated cholangitis. Daily FBC and U&E, calcium and glucose measurements should be performed. Surgery should be considered if haemorrhagic necrosis of the pancreas is suspected or diagnosed following imaging.

Chronic pancreatitis

Chronic pancreatitis is a chronic, irreversible inflammation and/or fibrosis of the pancreas, often characterized by severe pain and progressive endocrine and exocrine insufficiency. The main cause of chronic pancreatitis is alcohol misuse. Other causes include cystic fibrosis and haemochromatosis.

The patient is generally ill with weight loss and has recurrent abdominal pain radiating to the back. Steatorrhoea secondary to malabsorption from pancreatic insufficiency may occur. Diabetes may occur because of involvement of pancreatic islet beta cells, and there may be intermittent or persistent obstructive jaundice.

Investigations

These are as for those for acute pancreatitis, although serum amylase level is not helpful in the diagnosis as it is usually normal or only slightly raised. In addition plasma glucose test should be performed (level raised in diabetes).

Management

Alcohol should be avoided. A low-fat diet is advised because of malabsorption. Fat-soluble vitamins, calcium and pancreatic enzymes (e.g., Creon) are given. Complications such as diabetes should be managed. ERCP may be useful for strictures. Pancreatic duct stones may be treated using extracorporeal shockwave lithotripsy (ESWL). For recurrent attacks causing unremitting pain, pancreatic resection or pancreaticojejunostomy (a duct drainage procedure) may be considered.

Pancreatic cancer

Pancreatic cancer is the 11th most common cancer in the United Kingdom. Risk factors include smoking, poor nutrition, chronic pancreatitis and familial cancer syndromes (e.g., *BRCA1* and *BRCA2* mutations). The clear majority of pancreatic tumours are adenocarcinomas. Approximately three-quarters occur in the head of the pancreas, the rest occurring in the body or tail.

Clinical features

General features of malignancy may be present including anorexia, weight loss and lethargy. Local features include dyspepsia or epigastric pain radiating to the back, and obstructive jaundice with an enlarged palpable gallbladder (Courvoisier sign). There may be hepatomegaly from biliary obstruction or metastases. Pancreatitis may occur because of obstruction of the pancreatic duct. Thrombophlebitis migrans is a paraneoplastic feature in 10% of patients. Fever may occur. Pancreatitis may occur because of obstruction of the pancreatic duct.

HINTS AND TIPS

Pancreatic cancer should be suspected in any patient presenting with painless jaundice.

Investigations

FBC is required to test for anaemia and LFTs should be performed and, if a diagnosis of pancreatic cancer is suspected, the tumour marker cancer antigen 19-9 (CA19-9) should also be measured. Ultrasound examination may identify a mass and dilated bile ducts. CT scan is used to define resectability and tumour staging. MRCP and endoscopic ultrasound examination can provide valuable information regarding tumour characteristics and local involvement. ERCP allows biopsies to be taken; stents can be inserted for symptomatic control.

Management

Surgical resection is the only curative treatment, but most patients (85%–90%) present late in the disease after local invasion and spread have occurred (e.g., to portal vessels), making surgical intervention unsuitable. If the tumour is resectable, a Whipple procedure (pancreaticoduodenectomy) is the most commonly performed operation. Adjuvant chemotherapy is recommended for patients postoperatively. Management in unresectable disease is aimed at symptomatic control. Palliative chemotherapy with gemcitabine may be given. Despite interventions, prognosis is poor and the 5-year survival rate is less than 3%.

Liver disorders

Chronic liver disease

Chronic liver disease can be a result of many underlying disorders, several which are discussed in this chapter. Clinical features include leuconychia, clubbing, Dupuytren contracture, bruising, gynaecomastia, spider naevi and caput medusa. Liver size is not a reliable sign, as livers which have reached end-stage cirrhosis are often not palpable. Progression happens over years, but patients may present acutely with decompensated liver failure; the symptoms of which include variceal bleeding, ascites, encephalopathy, coagulopathy and hepatorenal syndrome.

The principal problems in severe chronic liver disease are due to: (1) the degree of hepatocellular failure (causing hypoglycaemia, failure of synthesis of clotting factors and hypoalbuminaemia) and (2) the complications of portal hypertension.

Features of decompensation

Chronic liver disease is the result of cycles of destruction and regeneration of liver parenchyma resulting in scarring by means of fibrosis, eventually causing cirrhosis. Often patients may have no or few symptoms, but the degree of hepatocyte destruction reduces hepatic reserve, and minimal events may precipitate hepatic decompensation (Table 30.7), the features of which are discussed next.

Table 30.7 Factors that can precipitate hepatic decompensation

Constipation
Vomiting and diarrhoea
Gastrointestinal bleeding
Intercurrent infection
Alcohol
Morphine
Surgery
Electrolyte imbalance

Varices—Oesophageal varices result from portal hypertension: a portal–systemic shunt between the left gastric vein (portal) and lower oesophageal veins (systemic). The increased pressure in these varices makes them prone to rupture and consequently bleeding. The management of variceal bleeding was discussed previously in this chapter.

Ascites—Ascites is the presence of free fluid within the peritoneal cavity. Factors leading to the formation of ascites include salt and water retention because of cirrhosis, hypoalbuminaemia resulting in decreased plasma oncotic pressure, portal hypertension and increased hepatic lymph production.

Clinically, there may be abdominal distension, shifting dullness and a fluid thrill, if the ascites is tense. Associated features include hernias, divarication of the recti, abdominal wall venous distension, ankle oedema and distension of the neck veins.

Investigations include diagnostic paracentesis (ascitic tap). Ascitic fluid is analysed by appearance and biochemistry. The ascites is clear and yellow unless it is infected, when it appears cloudy/turbid indicating possible bacterial peritonitis (SBP). If the tap is nontraumatic, blood signifies intraabdominal malignancy or haemorrhagic pancreatitis (where it is accompanied by Grey-Turner's sign – see Chapter 9). Milk-coloured fluid indicates lymphoma, TB or malignancy. Biochemical analysis can help narrow the differential diagnosis. A glucose level higher than serum glucose level indicates TB or malignancy. A raised amylase level suggests pancreatitis. The protein content is usually less than 15 g/L. Higher values indicate infection, hepatic venous obstruction or malignancy. To further narrow the differential diagnosis, the serum ascitic albumin gradient (SAAG) is used, which indirectly measures portal pressure and can be used to determine if ascites is due to portal hypertension. A high SAAG suggests that the fluid is a transudate, indicating the presence of portal hypertension, while a low SAAG suggests that the fluid is an exudate and the cause of ascites is more likely due to infection, pancreatitis or malignancy. Fluid should also be sent for cytology, microscopy and culture.

RED FLAG

Spontaneous bacterial peritonitis (SBP) is one of the most frequently encountered bacterial infections in patients with cirrhosis, and is most commonly seen in patients with end-stage liver disease. It is an infection of ascitic fluid that cannot be attributed to any intraabdominal, ongoing inflammatory or surgically correctable condition. Diagnostic paracentesis should be carried out without a delay as part of the septic screen to rule out SBP in all cirrhotic patients with ascites on hospital admission. Ascitic neutrophil >250/mm count remains the gold standard for the diagnosis of SBP. Cultures should also be performed. The most common organisms isolated in patients with SBP include Escherichia coli, Gram-positive cocci (mainly *Streptococcus species*) and enterococci. Empirical antibiotic therapy must be initiated immediately after the diagnosis of SBP.

General management of ascites includes restricted salt and fluid intake. The first-choice diuretic is spironolactone. This can cause painful gynaecomastia in men, and other diuretics can be used instead. If there is a poor response to spironolactone, furosemide may be added. Fluid balance, weight and U&E levels should be monitored daily. Ascites can also be treated with therapeutic paracentesis and albumin infusion. Overdiuresis may result in dehydration, uraemia and hyponatraemia and may precipitate hepatic encephalopathy, oliguria and hepatorenal syndrome. Transjugular intrahepatic portosystemic shunt (described previously in this chapter) is an alternative in patients requiring ascitic taps frequently.

Hepatic encephalopathy—Hepatic encephalopathy can either be reversible and episodic or lead to coma and death (Table 30.8). Liver failure results in diminished hepatic metabolism of substances derived from the gut, which can cause neurotoxicity. Nitrogenous waste (ammonia) builds up in the circulation and passes to the brain, where it is cleared by means of processes involving conversion of glutamate to glutamine. This causes an osmotic shift at the blood–brain barrier, leading to cerebral oedema. Clinical features include impaired conscious level, personality disturbances, inversion of the normal sleep pattern, slurred speech, constructional apraxia, flapping tremor (asterixis), hepatic fetor, brisk tendon reflexes, increased muscle tone and rigidity and hyperventilation in deep coma.

Initial treatment aims to correct or remove the precipitating causes. These may include electrolyte abnormalities, sepsis, hypovolaemia, hypoxia, GI bleeding and constipation. Use of diuretics, sedatives and opiates should be stopped, and intracranial disease should be excluded, especially in patients with alcoholism. CT scanning of the brain may be appropriate to exclude subdural haematomas. Measures should then be instituted to

Table 30.8 Grading of conscious level in hepatic encephalopathy

Grade	Features
1	Confusion, altered behaviour, psychometric abnormalities
2	Drowsy, altered behaviour
3	Stupor, obeys single commands, very confused
4	Coma responding to painful stimuli

Table 30.9 Causes of acute hepatitis

Cause	Example
Infection	Hepatitis A virus, hepatitis B virus, hepatitis C virus, EBV, CMV
Drugs	Paracetamol, β-lactams
Toxins	Alcohol, carbon tetrachloride
Autoimmune	Autoimmune hepatitis, SLE
Metabolic disease	Wilson disease
Ischaemia	Portal vein thrombosis (70% of oxygen is delivered through portal vein)

EBV, Epstein-Barr virus; *CMV*, Cytomegalovirus; *SLE*, Systemic Lupus Erythematosus.

remove nitrogenous material and bacteria from the bowel. High doses of lactulose should be used. Antibiotics such as rifaximin can be helpful in reducing gut ammonia-producing bacterial load.

Hepatorenal syndrome—Hepatorenal syndrome is discussed in Chapter 31.

Hepatitis

Acute hepatitis

Acute hepatitis is inflammation of a previously healthy liver lasting less than 6 months. It has multiple causes (Table 30.9). Treatment and prognosis are dependent on the underlying cause (see later). However, certain comorbidities will affect overall recovery and disease progression. These include chronic infection with, for example, HIV or hepatitis C virus (HCV), long-term alcohol abuse, necessary drug therapy (e.g., methyldopa) or genetic disorders (e.g., haemochromatosis). Fulminant hepatic failure is a syndrome that is due to overwhelming hepatocyte necrosis, leading to severe impairment of liver function.

Acute viral hepatitis

Hepatitis A

Epidemiology—Hepatitis A virus (HAV) is a member of the picornavirus family. It is an RNA virus. Transmission is by the faecal–oral route. The incubation period ranges from 2 to 6 weeks. Fever, fatigue, abnormal liver function and jaundice occur in adults. Clinical disease is uncommon in infants and young children, and the infection may go unnoticed.

Serology—At the onset of symptoms, immunoglobulin M (IgM) anti-HAV antibody is present in serum. High titres persist for 3 to 12 months, so a positive test in a patient with acute hepatitis indicates recent acute infection. Previous infection, and therefore immunity, can be illustrated by the presence of IgG anti-HAV without IgM anti-HAV. IgG is detectable lifelong.

Prognosis—The disease is usually self-limiting and treatment is symptomatic. Relapses and cholestatic jaundice may occur but hepatitis A does not progress to chronic hepatitis.

Prevention and control—Prophylaxis can be obtained by immune serum immunoglobulin or active immunization. The latter induces higher levels of anti-HAV.

Hepatitis B

Epidemiology—Hepatitis B virus (HBV) is a DNA virus. The complete infectious virion (Dane particle) consists of the following:

- Hepatitis B surface antigen (HBsAg): the outer lipoprotein 'surface' envelope.
- Hepatitis B core antigen (HBcAg): the internal core, which surrounds the viral genome of DNA.
- Hepatitis B e antigen (HBeAg): a subunit of HBcAg; it can be detected in serum and is a useful marker of circulating virions and infectivity.

Transmission is parenteral through infected body fluids or blood, and the incubation period is 40 to 160 days. In developed countries hepatitis B usually occurs sporadically.

Those at risk are intravenous drug users, healthcare workers, people with haemophilia or patients on haemodialysis, babies of HBsAg-positive mothers, people who have moved from areas where it is endemic, those engaging in risky sexual behaviours and individuals resident in long-term care facilities. Infection is characteristically anicteric (not accompanied by jaundice), asymptomatic and chronic.

Serology—Following exposure to HBV, HBsAg can be detected throughout the prodromal phase and is not usually cleared from the serum until convalescence. Other early markers include anti-HBc and HBeAg. A positive IgM anti-HBc test typically distinguishes acute hepatitis B from chronic hepatitis B. The presence of HBeAg implies high infectivity.

The loss of HBeAg is a good prognostic sign, indicating that the patient will clear HBsAg and is unlikely to develop chronic infection. The disappearance of HBeAg is usually followed by the appearance of serum anti-HBe. Anti-HBs is the last marker to appear in serum (Fig. 30.1).

Prognosis—Acute infection rarely leads to fulminant hepatic failure. Treatment is normally supportive, and patients are advised to avoid alcohol. Between 8% and 20% of patients will develop cirrhosis without antiviral treatment within 5 years

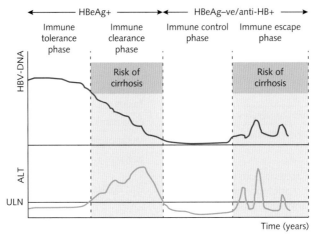

Fig. 30.1 Natural history of chronic hepatitis B virus (HBV) infection. ALT, Alanine aminotransferase; HBeAg, hepatitis B e antigen; ULN, upper limit of normal.

of infection. Patients with established cirrhosis should undergo hepatocellular carcinoma (HCC) surveillance.

Prevention and control—Infection can be prevented by active immunization. Management includes peginterferon alfa-2a. Treatment is continued for 48 weeks in patients with compensated liver disease.

Hepatitis C

Epidemiology—HCV is an RNA virus, and can be divided into many major types and subtypes. Hepatitis C is a slowly progressive liver disease with a varied clinical picture, ranging from asymptomatic to rapidly progressing cirrhosis with HCC. Transmission is parenteral through blood and bodily fluids. The incubation period is between 6 and 9 weeks.

Serology—Anti-HCV develops 1 to 3 months after the onset of clinical illness in most cases; however, it may take up to 9 months in some individuals. Identification of the viral RNA in serum is possible by polymerase chain reaction (PCR), and signifies ongoing infection. HCV antigens cannot be detected in serum.

Prognosis—The acute disease is often asymptomatic, and leads to chronic infection in around 80% of patients. In about 20% of patients, cirrhosis may develop insidiously within 10 years, and patients may develop a clinical picture resembling autoimmune hepatitis. Systemic manifestations include cryoglobulinaemia, porphyria cutanea tarda and mesangiocapillary glomerulonephritis. Untreated HIV infection accelerates the progression of HCV-induced cirrhosis. Success of antiviral treatment differs with the viral genotype. NICE recommends a combination therapy of peginterferon alfa and ribavirin. Genotypes 2 and 3 of HCV tend to respond to this treatment better than genotype 1.

Prevention and control—Unlike for HAV and HBV there is no effective vaccination. Prevention of transmission is therefore the mainstay of infection control. Blood bank screening for anti-HCV and genetically engineered factor VIII preparations for people with haemophilia limit the occurrence of hepatitis C.

Hepatitis D—Hepatitis D (delta) virus (HDV) is an RNA virus. The virion particle is encapsulated by the coat protein of HBV (HBsAg). Thus infection by HDV occurs only in patients with hepatitis B. Transmission is as for HBV, and the incubation period is 35 days. Diagnosis is through IgM anti-HD, IgG anti-HD and hepatitis D antigen detection. The disease is not usually progressive, but outbreaks of fulminant hepatitis caused by HBV plus HDV can occur.

Hepatitis E—This RNA virus is transmitted via the faecal–oral route, with a peak of epidemic infection 6 to 7 weeks after primary exposure and low secondary attack rate. Serum IgG and IgM anti-HEV can be detected by ELISA. The condition is usually self-limiting, and progression to chronic hepatitis is rare. Mortality can be as high as 20% if the infection occurs while the patient is pregnant. Prevention and disease control are dependent on high standards of public sanitation and sewage elimination.

Other viruses—Viral hepatitis can be caused by nonhepatic, systemic viruses. Examples include EBV, CMV, herpes simplex virus, Q fever and arbovirus (yellow fever). Clinical features differ enormously from asymptomatic mild hepatitis to rapidly progressive fulminant fatal hepatitis. Diagnosis is through specific viral assays using techniques such as PCR or ELISA. If virology gives negative results, alternative causes such as autoimmune hepatitis or Budd–Chiari syndrome, see later, must be considered.

Clinical features—In the preicteric phase, symptoms are nonspecific and include malaise, fatigue, listlessness and lack of energy. Anorexia, nausea and vomiting may occur. Right upper quadrant pain, change in bowel habit, myalgia, fever and headaches may be present. The prodromal symptoms become less severe as jaundice appears. Dark urine and pale stools may occur.

The physical signs are usually minimal. Common findings include jaundice, hepatic tenderness, hepatomegaly, splenomegaly and lymphadenopathy. Rashes may be present.

Fulminant hepatitis leads to hepatic encephalopathy with severe jaundice, ascites and oedema and is usually accompanied by haemorrhage caused by coagulopathies. The disturbance of consciousness reflects a combination of hepatic coma, hypoglycaemia and cerebral oedema.

Investigations
- LFTs: alanine aminotransferase (ALT) and aspartate aminotransferase (AST) levels are markedly elevated. Bilirubin level is raised. During recovery, liver enzyme levels return to normal. A persistently raised ALT 6 months after the acute onset of hepatitis usually indicates progression of the disease.
- Prothrombin time: may be prolonged with fulminant hepatic failure.
- Serum albumin: level may be low and serum globulin level may rise.
- Hypoglycaemia: may occur with fulminant hepatic failure.
- Serum alpha-fetoprotein (AFP): levels increased transiently in patients with acute viral hepatitis.

Management—Specific management depends on the cause of the hepatitis. General measures include simple analgesia, alcohol avoidance and good nutrition. Cholestyramine may alleviate itching. Patients should be barrier nursed until the cause of hepatitis is identified. Use of all unnecessary drugs should be stopped.

Autoimmune hepatitis
Autoimmune hepatitis is caused by autoantibodies against hepatocytes, causing an inflammatory condition of the liver. It predominantly affects young and middle-aged women, and is associated with thyroiditis, diabetes mellitus, ulcerative colitis and fibrosing alveolitis. Clinical features may be insidious, and include fever, right upper quadrant pain, jaundice, epistaxis and gum bleeding, polyarthritis and urticaria.

Investigations reveal deranged LFT values (raised AST/ALT levels) and raised IgG levels. Autoantibodies anti-liver-kidney microsomal (anti-LKM), antinuclear (ANA), antimitochondrial (AMA) and anti-smooth muscle antibodies (ASMA)) may be present. Liver biopsy will show mononuclear cell infiltration of portal and periportal regions with piecemeal necrosis, fibrosis or cirrhosis.

Treatment includes orally administered prednisolone, reduced over time and maintained for 2 years. If treatment is stopped, autoimmune hepatitis relapse is likely. Azathioprine may need to be added. Rituximab or methotrexate can be considered. If decompensated liver failure secondary to cirrhosis is present, liver transplantation is indicated.

Alcoholic liver disease—Men who drink more than 50 units and women who drink more than 35 units of alcohol per week have a significant risk of developing cirrhosis. Ten to twenty percent of people with chronic alcoholism develop cirrhosis. Risk factors include genetics, female sex (women develop alcoholic hepatitis and cirrhosis younger, and after less intake, than men), poor nutrition (alcohol is better tolerated under optimal dietary conditions) and a synergistic effect with hepatotrophic viruses.

Pathology
Initially there are fatty changes within the liver. With alcoholic hepatitis, there is liver cell necrosis and generalized inflammation. Cells contain alcoholic hyaline or Mallory bodies. Later there is deposition of collagen around the central veins, which may spread to the portal tracts.

Cirrhosis may result, which is initially micronodular. Extensive fibrosis contributes to the development of portal hypertension. With continued cell necrosis and regeneration, the cirrhosis may progress to a macronodular pattern.

Clinical features
The patient may initially be asymptomatic. With alcoholic hepatitis, there may be fatigue, anorexia, nausea and weight loss. There may be signs of chronic liver disease (see Chapter 14).

Hepatic decompensation leads to encephalopathy and liver failure. Precipitating factors are listed in Table 30.7.

With advanced cirrhosis, there may be signs of malnutrition, ascites, encephalopathy and a tendency to bleed (thrombocytopenia and coagulopathy). Signs include bilateral parotid enlargement, palmar erythema, Dupuytren contractures and multiple spider naevi. Men develop gynaecomastia and testicular atrophy. Portal hypertension develops, leading to splenomegaly and distended abdominal wall veins. Oesophageal varices are often present. There may be signs of alcohol damage in other organs (e.g., peripheral neuropathy, cardiomyopathy, proximal myopathy or pancreatitis).

Investigations
Mean corpuscular volume and γ-glutamyltransferase level are sensitive indices of alcohol ingestion. Important variables for predicting outcome include indicators of synthetic liver function: clotting, glycaemic control, albumin level and LFT values.

Ultrasound examination will demonstrate fatty liver, and histology of liver biopsy specimens will show the pathological changes discussed earlier. Transient elastography (a type of ultrasound examination used to quantify liver fibrosis and steatosis) can be used to diagnose cirrhosis. Patients with an established diagnosis of alcohol-related liver disease should be offered 2-yearly cirrhosis retesting.

Management
Patients should be counselled to completely abstain from alcohol. General measures for the management of chronic liver

disease should be instigated. Patients may need nutritional support, including vitamins B and C. Liver transplantation is usually offered only to fully medically managed otherwise suitable candidates with persistent decompensated liver disease after abstinence from alcohol for at least 3 months.

Prognosis

If the patient abstains from alcohol, fatty liver alone carries a good prognosis. If the patient is encephalopathic and malnourished, mortality is up to 50%. Ascites, peripheral oedema, persistent jaundice, uraemia and the presence of collateral circulation are unfavourable prognostic signs.

The Child–Pugh classification (Table 30.10) is a scoring system that was originally used to estimate the risk of complications, especially in cirrhotic patients considered for liver transplantation; however, it has now been largely replaced by the newer Model for End-Stage Liver Disease score (Clinical Notes: MELD score).

CLINICAL NOTES

MELD SCORE

The Model for End-Stage Liver Disease score is used to evaluate liver disease severity and predict survival. It is often used to help determine if a patient could be considered for liver transplantation. It is calculated by the entering of the levels of bilirubin and creatinine and the international normalized ratio into a mathematical formula. The equation is adjusted if the patient has been receiving renal replacement therapy. A score of more than 40 corresponds to 3-month mortality of more than 70%.

Table 30.10 Child–Pugh score

Criteria	Points		
	1	2	3
Encephalopathy	Absent	Grade 1 or 2	Grade 3 or 4
Ascites	Absent	Mild to moderate	Severe
Bilirubin (mg/dL)	<2	2–3	>3
Albumin (g/dL)	>3.5	2.8–3.5	<2.8
Prothrombin time (s) or INR	<4 <1.7	4–6 1.7–2.3	>6 >2.3

Five or 6 points correspond to class A (low operative mortality), 7–9 points correspond to class B (moderate operative mortality) and 10–15 points correspond to class C (high operative mortality).
INR, International normalized ratio.

Nonalcoholic steatohepatitis

Nonalcoholic steatohepatitis (NASH) is an increasingly common condition because of the obesity epidemic. The condition is characterized by fatty deposit in the liver in association with inflammation. NASH without inflammation is termed 'nonalcoholic fatty liver disease' (NAFLD). It is typically asymptomatic, but occasionally a smooth hepatomegaly may be felt on examination. The diagnosis may be suspected because of chronically elevated aminotransferase levels, typically with an AST-to-ALT ratio less than 1. Alkaline phosphatase and γ-glutamyltransferase levels are usually raised. Liver ultrasound scan will show diffuse hyperechogenicity. Treatment is predominantly lifestyle-based: increased exercise and weight loss have been shown to reverse early disease. Tight glycaemic control is important as diabetic patients are at increased risk of NASH. NICE guidelines developed in 2016 advise that pioglitazone or vitamin E should be considered when advanced fibrosis is present. Prognosis is good if lifestyle changes are made, but NASH can progress to cirrhosis and HCC.

Haemochromatosis

Haemochromatosis occurs as a result of excess iron in the tissues. It was referred to as 'bronze diabetes' in the past due to the presenting features of skin discoloration and diabetes mellitus. It may be classified as hereditary ('primary') or secondary. Hereditary haemochromatosis is an autosomal recessive disorder of iron metabolism characterized by increased intestinal absorption of iron. Secondary haemochromatosis may result from excessive iron administration (e.g., blood transfusion or iron tablets). Affected organs include the liver, endocrine system, heart and joints. The prevalence ranges from 1 in 200 to 1 in 2000, and men are 5 to 10 times more likely to be affected than women, indicating that environmental and genetic factors modify disease expression. Alcohol may exacerbate the disease by influencing iron absorption and metabolism.

Total body iron is increased in haemochromatosis from 4 g to as much as 60 g. There is cellular damage and fibrosis, leading to a rusty colour of the liver, pancreas, spleen and abdominal lymph nodes. Complications include diabetes mellitus, cirrhosis, heart disease with arrhythmias and liver cancer.

Most patients are asymptomatic or have nonspecific symptoms such as arthralgia and lethargy, until the effect of iron overload becomes apparent in the fifth or sixth decade. Joints are involved by chondrocalcinosis, which is associated with synovial haemosiderin and loss of intraarticular space. In the early stages, pain and swelling of the second and third metacarpophalangeal joints is characteristic. Later, slate-grey skin pigmentation due to melanin and iron deposition is a feature. Symptoms include asthenia, abdominal pain, impotence, arthralgia and amenorrhoea. Signs include hepatomegaly, splenomegaly, jaundice and gynaecomastia. The disease may lead to cirrhosis.

Investigations

- Serum ferritin level is high (however, this is of low specificity as it can be raised in a number of other inflammatory conditions).
- Serum iron level is elevated, and saturation of plasma transferrin is high (however, these findings alone should not be used for diagnosis as they do not adequately reflect total body iron).
- Definitive diagnosis of haemochromatosis depends on histology of liver biopsy specimens.
- CT scanning and MRI can be used to detect increased tissue iron but are not routine.
- Genetic testing can be performed to look for the most common mutations (C282Y and H63D).

Management

Patients should be venesected regularly (400–500 mL weekly), until they develop a mild microcytic anaemia. Care is needed in patients with severe hepatic disease because vigorous bleeding may be complicated by hypoproteinaemia. Folate supplementation may be needed to optimize erythropoiesis. Seriously ill patients with overt cardiac haemochromatosis may require high-dose parenteral chelation therapy with desferrioxamine to reverse life-threatening disease.

Patients with established haemochromatosis should be investigated for cardiac involvement and pituitary, as well as target organ endocrine failure, and replacement therapy should be instituted when necessary. Patients should be reviewed to monitor diabetic control, to care for joint disease and to inspect them for the development of complications (e.g., HCC).

Life expectancy and hepatic and cardiac function in primary haemochromatosis are improved by iron depletion. The 5-year survival rate increases from 30% to 90% with treatment. Removal of iron does not prevent the development of cancer in patients with established cirrhosis.

Primary biliary cholangitis

Primary biliary cholangitis (PBC) is an autoimmune disorder primarily affecting the small intrahepatic bile ducts (canals of Hering) as a nonsuppurative, destructive cholangitis leading to bile duct damage, cholestasis, fibrosis, cirrhosis and death from liver failure. The UK prevalence is around 13 per 100,000. The average life expectancy is 10 years from diagnosis but differs considerably; if the serum bilirubin level is greater than 180 μmol/L, the life expectancy is 18 months without transplantation. It is associated with other autoimmune conditions (e.g., Sjögren syndrome, thyroid disease, Addison disease, Raynaud syndrome, systemic sclerosis and coeliac disease). It is also associated with malabsorption, extrahepatic malignancies, particularly of the breast and HCC. Around 50% of people with PBC develop renal tubular acidosis.

Women are nine times more likely to be affected. PBC usually presents in middle age with lethargy and pruritus. Pigmentation and xanthomata may be present, jaundice may develop and

portal hypertension may lead to ascites or oesophageal varices. There may be stigmata of chronic liver disease. Approximately 25% have hepatomegaly at presentation, and 15% have splenomegaly. The patient may be asymptomatic at presentation, or may present with liver failure. Investigations will show deranged LFT values (obstructive pattern with raised alkaline phosphatase, γ-glutamyltransferase and bilirubin levels in late disease). Immunologically, HLA-B8 and HLA-DR3 are associated with a threefold increase in the risk of PBC. Serum immunoglobulin levels are raised, especially IgM level. There is antimitochondrial antibody positivity in 90% to 95% of cases. Ultrasound examination of the liver is important to exclude obstruction. It can also show evidence of portal hypertension and splenomegaly. Histology of the liver will confirm the diagnosis. Initially, there is asymmetrical destruction of bile ducts and surrounding lymphocytic infiltrate. Granulomas may be present. Increasing fibrosis, and eventually cirrhosis, develops.

There is no evidence of benefit from the use of immunosuppressive agents. Bile salts (e.g., ursodeoxycholic acid) may help with cholestasis, and improve biochemical blood results, and slow progression in early disease. Liver transplantation is indicated for intractable symptoms or end-stage disease. Patients with jaundice should receive supplementation with fat-soluble vitamins A, D and K. Diarrhoea is treated with a low-fat diet and pancreatic supplements.

Primary sclerosing cholangitis

Primary sclerosing cholangitis is characterized by inflammation, scarring and narrowing of the intrahepatic and extrahepatic bile ducts. The cause is unknown, but the condition is associated with IBD (usually ulcerative colitis, rarely Crohn disease) and HIV infection. Immunologically, there is an association with HLA-A1, HLA-B8 and HLA-DR3. The clinical features are due to chronic biliary obstruction, and include jaundice, hepatomegaly, pruritus, fatigue and abdominal pain. Patients are at increased risk of ascending cholangitis, cholangiocarcinoma and autoimmune hepatitis.

Blood tests reveal elevated alkaline phosphatase or γ-glutamyltransferase and bilirubin levels. Tests for antinuclear antibodies, p-ANCA and anticardiolipin antibodies may be positive. MRCP is the imaging method of choice, and shows multiple bile duct strictures with a characteristic beaded appearance. ERCP allows stricture dilation and stenting. Liver biopsy shows fibrous, obliterative cholangitis. Management is symptomatic; ursodeoxycholic acid is used to relieve cholestasis. Liver transplantation is indicated for end-stage disease

Wilson disease (hepatocellular degeneration)

Clinical features

This is an autosomal recessive disorder (gene on chromosome 13) of copper metabolism leading to deposition of copper in;

- Liver: cirrhosis with its ensuing complications.
- Basal ganglia: tremor and choreoathetosis.
- Cerebrum: dementia and fits.
- Eyes: Kayser–Fleischer rings (a brown pigmentation of the periphery of the iris best seen with a slit lamp).
- Renal tubules: renal tubular acidosis.
- Bones: osteoporosis and osteoarthritis.
- Red blood cells: haemolytic anaemia.

Clinical features are usually due to hepatic or central nervous system involvement.

Investigations
There is a high concentration of copper in the blood, and a low concentration of caeruloplasmin, a copper-binding protein.

Management
The dietary intake of copper should be reduced, and penicillamine should be given to aid the elimination of copper ions. Regular blood counts are mandatory because of potential agranulocytosis and thrombocytopenia with treatment. Other side effects of penicillamine treatment include oedema, proteinuria, haematuria, rashes, loss of taste and muscle weakness. Relatives should be screened. The prognosis is generally good.

Hepatic tumours

Benign tumours
Benign tumours of the liver are often an incidental finding on CT or ultrasound scan. Haemangiomas are the most common. Cysts, adenomas, fibromata, focal nodular hyperplasia and leiomyomas are further types of benign liver tumours. Haemangiomas should not be biopsied because of bleeding risk. Unless they are symptomatic, tumours are managed conservatively.

Malignant tumours—The most common malignant liver tumours are metastases. Primary tumours that tend to metastasize to the liver include colon, stomach, lung, uterus, breast, pancreas and carcinoid tumours. Lymphoma and leukaemia may also spread to the liver. Primary carcinomas of the liver are less common, although they are increasing in incidence, and include HCC, angiosarcoma, cholangiocarcinoma and fibrosarcoma.

HCC is by far the most common primary liver tumour accounting for 90% of malignant tumours, and is associated with viral hepatitis, cirrhosis (and therefore alcohol excess), parasite infection and anabolic steroid use. Clinical features of malignant liver cancer, primary or secondary, include weight loss, anorexia, malaise and right upper quadrant pain. The pain is capsular in nature and is clinically difficult to treat. Jaundice is a late feature, if at all, except in the case of cholangiocarcinoma. Investigations include FBC and blood film, LFTs, hepatitis serology, AFP measurements (AFP level is elevated in 75% of patients with HCC) and CT or MRI scanning. Liver biopsy allows tissue diagnosis. Treatment and prognosis in metastatic liver cancer depends on the cause and the extent of the disease. Treatment of HCC is surgical resection if the tumour is solitary and smaller than 3 cm or liver transplantation. Percutaneous ablation, chemotherapy and tumour immobilization are also used.

Miscellaneous conditions

α_1-Antitrypsin deficiency
α_1-Antitrypsin (A1AT) is a serine protease inhibitor, synthesized in the liver, important in the correct functioning of the inflammatory cascade. A1AT deficiency is an autosomal recessive disorder (chromosome 14), and causes emphysema, cirrhosis and potentially HCC. The diagnosis is made by measurement of protease inhibitor concentrations and can be screened for prenatally with oligonucleotides. There is no cure, and management is symptomatic. Pneumococcal and flu vaccination should be offered. Liver transplantation is performed for end-stage liver failure.

Liver abscess
Liver abscesses are relatively rare in the United Kingdom but are common in the developing world. The infectious organism can be bacterial, parasitic, protozoal or helminthic. Entry to the liver can be direct (penetrating injury), through the portal circulation, through the systemic circulation or by ascending the biliary tree. The clinical feature is predominantly swinging pyrexia and night sweats with right upper quadrant pain. Tender hepatomegaly is often present, and if subacute, it can be associated with cachexia. A blood test may show raised levels of inflammatory markers and deranged LFT values. Blood cultures are positive in 50% of cases, and may yield the causative organism. Liver ultrasound examination will show defined areas of hypoechogenicity. CT is an alternative/additional imaging modality. Treatment can be conservative with antibiotics or specific agents against the suspected or proven microorganism. CT- or ultrasound-guided drainage is an alternative option.

Budd–Chiari syndrome
This condition is characterized by hepatic vein obstruction, through either thrombosis or compression, causing hepatomegaly, ascites and abdominal pain. It has multiple causes, including hypercoagulability states, myeloproliferative disorders, hepatocellular tumours and radiotherapy, although 30% of cases are idiopathic. The investigations of choice are ultrasound examination with Doppler or CT scans to show hepatic vein thrombosis and ascites. Management involves treating the underlying cause and draining the ascites. Angioplasty or a surgical shunt may be required to bypass the obstruction. Anticoagulation is indicated in the absence of varices. In fulminant liver failure, transplantation should be considered.

Chapter Summary

- Barrett oesophagus increases the risk of oesophageal adenocarcinoma.
- *Helicobacter pylori* infection and chronic nonsteroidal antiinflammatory drug use are the biggest causes of peptic ulcer disease.
- Acute gastrointestinal bleeding is a medical emergency. If severe, oesophagogastroduodenoscopy should be performed urgently. If the cause is known to be oesophageal varices, terlipressin should be used, alongside high-dose intravenous proton pump inhibitor and intravenous broad-spectrum antibiotics.
- Gastric cancer is treated surgically, and chemotherapy is not used with curative intent.
- Colorectal cancer is the third commonest cancer in the United Kingdom. A national screening program for colorectal cancer is available in the United Kingdom.
- Diverticulitis can lead to serious complications such as perforation and peritonitis.
- *Clostridium difficile* infection is most commonly associated with the use of cephalosporins, β-lactam inhibitors, clindamycin, macrolides and fluoroquinolones.
- Ulcerative colitis and Crohn disease are debilitating conditions associated with serious complications. Colon cancer surveillance is an important part of management.
- Charcot triad is typical for acute cholangitis, and includes right upper quadrant pain, jaundice and pyrexia.
- Murphy sign is positive in cholecystitis.
- Alcohol abuse is the leading cause of liver disease.
- Acute pancreatitis is a well-known cause of acute respiratory distress syndrome. Causes can be recalled using the mnemonic GET SMASHED.
- Alcohol is the most common cause of chronic pancreatitis.
- The 5-year survival rate in pancreatic cancer is less than 3%.
- Chronic liver disease increases the risk of developing liver cancer.
- Hepatitis B virus and hepatitis C virus lead to chronic infection and can result in cirrhosis.
- Hepatitis D virus cannot exist in the absence of hepatitis B virus.
- Nonalcoholic steatohepatitis is defined as nonalcoholic liver disease with evidence of inflammation.

UKMLA Conditions
Acute cholangitis
Acute pancreatitis
Alcoholic hepatitis
Anal fissure
Ascites
Cholecystitis
Coeliac disease
Colorectal tumours
Diverticular disease
Gallstones and biliary colic
Gastric cancer
Gastro-oesophageal reflux disease
Haemorrhoids
Hepatitis
Hiatus hernia
Infectious colitis
Inflammatory bowel disease
Irritable bowel syndrome
Liver failure

UKMLA Presentations
Abdominal distention
Abdominal mass
Acute abdominal pain
Ascites
Bleeding from lower GI tract
Bleeding from upper GI tract
Change in bowel habit
Change in stool colour
Chronic abdominal pain
Cirrhosis
Constipation
Decreased appetite
Diarrhoea
Gastrointestinal perforation
Jaundice
Melaena
Nausea
Perianal symptoms
Swallowing problems

Continued

Chapter Summary—cont'd

UKMLA Conditions
Malabsorption
Malnutrition
Oesophageal cancer
Pancreatic cancer
Peptic ulcer disease and gastritis
Perianal abscesses and fistulae
Peritonitis

UKMLA Presentations
Vomiting
Weight gain

Renal, genitourinary and sexual health medicine

31

INTRODUCTION

In this chapter, we discuss the basics of renal medicine, focusing on proteinuria; approach and importance of acute kidney injury (AKI); classification of stages of chronic kidney diseases (CKD); indications for initiating renal replacement therapies (RRTs); classification and management of glomerulonephritis and how not to miss the nephrological emergency of a rapidly progressive glomerulonephritis. We go on to describe management of urinary tract infections; renal calculi, urothelial tract malignancies and gender medicine. This chapter concludes with a summary of common sexually transmitted diseases, chlamydia, gonorrhoea, syphilis and genital herpes.

HAEMATURIA AND PROTEINURIA

Haematuria and proteinuria are common presentations of renal disease and are often incidental findings on urine dipstick testing. Isolated haematuria is covered in Chapter 15.

Proteinuria

Albuminuria is defined as an albumin-to-creatinine ratio (ACR) >3 mg/mmol (30 mg of albumin loss per 24-hour urine collection). ACR specifically measures albumin loss, which indicates damage to the glomerulus. It is very sensitive at detecting early-stage proteinuria (e.g., with diabetic nephropathy). You will also see protein: creatinine ratio (PCR) measured, this includes all protein leak, including non-albumin-containing proteinuria, which will be present when damage occurs at other sites of the kidney (e.g., with renal tubular damage).

Low-level proteinuria can occur in nonrenal disease, such as urinary tract infections (UTI) and in the presence of vaginal mucus. Significant proteinuria, ACR >70 mg/mmol or PCR >100 mg/mmol (1 g protein leak per 24 hours), usually indicates glomerular damage (Table 31.1).

CLINICAL NOTES

The leading cause of death in renal disease is cardiovascular disease (CVD). Albuminuria correlates with CVD risk, even low levels of albuminuria correlate with higher CVD risk.

Table 31.1 Levels of proteinuria

Type	ACR (mg/mmol)	PCR (mg/mmol)	Protein leak (g/day)
Normal	<3	<15	0.02
Microalbuminuria	<30	<50	0.03–0.3
Significant	>70	>100	>1.0
Nephrotic range		>300	>3.0

ACR, *Albumin-to-creatinine ratio;* PCR, *protein-to-creatinine ratio.*

Benign proteinuria

- Functional: pyrexia, strenuous exercise, congestive cardiac failure, acute illnesses, pregnancy.
- Orthostatic: present when upright but normal when supine. Relatively common in adolescents, rare over the age of 30 years.

Pathological proteinuria

This can result from:

- Any glomerular disease associated with damage to the basement membrane (diabetes mellitus, glomerulonephritis, other causes of nephrotic syndrome (see Table 31.2)).
- Tubular or interstitial damage may cause tubular proteinuria (failure of the tubules to reabsorb some of the plasma proteins that have been filtered by the normal glomerulus). This protein loss is lower level (i.e., ACR <70 mg/mmol or PCR <100 mg/mmol).

CLINICAL NOTES

Nephrotic syndrome is the triad of proteinuria (>3 g/day), hypoalbuminaemia (<30 g/L) and oedema. It is associated with high cholesterol levels and individuals are at increased risk of thromboembolic disease and infections.

Overflow proteinuria

This is when abnormal amounts of low-molecular-weight protein, filtered at the glomerulus, are neither reabsorbed nor catabolized completely by the renal tubular cells. This results in increased protein filtration (e.g., urinary light chains in multiple myeloma (Bence Jones protein)).

Table 31.2 Causes of nephrotic syndrome

Cause	Examples
Renal disease	Glomerular disorders:[a] primary; secondary to a systemic disease
Systemic disease	Amyloidosis[a] Systemic lupus erythematosus[a]
Metabolic disease	Diabetes mellitus[a]
Infection	HIV infection Hepatitis B
Malignancy	Membranous associated
Drugs	Gold Penicillamine Heroin Heavy metals
Familial disorders	Familial FSGS

[a]Common cause.
FSGS, *Focal segmental glomerulosclerosis.*

Clinical features

When you are taking a focused history in a patient presenting with proteinuria, with or without haematuria, key questions are vital in forming your differential diagnosis. Chapter 15 covers important aspects of the history and examination of a patient with urinary symptoms and haematuria. Later in this chapter, important parts of the history are covered as relevant to AKI, CKD and glomerular injury. In general, always consider:

- Urinary symptoms (e.g., frequency, haematuria, volume).
- Other relevant symptoms (e.g., oedema, hypertension, orthopnoea) or systemic features associated underlying causes (e.g., arthralgia/nasal crusting/epistaxis in vasculitis, acute illness in poststreptococcal glomerulonephritis, weight loss in malignancy).
- Any systemic chronic diseases (diabetes mellitus, rheumatoid arthritis, systemic lupus erythematous (SLE), previous calculi, recurrent urine infections).
- Past and current medications (particularly nephrotoxic agents)
- Family history (e.g., Alport syndrome, sickle cell disease)

Investigations

An algorithm for the investigation of the patient with haematuria and proteinuria is given in Fig. 31.1.

Urine

- Gross appearance: visible haematuria (if painless consider malignancy), Coca-Cola coloured urine (think rhabdomyolysis).
- Urinary dipstick: provides initial information about the presence or absence and degree of proteinuria and

haematuria; also test for nitrites/leucocytes/ketones/pH and glucose.
- Microscopy and culture: infection.
- PCR/ACR: this quantifies urinary protein loss. If there is a large gap between the two readings, this suggests that there is high loss of nonalbumin protein. This may be the case in myeloma with light chain excretion.

HINTS AND TIPS

Albumin-to-creatinine ratio (ACR) or protein-to-creatinine ratio (PCR) measurement is taken from a spot urine sample and it correlates well with the results from a 24-hour urine collection and is far easier for the patient to do. Note, an ACR of 70 mg/mmol or PCR of 100 mg/mmol is equivalent to 1g of proteinuria in 24 hours. When proteinuria is heavy, i.e., ACR is greater than 70 mg/mmol, then PCR is used. A PCR of 300 mg/mmol is equivalent to 3 g in 24 hours, and a PCR above this value is defined as nephrotic syndrome.

CLINICAL NOTES

Urine dipsticks are very sensitive to haematuria. Nonvisible haematuria is significant only if it is persistent (i.e., seen on two of three dipsticks in the absence of infection).

Blood tests

The following blood tests should be performed:

- Full blood count (FBC): leucocytosis with infections, anaemia with chronic renal failure.
- Renal profile: urea, creatinine, estimated glomerular filtration rate (eGFR), potassium and sodium.
- Bone profile: calcium, phosphate, magnesium, parathyroid hormone (PTH).
- Erythrocyte sedimentation rate (ESR) and C-reactive protein (CRP) (e.g., vasculitis).
- Clotting studies: bleeding diathesis.
- Blood glucose, glycated haemoglobin (HbA1c): diabetes mellitus.
- Bicarbonate.
- Creatine kinase: myoglobinuria.
- Uric acid: gout, tumour lysis syndrome.
- Blood cultures: infective endocarditis.

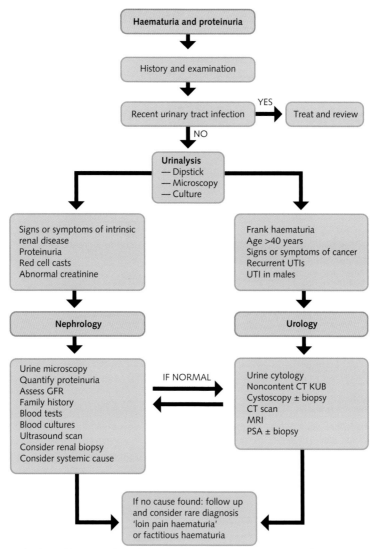

Fig. 31.1 Algorithm for investigation of haematuria and proteinuria. *AXR*, Abdominal X-ray; *CT*, computed tomography; *GFR*, glomerular filtration rate; *KUB*, kidneys ureter and bladder; *MRI*, magnetic resonance imaging; *PSA*, prostate-specific antigen; *UTI*, urinary tract infection.

- Specialized investigations according to clinical suspicion (e.g., serum complement – C3 and C4, antinuclear antibodies (ANA), antineutrophil cytoplasmic antibodies (ANCA), antistreptococcal titres, anti-GBM(glomerular basement membrane) antibody and anti-phospholipase A2 receptor antibody (anti-PLA2R).
- Protein electrophoresis, serum free light chains and urinary Bence Jones protein (myeloma).
- Blood film, lactate dehydrogenase (LDH), haptoglobins and reticulocytes if haemolysis is considered (i.e., microangiopathic haemolytic anaemia (MAHA)).

- HIV and hepatitis serology: potential causes of nephrotic syndrome.
- Cryoglobulins.

Imaging

A renal ultrasound scan is the first-line imaging study; it will confirm whether two kidneys are present, and if there are size or structural abnormalities. It may guide further imaging (e.g., CT; noncontrast CT kidney, ureter, bladder (KUB) is used for investigation of renal calculi).

Histological diagnosis

Renal biopsy may provide the best diagnostic information but is invasive and not without risk (1% of patients have significant bleeding, 1 in 100 need blood transfusion and 1 in 1000 need emergency nephrectomy). Careful thought needs to be given as to how the biopsy result will alter the management.

CLINICAL NOTES

A renal ultrasound scan must be performed before a renal biopsy is performed. Blood pressure control and coagulation need to be optimized before the procedure.

ACUTE KIDNEY INJURY

Acute kidney injury (AKI) was previously known as 'acute renal failure' and is a decline in glomerular filtration rate (GFR) over hours to days. Occurrence of an AKI is associated with increased morbidity, mortality and risk of developing long-standing chronic kidney disease (CKD). Many cases can be prevented if we recognize those people at risk. The Acute Kidney Injury Network classification is the most widely used system for staging AKI (Table 31.3)

Aetiology

AKI causes are often termed prerenal, renal and postrenal (Table 31.4). Prerenal causes are commonly due to relative hypotension. If poor renal perfusion persists, acute tubular necrosis results and is the most common cause of intrinsic renal failure. The cause of an AKI is often multifactorial, for example, in postsurgical AKI, fluid depletion, systemic inflammatory response syndrome and nephrotoxic drugs may all play a role. Many cases of AKI are avoidable.

Table 31.3 Acute Kidney Injury Network staging

Stage	Serum creatinine level	Urine output
1	1.5–2 times baseline level or increase of ≥26.5 μmol/L	<0.5 mL/kg/h for 6–12 h
2	2.0–3 times baseline level	<0.5 mL/kg/h for ≥12 h
3	>3.0 times baseline level	<0.3 mL/kg/h for ≥24 h or anuria for ≥12 h

Modified from Mehta RL, Kellum JA, Shah SV, Molitoris BA, Ronco C, Warnock DG, Levin A. Acute Kidney Injury Network: report of an initiative to improve outcomes in acute kidney injury. Critical Care 2007; 11(2): R31.

Table 31.4 Causes of acute kidney injury

Prerenal (ischaemic)	Extracellular volume loss: gastrointestinal loss (e.g., severe diarrhoea or vomiting), urinary loss (polyuria with salt-losing kidneys), burns
	Intravascular volume loss or redistribution: sepsis, haemorrhage (e.g., postpartum or at operation), hypoalbuminaemia
	Decreased cardiac output: heart failure (e.g., after myocardial infarction), cardiac tamponade, cardiac surgery
	Miscellaneous: hepatorenal syndrome
Renal	Postischaemic acute tubular necrosis: shock, trauma, sepsis, hypoxia
	Nephrotoxic acute tubular necrosis: antibiotics, analgesics, contrast media, heavy metals, solvents, proteins
	Glomerulonephritis
	Acute pyelonephritis
	Acute interstitial nephritis: antibiotics, analgesics, leptospirosis, viral infections
	Vasculitis
	Intratubular obstruction: myeloma (Bence Jones protein), urate, rhabdomyolysis
	Coagulopathies: acute cortical necrosis, haemolytic uraemic syndrome, thrombotic thrombocytopenic purpura, postpartum renal failure
	Miscellaneous: malignant hypertension, hypercalcaemia
Postrenal	Renal tract obstruction: stones, tumour (prostatic or pelvic), prostatic hypertrophy, surgical mishap (e.g., accidental ligation of ureters), periureteric fibrosis, bladder dysfunction
	Major vessel occlusion: renal artery thrombosis, renal vein thrombosis

CLINICAL NOTES

A thorough drug history is very important in AKI; pay attention to drugs that interfere with renal perfusion, e.g., NSAIDs, renin–angiotensin system antagonist (RAS blockers) which include angiotensin-converting enzyme inhibitors (ACEi) and angiotensin II receptor blockers (ARBs); or contrast medium from recent CT. Ask about new medications (e.g., antibiotics) and any over-the-counter medications (e.g., herbal medicines).

Clinical features

AKI is commonly detected with routine blood tests and symptoms are often nonspecific. A full history should be taken focusing on any recent infections, surgery, any possible hypovolemic episodes (e.g., diarrhoea or vomiting) and any urinary symptoms. Ask about risk factors for AKI, including any previous renal disease, diabetes and hypertension. Take a thorough drug history, focus on NSAIDs and ACEi/ARBs and ask about use of these drugs in relation to any recent illness/surgery.

Your examination should focus on the cause and consequences of the renal impairment. The most important initial assessment is the patient's volume status. Skin turgor, jugular venous pressure, postural blood pressure, heart rate, urine output and the presence of peripheral or pulmonary oedema should be noted. In an inpatient, a fluid balance chart may be available. You may be able to palpate your patient's kidneys if the patient has polycystic kidney disease or hydronephrosis. There may be tenderness in the renal angle in any disease that stretches the renal capsule, such as renal colic or pyelonephritis. You may be able to palpate the bladder, with associated suprapubic discomfort, in the presence of outflow obstruction. Examine the skin and look for evidence of purpuric rash (e.g., in vasculitis) or features of active lupus (e.g., malar butterfly rash).

Complications of AKI should be elicited as they may indicate the need for dialysis or haemofiltration. Uraemia manifests itself as pericarditis, uraemic flap, twitching and hiccups and causes itch (look for skin excoriations). Kussmaul respiration (deep, sighing breaths) may indicate acidosis. Respiratory examination may be consistent with pulmonary oedema.

CLINICAL NOTES

When assessing a patient with acute kidney injury, ask yourself:

- Are there any life-threatening complications?
- What is the patients' baseline renal function?
- What is the cause of the renal impairment? Is it prerenal, intrinsic renal disease or postrenal?
- Review the drug chart, do any of the drugs need stopping or the dose changing in light of their current level of renal function?

COMMUNICATION

ACE-inhibitors and ARBs act to dilate the efferent renal arteriole to reduce glomerular filtration pressure. Due to this mechanism they are commonly prescribed to reduce proteinuria and prevent progressive renal disease. They are renoprotective medications.

However, in the context of systemic illness, and hypovolaemia, this reduced glomerular filtration pressure can lead to a dangerous lack of renal perfusion and cause an acute kidney injury. Patients should be told to stop taking ACEi/ARBs during intercurrent illness (e.g., diarrhoea/vomiting and fever).

Investigations

Urine

- Urine analysis for blood, protein, nitrites, leucocytes. Aim to have urine analysis results before catheterization.
- A midstream urine sample (MSU) should be sent for microscopy, culture and sensitivity testing. The presence of red cell casts on microscopy is pathognomonic of glomerulonephritis but is rarely looked for in clinical practice.
- Send urine to the laboratory for a spot ACR to quantify urinary protein loss.
- Assessment of urinary biochemistry may help in distinguishing prerenal failure from established acute tubular necrosis. In prerenal failure, the kidney avidly retains salt and water, and hence urinary sodium level is below 20 mmol/L

and the urine is concentrated. In established acute tubular necrosis, the patient cannot concentrate the urine or conserve sodium, therefore a urinary sodium level is more than 40 mmol/L and the urine is dilute. These parameters are less reliable if the patient is taking diuretics.

CLINICAL NOTES

Be suspicious–the first presentation for myeloma can be with an acute kidney injury. Request urinary electrophoresis for Bence Jones protein if you are considering an underlying myeloma.

RED FLAG

Blood and protein (in the absence of infection) on urine analysis suggests underlying glomerular disease. Consider rapidly progressive glomerulonephritis if this is occurring with an AKI.

Blood tests

- Full set of blood tests: FBC, renal and bone profile, liver function tests (with attention to albumin), CRP and bicarbonate. The renal profile and bicarbonate level should be monitored at least daily.

HINTS AND TIPS

It is important to ascertain a patient's baseline renal function. This may require detective work (i.e., calls to GP, access to old notes). Look for whether the patient has previously had an acute kidney injury and in what context.

RED FLAG

In any patient with renal failure pay careful attention to the potassium level; a high potassium level is life-threatening. Be concerned about a potassium level above 5.8 mmol/L; a potassium level above 6.5 mmol/L can lead to arrhythmias and cardiac arrest. Worry most about a short-term rise from the patient's normal potassium level.

Other tests

For specific blood tests, see Investigations in Haematuria/Proteinuria.

- Electrocardiogram (ECG) can show the precipitating cause (e.g., myocardial infarction) or complications such as pericarditis (saddle-shaped ST segments) or hyperkalaemia (peaked T waves).
- Chest X-ray (CXR) if fluid overload is suspected; look for underlying infection or pulmonary haemorrhage.
- Renal ultrasound scan to rule out hydronephrosis (i.e., postrenal cause); pay attention to kidney size; large size (i.e., >14 cm) in polycystic kidney disease, and often with diabetes or HIV; small size (<10 cm) suggests chronic renal impairment.
- Renal Doppler scan can establish if there is underlying renal artery stenosis, a cause of prerenal failure. Magnetic resonance angiography (MRA) is less operator dependent and is often used.
- Renal biopsy. This invasive test is often performed to establish an underlying diagnosis if intrinsic renal disease is suspected.

CLINICAL NOTES

MRA uses a gadolinium-based contrast agent. This is different from the iodinated contrast agent used with a CT scan. The gadolinium is not nephrotoxic like the contrast agent used with the CT scan, but does have a potential to cause nephrogenic systemic fibrosis, which is seen more commonly in patients with renal dysfunction; this is a rare but serious condition.

Management

Once the presence of an AKI has been established, treatment is supportive. Attention should be placed on confirming the underlying cause of AKI and minimizing ongoing injury. Pay attention to careful fluid management and avoidance of nephro-toxic medications; aim to avoid contrast imaging, prevent hypotension, treat obstruction and the underlying cause (e.g., sepsis, cardiac or liver failure).

CLINICAL NOTES

The prognosis of patients with an AKI depends on the cause, the presence of any other organ impairment and the patient's premorbid state. They are at risk of further AKIs and developing CKD.

Renal replacement therapies

Emergency dialysis can include use of intermittent haemodialysis, emergency peritoneal dialysis (less frequently used, see the discussion on CKD later) and haemofiltration.

- Haemodialysis is an intermittent treatment, generally lasting 3 to 4 hours and can be performed on the ward (it is also used in an outpatient setting in chronic dialysis). Fast electrolyte shift and fluid removal can result in haemodynamic compromise.
- Haemofiltration is performed in a high-dependency or critical care environment; it is slow and continuous and results in less haemodynamic compromise.

All RRTs correct the electrolyte imbalances, remove toxins and can remove fluid, albeit at different rates. Haemodialysis treatments require central venous access using a specifically designed large-bore dual lumen central venous catheter; peritoneal dialysis requires insertion of a peritoneal catheter (a Tenckhoff catheter) into the peritoneal space.

CLINICAL NOTES

Indications for urgent dialysis:
- resistant hyperkalaemia
- pulmonary oedema
- uraemic pericarditis
- severe acidosis

Hyperkalaemia

Hyperkalaemia is life-threatening if potassium level is greater than 6.5 mmol/L. Medical management with insulin/dextrose and salbutamol nebulizers (with calcium gluconate for myocardial irritability) is covered in Chapter 32. The use of insulin/dextrose and salbutamol nebulizers are holding measures and act by shifting potassium intracellularly. However, potassium wasting can be achieved through use of diuretics, to increase renal potassium loss (e.g., with furosemide). This can be used if the patient is still passing urine. Calcium Resonium (a calcium polystyrene sulfonate resin) taken with regular lactulose, removes potassium via the gastrointestinal tract; however, this has a slow effect, and it should not be used as a therapy in the acute setting. Calcium Resonium is now rarely used with the advent of novel potassium binders, such as Patiromer and Lokelma, which act to increase faecal potassium excretion. Following acute management, potassium measurements should be repeated every 4 to 6 hours. Hyperkalaemia resistant to medical treatment is an indication for dialysis.

Acidosis

A persistent severe acidaemia is an indication for dialysis. Sodium bicarbonate replacement can be used in the first instance to help correct the acidosis; it will also lower the potassium level in the context of an acidaemia. Venous blood gases are a rapid way to check pH.

Pulmonary oedema

This may be life-threatening, particularly in patients with a reduced urine output. Conventional therapies may be used: high-flow oxygen, diuretics (high doses may be necessary), nitrates and opiates (caution: use low doses as these drugs are excreted renally). Noninvasive positive pressure ventilation may be helpful. In the absence of a reasonable urine output, RRT will be required.

COMMON PITFALLS

Diuretic use to drive urine output does not improve renal function. Diuretics can help with the management of pulmonary oedema and hyperkalaemia in the patient with salt and fluid overload, if urine is still being passed.

Summary

- AKI is often predictable, avoidable and multifactorial.
- Pay attention to fluid status, drugs, contrast agent and relative hypotension.
- Perform a urine dipstick test to establish whether there is intrinsic renal disease.
- If you are considering obstruction, a renal ultrasound scan should be performed within 24 hours to rule out hydronephrosis; if you are considering pylonephrosis (infected and obstructed kidney), a noncontrast CT KUB should be performed within 6 hours.
- Hyperkalaemia is an emergency and needs prompt recognition and treatment.

CHRONIC KIDNEY DISEASE

CKD describes an irreversible reduction in renal function. It is classified in stages related to the eGFR and ACR (Fig. 31.2). CKD is a risk factor for cardiovascular disease, which is the leading cause of death in those with renal impairment. As a rough guide, patients start to need activated vitamin D, phosphate control and anaemia management at CKD stage IV. At CKD stage V the patient may start getting symptoms of uraemia, and RRT is started.

Most patients with CKD are managed in primary care, with the management focused on prevention of cardiovascular disease and blood pressure control. The following groups of patients need to be referred to secondary care:

				Persistent albuminuria categories Description and range		
				A1	A2	A3
				Normal to mildly increased	Moderately increased	Severely increased
				<30 mg/g <3 mg/mmol	30–300 mg/g 3–30 mg/mmol	>300 mg/g >30 mg/mmol
GFR categories (ml/min/1.73 m²) Description and range	G1	Normal or high	≥90			
	G2	Mildly decreased	60–89			
	G3a	Mildly to moderately decreased	45–59			
	G3b	Moderately to severely decreased	30–44			
	G4	Severely decreased	15–29			
	G5	Kidney failure	<15			

Fig. 31.2 Prognosis of CKD by GFR and albuminuria category. *CKD*, Chronic kidney disease; *GFR*, glomerular filtration rate; *KDIGO*, Kidney Disease: Improving Global Outcomes. Green: low risk; Yellow: moderate risk; Orange: high risk; Red: very high risk. (From KDIGO. *Definition and Classification of CKD. Clinical Practice Guideline for the Evaluation and Management of Chronic Kidney Disease*. Kidney international supplements. Volume 3, issue 1, page 10; 2013.)

- Severe renal failure (eGFR <30 mL/min per 1.73 m²).
- ACR of 70 mg/mmol or ACR >30 mg/mmol with haematuria.
- Progressive loss of renal function: sustained decrease of GFR of 15 mL/min/1.73 m² or more within 12 months, or a sustained decrease in GFR of 25%.
- Hypertension that remains poorly controlled despite the use of at least four antihypertensive drugs at a therapeutic dose.
- Suspected rare or genetic causes of CKD.
- Suspected renal artery stenosis.

CLINICAL NOTES

You should pay great attention to whether your patient has proteinuria. The ACR is used to prognosticate. The greater the proteinuria, the higher the risk of progressive renal failure, and the presence of proteinuria increases the risk of cardiovascular death (Fig. 31.2).

Aetiology

Identifying the cause of CKD is important to guide specific treatments, establish the risk to other family members and establish the risk of recurrence after renal transplantation. Common causes include:

- Diabetes mellitus.
- Hypertension.
- Glomerulonephritis: both primary and secondary (see later).
- Nephropathies: infective, obstructive and reflux.
- Renovascular causes (e.g., renal artery stenosis).
- Interstitial nephritis: generally from drugs (including NSAIDs, proton pump inhibitors and antibiotics).
- Inherited disease (e.g., autosomal dominant polycystic kidney disease) and Alport disease (type IV collagen defect associated with sensorineural deafness).
- Multisystem diseases (e.g., SLE).
- Hypercalcaemia.
- Neoplasms (e.g., myeloma).
- Amyloidosis.

HINTS AND TIPS

Is it an acute kidney injury or chronic kidney disease?

The single best test to help is a renal ultrasound scan. In acute kidney injury (AKI) the kidneys generally have a normal appearance whereas small scarred kidneys suggest chronic kidney disease (CKD).

Look for historical blood test results; this may involve a degree of detective work.

If your patient has a long-standing history of malaise, fatigue, poor appetite, itch and cramps, this suggests CKD. Anaemia also points towards a more chronic picture, as do biochemical disturbances, including calcium and phosphate level derangements, although these can still be seen with an AKI.

Clinical features

Progressive loss of renal function per se does not cause symptoms until the eGFR falls to very low levels (<30 mL/min/1.73 m^2; i.e., stage IV or stage V CKD). These patients should be managed in renal clinics. Under these circumstances, patients may develop fatigue, nausea, taste disturbance, cramps, itching and inability to concentrate their urine overnight (i.e., increased nocturnal micturition and fluid balance disorders, e.g., leg oedema). Symptom relief can be given for itch and cramps, and fluid imbalances can be corrected through reduction of salt intake, fluid restriction and use of diuretics.

Progressive stage IV or stage V CKD, requires preparations to be made for the patient's chosen RRT (e.g., peritoneal dialysis, haemodialysis or transplantation). This should include patient education, counselling and the involvement of the multidisciplinary team if they have not already been introduced to the patient.

When examining the CKD patient, focus your examination on:

- The underlying cause of renal dysfunction (e.g., vascular or diabetic complications, signs of hypertension, features of active lupus or vasculitis).
- Reversible causes: assess fluid status, renal bruit indicative of renal artery stenosis, renal outflow obstruction (e.g., palpable bladder).
- Indications of progressing towards need of RRT/reaching end stage renal disease: such as disorders of fluid balance with salt and fluid overload, (ask about paroxysmal nocturnal dyspnoea and orthopnoea), fatigue, weight loss,

poor appetite, vomiting, severe itch, uraemic flap and pericarditis.

Investigations

The same initial investigations used in AKI should be requested (see earlier).

CLINICAL NOTES

If renal function declines faster than anticipated, consider reversible causes (e.g., infection or obstruction). You should repeat a renal ultrasound scan to exclude acute hydronephrosis.

Management

The aim of treatment is to minimize further deterioration in renal function and to prevent or treat the complications of renal failure. Use of nephrotoxic drugs should be discontinued, and use of drugs that are excreted renally may need to be stopped or their dose reduced.

RED FLAG

Pay attention to diabetic medications. As renal impairment advances, your patient is likely to need less insulin – ask about hypoglycaemia. Stop metformin at an eGFR of <30 mL/min/1.73 m^2 as there is a risk of lactic acidosis. Pay attention to opiate medications as these are excreted renally and may accumulate, causing drowsiness or even a reduced Glasgow Coma Score (GCS).

Prevention of decline in renal function

Blood pressure, glucose level and acidosis should be tightly controlled as these factors can affect the rate of deterioration of kidney function. Keep the blood pressure below 140/90 mmHg (if there is proteinuria or if the patient is diabetic the target is <130/80 mmHg). Keep the haemoglobin A1c level (HbA1c) between 48 and 58 mmol/L. If there is proteinuria or if diabetes is present, then ACEi/ARBs should be the drug of choice. Following this, sodium-glucose transport inhibitors (SGLT2-i) are used, if eligible (see Clinical Note), to further reduce rate of decline. Watch out for intercurrent infection and any nephrotoxic medications as these can hasten the deterioration in kidney function.

Prevention of complications

Cardiovascular

Control of hypertension is the mainstay of reducing the rate of progression of renal failure and preventing cardiovascular complications. All patients should receive lifestyle advice, including smoking cessation and exercise advice. High cholesterol levels should be aggressively treated. All patients with CKD should be offered atorvastatin according to National Institute for Health and Care Excellence (NICE) guidelines.

Renal osteodystrophy

Renal bone disease is due to a combination of disturbed vitamin D metabolism, decreased ability to renally excrete phosphate and secondary hyperparathyroidism. Serum phosphate levels are raised and vitamin D is unable to be activated in the kidney, resulting in a fall in serum calcium level, and an appropriate rise in PTH level. Treatment involves giving synthetic vitamin D analogues (increases calcium and phosphate levels, lowers PTH level), and reducing phosphate level to the normal range through diet modification and phosphate binders taken with meals. If attention is not given to giving synthetic vitamin D and controlling serum phosphate level, then tertiary hyperparathyroidism (i.e., autologous PTH production) can ensue. Cinacalcet (a calcium mimetic) or parathyroidectomy may be required to treat this.

Acidosis

Systemic acidosis accompanies declining renal function. It increases myocardial excitability, accelerates renal bone disease and may contribute to increased potassium levels. Sodium bicarbonate supplements will help to maintain serum bicarbonate levels within the normal range (>22 mmol/L). Correction of acidosis may help prevent loss of renal function.

Anaemia

In renal failure, there is a normochromic normocytic anaemia due to the kidneys' inability to produce erythropoietin. However, be suspicious of blood loss if the anaemia is disproportionate to the degree of renal impairment. Ferritin, vitamin B_{12} and folate deficiency should be corrected. Recombinant human erythropoietin (epoetin) is generally required in CKD stage IV/V and the dose should be adjusted to maintain a target haemoglobin level of 100 to 120 g/L. This can relieve symptoms related to anaemia and decrease the need for blood transfusions, but epoetin can cause hypertension.

Hyperkalaemia

Correction of acidosis and dietary restrictions help to control potassium levels. Chocolate, crisps and fresh fruits (e.g., bananas and oranges) are examples of foods high in potassium. Always pay attention to serum potassium level in CKD. High-risk groups are those with CKD stage IV/V, diabetes and those taking ACE-i/ARBs and aldosterone antagonists (e.g., spironolactone). The novel potassium binders are licenced for use in these settings, if diet alone is not sufficient for potassium control.

End-stage renal failure

End-stage renal failure (ESRF) is identified on biochemical and clinical grounds as the point when, despite conservative measures, the patient will die without the institution of RRT. When RRT is initiated in a patient with CKD stage V, the patient is defined as having reached ESRF.

Specific indications for starting dialysis include:

- symptomatic uraemia
- hyperkalaemia
- metabolic acidosis

- pericarditis
- inability to control fluid status and blood pressure with advanced renal failure

The need for dialysis is generally predictable, allowing the creation of access (e.g., fistula creation/peritoneal tube insertion) and education, counselling and home adjustments before it is required. Problems with dialysis include loss of vascular access, infection, hypotension and the maintenance of fluid and electrolyte balance.

Renal replacement includes:

- Peritoneal dialysis: where a Tenckhoff catheter is placed into the abdomen to allow fluid to flow in and out, and uses the peritoneal membrane as the dialysis membrane. Peritoneal dialysis can allow manual exchanges of fluid (continuous ambulatory peritoneal dialysis), or night-time automated exchanges (automated peritoneal dialysis).
- Haemodialysis: where either a fistula or an indwelling dual-lumen central venous catheter is used. A fistula is favoured as it is associated with fewer infections and improved survival. Haemodialysis generally occurs in a hospital/community-based dialysis unit, with individuals attending for 4 hours, three times a week. Home haemodialysis, with the option of overnight dialysis, is also growing in popularity for certain motivated patient groups.

Renal transplantation is associated with the greatest survival advantage. The patient needs to be fit enough for the surgery and to tolerate the immunosuppressive regimen. Generally, a triple regimen of a calcineurin inhibitor (e.g., tacrolimus), an antiproliferative agent (e.g., mycophenolate mofetil (MMF)) and a steroid (e.g., prednisolone) is used. The purpose is to prevent rejection but predisposes the individual to infection and malignancies. Nephrologists tread a fine line; balancing under-immunosuppression (which can result in graft rejection), and over-immunosuppression (risking nephrotoxicity from high levels of calcineurin inhibitor, opportunistic infections and malignancies). Other complications of transplantation include transplant renal artery stenosis, graft thrombosis, obstruction of the ureteric anastomosis, de novo glomerulonephritis, recurrence of original disease and gradual loss of function with time (chronic allograft nephropathy, thought to be due to chronic rejection and calcineurin inhibitor use).

GLOMERULAR DISEASE

Glomerular disease may be primary or secondary (i.e., a manifestation of systemic disease) (see Clinical Notes). It may present acutely with an AKI or be picked up incidentally and cause CKD.

CLINICAL NOTES

Systemic disorders that can involve the glomerulus:

- diabetes
- amyloidosis
- systemic lupus erythematosus
- rheumatoid arthritis
- neoplasia
- myeloma
- vasculitic syndromes
- liver disease
- sarcoidosis

Clinical features

Glomerular disease is associated with the presence of blood and protein on urine analysis and often hypertension (Table 31.5). Glomerulonephritis is often categorized as nephritic and nephrotic syndromes.

Nephritic syndrome

Nephritic syndromes include diseases which cause damage to the glomerulus, mesangium, glomerular endothelium or basement membrane. They are associated with nonvisible haematuria, protein leak below the nephrotic range (<3 g/day), impaired renal function and often hypertension. They include diseases that can range from slow grumbling glomerulonephritis to a rapidly progressive glomerulonephritis, a renal emergency.

RED FLAG

Blood and protein with an acute kidney injury should raise alarm bells. Is this a rapidly progressive glomerulonephritis? If it is and it is left untreated, the patient could have end-stage renal failure within days.

Nephrotic syndrome

Nephrotic syndrome is the triad of significant proteinuria (protein >3 g/day), hypoalbuminaemia (albumin <30 g/L) and peripheral oedema. It is caused through dysfunction of podocytes, resulting in heavy protein leak but generally with a preserved excretory renal function (i.e., normal creatinine level). However, proteinuria is nephrotoxic and will lead to renal impairment if left untreated. Many cases are due to primary glomerulonephritis, e.g., minimal change disease, membranous glomerulonephritis and focal segmental glomerulosclerosis (FSGS).

Table 31.5 Relationship between glomerular diseases and clinical presentations

	Proteinuria/nephrotic syndrome	Haematuria/nephritic syndrome	Renal pain	AKI	CKD	Hypertension
Minimal change	+	–	–	±	–	–
FSGS	+	–	–	±	+	+
Membranous	+	–	±	–	+	+
IgA nephropathy	±	+	±	±	+	+
MCGN	+	+	–	+	+	+
Diffuse/proliferative	–	+	–	+	–	+
RPGN	–	+	–	+	–	+

Any given disease may present in a number of ways and, conversely, a particular clinical presentation may have a number of possible causes.
AKI, *Acute kidney injury;* CKD, *chronic kidney disease;* FSCS, *focal segmental glomerulosclerosis;* MCGN, *mesangiocapillary glomerulonephritis;* RPGN, *rapidly progressive glomerulonephritis.*

Examples of secondary causes include diabetes, amyloid, HIV and SLE.

Other clinical features include hyperlipidaemia due to increased hepatic synthesis, a prothrombotic tendency due to urinary loss of antithrombin III, protein C and protein S, and increased risk of infection due to urinary loss of immunoglobulins. Renal biopsy is indicated in most adults to establish a histological diagnosis. Treatment is aimed at inducing remission and preventing relapse. ACE inhibitors and ARBs are often prescribed to help reduce proteinuria.

History

With patients with suspected glomerular injury, arising in the nephritic or nephrotic syndrome, it is important to ask about:

- Urinary symptoms including any change in volume, any visible haematuria or frothy urine (suggests heavy protein leak).
- Other symptoms that can help point towards the underlying disease (e.g., rapidity of onset (rapid-onset renal failure in anti-GBM disease, with often minor symptoms; in minimal change disease, there is often rapid onset of oedema)).
- An associated upper respiratory tract illness: poststreptococcal glomerulonephritis classically presents around 2 weeks following a streptococcal infection; visible haematuria tends to occur few days after an upper respiratory tract infection in IgA disease.
- Any rashes, haemoptysis, epistaxis nasal crusting or hearing abnormalities: these are typical features of granulomatous with polyangiitis vasculitis.
- Any medical history of nephritis, UTIs or renal stones.
- Any associated systemic diseases (e.g., diabetes, hypertension, arthritis, valvular abnormalities or evidence of malignancy).
- Drug history: pay attention to NSAID use.

- Hearing impairment: present in Alport syndrome.
- Family history of renal disease.
- Travel and associated infectious diseases (e.g., HIV infection, hepatitis B and hepatitis C).

CLINICAL NOTES

Take a thorough drug history and *when* drug treatment was started in relation to any deterioration in renal function. Ask directly about recreational drugs, over-the-counter medication and herbal remedies.

Investigations

The following investigations are important in the patient with glomerular disease.

Urine
- Urine dipstick and spot ACR/PCR.
- Urine microscopy for red blood cell casts and dysmorphic red cells indicating glomerular disease (this is rarely performed in clinical practice).
- Urine for Bence Jones protein.

Blood tests
- FBC, urea and electrolytes, liver function tests and bone profile.
- Blood glucose and HbA1c: to exclude diabetes mellitus.
- Inflammatory markers: ESR, CRP.
- ANCAs are classically present in microscopic polyangiitis and granulomatosis with polyangiitis (formally called 'Wegener granulomatosis') and eosinophilic polyangiitis (formerly 'Churg–Strauss syndrome').

- Anti-double-stranded DNA and antinuclear antibodies (ANA) in SLE.
- Anti-GBM antibodies for the diagnosis of Goodpasture disease.
- Hepatitis B and C serology, HIV.
- Antistreptolysin O titre: recent streptococcal infection.
- Serum immunoelectrophoresis to exclude myeloma. Perform alongside urine analysis for Bence Jones protein.
- Cryoglobulins and rheumatoid factor.
- Blood cultures if the patient reports having fevers.
- Serum complement levels: C3 and C4 levels are classically reduced in active SLE, as well as in cryoglobulinaemia.
- Anti-phospholipase A2 receptor antibody (anti-PLA2R) associated with primary membranous glomerulonephritis.

CLINICAL NOTES

Hepatitis B can cause a membranous glomerulonephritis. Hepatitis C mainly causes a glomerulonephritis through formation of cryoglobulins. In both instances it is important to treat the underlying virus.

Imaging
- CXR: this may show pulmonary oedema, malignancy, pulmonary haemorrhage (e.g., with ANCA-associated vasculitis or anti-GBM disease) or it may show features of sarcoidosis.
- Renal ultrasound scan to ensure no hydronephrosis, assess renal size/symmetry and ensure no contraindication for renal biopsy.

Renal biopsy
To be considered to make a histological diagnosis if intrinsic renal disease is suspected. It can ascertain the likely disease process, the degree of activity of the disease and background scarring. This can help guide how aggressively to treat the disease and help give a prognosis for renal recovery.

HINTS AND TIPS

There will be a raised transfer factor level on lung function testing in the presence of pulmonary haemorrhage.

Management

All patients with suspected glomerulonephritis should be seen by a nephrologist. The correct treatment will be specific to the underlying cause of the glomerulonephritis.

Certain general principles apply: tight blood pressure control and if ACR >70 mg/mmol or PCR >100 mg/mmol, ACEi/ARBs should be used to help reduce proteinuria. Depending on the presumed underlying cause SGLT2i may also be used to further reduce proteinuria.

The general principle of treating nephrotic syndrome is to diurese the patient and turn off the protein leak by treating the underlying cause (e.g., with immunosuppression). Fluid removal is achieved through reducing salt intake, restricting fluid intake and administering diuretics. Often intravenous diuretics are required at a high dose, and a combination of different classes of diuretic agents is used to achieve sequential nephron blockade. Patients with nephrotic syndrome are at higher risk of an AKI, intercurrent infection, thrombosis and should be started on lipid-lowering treatment if remission is unlikely to be achieved timely.

HINTS AND TIPS

When diuresing a patient with nephrotic syndrome aim to achieve a maximum fluid loss of 1 kg/day and ensure monitoring of urea and electrolyte levels daily.

RED FLAG

Patients with nephrotic syndrome are highly coagulopathic. Warfarin or low-molecular-weight heparin is generally started when the albumin level is less than 20 g/L. In patients with nephrotic syndrome, loin pain and an acute kidney injury – rule out renal vein thrombosis.

Important primary and secondary glomerular diseases

Rapidly progressive glomerulonephritis
Rapidly progressive glomerulonephritis (crescentic glomerulonephritis) is usually an aggressive process and presents with renal failure, haematuria, oliguria and hypertension. It is a medical emergency. Renal biopsy shows severe acute inflammation in the glomerulus with necrotizing 'crescent' formation. It may occur in SLE, anti-GBM disease, ANCA-associated vasculitis and occasionally with IgA nephropathy. Treatment is with immunosuppression, commonly high-dose hydrocortisone, cyclophosphamide and in selected cases plasma exchange. Unless treatment is instituted sufficiently early, the renal prognosis is usually poor.

Antineutrophil cytoplasmic antibody - positive vasculitis

This is typically either

- granulomatosis with polyangiitis (cytoplasmic ANCA (cANCA) against proteinase 3 (PR3), formerly known as 'Wegner's granulomatosis'); it causes granulomatous lesions and commonly has upper airway involvement. Ask about nasal crusting, epistaxis, hearing changes and haemoptysis;
- microscopic polyangiitis (perinuclear ANCA (pANCA) against myeloperoxidase (MPO)); or
- eosinophilic granulomatosis with polyangiitis (previously known as Churg–Strauss syndrome, a triad of raised levels of eosinophils, asthma and renal failure and generally pANCA with antibodies directed against MPO).

They are small vessel vasculitides. They may affect only the kidney (renally limited disease) or may affect any other organ, including lungs, skin, gut, heart and the neurological system. All forms of vasculitis can cause a rapidly progressive glomerulonephritis.

Symptoms can be nonspecific, including malaise and poor appetite. Any organ system may be affected, and the patient may have been seen in many different specialty clinics already. CXR may show pulmonary haemorrhage.

Diagnosis is made serologically with the presence of ANCA. A renal biopsy is performed to establish the degree of active glomerulonephritis and background scarring. Vasculitis has high associated mortality and risk of ESRF if not treated aggressively. High-dose immunosuppression is given to induce remission, followed by a maintenance dose to prevent recurrence. Initial treatment involves high-dose steroids, cyclophosphamide and consideration of plasma exchange. Maintenance treatment classically involves lower-dose steroids and azathioprine. Dialysis therapy may be required. Rituximab (a CD20 monoclonal antibody) is also used to both introduce remission and for maintenance therapy.

Antiglomerular basement membrane disease

Anti-GBM disease (also known as 'Goodpasture disease') is associated with the presence of circulating antibodies against collagen, resulting in damage to the alveolar and glomerular basement membranes. It can be limited to causing just lung injury or renal injury or can cause both. Other 'pulmonary–renal syndromes' include SLE, granulomatosis with polyangiitis and microscopic polyangiitis. Anti-GBM disease classically has a very rapid onset. Treatment is very aggressive, but once remission is achieved, relapse is very rare.

Treatment includes plasma exchange and immunosuppressive therapy.

IgA nephropathy

IgA nephropathy (Berger disease) is the most common glomerulonephritis worldwide. This condition is classically associated with 'synpharyngitic' haematuria (i.e., macroscopic haematuria 1 to 2 days after an upper respiratory tract infection). In contrast, poststreptococcal glomerulonephritis (see later) usually follows a delay of 1 to 2 weeks. Other presentations include nonvisible haematuria, proteinuria and renal impairment. Individuals with nonvisible haematuria, normal renal function, no proteinuria and normal blood pressure are at low risk of progressive renal disease. In this group a renal biopsy is rarely performed. Follow-up is in general practice with annual blood pressure and electrolyte monitoring. Individuals with proteinuria, renal impairment or hypertension are at a higher risk of progressive renal disease. IgA may very occasionally cause a rapidly progressive glomerulonephritis, and, in this instance, would be treated with aggressive immunosuppression. Typically, IgA nephropathy follows a slow grumbling course. Treatment is aimed at reducing blood pressure with medications that also reduce proteinuria, including ACEi/ARB and SGLT2 inhibitors. Henoch–Schönlein purpura causes an IgA glomerulonephritis in the kidney and is more common in children and adolescents.

Lupus nephritis

SLE is a multisystem disease, with the kidneys commonly affected. The changes are classified by the World Health Organization from I to V on the basis of histology. The different types lead to presentations ranging from nephritis to nephrotic syndrome. Typically, the anti-double-stranded DNA titres are raised and C3 and/or C4 levels are low in active lupus. Treatment includes immunosuppression, which may consist of steroids, cyclophosphamide, MMF and in some centres, rituximab.

CLINICAL NOTES

Lupus nephritis follows a relapsing and remitting course. It often affects women of childbearing age. Pregnancy can both affect which medications can be safely used to manage the condition and put extra strain on the kidneys. Lupus often affects patients differently, and classically presents in a similar way in each patient. Ask the patient how their lupus affects them.

Minimal change nephropathy

This accounts for 80% of children and 20% of adults in the United Kingdom who present with nephrotic syndrome. It classically presents with sudden-onset swelling. Renal biopsy is not always indicated in children. Light microscopy findings are normal (hence the name) but electron microscopy shows podocyte foot process effacement. There is nephrotic range proteinuria, which responds to corticosteroid therapy in 90% of paediatric patients and 75% of adult patients. Relapsing episodes are treated with cyclophosphamide or a calcineurin inhibitor, commonly tacrolimus. The development of renal failure is rare (<1%), and is more likely to occur when disease remission is hard to obtain.

Focal segmental glomerulosclerosis

This also causes nephrotic syndrome but classically with less oedema. Nonvisible haematuria is generally found. It is diagnosed on renal biopsy, where areas of the kidney show focal sclerosis. It can be idiopathic or familial but is also associated with a wide range of systemic diseases (e.g., HIV infection), pamidronate and sickle cell disease. HIV-associated nephropathy is increasingly common and causes a characteristic 'collapsing' FSGS.

Treatment is directed at the underlying cause. FSGS requires prolonged treatment with high-dose steroids. If proteinuria cannot be controlled, then progression to ESRF is common. It is thought that some steroid-resistant minimal change disease may in fact be missed cases of FSGS.

FSGS commonly reoccurs after transplantation (quoted at 30%); inherited forms, however, are unlikely to reoccur.

CLINICAL NOTES

'Secondary focal segmental glomerulosclerosis' is a term used for focal sclerosis seen on renal biopsy. In this case, the underlying process is not immune mediated, but is from increased pressure on the glomeruli. This is seen with obesity, hypertension or where there are fewer nephrons (e.g., a single kidney or small kidneys). Treatment in this instance is by blood pressure control, medications that reduce proteinuria (ACEi/ARBs and SGLT2i) and weight loss.

Membranous glomerulonephritis

This is the most common cause of nephrotic syndrome in adults. Renal biopsy will show a characteristic diffuse thickening of the GBM and immune complexes deposited in the subepithelial space causing a spike formation. The condition if primary can be associated with a circulating phospholipase A_2 receptor antibody (anti-PLA2R). Secondary causes may include an underlying malignancy, drugs (e.g., gold), autoimmune conditions (such as class V SLE or rheumatoid arthritis) and infections (hepatitis B).

Initial treatment is with ACEi/ARB, and if secondary, treating the underlying cause. In cases of presumed primary membranous, or with PLA2R-associated disease, immunosuppression is initiated if the patient does not go into remission despite a 3- to 6-month period of maximal tolerated ACEi/ARB therapy. Approximately 30% of cases of membranous glomerulonephritis will resolve spontaneously, 30% will have a partial response and 30% will progress to ESRF.

RED FLAG

Membranous disease may be the first presentation of an underlying malignancy. Perform a thorough clinical investigation to exclude underlying neoplasm with low threshold for cross-sectional imaging. These patients are at very high risk of thromboembolic disease.

Membranoproliferative glomerulonephritis

This condition, also known as 'mesangiocapillary glomerulonephritis', is characterized by immunocomplex deposits in the glomerular mesangium and basement membrane thickening. It is uncommon, and is associated with a nephritic or nephrotic syndrome and low C3 and/or C4 levels. Secondary forms are associated with chronic infections, SLE, cryoglobulins and hepatitis C. Treatment of membranoproliferative glomerulonephritis focuses on treating the underlying disease. If a patient presents with nephrotic syndrome and progressively declining renal function, aggressive immunosuppression should be given. Prognosis is poor – 50% of patients develop ESRF at 10 years.

Poststreptococcal glomerulonephritis

This condition, also known as 'diffuse proliferative glomerulo-nephritis', is a complication of streptococcal pharyngitis (strep throat) or impetigo. Clinically, it is characterized by sudden onset nephritic syndrome (haematuria, proteinuria, oedema and hypertension). There is commonly a latent period after the infection; 1 to 2 weeks for strep throat and typically 6 to 8 weeks for impetigo. Treatment is symptomatic (i.e., treat hypertension, oedema and hyperkalaemia). Immunosuppression is not indicated. Prognosis is good in children; a small proportion of adults may develop renal impairment.

URINARY TRACT INFECTIONS

UTIs are one of the most common infections encountered in medical practice. In the elderly population, they can present atypically and can rapidly cause sepsis. Women are more prone to UTIs than men, except during the first few months of life and in old age. Approximately 25% to 35% of all women describe symptoms of a UTI at some stage in their lives.

'Urinary tract infection' is a general term referring to the presence of microorganisms in the urine. Significant bacteriuria is defined as urine that yields a pure growth of more than 100,000 organisms per millilitre on culture. Broadly speaking, UTIs are divided into those affecting the lower urinary tract (urethra, prostate and bladder) and those affecting the upper urinary tract (kidneys). A further distinction is made between uncomplicated (normal renal tract and function) and complicated (abnormal renal or genitourinary tract, impaired host defences or virulent organism) UTIs. Predisposing factors for UTI are given in the Clinical Notes box.

> **CLINICAL NOTES**
>
> Predisposing factors of urinary tract infection:
> - stones
> - obstruction
> - polycystic kidneys
> - papillary necrosis
> - diabetes mellitus
> - analgesic nephropathy
> - sickle cell disease
> - sexual intercourse
> - pregnancy
> - bladder catheterization

Lower urinary tract infections

Lower UTIs may take the following forms:

- Cystitis: a symptomatic infection of the bladder with significant bacteriuria.
- Asymptomatic bacteriuria: the patient has no symptoms, but urine culture yields a growth of more than 100,000/mL.
- Acute urethral syndromes: symptomatically like cystitis, but the urine culture may be sterile.

Upper urinary tract infections

Upper UTIs may take the following forms:

- Acute pyelonephritis: an inflammatory process within the renal parenchyma, most commonly caused by bacterial infection.
- Chronic pyelonephritis: more common in children and usually the result of long-standing or recurrent bacterial infection, with eventual parenchymal scarring characteristic of chronic pyelonephritic kidneys. Vesicoureteric reflux and obstruction also contribute. Hypertension and chronic renal failure may ensue.

Infection usually occurs by ascent of the invading organism from the urethra into the bladder. Colonization of the ureters may occur, and from there to the kidneys. The haematogenous route of infection is less common but may occur secondarily to bacteraemia, septicaemia or endocarditis.

Clinical features

Symptoms of lower UTIs include suprapubic pain, frequency, nocturia and dysuria (classically 'burning'). Upper UTIs such as acute pyelonephritis or renal abscesses present with fever, rigors, loin pain, vomiting and weight loss. Macroscopic haematuria can occur in one-third of severe cases. In the elderly, the presentation may be very nonspecific with mild cognitive, behavioural and mobility changes.

Investigations

A clean, MSU sample should be obtained and it should be sent to the laboratory for microscopy and culture. White cell count and CRP are generally raised in infection. Obvious predisposing factors such as pregnancy, diabetes or an indwelling catheter should be considered.

Indications for further investigations include childhood onset, male sex, urological symptoms, persistent haematuria (especially if aged >40 years), unusual organisms (such as *Pseudomonas*) and recurrent infections.

A renal ultrasound should be performed for UTI in children and men, if more than two episodes per year, failure to respond to treatment, pyelonephritis, unusual organisms or persistent haematuria. If pyelonephritis is suspected the imaging modality of choice is a CT scan. A CT is better at detecting renal calculi and a pyonephrosis (infected obstructed kidney, which will require decompression to avoid overwhelming sepsis). In recurrent urinary infections, a dynamic test such as micturating cystogram (MCUG) can show evidence of reflux, and a dimercaptosuccinic acid scan (DMSA) can be performed to assess the patient for split renal function and scarring.

CLINICAL NOTES

A urine dipstick suggests urinary infection if positive for leucocytes and nitrites. However, this is unreliable in the elderly, as they may have asymptomatic bacteriuria which does not require treatment unless symptomatic.

HINTS AND TIPS

Sterile pyuria is bacteriuria with no growth. Causes include:

- tuberculosis of the urinary tract
- partially treated UTI
- neoplasia
- urethritis (e.g., chlamydia, gonorrhoea)

Management

Treatment should be started *after* urine has been sent for culture and antibiotic sensitivity testing but, commonly, before results are available. Broad-spectrum antibiotics may then be changed if necessary according to the results. High fluid intake should be encouraged. More than 80% of lower UTIs respond to a short course of an antibiotic such as trimethoprim, nitrofurantoin or amoxicillin. For complicated UTIs, a 5- to 10-day course of therapy is indicated. Patients with acute pyelonephritis usually require admission to hospital for treatment with intravenous fluids and antibiotics.

Patients with recurrent infections require a high fluid intake; frequent and complete voiding should be encouraged. Long-term, low-dose prophylaxis using rotating antibiotics may be of

benefit but the need for continued treatment should be reassessed after 6 months.

If infection is related to sexual intercourse, the patient should void after intercourse and may benefit from a single dose of an antibiotic.

COMMON PITFALLS

- Do not treat asymptomatic bacteriuria except in pregnancy.
- You will not be able to clear bacteriuria with the presence of a catheter.
- It will be hard to clear infection if there is an underlying renal calculus.
- Nitrofurantoin is not effective in chronic kidney disease of stage III or above; trimethoprim impairs creatinine secretion and can cause a rise in serum creatinine level despite not worsening renal function.

RENAL CALCULI

Renal calculi (kidney stones) are common. They are more common in men, with the initial presentation usually in the third and fourth decades of life. Most common is calcium oxalate, followed by calcium phosphate. Struvite (also known as 'triple phosphate') is most commonly associated with *Proteus* infection. These are all radio-opaque and can be seen on a plain X-ray. Twenty percent of stones are radiolucent, including urate, cystine (only partially lucent) and xanthine.

Bladder calculi form 5% of all urinary tract stones; risks for formation include foreign bodies (e.g., indwelling catheter), obstruction or infection.

General overview

Predisposition to forming renal calculi:

- Poor urinary drainage (i.e., urinary stasis)
- Low urinary output (e.g., dehydration)
- High solute concentration (e.g., high oxalate concentration, hypercalcaemia)
- Urinary pH (acidic pH favours uric acid stone formation, whereas alkali pH favours calcium oxalate stone formation)

Clinical features

The classic presenting symptom of renal calculi is severe, colicky, loin to groin pain. The patient is unable to lie still and it is often associated with nausea and vomiting. Frank haematuria may occur, but more commonly haematuria is not visible. There may be renal angle tenderness, with pain referred to the testes, although these should not be tender on palpation.

> **RED FLAG**
>
> Do not assume renal colic. Ensure a thorough investigation to exclude an abdominal aortic aneurysm (AAA), appendicitis or ectopic pregnancy. If it is the first presentation of renal colic in an individual older than 60 years, or an individual with peripheral vascular disease, consider an AAA; it can also present with loin to groin pain.

Investigations

Renal colic is a typical 'end of the bed' diagnosis. Diagnosis is based on a suggestive history, examination and classically haematuria on urine dipstick testing. A noncontrast CT scan of the kidneys, ureter and bladder (CT-KUB) is the first-line investigation. This will identify the site/size of the stone and importantly if there is hydronephrosis, or an alternative diagnosis. The size of the calculi will help guide management.

Management

Only one-third of stones greater than 5 mm in diameter and positioned in the upper third of the ureter, will pass spontaneously. Most stones, typically those smaller than 4 mm, pass spontaneously. Renal calculi that are unlikely to pass spontaneously need to be urgently referred to a urologist, as they may result in ureteric obstruction. It is important to be aware that a kidney can be obstructed without the presence of hydronephrosis on imaging. Immediate treatment is analgesia with NSAIDs (typically diclofenac, but consider the renal function) and fluids. Surgical treatments involve ureteroscopy or lithotripsy. To avoid future stones, the patient should maintain a high urine output through high fluid intake and follow a low-sodium diet. Patients who form recurrent stones need a metabolic study to guide directed treatment.

> **RED FLAG**
>
> An infection in the context of obstruction (i.e., pyonephrosis) is a medical emergency, and needs urgent decompression with a nephrostomy and intravenous antibiotics. A nephrostomy is generally performed by an interventional radiologist.

> **RED FLAG**
>
> Renal calculi in patients with a single kidney or underlying renal failure needs to be managed with great caution.

> **COMMUNICATION**
>
> Ask the patient to collect the urine in a clear container to try to collect a stone. Analysis of the composition of the stone can guide directed preventative strategies.

URINARY TRACT MALIGNANCIES

Renal cell carcinoma

Renal cell carcinoma is the commonest renal tumour in adults; it is twice as common in men, with the peak age of onset between 50 and 60 years. Most renal cell carcinomas are clear cell type, named after their distinctive clear cytoplasm on microscopy. Risk factors include smoking, obesity and genetic disease (e.g., von Hippel Lindau, polycystic kidney disease). They are commonly identified incidentally; however, the 'classic triad' is haematuria, loin pain and a palpable mass, although this is rarely seen. Other features may include pyrexia, weight loss, polycythaemia, visible haematuria, bone pain with hypercalcaemia and left-sided varicocele associated with left renal vein obstruction. Spread is into adjacent structures (e.g., adrenal glands, local lymph nodes), and it may extend into the renal vein and the inferior vena cava. Metastases are common, with 'cannon ball' lung metastases being a classic feature. Other sites of metastases include bone. The overall 5-year survival rate is approximately 60%, but is greater if the tumour is confined to the renal parenchyma and lower if there are metastases or lymph node involvement.

Initial identifying investigations may include urinary cytology, ultrasound scan and CXR (cannon ball metastasis). All patients will require a CT chest, abdomen and pelvis (CT CAP) to assess the renal mass, identify metastatic disease and for staging purposes. Other less common investigations may include a bone scan and magnetic resonance imaging (MRI) of the abdomen.

Treatment is with radical nephrectomy where possible in local disease. It is also occasional used in metastatic disease as metastases may regress after the primary tumour is removed. Targeted therapy (tyrosine kinase inhibitors, e.g., sunitinib, pazopanib) and immunotherapy (e.g., ipilimumab/nivolumab, pembrolizumab) may be used in metastatic disease, either separately or in combination. Radiotherapy may be used as a palliative therapy for bone pain or for brain metastases.

> **CLINICAL NOTES**
>
> Tumours presenting with polycythaemia include renal cell carcinoma, hepatoma and cerebellar haemangioblastoma.

Transitional cell carcinoma

Transitional cell carcinomas (TCCs) occur mainly in those older than 40 years and most commonly affects the bladder, although the ureter and renal pelvis are other sites. It is three times more common in men than women. Predisposing factors include cigarette smoking, exposure to industrial carcinogens (e.g., aniline dyes), exposure to drugs (e.g., cyclophosphamide) and chronic inflammation (e.g., schistosomiasis).

Patients usually present with painless haematuria, although pain may occur. There may be symptoms like in UTIs. Investigations include urine cytology, cystourethroscopy and a CT scan.

Treatment options include local resection with regular follow-up cystoscopy, bacillus Calmette–Guérin (BCG) intravesical immunotherapy, cystectomy, radiotherapy and local or systemic chemotherapy.

Prostate carcinoma

Prostate carcinoma (most commonly adenocarcinoma) is the second most common malignancy in men; the incidence increases with age and it may be indolent. Patients are often asymptomatic but may present with lower urinary tract symptoms (frequency, urgency, nocturia, poor flow). Symptoms may arise from metastatic spread, classically to bone, presenting with back pain. A hard irregular prostate may be palpable on rectal examination.

Investigations include prostate-specific antigen (PSA), transrectal ultrasound (TRUS) examination and prostate biopsy, or prostatic MRI. A Gleason score is used to grade prostate cancer from biopsy. A CAP and bone scan are used to identify local invasion, nodal spread and metastases for staging purposes.

Treatment of local disease may be observation alone, transurethral resection of the prostate (TURP), radical prostatectomy or radiotherapy. Radical prostatectomy can lead to incontinence and impotence.

Testosterone is a growth factor for prostate cancer and therefore prostate cancer responds well to antagonizing the effect of testosterone (androgen-deprivation therapy (ADT)). This can be achieved with orchidectomy, luteinizing hormone-releasing hormone (LHRH) analogues (e.g., goserelin), gonadotrophin-releasing hormone (GnRH) antagonists (e.g., degarelix) and anti androgens (e.g., bicalutamide). In those that stop responding to ADT, or in metastatic disease, novel ADT agents (e.g., enzalutamide, abiraterone) or chemotherapy (e.g., docetaxel) may be considered by oncologists. Prognosis, even with metastases, may be excellent if the tumour responds to hormonal treatment.

PSA is very useful as a tumour marker to assess response to therapy in prostate malignancy. However, how to screen patients for prostate cancer and how to follow up abnormal PSA test results is a cause of much debate for urologists and public health authorities. Currently, it does not meet the criteria for a national screening programme.

> **CLINICAL NOTES**
>
> Prostate-specific antigen level will increase after catheterization, with urinary infections and even after rectal examination.

> **RED FLAG**
>
> In an elderly man with back pain and hypercalcaemia, check the PSA level and send a myeloma screen.

Testicular cancer

Testicular cancer is the most common malignancy to affect males in their second to fourth decade. Typical presentation is a painless testicular mass. Risk factors include a maldescended testicle, infant hernia, family history of infertility and previous testicular malignancy. Ninety-five percent are germ cell origin, 50% of these are seminomas and 50% are nonseminomas. Nonseminomas include teratomas and yolk sac tumours. Rarer tumours include Leydig and Sertoli tumours. Investigations include ultrasound scan and histological assessment either from biopsy or after orchidectomy. All patients must have a CT scan to rule out metastases. Tumour markers include alpha-fetoprotein (AFP), and β-human chorionic gonadotropin (β-HCG), which are particularly helpful in monitoring response to treatment.

Ninety percent of patients achieve complete remission with treatment; even metastatic disease is potentially curable. Treatment is with orchidectomy; before this, patients should be offered sperm storage and the option of a testicular prosthesis. In stage 1 disease (confined to testicle) this may be followed by surveillance alone. Depending on stage or risk seminomas may subsequently be treated with chemotherapy and radiotherapy. Nonseminatous germ cell tumours respond well to combination chemotherapy (BEP – **b**leomycin, **e**toposide and cis**p**latin). Younger patients may suffer from long-term toxicity of treatment.

> **COMMUNICATION**
>
> Tell all your male patients to examine themselves for lumps in their testes.

MISCELLANEOUS CONDITIONS

Adult polycystic kidney disease

This is an autosomal dominantly inherited disease; the genes, *PKD2* and *PKD1*, lie on chromosomes 4 and 16, respectively. Patients are usually aged between 30 and 50 years. There is not always a family history, and the disease can present de novo. Cysts develop in the kidney parenchyma, the number and size increase with age and they can lead to progressive renal failure. Approximately 40% of patients also have cysts in the liver. Haematuria, cyst infection and cyst rupture are common presenting features. The disease tends to affect families similarly (e.g., age of onset and of reaching ESRF). There is an association with subarachnoid haemorrhage, and this tendency runs in families.

Examination may reveal large irregular palpable kidneys, and the patient is often hypertensive. Mitral valve prolapse, diverticular disease and hernias may also be associated features. Diagnosis is based on an ultrasound scan showing enlarged kidneys with multiple cysts. There are diagnostic criteria for this (see Table 31.6), as cysts can be a normal finding (more common with ageing). A family history or genetic testing will help confirm the diagnosis.

Management includes tight blood pressure control and avoidance of dehydration and nephrotoxins. Renal function declines progressively over time with cyst growth. Tolvaptan, a competitive vasopressin receptor antagonist, has been licensed by NICE to slow the progression of cyst development and renal insufficiency in those with rapidly progressive disease. Patients with polycystic kidney disease tend to be excellent candidates for renal transplantation, occasionally with the polycystic kidney needing to be removed to make space for the transplant.

> **CLINICAL NOTES**
>
> First-degree relatives of those with adult polycystic kidney disease should be offered screening.

Hepatorenal syndrome

Hepatorenal syndrome (HRS) is defined as renal failure in patients with severe liver disease. The underlying problem is with the liver. It is a diagnosis of exclusion: exclude sepsis, hypovolaemia, nephrotoxic drugs and glomerulonephritis. In HRS the problem is of renal perfusion, with liver failure leading to splanchnic vasodilatation and subsequent activation of the sympathetic nervous system and the renin–angiotensin–aldosterone system, resulting in intrarenal arteriolar vasoconstriction. Expect the results of urine analysis to be bland (i.e., no blood or protein). There are two types:

- HRS 1: rapidly progressive renal failure often in tandem with acute liver failure, alcohol-related hepatitis or decompensation of chronic disease.
- HRS 2: renal failure is more slowly progressive, often over months.

HRS occurs in about 20% of patients with cirrhosis in the presence of ascites. Treatment is mainly supportive. You should have a high clinical suspicion for infection, which often presents atypically, and treat it aggressively when recognized. Renal function recovers if the liver recovers, including after liver transplantation. Splanchnic vasoconstrictors are used, including terlipressin in combination with albumin. Octreotide or noradrenaline may also be used to improve renal haemodynamics. Prognosis is poor.

Thrombotic microangiopathies

Thrombotic microangiopathies (TMA) are a group of pathologies causing small vessel injury and microvascular thrombosis. It encompasses haemolytic uraemic syndrome (HUS) and thrombotic thrombocytopenic purpura (TTP). They are diseases attributed to disordered complement activation, leading to endothelial damage.

Table 31.6 Criteria for diagnosing polycystic kidney disease on ultrasonography

Age (years)	Family history	No family history
<30	Two cysts bilaterally (or unilaterally)	Five cysts bilaterally
30–60	Four cysts bilaterally	Five cysts bilaterally
>60	Eight cysts bilaterally	Eight cysts bilaterally

From Kumar A, Hamid S, Bali SK, Akhter M, Hamid S. A prospective study on clinical profile of autosomal dominant polycystic kidney disease (ADPKD) in Jammu for a period of 1 year. *Open Journal of Nephrology* 2012; 2(4): 123.

TTP rarely results in renal failure; classically it is associated with a very low platelet count and has associated neurological features. TTP is associated with ADAMTS13 deficiency and if suspected, treatment is with urgent plasma exchange otherwise the prognosis is very poor. Platelet transfusion should be avoided as this fuels the inflammatory process.

HUS is characterized by MAHA, AKI and thrombocytopenia. It can be divided into typical and atypical forms. Typical HUS is associated with diarrhoea; it is often triggered by *Escherichia coli* O157:H7. Test stool for Shiga toxin to support the diagnosis. Treatment is supportive, and dialysis may be required. Generally, most patients recover normal renal function. Atypical HUS is a diagnosis of exclusion. It is associated with underlying complement mutations. Renal biopsy shows a thrombotic microangiopathy. If the clinical picture is suggestive of atypical HUS and there is no ADAMST13 deficiency, then it can be treated with eculizumab. This is a monoclonal antibody and a terminal complement inhibitor. It is very effective but extremely expensive, needs to be taken indefinitely and can increase the risk of encapsulated bacterial infections (e.g., meningococcal sepsis).

> **RED FLAG**
>
> If there are low platelet levels, acute kidney injury and diarrhoea, think of haemolytic uraemic syndrome. Look for evidence of haemolysis by sending a blood film (to look for red cell fragments). If haemolysis is present, the levels of reticulocytes and LDH will be raised and the levels of haptoglobins will be low.

SEXUALLY TRANSMITTED DISEASES

Sexually transmitted infections (STIs) are often asymptomatic and can lead to long-standing problems with fertility, chronic abdominal pain and multiple organ disorders. Those with an STI may be coinfected with other STIs. Take the opportunity to screen patients for these. STIs are best managed in a sexual health clinic, where a full screen for other STIs, repeat testing and partner notification can be performed. HIV infection is discussed in Chapter 38.

Chlamydia

Chlamydia trachomatis is a gram-negative bacterium that infects human columnar and transitional epithelium. It is the most common STI in the United Kingdom, with 75% of infections in individuals younger than 25 years. It is the most common preventable cause of infertility. It is asymptomatic in about 50% of men and 70% women. Most cases are detected through screening

or investigation of other genitourinary infections. Symptoms include vaginal discharge, dysuria, intermenstrual bleeding and dyspareunia. In men the most common symptom is urethritis with dysuria, or testicular pain. Diagnosis is by vulvovaginal swab in women and first-catch urine in men (this can also be used in women but is less sensitive). Treatment is with doxycycline for 7 days or a single dose of azithromycin. If left untreated, it can lead to pelvic inflammatory disease (PID), ectopic pregnancy, infertility in women and epididymitis and epididymo-orchitis in men.

> **HINTS AND TIPS**
>
> Remember to give antibiotic treatment to the index case, screen the patient for other sexually transmitted infections and notify the patient's partner(s). This is best done by a sexual health clinic.

> **COMMUNICATION**
>
> The patient should be advised to abstain from sex (even if the patient is using barrier contraception) whilst receiving treatment.

> **CLINICAL NOTES**
>
> Reiter syndrome, a triad of urethritis, arthritis and conjunctivitis, can be triggered by chlamydia.

Gonorrhoea

This is caused by *Neisseria gonorrhoeae*, a gram-negative diplococcus. It infects mucous membranes of the urethra, endocervix, rectum, pharynx and conjunctiva. Symptoms will be local to the infected mucous membrane site, and the condition is diagnosed through swabs of the infected site. Gonorrhoea is increasing in prevalence, particularly in men who have sex with men, with the incidence of drug-resistant strains rising. Coinfection with other STIs is common. Ninety-five percent of men will have symptoms, compared with only 50% of women. Symptoms are related to the site of infection, and may include penile/vaginal discharge, dysuria and anal bleeding/pruritus. Examination findings are generally normal but may reveal discharge, contact bleeding of the endocervix or epididymal tenderness. Diagnosis involves a nucleic acid amplification test of endocervix/urethral, pharyngeal and rectal swabs or urine culture (the latter being less sensitive). The organism will then be cultured to detect the strain and antibiotic sensitivities. Treatment is with a single dose of ceftriaxone intramuscularly (1 g). Complications of gonorrhoea include urethral strictures in men, which can lead to bladder outflow obstruction and PID, and infertility in women.

The general principles of partner notification and screening for other STIs applies.

HINTS AND TIPS

Intramuscular injections of ceftriaxone are often painful and patients are likely to remember being given the injection! This can be a useful prompt in your history taking.

Syphilis

Syphilis is caused by *Treponema pallidum*, and can be acquired or congenital. It is divided into stages. In the first stage, primary syphilis, there is local infection (e.g., a small painless papule which forms an ulcer, the chancre). Secondary syphilis develops in 25% of untreated primary infections, and is associated with generalized infection. Symptoms of secondary syphilis classically include a generalized polymorphic rash affecting the palms, soles and face, with generalized lymphadenopathy. The papules of the rash enlarge into condylomata lata (pink-grey discs) and then disappear. There is then a latent phase, during which infectious relapses can occur. During these phases, although patients are asymptomatic, serological testing will confirm syphilis. Tertiary syphilis can then develop and cause cardiovascular syphilis (aortitis, ascending aortic aneurysm and aortic regurgitation), neurosyphilis (tabes dorsalis and dementia) and gummatous syphilis (fibrous nodules affecting bone and skin). The incidence of syphilis is increasing rapidly, particularly among men who have sex with men. Testing includes treponemal enzyme immunoassay, which can detect IgM in early disease. The Venereal Disease Reference Laboratory (VDRL) test can be used as an indication for the stage of syphilis, with false negatives occurring in secondary disease. Treat primary disease with high-dose penicillin (benzathine penicillin intramuscularly); this is given as a single dose in primary disease and for up to 14 days in neurosyphilis.

HINTS AND TIPS

Jarisch–Herxheimer reaction is an acute febrile illness that occurs after the patient commences antibiotic treatment. It is thought to be caused by endotoxin-like products being released during the death of the *Treponema*.

Genital herpes

Herpes is caused by *Herpes simplex virus (HSV)* 1 and 2. HSV-1 causes oral herpes and both HSV-1 and HSV-2 cause genital herpes, which is an STI transmitted via contact. Initial infection is commonly asymptomatic, but may have multiple painful blisters/ulceration of the genitalia or peri anal region leading to dysuria and possible discharge. Individuals may also have nonspecific systemic symptoms such as fever and myalgia or inguinal lymphadenopathy. Following primary infection, the virus enters a latent phase and may then reactivate at various intervals. Diagnosis is by HSV detection from swabs taken from the base of the ulceration. Treatment is with anti viral drugs (aciclovir, famciclovir or valciclovir) in both the primary and recurrent episodes, to reduce duration and severity. Symptomatic treatments include saline baths and topical anaesthetic agents.

HINTS AND TIPS

Genital herpes in women can be particularly painful when urinating and may precipitate urinary retention. In women presenting with urinary retention, consider examination of the labia for genital herpes.

GENDER MEDICINE

Sex and gender are often incorrectly used interchangeably but are separate concepts. Sex refers to the biological characteristics of an individual (anatomy, chromosomes, assigned at birth), whereas gender is a social construct relating to behaviours and attributes. Gender is increasingly being recognized as a spectrum and commonly used terms an individual may identify with are cisgender (gender aligns with sex assigned at birth), transgender (gender differs with sex assigned at birth) and nonbinary (gender does not identify with male/female). Individuals may undergo gender transition to align their bodies with their gender identity – this may include medical interventions such as hormone therapy or surgery (gender confirmation surgery). Gender medicine is the study of how biological, socioeconomic and cultural differences influence health. There is growing research into gender medicine and the impact this has on how medical conditions develop, present and progress and therefore how treatments may have differing impacts.

It is important to consider that there are conditions which are specific to males/females which are shown in Table 31.7. When reviewing a patient who is not cisgender, it is important to consider these conditions to ensure they are not missed. It

Table 31.7 Conditions which are specific to male/females

Male	Malignancy – prostate, testicular
	Genetic – haemophilia, Klinefelter syndrome, Alport syndrome
	Other – androgen insensitivity syndrome
Female	Malignancy – ovarian, endometrial, cervical, breast (predominantly)
	Gynaecological – endometriosis, fibroids
	Genetic – turners syndrome

must also be considered the impact hormone-based therapy may have on a specific disease process as this may increase or reduce risk of certain conditions (i.e., bone density in increased/reduced testosterone, breast cancer with oestrogen replacement/mastectomy, cardiovascular risk). In those who have undergone gender confirmation surgery, indwelling biological organs (e.g., prostate, cervix, ovaries) may still be in situ and this needs to be factored into consideration of diseases and screening.

● Chapter Summary

- In an individual with an acute kidney injury (AKI), always perform a urine dipstick test. If protein is present in the absence of infection, quantify this loss with a spot ACR measurement. If there is blood and protein on the urine dipstick and an AKI, ask yourself whether this is rapidly progressive glomerulonephritis.
- AKI is largely predictable and avoidable. Take care to identify groups at higher risk of AKI. Individuals with AKI have longer hospital stays and greater risk of death.
- Chronic kidney disease is divided into five stages. The rate of progression is determined largely by the heaviness of proteinuria and hypertension. Ensure tight control of blood pressure and aim to start ACEi/ARB and then SGLT2i for renoprotection if proteinuria.
- Indications for emergency haemodialysis include resistant hyperkalaemia, pulmonary oedema, uraemic pericarditis and severe acidosis.
- Renal obstruction and sepsis, a pyonephrosis, is an emergency and needs prompt antibiotic treatment and decompression.
- Patients with a sexually transmitted infection need to be screened for other coexisting sexually transmitted infections. This is best performed in a sexual health clinic, where partner notification can be conducted.

UKMLA Conditions
Acute kidney injury
Bladder cancer
Chlamydia
Chronic kidney disease
Dehydration
Diabetic nephropathy
Gonorrhoea
Haematuria
Herpes simplex virus
Nephrotic syndrome
Polydipsia
Prostate cancer
Testicular cancer
Urinary symptoms
Urinary tract calculi
Urinary tract infection

UKMLA Presentations
Abnormal urinalysis
Acute kidney injury
Chronic kidney disease
Dehydration
Electrolyte abnormalities
Gonorrhoea
Haematuria
Oliguria
Peri anal symptoms
Scrotal/testicular pain and/or lump/swelling
Urethral discharge and genital ulcers/warts
Urinary symptoms
Vaginal discharge
Vulval itching/lesion

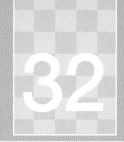

Fluid balance and electrolyte disturbances

32

INTRODUCTION

Understanding fluid balance and electrolyte disturbance will be essential in your medical career. From the first day as a Foundation doctor, you will use this understanding when checking blood test results and prescribing fluids. In this chapter, we will review appropriate intravenous fluid prescribing and the approach to management of sodium, potassium and calcium electrolyte disturbances.

It is worth taking time to appreciate the following concepts:

- In a 70-kg man, the total fluid volume is 42 L (60% of the body weight).
  - Intracellular fluid volume is 28 L – two-thirds of the total body fluid.
  - Extracellular fluid volume is 14 L – one-third of the total body fluid.
  - The intravascular component is 3 L.
- The average total fluid intake in 24 hours is 2500 mL (1500 mL drunk, 800 mL in food and 200 mL via the metabolism of food), and output usually matches this via urine, insensible loss and stool.
- Sodium ingestion is approximately 2 mmol/kg in 24 hours.
- Potassium ingestion is approximately 1 mmol/kg in 24 hours.

Understanding the aforementioned requirements will help you in prescribing fluids in a sensible and appropriate manner. Generally speaking, fluids can be divided into crystalloids (e.g., 0.9% 'normal' saline or Hartmann solution) and colloids (e.g., albumin); see Table 32.1.

SODIUM AND WATER BALANCE

Fluid balance is achieved in the body by ensuring that the amount of water consumed in food and drink (and generated by metabolism) equals the amount of water excreted. Consumption is regulated by behavioural mechanisms, including thirst and salt cravings. Approximately 1 L is lost each day through insensible losses, and the kidneys can regulate the remaining excretion of water. This is achieved through the action of antidiuretic hormone (ADH; also known as 'vasopressin') on the distal collecting duct controlling water reabsorption (see Chapter 15).

In addition to regulation of total volume, the osmolality of bodily fluids is also tightly regulated. Regulation of osmolality is achieved by balancing the intake and excretion of sodium with that of water. Fluid status and sodium level are interdependent. Sodium balance can be controlled through the action of the renin–angiotensin system. Disorders of sodium homeostasis are common.

HYPONATRAEMIA

Hyponatraemia (serum sodium level <135 mmol/L) is very common, and the development of hyponatraemia is a poor prognostic marker. In hospital, it is usually the result of neurohumoral changes in acute illness and the type, volume and route of fluid administered. Consider what intravenous fluids to prescribe carefully. To evaluate hyponatraemia, these questions should be answered:

- How low is the sodium level and how quickly has it fallen?
- What is the patient's volume status?
- What is the urine osmolality?
- What is the urinary sodium value?

For example, in hypovolaemia secondary to dehydration or diarrhoea, the kidneys retain salt and water, resulting in low urinary sodium level (<20 mmol/L). Diuretics or mineralocorticoid (principally aldosterone) deficiency will cause hypovolaemia with a high urinary sodium level (>20 mmol/L). With this information, the diagnostic algorithm shown in Fig. 32.1 can be followed.

Any symptoms will depend on the chronicity of the hyponatraemia as well as the actual sodium level. The more chronic the hyponatraemia, the better tolerated it is. In general, a mild hyponatraemia may be asymptomatic but may give symptoms of fatigue and confusion. As this becomes more severe, the patient is likely to get more confused and drowsy. In acute or severe hyponatraemia (i.e., sodium level <115 mmol/L), seizures can occur.

Investigations

When investigating the patient with hyponatraemia, start by examining the patient for an accurate fluid assessment (see Chapter 15). Sending a urine sample to biochemistry for a spot urinary sodium is the most useful preliminary investigation. Paired serum and urine osmolalities should also be measured. This involves a blood and urine sample taken at approximately the same time to be sent to biochemistry. Ensure review of serum potassium, glucose and lipid levels. Checking thyroid function test results and an early morning cortisol level is also useful. If the serum 9 a.m. cortisol level is low, this suggests adrenal insufficiency (such as Addison

Table 32.1 Composition of common intravenous fluids

Fluid type	Use	Sodium (mmol/L)	Chloride (mmol/L)	Potassium (mmol/L)	Lactate (mmol/L)	Glucose (g/L)
Normal saline (0.9% NaCl)	Crystalloid Maintenance and resuscitation fluid	154	154	0	0	0
Hartmann solution	Crystalloid Maintenance and resuscitation fluid	131	111	5	29	0
Dextrose, 5%	Maintenance	0	0	0	0	50
Human serum albumin, 5%	Colloid	130	130	0	0	0

The daily requirements for a 70-kg man are approximately 140 mmol sodium and 70 mmol potassium.

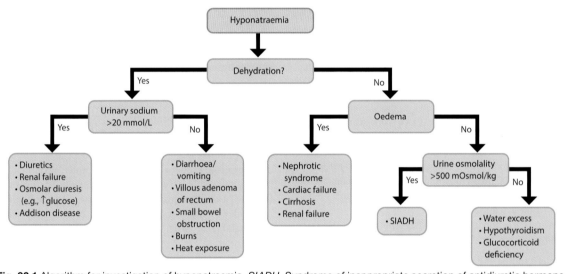

Fig. 32.1 Algorithm for investigation of hyponatraemia. *SIADH*, Syndrome of inappropriate secretion of antidiuretic hormone.

disease) and will require a short Synacthen test (see Chapter 33) to confirm.

Management

Treatment depends on the cause. If the patient is dehydrated, then volume replacement with normal saline is required. If the patient is hypervolaemic, treat the underlying cause (e.g., cardiac, liver or renal failure). This tends to involve strict fluid restriction. In the case of SIADH, stop any possible causative medications and restrict the patient's fluid intake. Often, restriction starts with a 1 L restriction, and if this is not effective, then the amount allowed is decreased (750 mL then 500 mL). If this is still not effective, then tolvaptan (an aquaretic) can be used. This is used under endocrine guidance and with great caution that sodium levels do not rise too rapidly.

Acute symptomatic hyponatraemia is a **medical emergency**. Treatment involves carefully raising the sodium level: the more chronic the hyponatraemia, the slower the correction should be. In the case of a sodium level below 115 mmol/L or severe symptoms, the patient should be admitted to a critical care environment. The sodium level should be corrected very slowly, not faster than 1 mmol/L per hour, and not more than 10 mmol/L in the first 24 hours as central

Table 32.2 Examples of causes of syndrome of inappropriate antidiuretic hormone secretion

Groups	Examples
Central nervous system	Stroke
	Subarachnoid haemorrhage
	Head trauma
	Brain tumour
	Meningitis
Pulmonary	Neoplasms
	Tuberculosis
	Pneumonia
Malignancies	Small cell lung cancer
	Pancreatic
	Lymphoma
Drugs	Antidepressants – SSRIs
	Neuroleptics
	Chlorpropamide
	Carbamazepine
	Proton pump inhibitors (e.g., omeprazole)

SSRI, *Selective serotonin reuptake inhibitor.*

pontine myelinolysis (osmotically induced demyelination), can ensue.

SIADH is characterized by hyponatraemia, (serum sodium level <135 mmol/L), low plasma osmolality with an inappropriately high urine osmolality (>100 mOsmol/kg) and high urinary sodium level (>30 mmol/L). SIADH is a diagnosis of exclusion and can be diagnosed only if the patient is euvolaemic and cardiac, adrenal, thyroid and renal dysfunction have all been excluded. Causes are shown in Table 32.2.

COMMON PITFALLS

Consider your intravenous fluid prescription. If you use 5% dextrose too frequently, you will induce hyponatraemia.

HINTS AND TIPS

Is this true hyponatraemia? Falsely low sodium readings can occur in the presence of hyperglycaemia and hypercholesterolaemia.

RED FLAG

Patients with serum sodium levels below 120 mmol/L are best managed in a critical care environment. Care needs to be taken to establish the underlying cause and to carefully increase the sodium level at a slow rate. The rate of correction is dependent on the chronicity of the hyponatraemia. Acute causes of hyponatraemia are likely to give more symptoms and can be corrected faster.

HYPERNATRAEMIA

Hypernatraemia (serum sodium level >145 mmol/L) most often occurs due to dehydration (e.g., with thirst impairment in patients who have dementia and diabetes insipidus). A common iatrogenic cause is due to inappropriate fluid prescribing (0.9% saline). Table 32.3 summarizes causes of hypernatraemia. Hypernatraemia leads to central nervous system dysfunction, leading to symptoms including lethargy, weakness, confusion and even seizures. In the case of diabetes insipidus, the patient will have polydipsia and polyuria (see Chapter 15).

Investigations

Investigations include checking renal function, electrolyte levels, bone profile (pay attention to calcium) and plasma glucose level. Paired serum and urine osmolalities (described earlier) should also be measured. In diabetes insipidus, you would expect to find a high serum osmolality and low urine osmolality.

Management

Treatment is directed at the underlying cause. Review medications, stop the use of any diuretics or laxatives, and ensure appropriate fluid replacement. The sodium level should be reduced no faster than 1 mmol/L per hour to avoid rapid fluid shifts and cerebral oedema. Giving fluid replacement by the enteral route if possible is best. If intravenous treatment is used, adjust the fluid prescription in relation to the serum sodium level and monitor this level regularly.

CLINICAL NOTES

Try to establish how chronic the hypernatraemia is. The more long-standing it is, the slower the correction needs to be.

Table 32.3 Causes of hypernatraemia

Total body sodium	Causes
Low total body sodium level	Extrarenal: e.g., sweating, diarrhoea Renal: osmotic diuresis
Normal total body sodium level	Diabetes insipidus
High total body sodium level	Steroid excess: e.g., Cushing disease, Conn syndrome Iatrogenic: e.g., hypertonic sodium infusions Self-induced: e.g., ingestion of sodium chloride tablets

Table 32.4 Causes of hypokalaemia

Cause	Examples
Losses	Gastrointestinal: diarrhoea and vomiting, chronic laxative abuse, villous papilloma of the colon Renal: diuretics (e.g., thiazides and furosemide), hyperaldosteronism, glucocorticoid excess (including treatment with steroids, and ACTH-secreting tumours), renal tubular acidosis, Bartter syndrome Inadequate replacement: postoperative, diuretic phase of acute kidney injury
Redistribution of potassium	Alkalosis, insulin overdose, familial periodic paralysis
ACTH-secreting tumour	
Secretion of atrial natriuretic peptide	Paroxysmal SVT

ACTH, Adrenocorticotrophic hormone; SVT, supraventricular tachycardia.

ETHICS

Patients with end-stage dementia often have hypernatraemia caused by impairment of thirst. There is often a debate whether these patients should be given intravenous fluid replacement. This needs careful consideration with the patient's next of kin and the multidisciplinary team.

HYPOKALAEMIA

Hypokalaemia (serum potassium level <3.5 mmol/L) causes are given in Table 32.4. The clinical features of hypokalaemia tend to occur at a serum potassium level of less than 3.0 mmol/L, and include muscle weakness, confusion and constipation. Levels below 2.5 mmol/L can cause severe muscle weakness and paralysis. However, any degree of hypokalaemia can result in increased cardiac excitability and augment digoxin toxicity. Rarely, prolonged hypokalaemia can cause a nephrogenic diabetes insipidus.

Investigations

The key is to identify the underlying cause. A spot urinary potassium level can greatly help in differentiating the cause, alongside serum pH and chloride level. A high urine potassium level (i.e., >20 mmol/L) in the face of a low serum potassium level suggests renal losses (e.g., from diuretic therapies), renal tubular disorders, glucocorticoid or mineralocorticoid excess.

Perform an electrocardiogram (ECG) to detect whether the hypokalaemia is affecting cardiac function. ECG findings of hypokalaemia include flattened T waves, ST depression and U waves. Hypokalaemia can lead to life-threatening arrhythmias such as ventricular tachycardia and ventricular fibrillation.

Management

The underlying cause should be identified and treated. Review any drugs that could be contributing (e.g., diuretics and laxatives). If hypokalaemia is mild, oral potassium supplements can be given and food rich in potassium should be encouraged, such as bananas and fresh orange juice. If the hypokalaemia is severe, potassium should be administered intravenously (the maximum rate of administration is 10 mmol/h) via a peripheral line. If a more concentrated preparation is required, this needs to be through central venous access and while the patient is having continuous cardiac monitoring, usually requiring admission to a critical care environment.

CLINICAL NOTES

To correct hypokalaemia effectively you must correct any coexisting hypomagnesaemia.

HYPERKALAEMIA

Hyperkalaemia (serum potassium level >5 mmol/L) causes are given in Table 32.5. Symptoms are rare, and it is usually identified on blood tests. It is worth noting, if the blood sample was haemolysed, the serum potassium level can be spuriously raised because of mixing with intracellular potassium. However, do not assume it is a false reading: perform an ECG and repeat measurement of the potassium level urgently. Significant hyperkalaemia is commonly associated with typical ECG changes (Fig. 32.2). These changes are tented T waves, flattened P waves and shortened PR interval. Later signs are a broadened QRS complex, which can become sinusoidal, with ventricular tachycardia and ventricular fibrillation ensuing. Hyperkalaemia can also cause an atrioventricular block, resulting in bradycardia. Hyperkalaemia must therefore be treated promptly when identified.

HINTS AND TIPS

A venous blood gas sample, analysed in a blood gas machine (generally found in the emergency department and intensive care unit) can give you a quick reading of potassium.

Table 32.5 Causes of hyperkalaemia

Cause	Examples
Excess oral intake	Potassium supplements, dietary
Diminished renal excretion	Renal impairment Drugs (e.g., potassium-sparing diuretics, ACE inhibitors, ARBs, NSAIDs)
Redistribution of potassium from intracellular compartment	Haemolysis Tissue necrosis (e.g., burns)
Artefact	Delay in separation of plasma or serum

ACE, Angiotensin-converting enzyme; ARB, angiotensin receptor blocker; NSAID, nonsteroidal antiinflammatory drug.

Investigations

Along with the potassium level, check serum creatinine and bicarbonate levels. Look at the patient's previous blood test results. Do they show high baseline potassium levels? More chronically high potassium level will be better tolerated by the patient. If the potassium level is greater than 6.0 mmol/L perform an ECG urgently.

Management

Rapidly reducing extracellular potassium levels is best achieved by utilizing physiological mechanisms. Potassium can be temporarily redistributed into cells with use of an infusion of dextrose and insulin, and nebulized salbutamol (see Red Flag box). This can be repeated if needed. If the patient is acidotic, the use of bicarbonate can help this. Remember that these interventions only redistribute potassium between compartments and provide a window of opportunity for definitive therapy to excrete potassium from the body. The only way of achieving potassium excretion acutely is in the urine. Therefore oligoanuric patients with severe hyperkalaemia require urgent dialysis to achieve potassium removal.

ECG changes can be reversed temporarily by boluses of 10% calcium gluconate, which acts to stabilize the myocardial membrane.

Calcium Resonium (a calcium polystyrene sulphonate resin), taken with regular lactulose, removes potassium via the gastrointestinal tract; however, this has a slow onset, and it should not be used as a therapy in the acute setting. Calcium Resonium is now rarely used with the advent of novel potassium binders, such as patiromer (sodium polystyrene sulphonate (SPS)) and Lokelma (sodium zirconium cyclosilicate (SZC)), which act to increase faecal potassium excretion. Novel potassium binders need to be used in conjunction with acute management due to delayed onset of action (Lokelma 1–2 hours, patiromer 4–6 hours).

Following acute management, potassium measurements should be repeated every 4 to 6 hours. Hyperkalaemia resistant to medical treatment is an indication for dialysis (see Chapter 31).

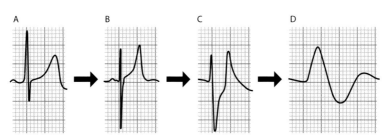

Fig. 32.2 ECG changes in hyperkalaemia. *ECG,* Electrocardiogram.

CLINICAL NOTES

Ensure to closely monitor blood sugars following treatment with insulin/dextrose due to risk of hypoglycaemia.

CALCIUM BALANCE

The normal range for calcium is between 2.2 and 2.6 mmol/L. About 40% of plasma calcium is bound to albumin, and it is the unbound ionized calcium that is important physiologically. The serum pH is also important because albumin acts to buffer free hydrogen ions. In the patient who is acidotic, hydrogen ions will be bound to albumin, increasing the concentration of unbound ionized calcium. This fact is important to remember clinically, as correcting acidosis will result in more ionized calcium being bound to albumin and may potentiate a hypocalcaemia. Calcium homeostasis is regulated by the parathyroid glands, which have calcium receptors on their surface, and vitamin D (Fig. 32.3).

HYPOCALCAEMIA

The causes of hypocalcaemia are shown in Table 32.6. It is often asymptomatic, but symptoms may include perioral numbness, cramps, tetany and seizures. Signs of hypocalcaemia include

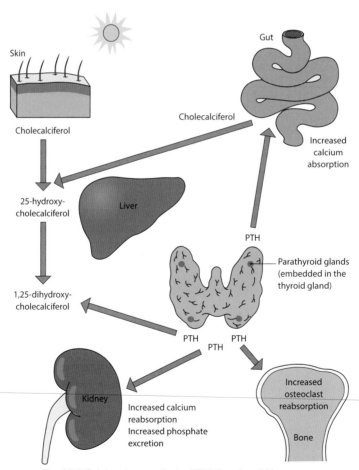

Fig. 32.3 Calcium homeostasis. *PTH*, Parathyroid hormone.

Chvostek sign (twitching of the facial muscles when the facial nerve is tapped) and Trousseau sign (carpopedal spasm when the brachial artery is occluded with a blood pressure cuff).

Investigations

When you are investigating hypocalcaemia, check serum magnesium, phosphate, parathyroid hormone (PTH) and vitamin D levels. Other tests include measurement of serum folate level and screening the patient for coeliac disease. Calcium and folate are absorbed in the duodenum, and coeliac disease can result in impaired absorption. High urinary calcium level suggests urinary calcium loss, as seen with loop diuretic use. ECG features of hypocalcaemia include a prolonged QT interval.

Management

Treatment of hypocalcaemia should be directed at the underlying cause. Stop the use of any medications that could be contributing (e.g., loop diuretics or bisphosphonates) and replace with orally administered calcium and vitamin D. In severe hypocalcaemia, intravenous replacement is required (10 mL of 10% calcium gluconate). Monitor the response to treatment, and repeat as needed.

> **CLINICAL NOTES**
>
> If there is hypomagnesaemia, this will need to be corrected along with the hypocalcaemia otherwise the calcium level will not normalize.

Table 32.6 Causes of hypocalcaemia

Mechanism	Example
Reduced calcium intake	Dietary deficiency, malabsorption
Reduced vitamin D intake/ production	Dietary deficiency, malabsorption, reduced sunlight exposure
Reduced activation of vitamin D	Renal disease, liver disease
Increased inactivation of vitamin D	Enzyme induction by anticonvulsants
Reduced production of PTH	Surgical removal of parathyroid glands, autoimmune, congenital (DiGeorge syndrome)
Resistance to PTH	Pseudohypoparathyroidism
Hypoalbuminaemia	Shock

PTH, *Parathyroid hormone.*

> **RED FLAG**
>
> Severe hypocalcaemia (serum calcium <1.9 mmol/L and/ or symptoms) is a medical emergency and requires urgent IV replacement with 10 mL of 10% calcium gluconate.

HYPERCALCAEMIA

The causes of hypercalcaemia are shown in Table 32.7. The two most common causes are primary hyperparathyroidism and malignancy. Symptoms of hypercalcaemia include abdominal pain, constipation and vomiting. Polyuria and polydipsia are common and may be severe. Depression and confusion may occur. Renal stones may form with chronic hypercalcaemia, and this may result in renal nephrocalcinosis. There may be features of the underlying cause.

Table 32.7 Causes of hypercalcaemia

Mechanism	Example
Increased calcium intake	Milk–alkali syndrome
Increased vitamin D intake	Self-administered, iatrogenic
Increased activity of vitamin D	Sarcoidosis, lymphoma, Addison disease
Increased production of PTH	Primary hyperparathyroidism (adenoma, hyperplasia, carcinoma), tertiary hyperparathyroidism (hyperplasia)
Production of PTH-related peptide	Squamous cell carcinoma, renal cell carcinoma
Increased osteoclastic activity	Osteolytic metastases, multiple myeloma
Increased bone turnover	Hyperthyroidism
Increased renal tubular calcium reabsorption	Familial hypocalciuric hypercalcaemia (autosomal dominant)

PTH, *Parathyroid hormone.*

> **HINTS AND TIPS**
>
> The causes of hypercalcaemia can be remembered with the mnemonic 'bones (bone pain), stones (renal stones), groans (abdominal pain) and moans (psychiatric disease)'.

Investigations

When you are investigating hypercalcaemia, check the PTH level. Is it appropriately suppressed? If it is in normal range, this is not appropriate. Also check renal function, the rest of the bone profile (i.e., phosphate, magnesium, alkaline phosphatase) and a vitamin D level. Consider investigations for an underlying malignancy. Myeloma commonly causes high calcium level and other tumours that have a predilection for metastasizing to bone (e.g., breast, kidney, lung, prostate, renal and thyroid cancers). Sarcoidosis can also give a high calcium level. Review medications that may cause or exacerbate hypercalcaemia including thiazide diuretics, calcium replacement and vitamin D tablets.

Management

Hypercalcaemia is a medical emergency. The mainstay of treatment is fluid resuscitation. Only after adequate hydration should treatment with intravenous bisphosphonate (e.g., pamidronate) be used. Following this, treatment should be directed at the causative factor. High-dose steroid is effective for treatment of hypercalcaemia secondary to myeloma and sarcoidosis.

● **Chapter Summary**

- Electrolyte imbalances are common, and if not treated can cause life-threatening arrhythmias. If long-standing, they are likely to be better tolerated by the patient, and the abnormality needs to be corrected more slowly.
- Check medications carefully, including intravenous fluids, as these can be causative or contributing to the abnormality. If electrolyte levels are severely low, correction should be undertaken in a critical care environment, where careful monitoring can be performed, allowing controlled correction.
- With any electrolyte disturbance:
  - Consider urgency. Extreme electrolyte abnormalities need urgent correction. Remember to go back to the ABCDE approach.
  - Assess the patient's fluid status (particularly relevant with hypercalcaemia and sodium abnormalities).
  - Is the patient symptomatic? Symptoms can be very nonspecific, such as confusion, dizziness, irritability and aggression.
  - Are there electrocardiogram abnormalities?
  - Consider the time frame. Is this an acute or chronic disturbance?
  - Think about the cause; iatrogenic, acute infection, systemic disease.
  - Treat the abnormality. Remember omitting a causative drug is a treatment intervention.
  - Monitor the rate of correction. Ensure you repeat blood tests to guide response to your treatment. How frequently this needs to be done will depend on the severity of the electrolyte disturbance and the treatment you are giving.

UKMLA Conditions
Acid–base abnormality
Acute kidney injury
Addison disease
Adverse drug effects
Arrhythmias
Breast cancer
Cardiac arrest
Chronic kidney disease
Coeliac disease
Decreased/loss of consciousness
Dehydration
Delirium
Dementias
Depression
Deteriorating patient
Diabetes insipidus

UKMLA Presentations
Abnormal urinalysis
Acute kidney injury
Altered sensation, numbness and tingling
Bone pain
Coeliac disease
Confusion
Decreased/loss of consciousness
Dehydration
Diarrhoea
Electrolyte abnormalities
Fits/seizures
Polydipsia (thirst)
Postsurgical care and complications
Vomiting

● **Chapter Summary—cont'd**

UKMLA Conditions
Diarrhoea
Fits/seizures
Hypercalcaemia of malignancy
Hyperlipidaemia
Hyperparathyroidism
Hypoparathyroidism
Hypothyroidism
Incidental findings
Lung cancer
Malabsorption
Malnutrition
Metastatic disease
Multiple myeloma
Polydipsia (thirst)
Prostate cancer
Sarcoidosis
Squamous cell carcinoma
Urinary tract calculi

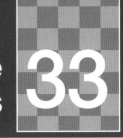

Metabolic and endocrine disorders 33

DIABETES MELLITUS

Diabetes mellitus is a persisting state of hyperglycaemia due to diminished availability or effectiveness of insulin. Approximately 422 million people worldwide have diabetes according to the latest World Health Organization (WHO) data, with 90% of cases being people with type 2 diabetes. This is projected to almost double by 2030. In the United Kingdom, it is estimated that around 4.5% of the population have diabetes. The rising tide of obesity is responsible for much of this.

Aetiology and Pathophysiology

Type 1 diabetes mellitus (DM) usually presents in childhood, with a peak age of incidence of 10 to 15 years, although it can occur at any age. The signs and symptoms develop quickly over days to weeks. Type 1 DM is due to autoantibodies directed against the insulin-producing beta cells of the pancreatic islets of Langerhans, causing a low concentration of circulating insulin. These patients always require insulin replacement therapy, and there is an association with other autoimmune diseases.

Patients with type 2 DM are usually older and overweight, and the onset is more insidious. It is increasingly being seen in children, however, and may be linked with rising levels of childhood obesity. Type 2 DM is due to a combination of reduced sensitivity of peripheral tissues to circulating insulin (insulin resistance) and failure of the beta cells to produce enough insulin to overcome this resistance. Patients may require insulin if hyperglycaemia persists despite maximal doses of oral hypoglycaemic agents, or in times of physiological stress such as severe infections or after myocardial infarction. There is approximately 80% concordance between identical twins, suggesting that inherited factors have a significant role. A very small proportion of patients with type 2 diabetes have a familial autosomal dominant form and present at a young age. This form is often referred to as 'maturity onset diabetes of the young' (MODY).

Secondary DM may be caused by:

- Drugs (e.g., steroids).
- Pregnancy (gestational diabetes): patients develop impaired glucose tolerance or frank diabetes during pregnancy.
- Pancreatic disease (e.g., pancreatectomy, carcinoma of the pancreas, pancreatitis, cystic fibrosis, haemochromatosis).
- Endocrine causes (e.g., Cushing syndrome, acromegaly, phaeochromocytoma).

DIAGNOSIS AND CLINICAL FEATURES

It can be difficult to differentiate between type 1 and type 2 DM at first presentation, and certain clinical features and biomarkers can help classify. Fig. 33.1 demonstrates some of the differences in presentation between type 1 and type 2 diabetes.

Type 1 DM is diagnosed on clinical grounds in a patient presenting with hyperglycaemia (random plasma glucose >11 mmol/L); they typically will have one or more of the following features:

- ketosis
- rapid weight loss
- age of onset <50 years of age
- BMI <25
- personal and/or family history of autoimmune disease

A diagnosis of type 1 DM should not be discounted in a patient presenting aged 50 years or above with a BMI of <25.

Type 2 DM on the other hand is diagnosed if an adult presents with persistent hyperglycaemia.

Persistent hyperglycaemia is defined as:

- HbA1c >48 mmol/mol.
- Fasting glucose >7 mmol/L

Table 33.1 Risk factors for developing type 2 diabetes mellitus

Obesity and inactivity	Overeating and inactivity exacerbate insulin resistance, with obesity accounting for 80%–85% of the overall risk for developing type 2 DM.
Family history	People with a family history are 2–6× more likely to develop type 2 DM than those without a family history.
Ethnicity	People of Asian, African and Afro-Caribbean heritage are 2–4× more likely to develop type 2 DM than European people.
History of gestational diabetes	Women with a history of gestational diabetes have a sevenfold increased risk in developing frank type 2 DM later in life.
Diet	A diet rich in high glycaemic index (GI) foods may increase the risk of being overweight or obese. High GI foods contain carbohydrates which are broken down rapidly and cause a rapid increase in blood glucose levels. Examples include sugary foods and drinks, white bread, white rice and potatoes.
Medications	Corticosteroids particularly increase risk of developing hyperglycaemia and type 2 DM.
Polycystic ovary syndrome (PCOS)	Increases the risk of nondiabetic hyperglycaemia and type 2 DM.
Metabolic syndrome	Insulin resistance is commonly associated with metabolic syndrome, defined as a combination of raised blood pressure, dyslipidaemia, fatty liver disease, central obesity and a tendency to develop thrombosis.
Low birth weight for gestational age	There is some evidence that preterm birth before 35 weeks of gestation is associated with an increased risk for type 2 diabetes developing in adult life.

- Random glucose ≥11.1 mmol/L in the presence of symptoms or signs of diabetes (see Clinical Notes box).

If the patient is symptomatic, a single abnormal HbA1c or fasting plasma glucose can be used. If asymptomatic then repeat testing, ideally with the same test is needed to make the diagnosis.

CLINICAL NOTES

Symptoms and signs of type II diabetes may include:

- Polydipsia, polyuria, blurred vision, unexplained weight loss, recurrent infections and tiredness.
- Acanthosis nigricans (a skin condition causing hyperpigmentation of skin folds, typically the axillae, groin and neck), which suggests insulin resistance.

CLINICAL NOTES

HbA1c should not be used to diagnose diabetes in children and young people <18 years of age, pregnant women, during concurrent illness, when taking medication that may cause hyperglycaemia, and in individuals with pancreatic or end-stage renal disease.

In situations where HbA1c is not reliable, then the diagnosis of type 2 DM should be made on the basis of a fasting plasma glucose level of 7.0 mmol/L or more.

CLINICAL NOTES

In cases where it is difficult to differentiate between type 1 and type 2 DM – for example, where type 1 DM is suspected, but there are atypical features, such as age 50 years or older, BMI >25, or slow evolution of hyperglycaemia then test for the presence of diabetes-specific autoantibodies, including antibodies to pancreatic islet cells (present in 90% of type 1 diabetics), glutamic acid decarboxylase or insulin. If antibody tests are negative, and classification is still uncertain, C-peptide levels can be used to differentiate between the two diagnoses. C-peptide is the part of proinsulin which is cleaved prior to cosecretion with insulin from pancreatic beta cells, and serves as a measure of insulin secretion. A C-peptide level of less than 0.2 nmol/L is associated with a diagnosis of type 1 DM.

A significant proportion of patients present for the first time with a diabetic emergency: diabetic ketoacidosis (DKA) in the case of type 1 DM or, more rarely, hyperosmolar hyperglycaemic state (HHS), in the case of type 2 DM. Some patients, particularly people whose type 2 DM has an insidious onset, may present with chronic complications of their diabetes.

The chronic complications of diabetes are summarized in Fig. 33.2. They can be considered in two broad groups: macrovascular and microvascular. 'Macrovascular' refers to complications

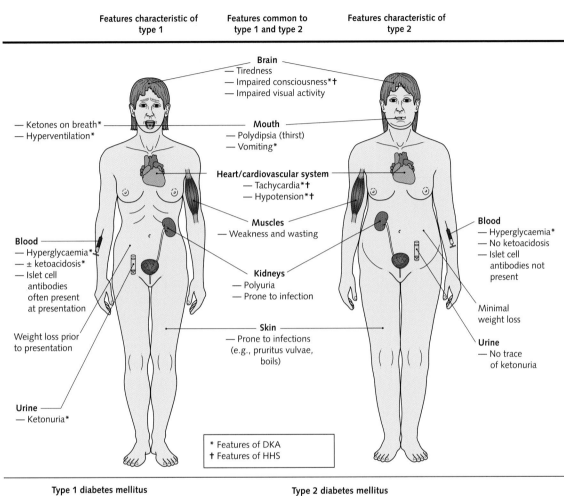

Features characteristic of type 1

Features common to type 1 and type 2

Features characteristic of type 2

Brain
— Tiredness
— Impaired consciousness*†
— Impaired visual activity

— Ketones on breath*
— Hyperventilation*

Mouth
— Polydipsia (thirst)
— Vomiting*

Heart/cardiovascular system
— Tachycardia*†
— Hypotension*†

Muscles
— Weakness and wasting

Blood
— Hyperglycaemia*
— ± ketoacidosis*
— Islet cell antibodies often present at presentation

Blood
— Hyperglycaemia*
— No ketoacidosis
— Islet cell antibodies not present

Weight loss prior to presentation

Kidneys
— Polyuria
— Prone to infection

Minimal weight loss

Skin
— Prone to infections (e.g., pruritus vulvae, boils)

Urine
— No trace of ketonuria

Urine
— Ketonuria*

* Features of DKA
† Features of HHS

Type 1 diabetes mellitus
• Patients usually thin
• Usually present with a short history of acute symptoms
• Treat with insulin

Type 2 diabetes mellitus
• Patients usually overweight (85% obese)
• Usually present with a longer history, with slowly progressing symptoms or with chronic complications
• May be asymptomatic, or have less severe but slowly progressing symptoms similar to type I diabetes, e.g., increasing tiredness
• Many cases are discovered only by routine testing
• Treat with diet and oral hypoglycaemic agents initially (may need insulin subsequently)

Fig. 33.1 Acute symptoms and signs of diabetes mellitus (types 1 and 2). *DKA,* Diabetic ketoacidosis; *HHS,* hyperosmolar hyperglycaemic state.

related to larger blood vessels (e.g., coronary artery, cerebrovascular and peripheral vascular disease). 'Microvascular' refers to complications related to smaller blood vessels (e.g., diabetic retinopathy, nephropathy and neuropathy). Some complications will arise because of both macrovascular and microvascular disease. Good control of hyperglycaemia is key to preventing complications.

Macrovascular disease

This is a cause of significant morbidity and mortality among people with diabetes. A person with diabetes has a risk of myocardial infarction equivalent to that of a nondiabetic person who has already had one previous infarction. Therefore it is of paramount importance to assess and address all cardiovascular risk factors when you are treating patients with diabetes (see later).

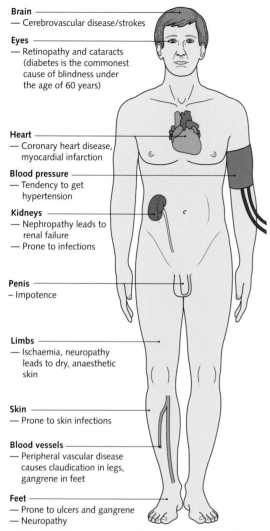

Brain
— Cerebrovascular disease/strokes

Eyes
— Retinopathy and cataracts
(diabetes is the commonest
cause of blindness under
the age of 60 years)

Heart
— Coronary heart disease,
myocardial infarction

Blood pressure
— Tendency to get
hypertension

Kidneys
— Nephropathy leads to
renal failure
— Prone to infections

Penis
– Impotence

Limbs
— Ischaemia, neuropathy
leads to dry, anaesthetic
skin

Skin
— Prone to skin infections

Blood vessels
— Peripheral vascular disease
causes claudication in legs,
gangrene in feet

Feet
— Prone to ulcers and gangrene
— Neuropathy

Fig. 33.2 Chronic complications of diabetes mellitus.

Microvascular disease

Diabetic retinopathy

Retinopathy occurs in virtually all patients with type 1 diabetes, and maculopathy occurs in up to 20% of patients. Patients with type 2 diabetes often have a degree of retinopathy at presentation. The stages of diabetic retinopathy are shown in Chapter 2 (see Table 2.17). Patients with maculopathy and preproliferative changes must be referred to an ophthalmologist; those with proliferative retinopathy require urgent referral for laser therapy as there is a risk of retinal haemorrhage and vision loss.

People with diabetes are also at elevated risk of early cataract formation. Rubeosis iridis is a late complication related to new vessel formation on the iris, and may result in glaucoma.

Diabetic nephropathy

The first sign of renal involvement is microalbuminuria. This is a poor prognostic marker, correlating with higher cardiovascular risk, and risk of progressive renal disease. The higher the albuminuria level, the greater the risk. A negative dipstick test does not exclude it, and therefore more sensitive tests must be used to screen people with diabetes: use the albumin-to-creatinine ratio (ACR) from a spot urine sample. An ACR ≥3 mg/mmol confirms microalbuminuria (equates to 30 mg of albumin in 24 hours). It affects 20% to 40% of people with diabetes 10 to 15 years after diagnosis. These patients can progress to macroalbuminuria/clinical nephropathy, where ACR is ≥30 mg/mmol (equating to more than 300 mg in 24 hours). Diabetic nephropathy can be a cause of nephrotic syndrome (see Chapter 31), and is the leading cause of end-stage renal failure in the United Kingdom.

CLINICAL NOTES

Diabetic nephropathy is almost always associated with the presence of retinopathy, and its absence should prompt a search for an alternative renal diagnosis. The pathological hallmark of diabetic nephropathy on histology from a renal biopsy sample is the Kimmelstiel–Wilson lesion (nodular glomerulosclerosis).

Diabetic neuropathy

Diabetic neuropathy can take several forms.

- Somatic neuropathies
- Somatic neuropathies may take the following forms:
  - Distal symmetrical polyneuropathy: this commonly affects the lower limbs first, with numbness and paraesthesia of the feet, spreading up the leg, before then affecting the hands ('glove and stocking' pattern). Symptoms are predominantly sensory with early loss of vibration sense and absent ankle jerks. In advanced cases the loss of pain sensation may lead to the development of punched-out chronic ulcers at pressure points in areas of thick callus, and may cause arthropathy (see later). The patient's foot may then become infected and eventually gangrenous.
  - Mononeuritis: may be due to entrapment or ischaemia. Commonly involved nerves include the third cranial nerve, ulnar nerve and lateral popliteal nerve. More than one nerve can be involved, causing mononeuritis multiplex.
  - Diabetic amyotrophy: painful asymmetrical weakness and wasting of the quadriceps muscles due to lumbosacral plexopathy and polyradiculopathy. The patient may recover.

Autonomic neuropathies

This may lead to symptoms of postural hypotension (i.e., dizziness on standing), impotence, diarrhoea and urinary retention. Gastroparesis causing vomiting can be a very troubling symptom for patients.

PATIENT SAFETY

Patients can have a lack of awareness of the symptoms of hypoglycaemia. Find out whether your patient has hypoglycaemic episodes and whether he or she is aware of them. This is particularly important to do before the start of treatment with any β-blockers, which can mask hypoglycaemic awareness.

Diabetic feet

Diabetic foot problems are due to a combination of neuropathy and peripheral vascular disease.

Sensory neuropathy causes ulcers over pressure points (e.g., metatarsal heads) and can cause joint deformity because of the lack of pain and proprioception (e.g., pes cavus, Charcot joints). Peripheral vascular disease, which may be due to small and/or large vessel occlusion, affects the toes primarily, and can lead to gangrene.

Diabetes predisposes patients to infection, which may affect the soft tissue and even bone (osteomyelitis) of ulcerated feet. This is a common reason for emergency presentation and admission. Amputations are common and preventable – key is early referral to diabetic foot care services, and optimization of diabetic control.

RED FLAG

The infected diabetic foot requires urgent and aggressive assessment and treatment with broad-spectrum antibiotics. Investigations need to be performed to assess the underlying blood supply (through Doppler studies and angiography) and to see whether there is an underlying osteomyelitis (MRI). If arterial perfusion is poor, medical treatment is rarely effective, and surgical debridement and amputation are often required.

COMMUNICATION

Explain to your patients the importance of inspecting their feet for any cuts or blisters which can become infected. Tell them to always wear well-fitting shoes, not to walk barefoot and to see a chiropodist regularly.

Skin

Complications occurring in the skin include:

- Lipoatrophy: this is loss of fat at insulin injection sites. It is much rarer now that human insulin has replaced bovine or porcine insulin. The patient should be advised to vary the injection sites because the absorption of insulin at sites of atrophy is unpredictable.
- Acanthosis nigricans: hyperpigmented velvety thickening of skin folds, predominantly in the neck, axilla and groin areas. It is common, and has a strong association with insulin resistance.
- Necrobiosis lipoidica: these are irregular, painless ovoid plaques with a yellow atrophic centre and red to purple edge. They are found on the skin of the tibia, and occur in approximately 1% of people with type 1 diabetes. Infections, such as boils and candida, are more common.

Infections

Common infections are of the urinary tract and skin, and candidiasis. Tuberculosis is also more common in people with diabetes. Susceptibility to infection is due to several factors, including a reduced immune response due to hyperglycaemia, tissue ischaemia secondary to vascular disease and increased portals of entry, such as ulcers.

Management

General

Living with diabetes is difficult. Education and access to dedicated care providers improve outcomes, and this is achieved through regular follow-up with a multidisciplinary team involving doctors, nurses, ophthalmologists, dietitians and chiropodists/podiatrists (see Clinical Notes box). The aims of continued assessment of diabetic patients are ongoing education, assessment of glycaemic control and assessment of complications. Alongside management of hyperglycaemia, lifestyle advice should be offered (e.g., smoking cessation, dietary advice), a statin should be started, and BP carefully monitored. Prepregnancy counselling should be offered where appropriate.

COMMUNICATION

Adolescent patients often find it especially difficult to achieve good control of their diabetes. Give these patients your special attention. Some hospitals offer transition clinics where there is an emphasis on multidisciplinary involvement and focus on addressing the patient's social needs. Peer support groups are often extremely valuable for patients.

The Diabetes Control and Complications Trial in type 1 diabetic patients and the UK Prospective Diabetes Study in type 2 diabetic patients demonstrated that tight control of blood glucose (aiming for a glycated haemoglobin (HbA1c) fraction of 6.5%–7.5%, 48–58 mmol/mol) reduces microvascular complications. This needs to be balanced against the increased risk of hypoglycaemic episodes. The UK Prospective Diabetes Study also demonstrated that tight control of blood pressure reduces both macrovascular and microvascular complications. This and other trials have suggested that the aim should be a blood pressure below 130/80 mmHg. This emphasizes the need for a global assessment of a diabetic patient's cardiovascular risk factors and aggressive management of all of them.

CLINICAL NOTES

Regular check-ups are vital to ensure that patients do not progress to develop other health problems. This involves monitoring of diabetic control, and screening for microvascular complications. HbA1c fraction should be tested every 3 months when newly diagnosed, and then every 6 months thereafter once stable. Many patients now also monitor their own blood glucose concentrations at home. Traditionally this was through use of blood glucose strips and an electronic meter, though technology has now evolved, and continuous glucose monitors are available which allows patients to check their blood sugar levels without having to prick their finger. A small sensor is worn day and night that reads blood glucose levels, and sends this information to an app for the patient to track.

Microvascular complications should be monitored as part of an annual diabetic health check, unless concerns arise earlier:

- Eyes – visual acuity checks together with examination of the optic fundi for retinopathy.
- Feet – the feet should be examined for neuropathy, ischaemic changes and infection.
- Kidneys - nephropathy should be sought by monitoring of urea and electrolyte levels, and by testing for albuminuria.
- Cardiovascular system – blood pressure and cholesterol levels should be monitored to assess CV risk.

Diet and lifestyle

Many patients with type 2 diabetes can successfully control their diabetes through exercise and diet alone. The diet should be low in fat (to help delay the progression of atherosclerosis) and low in refined sugars, but high in complex carbohydrates (such as starch) and high in fibre, which among other benefits helps to lower the incidence of postprandial hypoglycaemia. Patients should be encouraged to take regular exercise and reduce energy intake to help achieve and maintain ideal body weight. This often proves to be very difficult, and studies suggest that bariatric surgery for weight loss can be an effective and cost-effective treatment for type 2 diabetes in some patients, and may lead to remission.

Oral hypoglycaemic agents

Treatment with these is usually started when diet and lifestyle measures fail to offer adequate control. Individualized antidiabetic treatment should be offered, depending on the person's HbA1c treatment target, age, comorbidities, BMI, risks and benefits of treatment and polypharmacy.

First-line treatment

National Institute for Health and Care Excellence (NICE) recommends metformin (a drug of the biguanide class) as first-line therapy, unless contraindicated. It exerts its effect mainly by decreasing gluconeogenesis and increasing peripheral utilization of glucose; some residual islet cell function is required. Gastrointestinal side effects are common, including nausea and diarrhoea. There is a risk of lactic acidosis in the acutely unwell patient, and therefore metformin should be stopped during concurrent illness, and reviewed once better. This risk is greater in patients with underlying renal disease, heart failure and liver disease.

A patient's cardiovascular risk should be assessed, and based on this, if they either have chronic heart failure or chronic kidney disease, or are high risk of developing cardiovascular disease (CVD), an SGLT-2 inhibitor should be offered in addition to metformin as this has proven cardiovascular and nephroprotective benefit. These two medications should be started sequentially, with metformin first, and once tolerability established the SGLT-2 inhibitor can be introduced.

PATIENT SAFETY

Before starting SGLT-2 inhibitor, check whether the patient has ever had a DKA. They need to be aware to stop this drug when unwell as it can precipitate DKA.

Second-line treatment

If first-line therapy is ineffective, poorly tolerated, or contraindicated, one or more of the following second-line agents should be started:

- SGLT-2 inhibitor (if not already taken as first-line therapy)
- DPP-4 inhibitor
- pioglitazone
- sulphonylurea

Third-line treatment

If triple therapy with metformin and two other oral drugs is not effective, not tolerated or contraindicated, consider triple therapy by switching one drug for a GLP-1 mimetic.

This has weight loss properties and is chosen as add-on therapy in patients with a BMI >35 or have obesity-related comorbidities.

Insulin

All type 1 diabetic patients are treated with insulin from the outset, and many type 2 diabetic patients require insulin to achieve satisfactory glycaemic control. Mixtures of available insulin preparations may be required to maintain good control, and these will differ for individual patients. Requirements may be affected by variations in lifestyle, other medications and concurrent illness such as infection. Patients should aim for blood glucose concentrations between 4 and 10 mmol/L for most of the time, while accepting that on occasions they will be above or below these values. They should be advised to look for 'peaks' and 'troughs' of blood glucose and to adjust their insulin dosage only once or twice weekly.

In the United Kingdom, there are three types of insulin available: human insulin, insulin analogues and animal insulin. The preparations may be short-acting (Actrapid, Humulin S), intermediate-acting (Insulatard, Humulin I) or long-acting (Lantus). If possible, a 'basal-bolus' regimen is used: a once-daily injection of a medium-acting or long-acting insulin, with short-acting or rapid-acting insulin injection before or with meals. This most closely resembles the physiological changes in insulin levels, but requires education and commitment. In some patients twice-daily injections of 'biphasic insulin' (mixtures of a short-acting and an intermediate-acting insulin, e.g., Novomix or Humulin M3) are better (Fig. 33.3). Some patients may have an insulin pump, which gives them a continuous insulin infusion.

Pancreatic transplant may be performed if the patient meets the criteria, in patients undergoing renal transplant, in which case it is performed simultaneously, or if the patient has very labile and problematic diabetes, particularly hypoglycaemic unawareness.

Diabetes and surgery

Patients who have diabetes should be first on the operating list and should fast on the morning of surgery. Diet-controlled diabetic patients simply require careful monitoring of glucose levels. Oral agents should be avoided on the morning of surgery and can be recommended with the first meal postoperatively. If glucose levels are poorly controlled, if oral intake will be problematic postoperatively, or if the procedure is long, intravenous (IV) administration of insulin may be required (see later).

For patients already using insulin, IV administration of insulin is started early on the day of the operation, with use of a variable rate insulin sliding scale. Depending on the protocol, the patient's normal long-acting bolus medication may be continued. The IV insulin regimen usually consists of a 1 unit per millilitre infusion of soluble insulin in 0.9% saline (i.e., 50 units of Actrapid in 50 mL 0.9% NaCl). The capillary glucose level is checked on an hourly or 2-hourly basis, and the rate of insulin infusion is changed accordingly. While the patient is fasting, a 5% dextrose with 20 mmol/L KCl infusion must always be running concurrently with the insulin infusion and other fluid and electrolyte requirements should supplement this infusion. When patients start to eat and drink, their normal insulin regimen may be restarted.

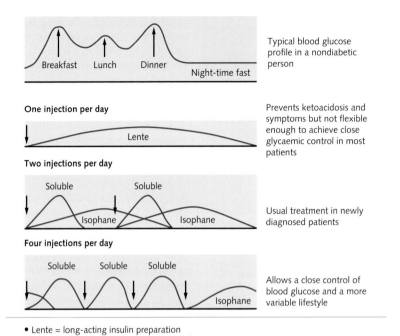

- Lente = long-acting insulin preparation
- Isophane = medium-acting insulin preparation
- Soluble insulin = short-acting insulin preparation

Fig. 33.3 Examples of different insulin regimens.

Diabetic emergencies

Hypoglycaemia

Symptoms of hypoglycaemia include sweating, hunger and tremor (autonomic symptoms) and very low glucose concentrations may cause drowsiness, seizures, transient neurological symptoms and loss of consciousness. Hypoglycaemia is very common in diabetic patients, but there are many causes:

- Drugs: excessive insulin or sulphonylureas.
- Alcohol binges, especially with decreased food intake.
- Endocrine causes: pituitary insufficiency, Addison disease and insulinomas.
- Liver failure.

Certain specific investigations can help differentiate between the causes:

- Measurement of insulin and C-peptide levels; C-peptide is produced from the breakdown of proinsulin, and its level will be raised only with endogenous hyperinsulinaemia, suggesting an insulinoma.
- Sulphonylurea levels.
- Short Synacthen (tetracosactide) test for Addison disease.

Management—This should be approached in relation to whether the patient is conscious or not. If the patient is conscious, give high-sugar-containing foods orally (e.g., Lucozade, biscuits or glucose gel), followed by complex carbohydrate. If the patient is unconscious, begin with an ABCDE approach, and then commence an IV infusion of glucose. This needs to be a glucose concentration of greater than 10%; typically 100 mL of 20% dextrose is used. If no IV access is possible, then 1 mg of glucagon can be given intramuscularly (IM). Recheck the blood glucose level every 10 minutes following treatment, and repeat treatment as needed. Treat the underlying cause. In diabetic patients, issues surrounding education and awareness of hypoglycaemia should be addressed when the patient has recovered from the acute event.

CLINICAL NOTES

Following treatment of a hypoglycaemic episode, do not omit the patient's next dose of insulin, although a dose reduction may be needed.

PATIENT SAFETY

Be careful with insulin prescribing. Careful handwriting is essential, write out the dose in full (i.e., '15 units' rather than '15 U'. If any short-acting insulin dose is greater than 25 units or any intermediate-acting/long-acting insulin dose is greater than 50 units, stop and check if this is correct.

Diabetic ketoacidosis

The hyperglycaemic complications of diabetes can be life-threatening, and requires emergency hospital assessment if suspected.

Diabetic ketoacidosis (DKA) occurs in type 1 diabetes. It may be the mode of first presentation of diabetes, or it may be precipitated by an inadequate insulin dose or an intercurrent illness (e.g., infection or myocardial infarction). There is usually a gradual deterioration over hours to days.

Symptoms include polyuria, polydipsia, abdominal pain and vomiting. There may be evidence of the underlying cause. Patients often hyperventilate to compensate for the metabolic acidosis (Kussmaul respiration), and their breath smells of ketones (like nail varnish remover). There are physical signs of dehydration. As the condition worsens, lethargy, confusion, drowsiness and ultimately coma may occur.

CLINICAL NOTES

The diagnosis of diabetic ketoacidosis requires all three of the following to be present:

- The patient to be known to have diabetes or be hyperglycaemic (serum glucose level >11 mmol/L)
- The presence of ketones (serum ketone level >3 mmol/L or 2 + on urine dipstick test)
- An acidosis (pH <7.3; reference range 7.35–7.45)

When investigating the cause of a patient's acidosis, ask yourself could this be DKA? How severe is it? What has triggered it (e.g., sepsis, myocardial infarction)?

Investigations include:

- Blood tests: full blood count (FBC), urea and electrolytes (U&Es), bone profile, liver function tests (LFTs), C-reactive protein (CRP), bicarbonate and glucose. If you are considering myocardial infarction, then include troponin.
- Arterial blood gas: perform an arterial measurement initially; following this venous blood gas can be taken to give the pH and potassium level quickly – this is important in monitoring response to treatment.
- Bedside capillary glucose and capillary ketones (only some hospitals will have facilities for bedside ketone measuring).
- Urine dipstick: look for ketones.
- Culture and sensitivity: blood, urine and swab of any wound/abscess.
- ECG (evidence of silent myocardial infarction).
- Chest X-ray (CXR): look for underlying pneumonia/pulmonary oedema.

Management—Correction of dehydration takes precedence. Make sure you have at least two wide-bore cannulas; using one cannula, fluid-resuscitate the patient and through the other run a slow fixed-rate insulin infusion. Patients with DKA are potassium-depleted overall but the serum concentration may be normal or high as the acidosis causes potassium to move out of the intracellular compartment. Therefore the serum potassium concentration can fall precipitously as acidosis is corrected, and it must be monitored closely and replaced. Between 6 and 9 L of IV fluid may be required, and the first 2 L can be given over the first hour. An IV infusion of insulin, 0.1 units/kg per hour is commenced. Once the blood glucose level drops to around 15 mmol/L, 0.9% saline is generally replaced with dextrose to prevent too precipitous a fall in the glucose level. The aim of insulin treatment is to suppress ketogenesis as well as reduce the blood glucose level. In children, fluid requirements need to be calculated more accurately as cerebral oedema may occur with overaggressive fluid administration.

The patient should be catheterized, and fluid balance needs to be monitored very carefully. A nasogastric tube may need to be inserted to reduce the risk of aspiration from the gastric stasis that occurs in this condition. Prophylactic low-molecular-weight heparin is given as there is a significant risk of venous thromboembolism.

If there is evidence of infection, broad-spectrum antibiotics are used, and attempts should be made to identify the precipitant. The levels of the inflammatory markers may rise in the absence of infection. The patient should be observed very closely, with a low threshold for admission to the high-dependency or intensive care unit. IV insulin administration should be continued until there are no detectable ketones, the acidosis is corrected and the patient is eating and drinking.

Hyperosmolar hyperglycaemic state

This occurs in type 2 diabetes. The patient is often elderly and may not be known to have diabetes. The precipitants are as for DKA but onset is more gradual, usually over days. By the time of presentation, blood glucose level is usually very high (higher than in DKA – typically above 30 mmol/L) and plasma osmolality is increased with significant hypernatraemia. Polyuria leads to severe dehydration. Neurological symptoms such as confusion, seizures and coma may occur. Ketoacidosis almost never occurs as there is enough endogenous insulin remaining to suppress ketone formation. However, an initial check for ketones should be performed.

When investigating, again look at the severity of the hyperosmolar state and look for an underlying precipitant. In your investigations include:

- Blood tests: FBC, serum glucose, U&Es, bone profile, LFTs, CRP, bicarbonate.
- Plasma osmolality, which should be calculated.
- Bedside capillary glucose (and ketones, if available at the bedside).
- Capillary and urine analysis for ketones.
- ECG (look for evidence of a myocardial infarction).
- Further investigations directed at finding the underlying cause (e.g., blood cultures, urine culture, CXR, troponin).

Management—Rehydration is usually achieved with normal saline. IV administration of insulin should only be commenced when the glucose level is not falling with IV fluids alone, and is given at a lower dose than for DKA. If the sodium concentration is very high, it may be tempting to give hypotonic saline. However, this is not used as it can cause cerebral oedema and myelinolysis by lowering the osmolality too quickly, and because these patients are so volume depleted their total body stores of sodium are low and require replacement (see Chapter 32). Invasive cardiovascular monitoring may be required. Patients are at very high risk of venous thromboembolism, so be suspicious and treat this if it is present or suspected; in other cases ensure a prophylactic dose of low-molecular-weight heparin is used. The mortality rate is up to 50%.

OBESITY AND METABOLIC SYNDROME

Obesity is a growing global health problem, with worldwide obesity rates having nearly tripled since 1975. According to the most recent WHO estimates, 39% of the adult population were overweight in 2016, and 13% were obese. In the United Kingdom, NICE estimated these figures as 36% and 27%, respectively. In children this trend is even more concerning, with an estimated 39 million children under the age of 5 overweight or obese in 2020. It constitutes an enormous public health issue, with widespread changes in dietary and exercise patterns required.

In adults, WHO defines obesity as a body mass index (BMI) greater than 30 kg/m², and overweight is a BMI greater than 25 kg/m². The normal range is 18.5 to 25 kg/m². Central adiposity – an increased waist circumference to height ratio – is associated with greater health risks, including type 2 diabetes mellitus, CVD, dyslipidaemia, hypertension, osteoarthritis and cancer. There are several definitions of metabolic syndrome, each comprising a combination of hypertension, low high-density lipoprotein (HDL) level, hypertriglyceridaemia, raised fasting glucose level, insulin resistance and obesity. In every consultation obesity should be addressed and patients should be given lifestyle and dietary advice. Those patients with a BMI greater than 28 kg/m² with comorbid conditions that may benefit from weight reduction and those with a BMI greater than 30 kg/m² are considered for drug therapy after exercise, diet and behavioural intervention have been tried. Drug therapy includes glucagon-like peptide 1 (GLP-1), e.g., semaglutide, or orlistat, which works by inhibiting the absorption of fat in the intestine. Orlistat is often poorly tolerated by patients due to side effects of steatorrhoea, urgency and oily spotting, and is therefore recommended as second-line therapy. Both medications are discontinued at 3 months if there has not been more than 5% of total body weight loss.

Morbidly obese patients with a BMI greater than 40 kg/m² (or greater than 35 kg/m² with comorbidity) in whom there has been a failure to lose weight despite all conservative measures may be considered for surgery. This takes two forms: malabsorptive surgery, where bypass procedures are performed (e.g., gastric bypass), or restrictive surgery (e.g., gastric banding or sleeve gastrectomy), where the size of the stomach is reduced. Endoscopic procedures which cause early satiety (e.g., placement of an intragastric balloon) have also been used but risk development of gastric ulcers.

CLINICAL NOTES

Following bariatric surgery, particularly following bypass procedures, patients are at high risk of nutritional deficiencies, so watch for iron, calcium, zinc, folate and vitamin D deficiency. Hyperoxaluria can occur, with reduced intestinal oxalate absorption. This can predispose to renal stone formation.

HINTS AND TIPS

Dumping syndrome is commonly asked about in examinations. It is a neurohormonal reaction triggered by sugar after a gastric bypass procedure and causes dizziness, flushing, palpitations and diarrhoea.

LIPID DISORDERS

Hypercholesterolaemia is widely prevalent in Western societies. In the United Kingdom, two-thirds of the adult population have a serum total cholesterol concentration above 5.0 mmol/L. There is an association between serum cholesterol and cardiovascular risk. Low-density lipoprotein (LDL) particles are the main carriers of cholesterol to the liver and peripheries; LDL levels are positively associated with cardiovascular risk. HDLs are involved in 'reverse cholesterol transport' from the peripheries to the liver, and levels are inversely related to cardiovascular risk.

When you are assessing patients, it is more important to assess their overall cardiovascular risk to guide your advice and management decisions rather than focus on individual risk factors (see later). In this way therapy may be targeted at those with most to gain.

Aetiology and pathophysiology

The genetics of hyperlipidaemia are complicated; most commonly it is polygenic, with high serum cholesterol concentrations and normal triglyceride concentrations. It is greatly influenced by dietary lipid intake. 'Monogenic' forms are less common; some of these are discussed next.

Primary hyperlipidaemia

Familial combined hyperlipidaemia has a prevalence of 1 in 100 and is associated with high cholesterol and/or high triglyceride concentrations. It is heterogeneous, and the causative gene has not been identified.

Familial hypercholesterolaemia is an autosomal dominant condition and is due to LDL receptor deficiency, resulting in an increase in the level of LDL particles in the circulation. The prevalence of heterozygotes is approximately 1 in 500. Homozygotes (prevalence of 1 in 250,000) can have serum cholesterol levels of up to 30 mmol/L or more and may develop coronary artery disease in their teenage years.

Familial hypertriglyceridaemia is also an autosomal dominant condition, and can cause pancreatitis. Patients may have eruptive xanthomata. Triglyceride levels may also be raised in diabetes, alcoholism and obesity.

Other types of dyslipidaemia are rare. Cases of primary hyperlipidaemia are generally managed by lipid specialists.

CLINICAL NOTES

Interpret the results along with the family history; consider the possibility of familial hypercholesterolaemia if the total cholesterol level is greater than 7.5 mmol/L and there is a family history of premature coronary heart disease.

Secondary hyperlipidaemia

Causes include DM, excess alcohol consumption, hypothyroidism, chronic kidney disease, cholestasis (such as in primary biliary cirrhosis), Cushing syndrome, nephrotic syndrome, obesity and synthetic oestrogens.

HINTS AND TIPS

On clinical examination look for arcus senilis, a white ring in the corneal margin, and tendon xanthomata, hard nontender nodular enlargements of the Achilles tendon or knuckles. These signs are associated with familial hypercholesterolaemia.

Investigations

Measure both total cholesterol and HDL cholesterol to achieve the best estimate of cardiovascular risk. Before starting any lipid modification therapy for primary prevention of CVD, perform a full lipid screen. This should include total cholesterol, HDL cholesterol, non-HDL cholesterol and triglycerides. This does not need to be a fasting sample.

CLINICAL NOTES

Investigate the patient for secondary causes: check thyroid function, liver function, serum glucose level and cortisol level, and if serum albumin level is low, look for evidence of proteinuria.

Management

Causes of secondary hyperlipidaemia should be treated. Dietary measures should be tried, including reduction of total energy and saturated fat intake. However, the average fall in total cholesterol concentration with a general lipid-lowering diet is only 2%. The use of lipid-lowering therapy is key to secondary prevention, and should form part of an integrated approach alongside interventions directed at smoking, lifestyle, obesity, blood pressure and use of anti-platelet therapy. Lowering of lipid levels appears to reduce cardiovascular risk regardless of baseline serum cholesterol levels, and all patients with established CVD should be advised to start lipid modification therapy. The absolute risk reduction is greater if the patient's risk of CVD is higher.

Statins

High-intensity treatment with atorvastatin 80 mg, a drug of the statin class, is first-line therapy. Therapy aims to achieve a total cholesterol level below 4 mmol/L and an LDL level below 2 mmol/L. Statins competitively inhibit 3-hydroxy-3-methylglutaryl coenzyme A reductase, an enzyme involved in cholesterol synthesis, especially in the liver. They should be used with caution in those with a history of liver disease, and LFTs results should be monitored within 3 months of starting treatment, and again at 12 months. Side effects include reversible myositis, and treatment should be stopped if there are symptoms of myopathy or a significantly raised creatine kinase level. Patients should therefore be advised to report unexplained muscle pain, tenderness and weakness. Other side effects include headache, altered LFT values (which occasionally necessitates stopping therapy) and gastrointestinal effects (e.g., abdominal pain, nausea and vomiting).

COMMUNICATION

Clinical judgement must always be used, and a patient-centred approach is essential as lipid-lowering medications, such as statins, are taken life long and are taken life-long and will only be effective if the patient takes the tablets.

COMMUNICATION

Tell patients to avoid drinking grapefruit juice with simvastatin/atorvastatin as drug levels can increase through the inhibition of cytochromes P450. Watch out for other drug interactions.

Other drugs

Ezetimibe—This drug reduces the intestinal absorption of cholesterol. It may be used when a statin is not tolerated or in addition to a statin to achieve target levels.

Fibrates—Their main action is to decrease serum triglyceride levels. Current clinical guidelines recommend fibrates as the treatment of choice for severe isolated hypertriglyceridaemia. However, where high triglyceride levels coexist with high cholesterol levels, statins are still first-line therapy. They can also cause a myositis, especially when taken in combination with a statin. They are not recommended in chronic kidney disease or diabetes.

Additional lipid-regulating drugs—Other drugs include cholestyramine, nicotinic acid and omega fish oils. These are not recommended by the NICE but may occasionally be used in specialist clinics. Plasmapheresis in combination with additional pharmacological treatment is proven in managing homozygous hyperlipidaemia.

Primary prevention

NICE recommends use of the QRISK2 assessment tool to estimate 10-year risk of developing CVD in patients up to and including age 84. A shared decision-making approach should be utilized, with atorvastatin 20 mg recommended for patients who have a 10% or greater 10-year risk of developing CVD. NICE also recommends considering offering lipid modification therapy to all people aged over 85, and those with type 1 DM,

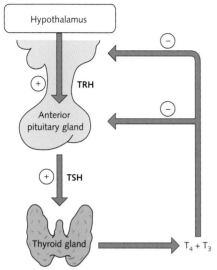

Fig. 33.4 Control of thyroid hormone production via the hypothalamus–pituitary–thyroid axis. *TRH*, Thyrotrophin-releasing hormone; *TSH*, thyroid-stimulating hormone.

CKD or familial hypercholesterolaemia, regardless of formal risk.

RED FLAG

Refer a patient for urgent specialist review if a patient has a triglyceride concentration greater than 20 mmol/L that is not the result of excess alcohol consumption or poor glycaemic control. Individuals with a total cholesterol level greater than 9 mmol/L or non-high-density lipoprotein cholesterol level greater than 7.5 mmol/L should be seen by a lipid specialist.

THYROID DISEASE

The control of thyroid hormone production and release is outlined in Fig. 33.4. Thyroid disorders are common, and include both overactive and underactive thyroid, and thyroid cysts, which may be benign or malignant. Some of these disorders will present with an enlarged thyroid gland (i.e., a goitre). Thyroid disease is discussed in detail in Chapter 17, and here we focus on the management of thyroid disease.

Hypothyroidism

Hypothyroidism results from deficiency of thyroxine (T_4) or tri-iodothyronine (T_3).

Management

Thyroxine sodium (normally levothyroxine, T_4 replacement) is the treatment of choice for maintenance therapy. Usual maintenance dosages are between 100 and 200 µg daily. The initial dose is usually 50 µg, increased as necessary over a few weeks, and even lower doses (25 µg) are started in elderly patients or patients with cardiac disease to avoid worsening angina or precipitating a myocardial infarction. Treatment is monitored by serum thyroid-stimulating hormone (TSH) level and serum T_4 level and is nearly always lifelong except in cases of subacute or silent thyroiditis. It is sometimes necessary to rule out adrenal insufficiency (e.g., in secondary hypothyroidism) before starting treatment, as giving thyroxine can precipitate an adrenal crisis if there is concomitant glucocorticoid deficiency.

CLINICAL NOTES

Subclinical hypothyroidism (i.e., raised thyroid-stimulating hormone level but normal thyroxine level) is treated with levothyroxine only if the patient is at high risk of progressing to overt hypothyroidism. These high-risk groups include individuals with thyroid antibodies, a history of previous radioiodine treatment or a thyroid-stimulating hormone level greater than 10 mU/L.

PATIENT SAFETY

Overtreating hypothyroidism with levothyroxine can result in atrial fibrillation and osteoporosis, and can worsen angina or cardiac failure in a patient with existing cardiac disease.

Hyperthyroidism

Thyrotoxicosis is the condition resulting from raised levels of circulating free T_4 and free T_3.

Management

Treatment options include drugs, radioiodine and surgery. Most patients younger than 50 years with Graves disease receive a course of an antithyroid drug as the initial treatment. There is a significant risk of relapse after drug treatment, and it is more likely in younger patients and those with a large goitre. Relapse after a period of drug therapy should be treated with iodine-131 (radioiodine) or subtotal thyroidectomy. Subtotal thyroidectomy is often recommended in young patients with large goitres to remove the neck swelling.

Toxic adenoma or toxic multinodular goitre is treated with radioiodine or surgery. All options should be discussed with the patient, and a joint decision should be made. β-Blockers are useful to ameliorate the symptoms of thyrotoxicosis.

Antithyroid drugs

In the United Kingdom, carbimazole is the most commonly used drug. It is metabolized to methimazole, the active agent. Propylthiouracil may be used in patients who have sensitivity reactions to carbimazole and is preferred in pregnancy. Both drugs act primarily by interfering with the synthesis of thyroid hormones.

The daily dose of carbimazole is adjusted according to response and then maintained until the patient becomes euthyroid, usually after 4 to 8 weeks. The dose may then be gradually reduced to a maintenance dose, again adjusted according to response. Patients are advised to report any infectious symptoms immediately as agranulocytosis is a rare complication. More common side effects of this drug include a rash and pruritus. If symptoms are profound, a combination of higher-dose carbimazole and exogenous T_4 daily may be used in a 'block and replace' regimen. A euthyroid state may be achieved more quickly with this regimen. Treatment with either of these regimens is usually for 18 months followed by long-term monitoring.

Iodine may be given 10 to 14 days before surgery, in addition to carbimazole, to assist control and to reduce vascularity of the thyroid.

The β-blocker, propranolol, is useful for the rapid relief of thyrotoxic symptoms before a euthyroid state is achieved. β-Blockers are also useful for the control of supraventricular arrhythmias secondary to thyrotoxicosis.

Radioiodine

This is commonly used for adenomas or toxic multinodular goitre. Radioactive sodium iodide ($Na^{131}I$) is concentrated by the thyroid and causes cell damage and cell death. Hypothyroidism may therefore develop at any stage after treatment, and so the patient should be under regular follow-up. Radioiodine is used increasingly for the treatment of thyrotoxicosis at all ages, particularly where medical therapy or adherence is a problem, in patients with cardiac disease and in patients who relapse after thyroidectomy. Contraindications include pregnancy and breast-feeding. Pregnancy is safe 4 months or more after treatment. Radioiodine may worsen the ophthalmopathy of Graves disease.

Subtotal thyroidectomy

This is more commonly performed for adenoma or multi-nodular goitre than for Graves disease, in which it is reserved for those with a large or obstructive goitre. The aim of surgery is to remove sufficient thyroid tissue to cure hyperthyroidism. One year later, approximately 80% of patients are euthyroid, 15% are hypothyroid and 5% have relapsed. Complications include hypoparathyroidism, recurrent laryngeal nerve damage and bleeding into the neck causing laryngeal oedema.

Thyroid emergencies

Thyrotoxic crisis ('thyroid storm')

This is an uncommon, life-threatening exacerbation of thyrotoxicosis with a mortality of up to 20% with treatment. Precipitating factors include thyroid surgery, radioiodine, withdrawal of antithyroid drugs, iodinated contrast agents and acute illnesses (e.g., stroke, infection, trauma and DKA). In addition to general symptoms, common features include hyperpyrexia, severe tachycardia and psychiatric symptoms, including anxiety, delirium or psychosis. It requires emergency treatment with oxygen, IV fluids because of profuse sweating, β-blockers for control of tachycardia (may need to be given IV), IV hydrocortisone (which inhibits peripheral T_4 conversion to T_3), oral administration of iodine solution (to block release of thyroid hormone) and propylthiouracil (to prevent new synthesis of thyroid hormones).

Myxoedema coma

This is uncommon. It is typically seen in the elderly, and is precipitated by infection, myocardial infarction, treatment with sedatives or inadequate heating in cold weather. Most patients have hypothermia and are hypotensive with heart failure, hyponatraemia, hypoxia and hypercapnia.

Treatment is with T_3 intravenously because of its rapid action. Hydrocortisone IV is also given, particularly if pituitary hypothyroidism is suspected. Supportive measures are also needed, including IV fluids, antibiotics, ventilation and slow rewarming. T_4 can be substituted after 2 to 3 days if there is a clinical improvement. Mortality is up to 20%.

PARATHYROID DISEASE

The parathyroid gland is located on the back of the thyroid gland and is generally made up of four small glands. These glands produce parathyroid hormone (PTH) from the chief cells. PTH is integral in the control of calcium and phosphate homeostasis in the body. Many conditions are associated with disorders of the parathyroid gland. These can be divided into those causing hypoparathyroidism and those causing hyperparathyroidism.

Table 33.2 Causes of hypocalcaemia

Mechanism	Example
Reduced calcium intake	Dietary deficiency, malabsorption
Reduced vitamin D intake/production	Dietary deficiency, malabsorption, reduced sunlight exposure
Reduced activation of vitamin D	Renal disease, liver disease
Increased inactivation of vitamin D	Enzyme induction by anticonvulsants
Renal calcium loss	Renal disease, drug-induced (loop diuretics)
Reduce calcium efflux from bone to circulation	Drug induced (bisphosphonates)
Reduced production of PTH	Surgical removal of parathyroid glands, autoimmune, congenital (DiGeorge syndrome), drug-induced (cinacalcet)
Resistance to PTH	Pseudohypoparathyroidism
Hypoalbuminaemia	Shock

PTH, *Parathyroid hormone.*

Hypoparathyroidism

Hypoparathyroidism results in hypocalcaemia and hyperphosphataemia. This occurs as a low PTH level, downregulates calcium release from the skeleton, downregulates activation of vitamin D in the kidney and suppresses phosphate excretion. In normal conditions the low serum calcium level and high serum phosphate level would trigger PTH production from the parathyroid gland.

Aetiology

Hypoparathyroidism is most commonly iatrogenic following surgery to the neck. Other causes are rare. Primary (idiopathic) hypoparathyroidism is an autoimmune disorder associated with vitiligo, Addison disease, pernicious anaemia and other autoimmune diseases, and it may be part of autoimmune polyendocrine syndrome (APS) (see later). Infiltration due to metabolic diseases such as Wilson disease and haemochromatosis can cause destruction of the parathyroid gland, but this is very uncommon. Rare mutations can cause inherited abnormalities of parathyroid development, such as in DiGeorge syndrome, when it is associated with intellectual impairment, cardiac abnormalities and thymic hypoplasia.

Pseudohypoparathyroidism is a rare syndrome genetic disorder of resistance to PTH. It is associated with intellectual impairment, short stature, a round face and short metacarpals and metatarsals.

Other causes of hypocalcaemia include chronic renal failure and osteomalacia. Acute pancreatitis and rhabdomyolysis can cause hypocalcaemia. Causes are summarized in Table 33.2.

Clinical features

These include the symptoms of hypocalcaemia, classically circumoral paraesthesiae and cramps (see Chapter 32).

Investigations

Serum calcium level is low, phosphate level is high and alkaline phosphatase level is normal. Additional tests include serum urea and creatinine levels, serum PTH level, parathyroid antibodies and vitamin D metabolite levels. Serum PTH level will be low in hypoparathyroidism but raised in pseudohypoparathyroidism. Investigations for other endocrinopathies may be required in certain cases.

X-rays of the hands show short fourth metacarpals in pseudohypoparathyroidism.

Management

Emergency treatment of hypocalcaemia is with 10 mL of 10% calcium gluconate IV, repeated as necessary (see Chapter 32). IV magnesium chloride may also be required if there is concurrent hypomagnesaemia. Calcium levels will be difficult to correct in the context of low serum magnesium levels.

Long-term treatment is with alfacalcidol or calcitriol. Serum calcium level should be monitored to prevent hypercalcaemia.

Hyperparathyroidism

Hyperparathyroidism results from excess circulating PTH. PTH acts to increase serum calcium levels by increasing mobilization of calcium from bone and increasing calcium reabsorption from the kidney. Also, in the kidney it increases the hydroxylation of vitamin D to active 1,25-dihydrovitamin D_3. This acts to increase calcium absorption from the small bowel. PTH also increases phosphate release from bone and increases renal phosphate excretion, with the overall effect of lowering phosphate concentrations.

Aetiology

Primary hyperparathyroidism (overproduction of PTH in the absence of other abnormalities) is usually due to a single benign adenoma. This is common, particularly in postmenopausal women. Less frequently it can be due to multiple adenomas, carcinoma or hyperplasia. It may be associated with other endocrine abnormalities as part of the multiple endocrine neoplasia (MEN) syndromes. Ectopic PTH production is very rare; more commonly, cancers of the lung or breast produce PTH-related protein, which causes a similar picture.

Secondary hyperparathyroidism occurs when PTH levels are persistently and appropriately raised to maintain calcium concentrations in the face of a disorder that lowers calcium levels. Causes include chronic renal failure and deficiency of vitamin D.

Tertiary hyperparathyroidism is the continued secretion of excess PTH after prolonged secondary hyperparathyroidism. The parathyroids act autonomously and cause hypercalcaemia, despite correction of the original cause of the secondary hyperparathyroidism. This can occur in patients with advanced renal failure.

Clinical features

Hyperparathyroid bone disease can cause osteopenia and osteoporosis. This may result in fractures causing bone pain. In addition, all the features associated with hypercalcaemia may be present (see Chapter 32).

Investigations

- In primary hyperparathyroidism, serum calcium level is raised. Serum phosphate level is low and alkaline phosphatase level is high, reflecting increased bone turnover.
- In secondary hyperparathyroidism of renal failure, serum calcium level is low or normal and phosphate level is normal or high, resulting in an appropriate rise in PTH production.
- In tertiary hyperparathyroidism, serum calcium level is high and PTH level is inappropriately high.

In patients with hyperparathyroidism a dual-energy X-ray absorptiometry (DXA) scan can show evidence of bone involvement. Pathognomonic X-ray features include subperiosteal resorption of the phalanges and salt and pepper degranulation of the skull. Imaging of the renal tract may show renal calculi. Imaging of the neck is used only to plan surgery and is not used for diagnosis.

CLINICAL NOTES

Perform a 24-hour urinary collection to look for familial benign hypocalciuric hypercalcaemia. This condition can present with a hypercalcaemia and an inappropriately raised parathyroid hormone level; in this case parathyroidectomy will be ineffective.

Management

Parathyroidectomy is indicated for symptomatic disease. The decision is more difficult in asymptomatic patients, many of whom will progress to overt disease. Guidelines suggest surgery when there is persistent hypercalcaemia with a calcium level greater than 0.25 mmol/L above normal, renal impairment, renal calculi, bone mineral density (BMD) *T* score below − 2.5, vertebral fracture or age younger than 50 years.

The parathyroid glands may be localized by computed tomography (CT) scan, single photon emission CT scan or a technetium (^{99m}Tc) sestamibi scan, which can detect adenomas. The operative procedure may be a full bilateral exploration (if multiple adenomas are present) or a minimally invasive endoscopic procedure with intraoperative PTH monitoring (when a single adenoma is seen on imaging). All abnormal glands are removed. If all the glands are hyperplastic, three and a half are usually removed, leaving the last half in situ.

COMMON PITFALLS

Serum calcium and magnesium levels should be monitored very carefully postoperatively as removal of the glands may lead to rapid and prolonged hypocalcaemia and hypomagnesaemia as the 'hungry bones' recover the minerals lost during the period of hyperparathyroidism. This often warrants frequent intravenous administration of calcium.

If surgery is contraindicated, bisphosphonates or calcimimetics (e.g., cinacalcet) may be useful.

PITUITARY DISORDERS

Hypopituitarism

The anterior pituitary produces six hormones: adrenocorticotrophic hormone (ACTH), growth hormone (GH), follicle-stimulating hormone (FSH), luteinizing hormone (LH), TSH and prolactin (PRL). Hypopituitarism may be associated with loss of all or some of these hormones. The clinical and biochemical presentation will depend on which hormones are deficient and to what extent.

Aetiology

The most common cause of hypopituitarism is from the mass effect of a pituitary adenoma (which, if functional, may cause features of hypersecretion of a specific hormone; see later), with additional loss of pituitary function after surgery and pituitary irradiation. Other causes include hypothalamic tumours and cysts, peripituitary tumours (e.g., gliomas and meningiomas, craniopharyngiomas), infiltrative diseases (e.g., sarcoidosis), pituitary infarction (Sheehan syndrome) or haemorrhage and metastatic lesions.

> ### RED FLAG
>
> Sudden haemorrhage or infarction of the pituitary causes headache, diplopia and hypopituitarism and is known as 'pituitary apoplexy'. This is an emergency and requires intravenous fluids and steroids.

Clinical features

These can be related to the size of the adenoma, which can cause headaches and affect vision, classically causing a bitemporal hemianopia through pressure on the optic chiasm (see later).

Otherwise, the features of hypopituitarism relate to which pituitary hormones are being affected. GH and gonadotrophins are often affected first:

- Suppressed GH: fatigue, increased abdominal adiposity and reduced muscle strength and exercise capacity.
- Suppressed LH and FSH: in women, there is oligomenorrhoea, infertility, dyspareunia, breast atrophy, loss of pubic and axillary hair and hot flushes; in men, there is loss of libido, impotence, infertility, flushes, regression of secondary sexual characteristics, soft testes and fine wrinkles on the face.
- Suppressed TSH: fatigue, muscle weakness, sensitivity to cold, constipation, apathy, weight gain and dry skin.
- Suppressed ACTH: fatigue, anorexia, weight loss, postural hypotension, weakness, nausea and vomiting, hypoglycaemia, apathy, reduced libido and loss of pubic and axillary hair.
- Suppressed prolactin: inability to lactate.

> ### CLINICAL NOTES
>
> The symptoms of hypopituitarism are nonspecific but must not be dismissed. A high index of suspicion may be required to make the diagnosis.

Investigations

Dynamic tests involving stimulation are occasionally needed to assess ACTH or GH levels; otherwise basal levels provide all the necessary information.

> ### HINTS AND TIPS
>
> Most pituitary hormones are secreted in a pulsatile fashion, and therefore random levels are not very useful.
>
> - Serum thyroxine (T_4) and thyroid-stimulating hormone: a low T_4 level together with a low or normal TSH level is suggestive of secondary hypothyroidism.
> - To assess adrenocorticotrophic hormone (ACTH), cortisol level should be measured between 8 a.m. and 9 a.m. If the level is low or intermediate, serum ACTH should be measured; the sample needs to be taken at 9 a.m. into a cold tube and immediately put on ice.
> - Follicle-stimulating hormone (FSH) and luteinizing hormone (LH): these should be measured in the morning with a simultaneous measurement of serum testosterone level in men and serum oestradiol level in women.
> - Growth hormone (GH): as basal levels of GH fluctuate greatly, if deficiency is suspected, an insulin tolerance test is required; the normal response is GH release as glucose levels decrease. Insulin-like growth factor 1 levels will also be low in GH deficiency.
> - Prolactin: raised levels would signify a prolactinoma.
> - Investigate with CT/magnetic resonance imaging (MRI)/visual field assessment: (see Investigations in Pituitary Tumours).

Management

Hormone replacement involves the use of multiple hormones. Hydrocortisone is given for adrenal failure, T_4 for hypothyroidism, testosterone for hypogonadal men and oestrogen for hypogonadal premenopausal women. Recombinant human GH is given by injection to patients with significant symptoms. Careful instruction and patient adherence are mandatory for long-term recovery.

Pituitary tumours

Pituitary tumours are generally benign and curable. They can result in problems by excessive hormone production, local effects of the tumour or inadequate hormone production by the remaining pituitary gland. Nonfunctioning and PRL-secreting tumours are the most common. Pituitary tumours account for around 20% of all intracranial neoplasms. PRL- and ACTH-secreting tumours occur most commonly in 25- to 35-year-olds, GH-secreting tumours occur most commonly in those aged 35 to 50 years, and nonfunctioning tumours usually present after the age of 60 years. They can also be classified by their size as microadenoma (<1 cm diameter) or macroadenoma (>1 cm).

Clinical features

Pressure effects cause headaches, and there may be compression of the optic chiasm causing bitemporal hemianopia. Seizures, other cranial nerve signs and hydrocephalus may occur with large masses. Extension into the hypothalamus affects appetite, sleep and temperature regulation.

The effects of functioning tumours depend on the hormone secreted. They may cause acromegaly via GH, amenorrhoea–galactorrhoea syndrome via PRL or Cushing disease via ACTH. Secondary thyrotoxicosis is rare. The features of hypopituitarism were described earlier.

Investigations

Endocrinological assessment is performed as described earlier. MRI scan is the best modality with which to assess the anatomy of the tumour. Formal visual field assessment is important as many of these tumours have effects on the visual pathways, particularly at the optic chiasm.

Management

Management may be medical, surgical or with radiotherapy. Aside from prolactinomas, surgical resection is the treatment of choice in most cases. The surgical approach is usually transsphenoidal, but with larger masses a transfrontal approach may be necessary. Drug therapy includes dopamine receptor agonists (e.g., cabergoline, bromocriptine) for prolactinoma; these inhibit PRL release and induce shrinkage of the tumour in more than 90% of cases. Somatostatin analogues inhibit GH release and induce tumour shrinkage in most GH-secreting adenomas. They are usually used after surgery in acromegaly.

ACROMEGALY

Acromegaly is an insidious disease resulting from excessive circulating levels of GH in adults. GH stimulates the production of insulin-like growth factor 1 (IGF-1), which is produced in the liver and is the main tissue mediator of the actions of GH. Diagnosis is often made years after symptoms first occur. Acromegalic gigantism results from acromegaly in young individuals before epiphyseal fusion, and is very uncommon.

Aetiology

The commonest cause is a benign pituitary tumour secreting GH. Pituitary carcinoma and carcinoid tumours that secrete hypothalamic GH-releasing hormone are uncommon causes.

Clinical features

The clinical features of acromegaly are summarized in Fig. 33.5.

- Cardiovascular problems are often the cause of death. Coronary artery disease, hypertension and diabetes are more common than in the normal population. Cardiomyopathy may occur.
- Headaches, visual field defects and cranial nerve palsies may occur because of the mass effect of the pituitary tumour.
- Hyperprolactinaemia (due to compression of the pituitary stalk and therefore loss of tonic inhibitory dopamine from hypothalamus) is common, and may present with milky nipple discharge and menstrual abnormalities – see later.
- Hypopituitarism can also occur.
- Sleep apnoea occurs in up to 50% of individuals because of an enlarged tongue and soft tissues of the upper pharynx.

HINTS AND TIPS

The diagnosis of acromegaly may become more obvious on comparison of old photographs of the patient with the present appearance. Ask the patient about changes in hat, glove or shoe size.

Investigations

IGF-1 is recommended as the initial screen for suspected acromegaly. If the level is raised, GH level is measured following a glucose tolerance test. In healthy individuals, GH level falls to below 1 ng/mL in the 2 hours following a 75-g glucose load. If the glucose load fails to reduce the GH concentration to below this level, a diagnosis of acromegaly can be made.

Other investigations include:

- Assessment of other pituitary hormones.
- Assessment of visual fields: bitemporal hemianopia.
- Skull X-ray and MRI of the brain.
- Hand X-ray: tufting of the terminal phalanges and increased joint spaces due to hypertrophy of the cartilage. The heel pad is usually thickened.
- CXR, ECG and echocardiogram: left ventricular hypertrophy and cardiomyopathy.
- CT scan to investigate the patient for ectopic GH production (e.g., from lung, ovarian, pancreatic or adrenal tumours).

Management

The aim of treatment is to relieve symptoms, reverse somatic changes and reverse metabolic abnormalities. Treatment is by surgery, radiotherapy or drugs.

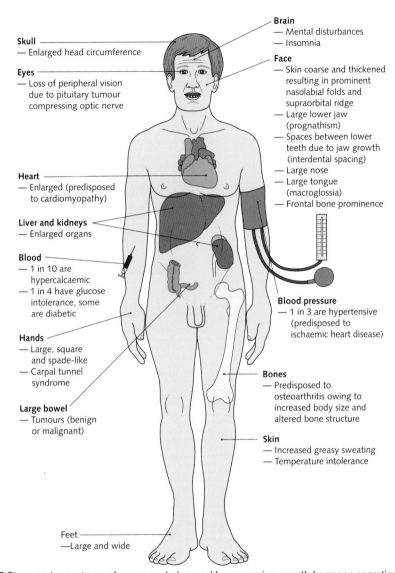

Fig. 33.5 Signs and symptoms of acromegaly (caused by excessive growth hormone secretion in adults).

Surgery

Surgery is the first-choice treatment. The transsphenoidal route is usually used. Up to 90% of microadenomas are cured, but the success rate is lower for larger tumours. Complications include hypopituitarism, meningitis and intraoperative bleeding.

Radiotherapy

This is often used for refractory disease, as an adjuvant for large invasive tumours and when surgery is contraindicated. The outcome is less good with radiotherapy. Hypopituitarism is a common complication.

Medical therapies

The most effective treatment is with octreotide, a somatostatin analogue. Somatostatin inhibits GH secretion. Side effects include colicky abdominal pain and diarrhoea, but this usually settles with continued treatment. Gallstones occur in approximately one-third of patients.

Table 33.3 Causes of hyperprolactinaemia

Cause	Examples
Physiological	Pregnancy, lactation, stress
Drugs	Antiemetics (e.g., metoclopramide, prochlorperazine), phenothiazines, tricyclic antidepressants
Primary hypothyroidism	
Pituitary tumours	Prolactinoma Growth hormone-secreting tumours Nonfunctioning tumours
Polycystic ovary syndrome	
Uncommon	Sarcoidosis
Hypothalamic lesions	Langerhans cell histiocytosis Hypothalamic tumours
Chest wall stimulation	Repeated self-examination of breasts After herpes zoster
Liver or renal failure	

Prognosis

Untreated, the mortality rate is approximately twice that in healthy individuals because of cardiovascular and cerebrovascular disease. There is also an increased risk of colon cancer and thyroid cancer.

PROLACTIN DISORDERS

Aetiology

Prolactin is the hormone most commonly secreted by pituitary tumours. They are generally benign tumours, and more common in women. Secretion of prolactin is under constant negative control by the action of dopamine produced in the hypothalamus and transported down the pituitary stalk. In this way, high levels of prolactin may be caused directly, by a prolactin-secreting tumour, or indirectly, by a nonsecreting tumour that prevents dopamine from reaching the normal prolactin-producing cells. Other causes of a raised prolactin level are summarized in Table 33.3.

CLINICAL NOTES

A prolactinoma may occur in association with the clinical syndrome multiple endocrine neoplasia type 1. This is an autosomal dominant genetic disorder where pituitary adenomas (most often prolactinomas) occur in association with tumours of the parathyroid and pancreatic islet cells.

Clinical features

In premenopausal women the most common symptoms are oligomenorrhoea and infertility (through raised prolactin level inhibiting gonadotrophin secretion of FSH and LH). Prolactinomas can also cause galactorrhoea and occasionally hirsutism. In men, symptoms include reduced libido, hypogonadism, impotence, infertility and galactorrhoea. Symptoms caused by large tumour size are more common in men and postmenopausal women, and include headache, visual field defects and cranial nerve palsies. Various degrees of hypopituitarism may be present.

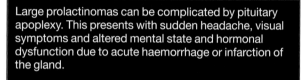

RED FLAG

Large prolactinomas can be complicated by pituitary apoplexy. This presents with sudden headache, visual symptoms and altered mental state and hormonal dysfunction due to acute haemorrhage or infarction of the gland.

Investigations

- Elevated PRL levels should be confirmed on repeated testing.
- Other blood tests include thyroid function tests, renal and LFTs and a pregnancy test in women.
- The drug history should always be taken carefully (antipsychotics such as haloperidol and chlorpromazine being the most common cause of drug-induced hyperprolactinaemia).
- Radiological assessment of the pituitary tumour should be performed with skull X-rays and MRI scan of the brain.
- Full assessment of pituitary function should be undertaken if an adenoma is suspected, and visual fields should be assessed.

Management

Microprolactinomas are smaller than 10 mm on MRI. Dopamine agonist therapy (bromocriptine, cabergoline) should be the first-line therapy as this is effective in most cases. Transsphenoidal surgery is usually successful for resistant cases, but there is a small recurrence rate. Prolactin levels are monitored and scans are repeated if there is evidence of tumour growth (e.g., headache, visual field defects).

Macroprolactinomas are larger than 10 mm on MRI. They can be treated with drugs, but if there are pressure effects, visual symptoms or pregnancy is considered (25% expand in pregnancy), surgery is usually performed.

Diabetes insipidus

This occurs from a primary deficiency in vasopressin (also called 'antidiuretic hormone' (ADH)) in the case of cranial

Table 33.4 Causes of acquired cranial diabetes insipidus

Cause	Example
Idiopathic	No known cause – likely to be autoimmune
Trauma	Head injury and neurosurgery
Tumours	Craniopharyngioma or secondary tumours
Granulomas	Tuberculosis, sarcoid, histiocytosis
Infections	Encephalitis or meningitis

Table 33.5 Causes of acquired nephrogenic diabetes insipidus

Metabolic: hypokalaemia, hypercalcaemia
Chronic renal failure
Lithium toxicity
Obstructive uropathy
Diabetes mellitus

thiazide diuretics are occasionally used to drive thirst or indomethacin, a nonsteroidal antiinflammatory, is used, which can reduce urine output by up to 50%. For patients with primary polydipsia, water restriction and treatment of any associated psychiatric disorder is required.

RED FLAG

In patients with cranial diabetes insipidus it is vital that they receive their desmopressin medication. Without this they are at risk of severe dehydration and hypernatraemia and ultimately death. Particularly vulnerable groups are those who have impaired thirst drive or access to water (e.g., elderly people, children, patients after a general anaesthetic or patients on the intensive care unit).

diabetes, or in a lack of response in the kidney to vasopressin, which is called 'nephrogenic diabetes insipidus'. A similar clinical picture can occur with primary polydipsia or excessive drinking. Clinically, the patient presents with polyuria, nocturia and polydipsia. Investigations are outlined in detail in Chapter 15, and include urine osmolality, serum osmolality, serum glucose and serum sodium. Cranial MRI may be indicated to investigate for cause of cranial diabetes insipidus (CDI).

Cranial diabetes insipidus

The causes of acquired CDI are given in Table 33.4. The most common type is idiopathic CDI, which may be due to an autoimmune process. Familial CDI is inherited as an autosomal dominant trait or as part of the DIDMOAD syndrome (diabetes insipidus, DM, optic atrophy and deafness).

Nephrogenic diabetes insipidus

Familial nephrogenic diabetes insipidus is X-linked recessive or autosomal recessive. It is rare and is due to mutations of the genes encoding arginine vasopressin receptor 2 (AVR2) or aquaporin 2 (AQP2) channel protein.

Causes of acquired nephrogenic diabetes insipidus are given in Table 33.5.

Management

For CDI, desmopressin (a vasopressin analogue) is the treatment of choice. It may be administered orally, intranasally or parenterally. For nephrogenic diabetes insipidus, any metabolic and electrolyte disturbances should be corrected, and any potential drug causes should be reviewed. In familial forms,

ADRENAL DISORDERS

Histologically, the adrenal glands are divided into the medulla, which secretes adrenaline and noradrenaline, and the cortex, which is divided into three zones:

- The inner zone, or *zona reticularis*, produces sex hormones.
- The middle zone, or *zona fasciculata*, produces cortisol. Production is stimulated by ACTH released by the pituitary gland. In a negative feedback loop, cortisol reduces both corticotrophin-releasing hormone (CRH) production in the hypothalamus and pituitary release of ACTH (Fig. 33.6).
- The outer *zona glomerulosa* produces aldosterone, which is regulated through the renin–angiotensin system.

Cushing syndrome

Cushing syndrome is the result of long-term exposure to excess glucocorticoid. This is most commonly iatrogenic, secondary to glucocorticoid administration given to treat inflammatory diseases (i.e., exogenous glucocorticoid). The causes of endogenous Cushing syndrome include:

- ACTH-dependent disease.
- Cushing disease: ACTH hypersecretion by a pituitary adenoma or corticotroph hyperplasia (70%).
- Ectopic ACTH syndrome caused by a variety of ACTH-secreting nonpituitary tumours such as small cell lung carcinoma (10%–15%).
- Non-ACTH-dependent disease (i.e., unregulated cortisol production).

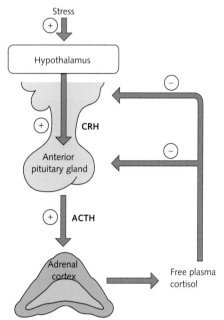

Fig. 33.6 Control of cortisol production via the hypothalamus–pituitary–adrenal axis. *ACTH*, Adrenocorticotrophic hormone; *CRH*, corticotrophin-releasing hormone.

- Primary adrenocortical tumours (15%–20%).

The annual incidence of spontaneous Cushing syndrome is approximately 1 in 100,000. Cushing syndrome due to adrenal tumours, or Cushing disease (from a pituitary tumour), is around four times more common in women.

> **CLINICAL NOTES**
>
> 'Cushing disease' describes excessive adrenocorticotrophic hormone production from the pituitary (e.g., from a pituitary adenoma). All other causes of raised cortisol levels are referred to as 'Cushing syndrome'.

Clinical features

The clinical features of Cushing syndrome are demonstrated in Fig. 33.7. Psychiatric disturbance may range from anxiety to psychosis, and cognitive problems such as short-term memory loss are common.

Investigations

The following investigations are important in Cushing syndrome:

- Plasma cortisol measurement: the level will vary throughout the day in normal individuals, being lowest at midnight and highest at 9 a.m. With Cushing syndrome both the midnight and the 9 a.m. cortisol level will be high and there will be loss of the normal diurnal variation.
- Twenty-four-hour urinary free cortisol measurement.
- Late-night salivary cortisol.
- Dexamethasone suppression tests and corticotroph function tests are outlined at the end of the chapter.
- Plasma ACTH measurement: this will be high in Cushing disease and ectopic ACTH production, and very low in adrenal cortisol hyperproduction.
- Imaging of the adrenal glands (with CT scan) and the pituitary (with MRI).

A 24-hour urinary free cortisol measurement or a low-dose dexamethasone suppression test is the best screening tool.

> **CLINICAL NOTES**
>
> Pseudo-Cushing syndrome is where the clinical features of Cushing syndrome occur along with high cortisol levels but without a pituitary–adrenal axis problem. Causes include poorly controlled diabetes, obesity, severe anxiety/depression and excess alcohol consumption.

Management

This is dependent on the cause of the raised cortisol level.

Cushing disease

Transsphenoidal surgery is the first line of treatment and is curative in approximately 80% of patients. Pituitary radiotherapy or drugs are used if surgery fails. Metyrapone inhibits steroidogenesis and is the drug of choice. Ketoconazole or mitotane may be used. Rarely, bilateral adrenalectomy is necessary, although there is a risk of causing Nelson syndrome, a rapidly enlarging pituitary tumour associated with hyperpigmentation.

Adrenocortical tumours

Surgical removal of a benign adrenocortical tumour is curative. Bilateral adrenalectomy necessitates replacement therapy with cortisol and fludrocortisone daily. Carcinomas may recur.

Ectopic adrenocorticotrophic hormone syndrome

Surgical resection of the tumour cures the hypercortisolism, although this is often not possible, and medical therapy is used to control cortisol levels.

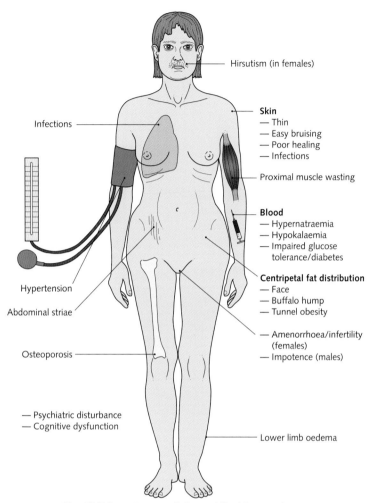

Fig. 33.7 Symptoms and signs of Cushing syndrome.

Hirsutism (in females)

Skin
— Thin
— Easy bruising
— Poor healing
— Infections

Infections

Proximal muscle wasting

Blood
— Hypernatraemia
— Hypokalaemia
— Impaired glucose tolerance/diabetes

Centripetal fat distribution
— Face
— Buffalo hump
— Tunnel obesity

Hypertension

Abdominal striae

— Amenorrhoea/infertility (females)
— Impotence (males)

Osteoporosis

— Psychiatric disturbance
— Cognitive dysfunction

Lower limb oedema

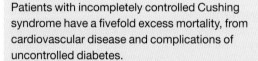

CLINICAL NOTES

Patients with incompletely controlled Cushing syndrome have a fivefold excess mortality, from cardiovascular disease and complications of uncontrolled diabetes.

Addison disease

Addison disease is primary adrenocortical failure. The annual incidence is about 1 in 10,000 people.

Aetiology

The causes of Addison disease include:

- Autoimmune adrenal destruction: this accounts for up to 90% of cases in developed countries. Women are affected two to three times more often than men. Up to 50% of patients have other autoimmune endocrine deficiencies (see later).
- Infections: worldwide, tuberculosis is a common cause.
- Adrenal haemorrhage/infarction: this may be associated with sepsis, particularly meningococcal septicaemia – Waterhouse–Friderichsen syndrome. The presentation is usually acute.
- Metastatic carcinoma: especially from the breast and lung.

- Infiltrative causes: sarcoidosis, amyloidosis and haemochromatosis.
- Inherited disorders: there are several familial disorders of adrenal function, which are all rare.
- Iatrogenic causes (e.g., following surgery, bilateral nephrectomies for renal cell carcinoma, long-term use of steroids (see Patient Safety box)).
- Trauma.

Clinical features

The symptoms and signs of Addison disease are predominantly caused by cortisol deficiency, although deficiencies of aldosterone and adrenal androgen will also be present to various extents (Fig. 33.8). The main symptoms are insidious and nonspecific: fatigue, weight loss, orthostatic dizziness and anorexia. Patients may present with gastrointestinal symptoms (e.g., abdominal pain, nausea, vomiting and diarrhoea). Hyperpigmentation of the skin and mucous membranes may occur because of high β-lipotrophin levels (see Hints and Tips box).

Addisonian crisis may occur with sudden onset adrenal failure (such as in haemorrhage) or increased cortisol requirements (such as in concurrent infection, surgery or trauma). There is hypovolaemic shock, often with acidosis and hypoglycaemia.

HINTS AND TIPS

The adrenocorticotrophic hormone (ACTH) precursor, proopiomelanocortin, is cleaved to ACTH and β-lipotrophin, which acts on melanocytes, increasing pigmentation.

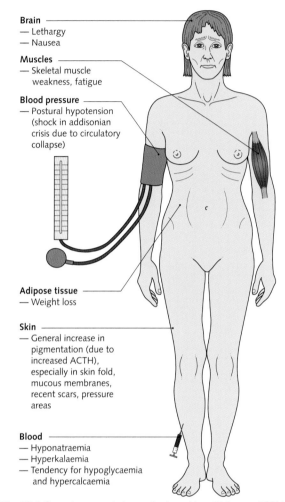

Brain
— Lethargy
— Nausea

Muscles
— Skeletal muscle weakness, fatigue

Blood pressure
— Postural hypotension (shock in addisonian crisis due to circulatory collapse)

Adipose tissue
— Weight loss

Skin
— General increase in pigmentation (due to increased ACTH), especially in skin fold, mucous membranes, recent scars, pressure areas

Blood
— Hyponatraemia
— Hyperkalaemia
— Tendency for hypoglycaemia and hypercalcaemia

Fig. 33.8 Symptoms and signs of adrenal insufficiency. *ACTH*, Adrenocorticotrophic hormone.

Investigations

The following are important investigations in patients with Addison disease:

- Serum cortisol concentration: low.
- Adrenal autoantibodies: these are detected in approximately 50% of patients (antibodies against steroid 21-hydroxylase).
- Serum ACTH levels: raised in Addison disease and low in secondary failure.
- Serum electrolytes: in an impending crisis there may be hyponatraemia, hyperkalaemia and raised blood urea level.
- Glucose level: bedside capillary blood glucose monitoring, watch for hypoglycaemia.
- Short and long Synacthen tests (described in 'Endocrine investigations' later).

- Screening for other autoimmune diseases such as autoimmune thyroid disease.

Management

Maintenance therapy is with hydrocortisone, usually in split doses throughout the day. The dose of hydrocortisone should be increased during intercurrent illnesses and during surgery. Enzyme-inducing drugs (e.g., phenytoin and rifampicin) may also increase patient requirements for hydrocortisone. Fludrocortisone is used to replace aldosterone because aldosterone taken orally undergoes first-pass metabolism in the liver. The dose is adjusted to maintain blood pressure and potassium levels.

Conn syndrome (primary hyperaldosteronism)

This is due to a unilateral adrenocortical adenoma in 75% of cases. Other causes include adrenal carcinoma or bilateral hyperplasia of the zona glomerulosa.

Clinical features

The clinical features are due to excess production of aldosterone. Resistant hypertension is the principal feature, along with hypokalaemia (although this is often not present). Sodium level tends to be mildly raised but there is usually no oedema.

Investigations

Measure serum electrolyte levels: serum potassium level is often low, serum sodium level may be raised and there is usually a metabolic alkalosis. Measure paired renin and aldosterone serum levels. In primary hyperaldosteronism aldosterone

level will be very high with a suppressed renin level (increased aldosterone-to-renin ratio). Imaging of the adrenals is required following a positive test result.

Secondary hyperaldosteronism is a result of high circulating renin levels. The most common cause is renal artery stenosis, although renin-producing tumours, coarctation of the aorta, congestive heart failure, liver cirrhosis and nephrotic syndrome are differentials.

Management

Tumours should be resected. Spironolactone is an aldosterone antagonist that can be given in primary or secondary aldosteronism.

Phaeochromocytoma

This is a rare tumour arising from the chromaffin tissues of the adrenal medulla, producing catecholamines. Similar tumours may arise from the cells of the sympathetic ganglia, and are often then referred to as 'paragangliomas'. It may be associated with medullary carcinoma of the thyroid, parathyroid adenoma and neurofibromatosis.

Clinical features

The symptoms and signs are due to the release of adrenaline and noradrenaline. The clinical features are very variable. The most common are headache, sweating and hypertension, which may be episodic. Others include pallor, tachycardia and palpitations, nausea, tremor, visual blurring and chest pain. The blood pressure may rise to very high levels and may precipitate a stroke, myocardial infarction or hypertensive encephalopathy.

Investigations

Urine is collected for 24 hours for measurement of adrenaline, noradrenaline and metanephrines. An abdominal CT scan may show the tumour. PET–CT or scintigraphy is occasionally used.

Management

This is by surgical removal of the tumour. The patient must be fully α-blocked with phenoxybenzamine or phentolamine, and β-blocked with propranolol before surgery to prevent the consequences of release of catecholamines during an operation. Changes in pulse and blood pressure should be monitored closely. α-Blockade must be achieved before β-blockade to prevent unopposed α-agonism causing severe hypertension.

Hypothalamus–pituitary–adrenal axis

Fig. 33.6 summarizes the control of cortisol levels via the hypothalamus–pituitary–adrenal axis. These tests are used to diagnose diseases of glucocorticoid excess (Cushing disease, ectopic ACTH production, adrenal hyperproduction of cortisol) and glucocorticoid deficiency (pituitary hypoproduction of ACTH and hypoadrenalism).

Dynamic tests for cortisol excess

Overnight dexamethasone suppression test—Dexamethasone (1 mg) is taken orally at midnight; plasma cortisol level is measured at 9 a.m. the next morning. In normal patients, ACTH and cortisol production will be suppressed by negative feedback. In all cases of Cushing syndrome there is absence of suppression of cortisol. In Cushing disease the feedback mechanism is less sensitive than normal (see High-dose dexamethasone suppression test). Ectopic ACTH production has no negative feedback mechanism. In adrenocortical tumours, ACTH will already be suppressed and cortisol level will remain high.

High-dose dexamethasone suppression test—This is used after positive results from tests to differentiate between Cushing disease and ectopic ACTH production. Plasma cortisol level is measured; 2 mg of dexamethasone is taken orally every 6 hours for 2 days. After 48 hours from the first dose, plasma cortisol level is measured again. In normal individuals, the plasma cortisol should be almost undetectable. In Cushing disease the less sensitive feedback mechanism should be overcome by the high dose, and the cortisol level should fall by at least half. Suppression should not be seen in ectopic ACTH production.

Corticotrophin-releasing hormone test—Plasma cortisol and ACTH are measured at several intervals shortly following administration of CRH. Ectopic ACTH production should not increase, whereas a pituitary adenoma will respond to the CRH, leading to a rise in ACTH and cortisol levels. This can be used with the high-dose dexamethasone test to increase diagnostic accuracy.

Tests for cortisol deficiency

Dynamic tests to demonstrate cortisol deficiency, e.g., Addison disease, include:

Short synacthen test—Plasma cortisol level is measured and 0.25 mg of Synacthen (which has the same biological action as ACTH) is given IM or IV. Plasma cortisol level is remeasured

after 60 minutes. In normal patients, cortisol level will rise by a minimum of 200 nmol/L to at least 500 nmol/L. The response will be poor in hypoadrenalism of any cause.

Long synacthen test—In this test, 1 mg of Synacthen is given by IM injection daily for 3 days. Hypoadrenalism due to adrenal gland atrophy because of long-term steroid treatment or secondary hypoadrenalism shows a response to this level of stimulation. No response will be seen in adrenal hypofunction.

Corticotrophin-releasing hormone test—This can be used to look for secondary hypopituitarism. There will be a poor response to CRH administration.

Pituitary function tests

If suspecting hypopituitarism or pituitary failure, initial blood tests should include measurement of TSH, T_4, T_3, prolactin, GH, IGF-1, LH, FSH, testosterone and cortisol levels. Pituitary fossa imaging is then undertaken (e.g., CT/MRI or lateral skull X-ray). Dynamic tests are sometimes needed:

- Insulin tolerance test: this is used to assess ACTH or GH deficiency. A bolus of insulin is given to cause hypoglycaemia and stimulate ACTH and GH release. A baseline blood sample for measurement of GH, cortisol and glucose levels is taken. A fast-acting insulin is then given, and further blood samples are taken at intervals. Glucose level below 2.2 mmol/L must be achieved. Cortisol and GH levels should rise.

HINTS AND TIPS

The insulin tolerance test needs test needs to be conducted in a very controlled fashion in a safe environment because of the risk of severe hypoglycaemia requiring correction with intravenously administration of glucose. Consult local guidelines and always follow these.

MISCELLANEOUS ENDOCRINE CONDITIONS

Multiple endocrine neoplasia

There are two main syndromes, both autosomal dominant and both rare. Tumours originate from two or more endocrine glands that produce peptide hormones.

- 'MEN type 1' refers to a predisposition to benign parathyroid adenomas, pancreatic islet cell/gastrointestinal adenomas and pituitary adenomas. Individuals with MEN type 1 are also at higher risk of developing other tumours such as thymus, carcinoid and adrenal.

- 'MEN type 2a' refers to the association of phaeochromocytoma, medullary carcinoma of the thyroid and parathyroid adenoma or hyperplasia. In MEN type 2b there is phaeochromocytoma and medullary carcinoma of the thyroid, but no parathyroid adenoma or hyperplasia. There are developmental abnormalities with a Marfanoid habitus and intestinal and visceral ganglioneuromas. Family members should be screened.

HINTS AND TIPS

Multiple endocrine neoplasia (MEN) features commonly in examination questions.
- MEN type 1 is three *P*s (*p*ituitary, *p*arathyroid and *p*ancreas),
- MEN type 2 is two *C*s (*c*atecholamines (i.e., phaeochromocytoma) and medullary *c*arcinoma of the thyroid) and parathyroid (for MEN 2a) or mucocutaneous neuromas (for MEN 2b).

Autoimmune polyendocrine syndrome

Autoimmune polyendocrine syndrome (APS) type 1 is an autosomal recessively inherited disorder characterized by hypoparathyroidism, adrenal insufficiency and candidiasis. It usually becomes clinically apparent in the second decade. Hypogonadism and gastrointestinal malabsorption also occur frequently. APS type 2 is more common and primary adrenal insufficiency is its principal manifestation, along with autoimmune thyroid disease and type 1 DM. Around half of cases are inherited, but this may be in a dominant, recessive or polygenic manner.

Congenital adrenal hyperplasia

These inherited deficiencies of enzymes involved in glucocorticoid synthesis lead to deficiency of cortisol and aldosterone, increased ACTH production and increased synthesis of sex hormones. In children, this may present as failure to thrive, ambiguous genitalia in females and early virilization in males. It may present later with precocious puberty, or in early adulthood with hirsutism and oligomenorrhoea.

METABOLIC BONE DISEASE

Vitamin D metabolism is shown in Fig. 33.9.

Osteoporosis

Bone normally consists of 60% mineral and 40% matrix or organic matter. In osteoporosis the deposition of calcium salts occurs normally, but there is a loss of bone matrix and a reduction in bone mass per unit volume of anatomical bone. The WHO has defined osteoporosis as a BMD of 2.5 standard deviations or more below the mean value for a young adult (*T* score). Osteopenia is defined as a *T* score between −1.0 and −2.5.

The prevalence of osteoporosis in white women aged 50 to 59 years is 4%, and the prevalence in those aged 80 years or older is around 25%. Osteoporosis predisposes patients to fractures, commonly of the hip, vertebrae or wrist. It is estimated that almost 200,000 osteoporosis-related fractures occur in the United Kingdom each year. These are associated with considerable morbidity and mortality.

Aetiology

Primary osteoporosis

Involutional bone loss commences at age 35 to 45 years in both sexes but is accelerated in women following the loss of sex steroids at menopause, explaining the higher incidence in postmenopausal women. Age-related bone loss is increased by smoking, alcohol consumption, inactivity, low BMI and impaired vitamin D production. Family history is also relevant; ask about a parental history of hip fracture.

Secondary osteoporosis

Causes include steroid therapy, hypogonadism, alcohol abuse, hyperthyroidism, hyperparathyroidism, anticonvulsants and some chronic diseases such as inflammatory bowel disease and cystic fibrosis.

Clinical features

Osteoporosis does not cause pain (or other symptoms) until a fracture occurs. The risk of fracture is related to the BMD but also to conditions predisposing to falls (e.g., stroke, parkinsonism, dementia, visual impairment). These must also be assessed.

CLINICAL NOTES

In patients with clinical risk factors for osteoporosis, the risk of fracture can be predicted using the FRAX score or QFracture calculator. These scores are utilized to determine need for DEXA scan or to start treatment.

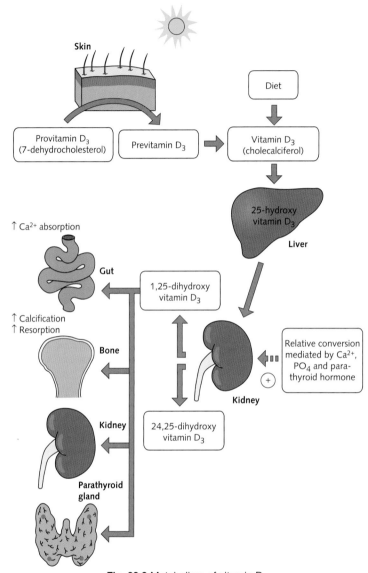

Fig. 33.9 Metabolism of vitamin D.

Investigations

- Blood tests: these results are normal with osteoporosis but look to identify treatable causes or rule out differential diagnosis (myeloma/osteomalacia), including a bone profile (calcium, phosphate, alkaline phosphatase), vitamin D level, PTH level, thyroid function tests, coeliac screen and serum electrophoresis. The results are normal with osteoporosis.
- BMD is estimated by DXA scan. There is no evidence to suggest any benefit of population-based screening. It is performed if there are risk factors and therapy is being considered (e.g., premature menopause, steroid therapy). It may also be done following a fragility (low trauma) fracture, an X-ray demonstrating osteopenia or for monitoring the effect of therapy. As well as the T score (see earlier), a Z score is calculated, which is an age-matched BMD score. The BMD of the vertebral body and femoral head is assessed.
- Thyroid function and LH, FSH and testosterone levels should be measured to exclude secondary causes. Fifty percent of males with hip fractures are hypogonadal.

Management

General principles

A holistic approach to the reduction of fracture risk is important. Fall risk should be assessed and interventions should be implemented. Alcohol excess, excess caffeine and smoking should be discouraged, and a good diet with regular weight-bearing activity should be encouraged. A diet adequate in calcium and vitamin D is essential, with a low threshold for supplementation.

Drug therapy use is guided by the FRAX or QFracture scoring systems. In general, for primary prevention treatment with a bisphosphonate will be commenced in postmenopausal women older than 65 years with confirmed osteoporosis. For secondary prevention (i.e., following an osteoporotic fracture), bisphosphonate therapy will be commenced in the postmenopausal woman regardless of age.

Drugs

Treatment options include bisphosphonates, strontium ranelate, denosumab, raloxifene (a selective oestrogen receptor modulator), calcitonin and intermittent PTH. Bisphosphonates are the first-choice therapy in most cases and are generally well tolerated. In patients who are unable to take them, strontium ranelate or denosumab is considered second-line therapy. Raloxifene may be considered for secondary prevention. Supplementation of calcium and vitamin D should be considered in all patients.

Patients taking steroids long term are particularly at risk, and a low threshold is needed for therapy.

PATIENT SAFETY

Be aware of side effects of bisphosphonates: severe dyspepsia, oesophageal erosion and the rare, but serious, complication of osteonecrosis of the jaw. Consider renal function in the choice of bisphosphonate.

Paget disease

In Paget disease there is uncontrolled bone turnover with areas of increased localized osteoclastic resorption. This is followed by disordered osteoblastic activity, leading to new bone formation that is structurally abnormal and weak (Fig. 33.10). The cause is unknown, although viruses have been implicated and genetic factors probably play a role. The highest prevalence is in the United Kingdom, United States, Australia and New Zealand, and is estimated to occur in 1% to 3% people older than 55 years.

Clinical features

The axial skeleton and femur are most commonly affected. The condition is most commonly asymptomatic, and is detected biochemically with a raised alkaline phosphatase level or by abnormal X-ray. Patients with symptoms complain of bone pain, tenderness and deformity such as an enlarged skull and bowed (sabre) tibia.

Complications include:

- Pathological fractures of long bones.
- Osteogenic sarcoma (patients need lifelong monitoring to screen them for this).
- Conductive deafness due to involvement of the ossicles.
- Progressive occlusion of the foramina of the skull, which can cause deafness due to eighth cranial nerve compression and visual impairment due to second nerve compression.
- Osteoarthritis of related joints.
- Rarely, high-output cardiac failure (with more than 20% skeletal involvement).

Investigations

Paget disease is generally diagnosed from raised serum alkaline phosphatase level (with normal calcium, phosphate and PTH levels) and X-ray abnormalities. There may be mild hypercalcaemia in immobile patients due to unopposed bone resorption.

X-rays of affected bones show a mosaic of osteolytic and sclerotic lesions, thickening of trabeculae and thick cortices with an enlarged irregular outline. Isotope bone scans will demonstrate the extent of skeletal involvement. A bone biopsy should be performed if malignant change is suspected.

Management

The objectives of treatment are control of pain and to treat active disease at a site where complications might occur. In addition to standard analgesia, the following treatments are given.

Bisphosphonates

Bisphosphonates are the mainstay of treatment (either orally, e.g., risedronate, or IV, e.g., zoledronic acid). They reduce bone turnover, reduce bone pain, promote healing of osteolytic lesions and restore normal bone histological features. Calcium deficiency and vitamin D deficiency need to be corrected before bisphosphonate therapy is started to avoid hypocalcaemia.

Calcitonin

Calcitonin is used as second-line therapy and is used only when bisphosphonates are not tolerated. It opposes many of the effects of PTH, and together with PTH regulates bone turnover and calcium balance. It has a risk of malignancy with long-term use.

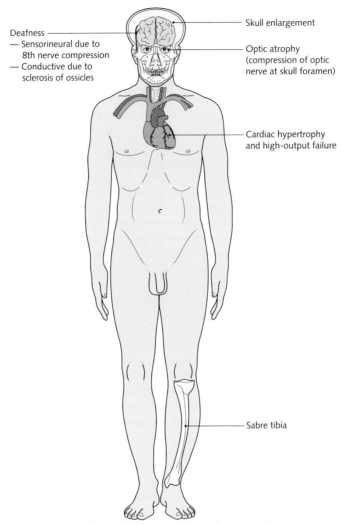

Deafness
— Sensorineural due to
  8th nerve compression
— Conductive due to
  sclerosis of ossicles

Skull enlargement

Optic atrophy
(compression of optic
nerve at skull foramen)

Cardiac hypertrophy
and high-output failure

Sabre tibia

Fig. 33.10 General features of Paget disease of the bone.

Surgery

Pathological fractures, bone deformity or nerve compression may require surgery. Bisphosphonates should be used preoperatively to try to reduce disease activity and reduce the risk of bleeding. Bone healing is often prolonged, and long rehabilitation is required.

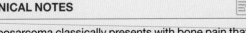

CLINICAL NOTES

Osteosarcoma classically presents with bone pain that is poorly responsive to medical treatment, local swelling and possibly a pathological fracture. Be on guard for this in your patient with Paget disease.

Osteomalacia

This disease occurs because of severe vitamin D deficiency. It results in inadequate mineralization of the bone matrix. If this occurs in adults (i.e., after fusion of the epiphyses has occurred), it is called 'osteomalacia'. If it occurs in children (i.e., during the period of bone growth before epiphyseal fusion), it gives rise to rickets.

Aetiology

The causes include factors that cause a low vitamin D level or cause low calcium/phosphate level. Vitamin D deficiency is most frequently caused by insufficient sunlight exposure and nutritional deficiency, but may be secondary to a wide range of other causes, for example:

- Intestinal malabsorption (e.g., gluten-sensitive enteropathy and postgastrectomy states) leading to reduced calcium and phosphate reabsorption.
- Vitamin D resistance: commonly this is due to ineffective conversion of 25-hydroxyvitamin D_3 to 1,25-dihydroxyvitamin D_3 in chronic renal disease. Inherited deficiency of renal 1α-hydroxylase and end-organ receptor abnormality are other causes.
- Drug induced: long-term anticonvulsant therapy may induce liver enzymes, leading to the breakdown of 25-hydroxyvitamin D_3.

Clinical features

Vitamin D deficiency is most commonly asymptomatic, so be suspicious. With osteomalacia, bone pain and tenderness are common. Fractures may occur, especially of the femoral neck. There is often a proximal myopathy, which may cause a waddling gait and difficulty in rising from a chair.

In rickets there are deformities of the legs (bow legs and knock knees), the chest (rachitic rosary) and the skull. There may also be features of hypocalcaemia (e.g., tetany); see Chapter 32.

Investigations

Biochemistry

Serum calcium, phosphate and magnesium levels: tend to be decreased but may be normal.

- Serum alkaline phosphatase activity: increased.
- Urinary calcium excretion: low.
- Vitamin D level (serum 25-hydroxyvitamin D) is most routinely measured; low.
- PTH level is generally high because of secondary hyperparathyroidism due to hypocalcaemia.

Imaging

Online X-rays of bone in rickets show cupped, ragged metaphyseal surfaces. In osteomalacia there is cortical bone loss and pseudofractures (Looser zones), which are small translucent bands perpendicular to the bone and extending inwards from the cortex. They are best seen on the lateral border of the scapula, on the femoral neck and in the pubic rami.

Isotope bone scans show a generalized diffuse increase in uptake of isotope.

Management

Dietary vitamin D deficiency can be prevented by taking an oral supplement of ergocalciferol daily. Vitamin D deficiency caused by intestinal malabsorption or chronic liver disease usually requires vitamin D in pharmacological doses, such as calciferol tablets daily. Calcium supplements may also be required, as may phosphate supplements in hypophosphataemic disease.

Hydroxylated vitamin D derivatives (alfacalcidol and calcitriol) should be used in patients with chronic renal impairment, as they are unable to hydroxylate vitamin D_3 to its active form.

> **CLINICAL NOTES**
>
> Ensure pregnant women and other high-risk groups (e.g., the elderly) are screened for vitamin D deficiency.

Renal osteodystrophy

The term 'renal osteodystrophy' is used to cover the various forms of bone disease that develop in chronic renal failure. These include:

- Delayed epiphyseal closure in children and young adults
- Rickets or osteomalacia
- Osteitis fibrosa cystica (brown tumours) due to secondary or tertiary hyperparathyroidism
- Generalized or localized osteosclerosis

The kidney does not excrete phosphate effectively as its function drops. This hyperphosphataemia stimulates PTH secretion. The impaired hydroxylation of 25-hydroxyvitamin D causes osteomalacia and hypocalcaemia, further stimulating the release of PTH (secondary hyperparathyroidism) and increasing osteoclast activity.

Management

Dietary phosphate intake is reduced, and oral phosphate binders are used to help control the hyperphosphataemia. Hydroxylated vitamin D supplements (e.g., alfacalcidol) are given to help normalize the calcium level and reduce the level of PTH further. If PTH is not suppressed, autonomous PTH production can result, causing tertiary hyperparathyroidism, which tends to require surgery (i.e., parathyroidectomy).

> **CLINICAL NOTES**
>
> In health, there is a balance between bone formation and reabsorption. If this natural turnover is underactive or overactive, the fracture rate increases. Parathyroid hormone level is used as a surrogate of bone turnover. The aim in renal osteodystrophy is to achieve a balance. See Chapter 30.

● Chapter Summary

- The prevalence of type 2 diabetes is dramatically increasing. Obesity is a major factor for this worldwide public health issue, which itself causes increased morbidity and mortality.
- Diabetes causes multiple organ dysfunction through microvascular and macrovascular changes. Type 2 diabetes may be controlled through diet and weight loss; generally hypoglycaemic agents and insulin therapy are required. Hypoglycaemic agents have multiple side effects, such as hypoglycaemia and weight gain.
- Type 1 diabetes is less common, is associated with other autoimmune diseases and typically presents earlier in life. These patients always require insulin. Insufficient insulin can result in ketone formation and lead to diabetic ketoacidosis, a medical emergency.
- Diabetic ketoacidosis is a triad of a raised glucose level, the presence of ketones and metabolic acidosis. Treatment involves aggressive fluid resuscitation and, following this, a fixed-rate intravenous insulin infusion. Attention needs to be paid to avoid hypokalaemia, and to identify and address the underlying precipitant.
- Hypoglycaemia (blood glucose level below 4 mmol/L) is another medical emergency. This is treated with orally administered carbohydrate, in the alert, conscious patient, otherwise with intravenously administered glucose or intramuscularly administered glucagon if there is no intravenous access.
- Bone is an active organ. Disorders of bone turnover can result in osteoporosis with loss of bone mass, osteomalacia with defective calcification or Paget disease with uncontrolled bone turnover. There is a close relationship between the parathyroid gland, vitamin D, calcium, phosphate and bone.
- Cortisol is produced from the adrenal gland. High levels of cortisol can lead to a Cushing syndrome. This is most commonly from exogenous glucocorticoid administration, and can lead to a Cushingoid appearance, with central adiposity, moon facies, proximal muscle wasting, easy bruising and skin thinning and can predispose to diabetes, hypertension and osteoporosis.
- Addison disease results in cortisol deficiency through primary adrenal failure. This condition can present as an Addisonian crisis. This can have nonspecific vague symptoms such as vomiting, nausea and abdominal pain. Signs include hypotension, hypothermia and increased pigmentation of skin and biochemically hypoglycaemia, hyponatraemia and hyperkalaemia may be present. Treatment is with hydrocortisone, with intravenous fluid resuscitation and by treating the underlying precipitant.
- Hypothyroid crisis (i.e., myxoedema coma) is another endocrine emergency. This can present with hypothermia, hypotension and reduced mental status. Treatment is with intravenous administration of thyroxine, intravenous fluid resuscitation, rewarming and identifying and treating the underlying precipitant. It is crucial to ensure that the patient has sufficient cortisol levels.
- Correcting thyroid function in the absence of sufficient cortisol levels can precipitate an Addisonian crisis.

● **Chapter Summary—cont'd**

UKMLA Conditions
Addison disease
Cushing syndrome
Diabetic eye disease
Diabetes in pregnancy
Diabetes insipidus
Diabetes mellitus type 1 and 2
Diabetic ketoacidosis
Diabetic nephropathy
Diabetic neuropathy
Hypercalcaemia of malignancy
Hyperlipidaemia
Hyperosmolar hyperglycaemic state
Hyperparathyroidism
Hyperthermia and hypothermia
Hypoglycaemia
Hypoparathyroidism
Hypothyroidism
Obesity
Osteomalacia
Osteoporosis
Pituitary tumours
Thyroid eye disease
Thyroid nodules
Thyrotoxicosis

UKMLA Presentations
Bone pain
Electrolyte abnormalities
Fatigue
Gradual change in or loss of vision
Gynaecomastia
Hoarseness and voice change
Menstrual problems
Nausea
Neck lump
Nipple discharge
Palpitations
Polydipsia
Weight gain
Weight loss

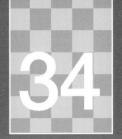
CEREBROVASCULAR DISEASE

Stroke and TIA

See Chapter 20.

Intracerebral haemorrhage

Intracerebral haemorrhage (ICH) is bleeding within the brain parenchyma or ventricular system. It is the cause of stroke in about 15% of cases. The signs and symptoms can differ but include headache, nausea, vomiting, neck stiffness, seizures, focal neurology and altered level of consciousness. Risk factors and causes are listed in Table 34.1. Management depends on the underlying cause. Patients receiving anticoagulants should have their effect reversed. For vitamin K antagonists, a combination of vitamin K and prothrombin complex concentrate is used. Idarucizumab is an antidote used to reverse the effect of dabigatran. Andexanet alfa reverses rivaroxaban and apixaban. Prothrombin complex concentrate can be used in cases associated with factor Xa inhibitor treatment. Protamine in heparin or low-molecular-weight heparin-induced bleeding. Systolic blood pressure should be 140 mmHg or lower within 1 hour of starting treatment and maintained for at least 7 days following the event unless early surgical intervention is planned, the patient has an underlying structural cause, the Glasgow Coma Scale score is below 6 or death is expected imminently.

Subarachnoid haemorrhage

Subarachnoid haemorrhage (SAH) is due to bleeding into the subarachnoid space (Fig. 34.1). It is the cause of acute stroke in 5% of cases. Around 85% of SAHs are due to rupture of an aneurysm in the circle of Willis and its adjacent branches (see Fig. 20.1); trauma, perimesencephalic vascular malformations, arteriovenous malformations, vasculitis or malignancy account for the remainder of cases.

The risk factors for aneurysm formation and rupture are summarized in Table 34.2.

Clinical features

The classic history is of a sudden onset severe headache that feels like a blow to the head or back of the neck. It is often referred to as a 'thunderclap headache'. Around 10% to 15% of significant SAHs are preceded by a prodromal less severe headache due to a small 'sentinel' haemorrhage. Severity is maximal at onset or in the following seconds. Associated signs and symptoms include neck stiffness, new confusion, blurred/double vision, altered consciousness, seizures, vomiting, hypertension and focal neurology.

On examination, there may be photophobia and features of meningism (see Chapter 16), although this usually takes about 6 hours to develop. There may be signs of raised intracranial pressure (ICP) or pressure effects on surrounding structures. Deficits appearing later may relate to vasospasm, rebleeding or hydrocephalus, and seizures may occur. Nonneurological complications include neurogenic pulmonary oedema, cardiac arrhythmia, cerebral salt wasting and the syndrome of inappropriate antidiuretic hormone secretion (SIADH).

Investigations

Computed tomography (CT) scanning is the investigation of choice for the detection of blood in the subarachnoid space; however, its sensitivity decreases with time from ictus. If CT findings are negative but the assessment is suggestive, lumbar puncture should be performed to detect xanthochromia (yellow discolouration of cerebrospinal fluid (CSF) due to the presence of bilirubin), which develops after approximately 12 hours and persists for several days. The gold standard investigation to identify a causative aneurysm is intraarterial angiography (digital subtraction angiography (DSA)). However, CT/magnetic resonance (MR) angiography is usually quicker and has fewer complications.

Management

Neurosurgical advice should be sought early. Up to one-sixth of patients rebleed, most within the first 8 hours. If untreated, the risk of rebleeding may be as high as 50% at 6 months. As such, occlusion of the aneurysm is the main aim of therapy unless neurosurgery is deemed of no benefit (e.g., damage is too extensive). Interventional treatment can be achieved by endovascular obliteration (coiling) or surgical clipping (requires craniotomy).

Nimodipine, a calcium channel blocker that acts preferentially on cerebral arteries, should be given at 60 mg every 4 hours or 30 mg every 2 hours to prevent vasospasm and cerebral ischaemia.

Subdural haemorrhage

Subdural haemorrhage (SDH) is the collection of blood in the subdural space (Fig. 34.3). Bleeding comes from torn bridging veins between the cortex and venous sinuses or damaged cortical artery. Head trauma and the associated rapid acceleration–deceleration force is the most common cause. SDH can be acute, subacute (3–7 days after injury) or chronic (2–3 weeks

Table 34.1 Risk factors and causes for ICH

Risk factors	Causes
Uncontrolled hypertension	Trauma
Age >55 years	Tumour
Male	Aneurysm rupture
Black ethnic group	Arteriovenous malformation
Previous stroke	Alcohol or drugs use
Anticoagulants	(especially cocaine and amphetamines)

Table 34.2 Risk factors for aneurysm formation

Risk factor
Hypertension
Family history of aneurysms
Age (>40 years)
Female
Black ethnic group
Smoking
Drug use (especially cocaine)
Linked genetic disorders (autosomal dominant polycystic kidney disease, Marfan syndrome, Ehlers–Danlos syndrome, fibromuscular dysplasia, neurofibromatosis type 1)

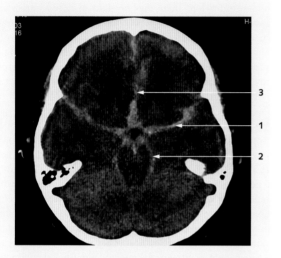

Fig. 34.1 Axial noncontrast CT brain with diffuse subarachnoid haemorrhage: Hyperdense acute haemorrhage in Sylvian fissures (*arrow 1*), basal cisterns (*arrow 2*) and interhemispheric fissure (*arrow 3*). (From Kelly B, Horton-Szar D, Bickle I. Crash Course: Imaging. Mosby Ltd.; 2007.)

after injury). SDH is more common in those with brain atrophy such as the elderly and people with alcoholism.

The signs and symptoms of SDH are often global and may develop insidiously. They include headache, confusion, personality change and a fluctuating level of consciousness (initially the patient appears well but as the haematoma develops, neurological deterioration occurs), focal neurology. Signs of raised ICP and secondary epilepsy.

A CT scan should show the haematoma (Fig. 34.4). As the clot breaks down, at around 7 days after the event it becomes transiently isodense to the brain, making it harder to identify on the scan. Neurosurgical advice should be sought. Some cases are managed conservatively, and small haematomas may resolve spontaneously. Neurosurgical intervention includes evacuation of the haematoma.

Extradural haemorrhage

Extradural haemorrhage (EDH) is a collection of blood in the potential space between the bone and the dura mater (Fig. 34.3).

It usually results from tearing of the middle meningeal artery or vein (or branches) following head injury. The classic picture is of a sudden brief loss of consciousness followed by a lucid interval. The signs and symptoms include headache, nausea, vomiting, reduced level of consciousness, seizure, focal neurology and signs of raised ICP. Skull X-rays may show bony abnormalities. Head CT shows a characteristic biconvex haematoma (Fig. 34.4). As for the management of SDH, neurosurgical input is required. Some cases may be treated conservatively. Surgical evacuation is recommended for any EDH with a volume greater than 30 cm^3.

HEADACHE

See Chapter 16 for the approach to a patient presenting with a headache. Specific types of headache are considered here.

> **COMMUNICATION**
>
> History taking is of paramount importance in patients reporting headache. Listen and allow the story to unfold. There may be hidden fears of an underlying tumour, stroke, etc.

Migraine

General overview

Migraine affects approximately 10% of the population and is more common in women than in men. About 80% of those who experience migraine have their first attack before the age of 30 years. It can be either episodic or chronic. Migraine can be classified into different types; the most common presentations are migraine with aura, migraine without aura and migraine aura without headache.

The mechanisms of migraine are not well understood. Human studies provide evidence that migraine aura is associated with a brief period of cortical hyperaemia followed by a

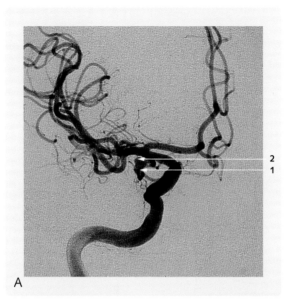

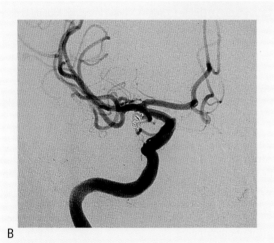

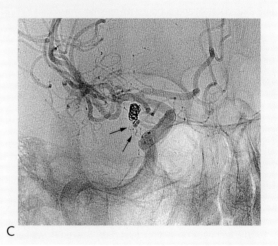

Fig. 34.2 Cerebral angiogram, intracerebral aneurysm (A) frontal view, right internal carotid artery, (B) aneurysm obliterated by coils (*arrow*), (C) same but unsubtracted image: Aneurysm in (A) arising at posterior communicating artery origin (*arrow 1*). Note rupture bleb (*arrow 2*). Coils in (B) and (C) clearly seen within the aneurysm (*arrows*). (From Kelly B, Horton-Szar D, Bickle I. Crash Course: Imaging. Mosby Ltd.; 2007.)

longer period of reduced blood flow. It is thought that this is linked to 'cortical spreading depression', a slowly expanding wave of depolarization followed by hyperpolarization. However, it is much debated as to whether this is the cause of the headache itself, which is thought to involve the activation of trigeminal nerve afferents from the dura and vascular structures, and the release of vasoactive neuropeptides.

The cerebral mechanism is responsive to mood, emotions, tiredness, relaxation, hormonal changes and peripheral stimuli (e.g., bright lights and noise). There is often a seasonal and/or diurnal pattern.

Clinical features

The frequency of headaches ranges from one to two per week to a few attacks scattered over a lifetime. Premonitory symptoms occur in 20% to 60% of those who experience migraine and may consist of yawning, euphoria, depression, irritability and food cravings.

In 25% of cases an aura is experienced before the headache. It is usually visual, consisting of teichopsia (flashes of light), scotomata and fortification spectra (zigzag lines). Objects may appear small (micropsia) or distorted (metamorphopsia). Paraesthesia or numbness that is usually unilateral can occur. In hemiplegic migraine hemiparesis sometimes dysphasia occurs.

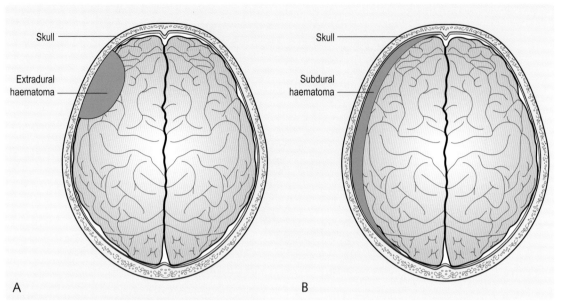

Fig. 34.3 Extradural (A) and subdural (B) haematoma. (From Kelly B, Horton-Szar D, Bickle I. Crash Course: Imaging. Mosby Ltd.; 2007.)

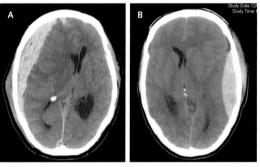

Fig. 34.4 (A) A subdural haematoma, which is concave in appearance. (B) An acute extradural haematoma. Note the characteristic biconvex collection. (Courtesy Steven Powell and Alex Roberts, Royal Liverpool University Hospital.)

The headache is severe and commonly unilateral (but can be bilateral). It is classically throbbing or pulsating. Commonly associated features include nausea and vomiting, photophobia and phonophobia. The headache is usually worse with movement. Migraine with aura is a risk factor for stroke.

Management

Identify and avoid precipitating factors. These can include stress, bright lights, loud noise, certain foods (cocoa, cheese, citrus fruits and alcohol), dehydration and sleep deprivation.

Acute attacks should be treated as early as possible. Simple analgesia (e.g., aspirin, nonsteroidal antiinflammatories or paracetamol) can be combined with a tryptan (see later). Antiemetics such as domperidone, metoclopramide or prochlorperazine can be added. If oral analgesics are not tolerated, an effective alternative is diclofenac suppositories.

Triptans (5-hydroxytryptamine receptor 1B/1D agonists), which inhibit the release of vasoactive neuropeptides, can be administered orally, intranasally or subcutaneously, and should be taken during the headache phase of migraine. Contraindications include coronary artery disease, cerebrovascular disease, coronary vasospasm or uncontrolled hypertension.

NICE does not recommend ergots and opioids for the treatment of migraine.

In certain patients, for instance those where attacks cause frequent disability, preventative treatment should be offered. Topiramate and propranolol are first-line drugs. Acupuncture and riboflavin (usually 400 mg once a day) are alternatives. The effectiveness and need for continuing therapy should be reviewed 6 months after the start of treatment.

Cluster headache

Cluster headache is the most common of the trigeminal autonomic cephalalgias (see later), and is more common in men than in women. Attacks usually start in adulthood. Headaches are unilateral and of agonizing severity around the eye or temple, and often occur at night. Attacks last from 15 minutes to several hours, up to eight times per day, and continue for around 2 weeks to 3 months. Total remission usually follows, and lasts until the next cluster, normally a year or two later.

The pain may radiate to the face, jaw, neck and shoulder. Autonomic symptoms are prominent: the eye may water and become red, the nostrils may run or feel blocked and there may be sweating. Miosis and ptosis are common and, in some patients, may persist permanently. Attacks can be precipitated by vasodilators (e.g., alcohol, nitrites and calcium channel blockers).

Acute attacks can be alleviated by high-flow oxygen and a subcutaneous or nasal triptan. Verapamil may be used to prevent attacks.

CLINICAL NOTES

TRIGEMINAL AUTONOMIC CEPHALALGIAS

Other than cluster headache trigeminal autonomic cephalalgias include paroxysmal hemicrania and short-lasting, unilateral, neuralgiform headache with conjunctival injection and tearing (SUNCT) syndrome, which also have prominent autonomic features.

Tension-type headache

Tension-type headache is the most common type of primary headache, and may be episodic or chronic. It is more common in women. The classic presentation is of intermittent bilateral attacks of diffuse tightness, and pressure or heaviness over the vertex, or in the neck or occiput, lasting from 30 minutes. Headache is not associated with other symptoms. The headache may be relieved by simple analgesia. Chronic tension-type headache may evolve from the episodic form, and simple analgesia is often of limited use when this occurs. The condition must be distinguished from medication-overuse headache (see Chapter 16).

Idiopathic intracranial hypertension

Raised ICP without hydrocephalus or a mass lesion, also known as 'pseudotumour cerebri'. Strictly speaking, this is not a headache syndrome, but it is an important cause of headache. It is thought to be related to impaired reabsorption of CSF from the subarachnoid space. Many medications have been associated with the condition, notably tetracyclines, levothyroxine, corticosteroids and vitamin A. It occurs mainly in overweight young women. Common symptoms include headache, visual disturbance and pulsatile tinnitus. There is often marked papilloedema, which, if long-standing, can lead to optic atrophy and infarction of the optic nerve, causing blindness.

RED FLAG

IDIOPATHIC INTRACRANIAL HYPERTENSION AND RISK OF BLINDNESS
In fulminant disease risk of blindness is high and patients must have their visual acuity recorded and be examined for the presence of papilloedema. Therapeutic lumbar puncture to release the pressure on the optic nerve can be vision saving.

MRI or CT may show a flattened sclera and an empty sella turcica. For the diagnosis to be made, other causes of raised ICP must be excluded. Lumbar puncture shows raised CSF pressure but normal composition. The mainstays of treatment are weight loss, acetazolamide and other diuretics; therapeutic lumbar punctures may be needed in certain patients. In resistant cases, or if visual acuity deteriorates, a CSF diversion utilizing lumboperitoneal or ventriculoperitoneal shunts may be necessary.

Trigeminal neuralgia

Trigeminal neuralgia is one of the most common causes of facial pain. It is thought to result from trigeminal nerve compression by an artery, vein, tumour or bone. It is more common in the elderly and women. It is unilateral in 97% of patients, and consists of paroxysms of stabbing extreme pain in the distribution of one or more branches of the trigeminal nerve. Maxillary and mandibular branches are the most commonly affected. Pain is often electric shock-like. It may be brought on by touching a specific trigger zone, and is thus provoked by factors such as eating, shaving or talking. If motor or sensory deficits are present, consider underlying structural disease (e.g., multiple sclerosis (MS), atriovenous malformation or cerebellopontine angle tumour). If left untreated, the condition usually progresses, with shorter periods of remission.

Carbamazepine is the first-line treatment. If carbamazepine is inappropriate, ineffective or not tolerated, a referral to a specialist pain service/relevant clinical speciality should be considered before any other medication is started.

CLINICAL NOTES

NEURALGIAS

Neuralgias other than trigeminal include glossopharyngeal neuralgia, precipitated by swallowing, and auriculotemporal neuralgia. Postherpetic neuralgia occurs in patients with previous herpes zoster (see Chapter 38).

Persistent idiopathic facial pain (atypical facial pain)

This refers to episodes of prolonged facial pain for which no cause can be found, and is therefore a diagnosis of exclusion. It is more common in women and may be preceded by facial surgery or injury. It is associated with depression and may respond to tricyclic antidepressants.

DEMENTIA

The approach to the confused patient and the differential diagnosis of dementia is covered in Chapter 19. Dementia is a syndrome of the progressive and irreversible decline of brain functioning not entirely attributable to normal ageing. The range of symptoms is broad and includes memory and cognitive impairment, psychiatric and behavioural disturbances and inability to perform activities of daily living. Disease onset before the age of 65 years is termed early-onset dementia. Dementia can result from several brain disorders. Many types have been identified (Fig. 34.5 and Table 34.3). Management is mainly supportive. Although research is being conducted to identify compounds that could aid treatment, no drugs have so far been effective in reversing or stopping the progression of the disorder.

For a more in-depth discussion of the topic, see *Crash Course: Neurology.*

EPILEPSY

General overview

Epilepsy refers to a group of conditions in which paroxysms of abnormal electrical activity of cerebral neurones result in recurring seizures. The incidence is estimated to be 4 to 10 per 1000. Antiepileptic drugs (AEDs) are used to control the disorder; satisfactory control is achieved in about two-thirds of patients. Flashing lights, exercise, strong emotions and hyperventilation (and subsequently alkalosis) can all trigger seizures in patients with epilepsy. The seizure threshold is also lowered by fever, certain medications, menstruation, lack of sleep and pregnancy.

> **RED FLAG**
>
> Do not confuse a single acute seizure with epilepsy and exclude the possible provoking factors (see Aetiology) in patients presenting with an isolated episode. The risk of developing epilepsy following a single seizure is about 3%.

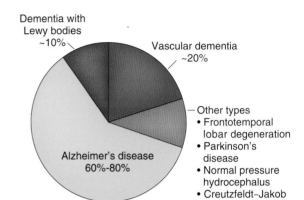

Fig. 34.5 Causes of dementia. (From Harding MM, et al. *Lewis's Medical-Surgical Nursing: Assessment and Management of Clinical Problems*, 12th ed. Elsevier; 2023.)

Table 34.3 Different types of dementia

Type of dementia	Clinical features
Alzheimer's disease	Short-term memory and episodic memory loss Loss of executive function Nominal dysphasia
Vascular dementia (multiinfarct dementia)	Stepwise deterioration in cognitive function Focal neurological signs Evidence of cerebrovascular disease
Dementia with Lewy bodies	Fluctuating course One or more motor symptoms of parkinsonism (rigidity, tremor, bradykinesia) Visual hallucinations Transient disturbances of consciousness
Frontotemporal dementia	Personality change Behavioural disturbance (e.g., sexual disinhibition, tactlessness, emotional blunting) Relative preservation of other cognitive functions

Classification

In 2017 the International League Against Epilepsy published an epilepsy classification (Fig. 34.6). This describes seizure type, followed by epilepsy type, followed by epilepsy syndrome.

Seizures can be of focal, generalized or unknown onset:

- Focal seizures arise in a single hemisphere and may be motor (e.g., atonic, clonic, hyperkinetic, myoclonic) or

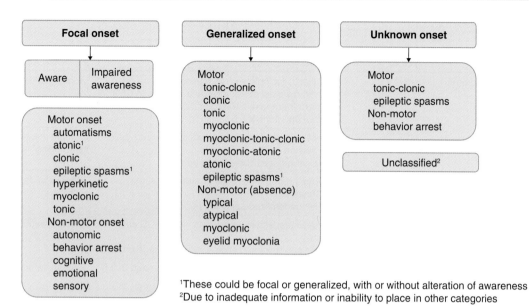

¹These could be focal or generalized, with or without alteration of awareness
²Due to inadequate information or inability to place in other categories

Fig. 34.6 International League Against Epilepsy Classification of Seizures. (From Goldman L, Schafer AI. *Goldman-Cecil Medicine*, 2-Volume Set, 26th ed. Elsevier; 2020.)

nonmotor in onset (e.g., autonomic, cognitive, sensory), with retained or impaired awareness.

- Generalized onset seizures arise in bilaterally located cortical and/or subcortical neuronal pathways and can be motor (tonic–clonic or other) or nonmotor (absence) in type.
- Seizures of unknown onset can be motor or nonmotor in type. They can also remain unclassified because of a lack of information, or an inability to classify them according to the type above.

Epilepsy can also be combined focal and generalized.

A seizure may be preceded by prodrome lasting hours to days where a change in mood or behaviour is present. This is not part of the seizure, unlike an aura (see later).

Some common syndromes are outlined in Table 34.4. A patient with epilepsy syndrome may experience several different types of seizures.

HINTS AND TIPS

Focal onset seizures may evolve to become bilateral tonic–clonic seizures.

Focal onset seizures

Focal onset seizures can be preceded by an aura. Aura reflects the initial seizure discharge; it can be sensory (any of the five senses can be affected) or experiential (involves higher functions, e.g., affect, memory). Abdominal aura, a rising feeling in the upper abdomen, is common. Gustatory and olfactory hallucinations are usually unpleasant.

CLINICAL NOTES

Other auras include a sense of 'Jamais Vu' a sudden feeling of unfamiliarity while the patient is in their environment and 'déjà vu' a vivid sense of familiarity with the current situation.

Normal awareness

Awareness is unimpaired, and these attacks are characterized by focal activity related to the site of abnormal neuronal stimulation. This may be motor, sensory (including special senses), autonomic (e.g., sweating, vomiting) or affecting higher consciousness. In motor seizures, the affected limb may experience a short-lived weakness after the attack (Todd paresis).

Impaired awareness

These seizures are often derived from the temporal lobes, but any part of the brain can be the origin. Hippocampal sclerosis may be present.

When awareness is lost, the patient may still appear awake, and automatisms may occur: semi-purposeful, stereotyped,

Table 34.4 Some of the common epilepsy syndromes

Epilepsy syndrome	Age of onset (years)	Features	First-line AEDs
Lennox–Gastaut syndrome	3–5	Generalized, multiple seizure types ≤2 Hz diffuse slow spike and wave pattern on EEG with intermittent fast (≥10 Hz) activity during sleep Cognitive impairment	Sodium valproate
Juvenile absence epilepsy	9–13	Absence seizures with occasional generalized tonic–clonic seizure 3–5-Hz generalized spike-wave on EEG	Sodium valproate, lamotrigine
Childhood absence epilepsy	4–10	Absences predominate, loss of awareness, may be many times/day 2.5–4-Hz generalized spike-wave on EEG	Ethosuximide, sodium valproate
Juvenile myoclonic epilepsy	10–24	Myoclonus (especially on awakening), GTCS and absences 3–5.5-Hz polyspike and spike-wave discharge on EEG	Sodium valproate
Genetic tonic-clonic seizures alone epilepsies	10–25	GTCS within 2 hours if awakening, generalized 3–5.5-Hz spike-wave or polyspike-wave on EEG	Sodium valproate

AED, *Antiepileptic drug;* EEG, *electroencephalogram;* GTCS, *generalized tonic–clonic seizures.*

repetitive movements such as lip smacking or picking at clothing. An abnormal posture may be adopted because of dystonia. The patient cannot remember these events after the attack.

Focal evolving to bilateral convulsive seizures

Initial focal involvement spreads widely, causing a generalized seizure.

Generalized onset seizures

Tonic–clonic seizures

Sudden onset seizure with loss of consciousness; initial generalized stiffening is followed by rhythmic muscular contractions (jerking). Teeth are clenched; cyanosis may occur. The patient is often drowsy and confused with a possible headache or amnesia following the event (postictal phenomena). Patients may describe a prodrome.

HINTS AND TIPS

Faecal (as opposed to urinary) incontinence and biting at the side of the tongue (as opposed to the tip) are helpful pointers toward the diagnosis of a seizure. This is because urinary incontinence can also be present in other causes of loss of consciousness such as syncope, whereas the side of the tongue biting is highly specific to generalized tonic–clonic seizures.

When a seizure becomes generalized it is generally associated with loss of consciousness.

Absence seizures

These often start in childhood. There are brief interruptions of consciousness, sometimes accompanied by rhythmical blinking of the eyelids (eyelid myoclonia). To an observer, the child may appear to be dazed or daydreaming. Recovery is immediate, and there are no sequelae. Electroencephalogram (EEG) shows generalized spike-wave activity (Fig. 34.7).

Myoclonic seizures

Sudden, brief, involuntary jerk-like movements occur. The patient often remains aware throughout. EEG shows polyspikes (Fig. 34.7).

Atonic or akinetic seizures

Sudden onset of loss of muscle tone.

COMMUNICATION

Take time to discuss and explain this condition to patients. They will often feel stigmatized by the diagnosis, and their concerns and worries need to be addressed.

Aetiology

Most seizures are idiopathic although it is increasingly understood that genetic disorders underlie a significant number of epilepsy syndromes. Structural causes, such as congenital

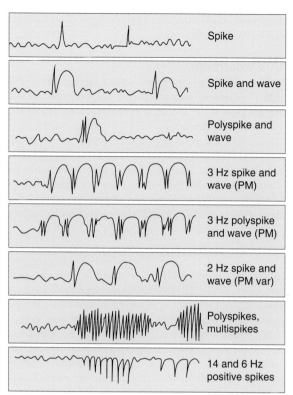

⟋ Spike	Spike
	Spike and wave
	Polyspike and wave
	3 Hz spike and wave (PM)
	3 Hz polyspike and wave (PM)
	2 Hz spike and wave (PM var)
	Polyspikes, multispikes
	14 and 6 Hz positive spikes

Fig. 34.7 EEG waveforms of epilepsy. *PM*, Petit mal (absence seizures). (From Khurana I, Khurana A. *Medical Physiology for Undergraduate Students*, 2nd ed. Elsevier; 2018.)

malformations or acquired lesions (stroke, space-occupying lesion, brain abscess, trauma), are also common. Other causes include:

- Metabolic: hypoxia, hyperglycaemia, hypoglycaemia, hypocalcaemia, uraemia, hyponatraemia, hypernatraemia, liver failure, pyridoxine deficiency, porphyria, aminoacidopathies.
- Infectious: tuberculosis, cerebral malaria, HIV, syphilis;
- genetic: both inherited or noninherited (e.g., Dravet syndrome).
- Immune: anti-NMDA receptor encephalitis, anti-LG11 encephalitis, acute disseminated encephalomyelitis;
- Drugs and toxins: alcohol (including alcohol withdrawal), lead, both prescription and recreational drugs (e.g., phenothiazines, monoamine oxidase inhibitors, tricyclic antidepressants, amphetamines, benzodiazepine withdrawal).
- Neurodegenerative disorders: Alzheimer's disease, Creutzfeldt–Jakob disease.
- Hypertension: in hypertensive encephalopathy.

HINTS AND TIPS

Reflex anoxic seizures following a faint are common, especially if the patient remains in an upright posture.

Investigations

Bedside

The diagnosis is clinical, and a good eyewitness account of the seizures is vital. Enquire what happened before, during and after the attack. Ask specifically for symptoms of aura or any potential triggers. Ask about the seizure itself (onset, duration, features). Blood tests including full blood count, urea and electrolytes, calcium and magnesium, liver function tests and glucose, should be performed. An arterial blood sample taken during or just after the seizure will often show metabolic acidosis with raised lactate, which will normalize rapidly after cessation of the seizure. It may be necessary to screen blood and urine for drugs/toxins. An ECG should be performed.

Imaging

Neuroimaging such as CT or MRI helps identify structural abnormalities that can cause seizures and should be offered if these are suspected. MRI is the modality of choice. It is especially important when epilepsy develops in adulthood or the very young (<2 years), for focal seizures and if first-line AEDs are not successful. Neuroimaging is not recommended in idiopathic generalized epilepsy or self-limited epilepsy.

Electroencephalogram

EEG is performed only to support the diagnosis and further identify the type of epilepsy, as 10% to 15% of the general population may have an abnormal EEG and approximately 15% of people with epilepsy never have specific epileptiform discharges. If a standard EEG is normal, a sleep EEG can be considered.

Genetic testing

This should be guided by a neurologist or geneticist.

Management

Patients should be referred for an assessment within 2 weeks following the first suspected seizure. Offer information about how to recognize further seizures, provide first aid, what to do to reduce the risk of having another episode and whom to contact for support. They should be informed not to drive until further assessment, and to refrain from high-risk activities such as climbing ladders and bathing unsupervised

Drug treatment

AEDs should be prescribed individually, at the lowest dose possible to obtain complete seizure control with minimum side effects. Use monotherapy where possible. If first-line single-drug treatment is unsuccessful, try another drug before adding a second agent. Approximately 20% of patients need more than one drug for acceptable control. Partial epilepsy is more likely to be refractory. After a drug has been chosen, the dose is gradually increased until control is achieved, the maximum dose is reached or toxic effects supervene. Treatment is first instituted according to the specific epilepsy syndrome; if this is not clear, it is started according to the seizure type. Sodium valproate is the drug of choice in generalized and unclassifiable epilepsies and lamotrigine in focal epilepsies. Buccally administered midazolam or rectally administered diazepam for use in the community is prescribed for patients with a history of prolonged or serial convulsive seizures. If treatment with a new drug is commenced, it is introduced and the dose is increased gradually while the use of the old drug is withdrawn slowly.

First-line drugs

Focal onset seizures—Levetiracetam and lamotrigine are the first-line therapies. Carbamazepine or oxcarbazepine can be offered as second-line monotherapy. Carbamazepine may cause central nervous system (CNS) side effects (e.g., dizziness, nausea, headaches and drowsiness), which may be avoided by a slow increase of the dose.

Generalized onset seizures—Sodium valproate is recommended as the first-line treatment. Lamotrigine or levetiracetam are second-line options. Lamotrigine, carbamazepine, gabapentin, phenytoin and pregabalin may exacerbate myoclonic or absence seizures. Common unwanted effects of sodium valproate include weight gain, hair thinning and tremor.

Absence seizures—Ethosuximide is the first-line treatment and sodium valproate second-line; if these are contraindicated, lamotrigine or levetiracetam can be used.

Myoclonic seizures—Sodium valproate is the first-line treatment; if contraindicated, levetiracetam or topiramate can be used.

Discontinuing drugs

Most patients are seizure-free within a few years of starting therapy, and 60% remain so after drug withdrawal. Therefore drug discontinuation is considered in some patients after a period of therapy if they have been seizure-free for at least 2 years. Assess patients' individualized risk of treatment termination. Withdrawal should be achieved over a period of at least 2 to 3 months, one medication at a time. Factors that increase the risk of seizure recurrence include abnormal EEG, abnormalities

on neurological examination or certain types of epilepsy (e.g., juvenile myoclonic epilepsy).

Other treatment

Resective surgery is sometimes needed for refractory, drug-resistant epilepsy. It is most effective for focal onset seizures when the focus of the abnormal electrical activity can be accurately localized and resected.

Behavioural and psychological interventions can be tried. A ketonic diet (high fat, moderate protein, low carbohydrate) diet may be considered in children and young adults when seizure control is difficult. Cognitive behavioural therapy or relaxation may be tried as adjuvant therapy. Vagus nerve stimulation can be used in patients who are refractory to AEDs and not suitable for surgery.

Convulsive status epilepticus

This is a medical emergency and is defined as prolonged generalized onset seizures lasting more than 5 minutes, or repeated seizures without intervening recovery of awareness. The clear majority of seizures are tonic–clonic in motor type. Both the risk of permanent brain damage and mortality are related to the length of the attack, and therefore seizures must be stopped as soon as possible. The most common causes include poor epilepsy control, metabolic abnormalities, alcohol excess or withdrawal, illicit drugs, stroke and hypoxia.

The ABCDE approach should be used initially:

- Secure the airway and administer high-flow oxygen.
- Lay the patient in the recovery position if the cervical spine has been cleared and the seizure type will permit it; remove false teeth.
- Gain intravenous (IV) access and take blood samples for arterial blood gas measurements, full blood count, urea and electrolytes, liver function tests, calcium, magnesium and clotting. Consider checking anticonvulsant levels if appropriate.
- Consider doing a toxicology screen and blood/urine cultures.
- Check capillary glucose level.
- Treat hypoglycaemia for example with 75 mL of IV 20% glucose over 10 to 15 minutes.
- Administer lorazepam IV (0.1 mg/kg) if IV access is available; rectal diazepam and buccally midazolam are alternatives.
- If seizures continue after two doses of a benzodiazepine second-line treatment is given (this can differ between hospitals but includes phenytoin, levetiracetam or sodium valproate).
- Third-line options if seizures persist are phenobarbital or general anaesthesia.
- After the seizure, investigations typically include chest X-ray, ECG, EEG, neuroimaging and lumbar puncture.

Pregnancy and epilepsy

There are several important issues to be considered for epileptic women of childbearing age. All women on AEDs planning a pregnancy or pregnant should be offered folic acid (5 mg once a day). AEDs such as carbamazepine, phenytoin and topiramate reduce the efficacy of hormonal contraceptives while the effectiveness of lamotrigine is impaired by oestrogen-containing medications. Several AEDs are teratogenic and can cause congenital malformations, neurodevelopmental impairments and foetal growth restriction, sodium valproate being the most dangerous one and contraindicated unless the patient is on a pregnancy prevention programme. Levetiracetam and lamotrigine are considered safest. Breastfeeding is encouraged in most cases.

COMMUNICATION

Counsel the patient about the effect of pregnancy on the mother's seizures and the risk to the foetus from maternal fits. Epileptic patients who are planning a pregnancy or pregnant should have a medications review to ensure the best possible and least risky drug regime is used to achieve seizure control.

Driving and epilepsy

Current regulations state that after a single unprovoked seizure with loss of consciousness, the patient must not drive for 6 months. If a diagnosis of epilepsy is made, the patient must be seizure-free for at least 1 year before driving can be recommended. Longer periods are necessary for drivers of large commercial vehicles.

Sudden unexpected death in epilepsy

Patients with epilepsy are at higher risk of sudden death, termed 'sudden unexpected death in epilepsy' (SUDEP). Certain features, mainly related to the severity of epilepsy (seizure frequency, disease duration) place patients at higher risk. Patients should be informed and counselled regarding SUDEP.

INTRACRANIAL TUMOURS

General overview

These can be primary or secondary. Primary brain tumours originate in the brain, whereas secondary brain tumours are cancers that have spread to the brain from somewhere else in the body (metastases). Primary brain, other CNS and intracranial tumours account for around 3% of all new cancer cases in

Table 34.5 The origins of brain tumours

Site	Example of tumour derived
Glia	Astrocytomas (including glioblastomas), oligodendrogliomas, ependymomas
Meninges	Meningiomas
Blood vessels	Angiomas, angioblastomas
Schwann cells of the cranial nerves	Acoustic neuromas
Pituitary gland	Craniopharyngioma
Lymphocytes	Primary CNS lymphoma

CNS, *Central nervous system.*

the UK. The incidence of these is rising, and it is estimated it will reach 22 per 100,000 by 2035 from 13 per 100,000 in 2011. Most benign neoplasms occur in the meninges, whereas most malignant tumours are in the brain tissue. Because of their location and threat to health, they are often classified as low-grade (slow-growing) or high-grade (rapidly growing and aggressive) tumours rather than benign or malignant. Certain familial conditions, such as neurofibromatosis, tuberous sclerosis, von Hippel–Lindau disease and Li–Fraumeni syndrome predispose to the development of primary brain tumours. Secondary intracerebral tumours are the most common, and occur in up to 30% of cancers; the main primary sites include the lung, breast, kidney, stomach, colon and rectum, skin, ovary, prostate and thyroid. The main types of primary brain cancers are shown in Table 34.5. More than 130 different types of brain, CNS and intracranial tumours have been identified. Astrocytomas are the most common and account for almost 35% of cases. Meningiomas are the second most common type (21%). The overall 1-year survival rate for patients with primary intracerebral tumours is 40%.

Clinical features

Symptoms depend on the location and rate of growth of the tumour but arise from the direct effects of the mass on surrounding structures, from raised ICP (see Chapter 16) and from the provocation of seizures. Similar symptoms may be produced by any mass lesion (e.g., haematomas, aneurysms, abscesses, tuberculomas, granulomas and cysts).

Direct effects depend on the site of the tumour:

- Frontal lobe: personality changes, social disinhibition, emotional instability and impairment of intellectual function. There may be anosmia, contralateral hemiparesis or expressive aphasia (Broca area).
- Parietal lobe: extinction phenomenon, contralateral homonymous field defects and hemisensory loss. There may be apraxia, agnosia and dysphasia/aphasia if the dominant

hemisphere is affected. Signs include 'parietal drift' or falling off the outstretched contralateral arm, astereognosis (inability to recognize an object placed in the hand) and sensory inattention.

- Temporal lobe: problems with memory, comprehension and emotion. Contralateral superior visual field defects, complex hallucinations. There may be receptive aphasia (Wernicke aphasia, anomic aphasia), and word agnosia if the dominant hemisphere is affected.
- Occipital lobe: homonymous hemianopia, visual hallucinations.
- Cerebellopontine angle: vertigo and progressive ipsilateral perceptive deafness (cranial nerve VIII), numbness of the ipsilateral side of the face (cranial nerve V), facial weakness (cranial nerve VII) and ipsilateral cerebellar signs.

Investigations

Generally, diagnosis relies on neuroimaging. MRI provides more detailed images than CT. More advanced techniques such as positron emission tomography, single photon emission CT, MR spectroscopy, MR angiography or imaging using labelled amino acid analogues may provide additional information about the extent and grade of the tumour; this is particularly useful in planning surgery. If metastases are suspected, investigations for the primary neoplasm should be performed. If a primary intracranial tumour is suspected, stereotactic biopsy provides a definitive diagnosis of the type and grade of the tumour. It will also rule out other causes, such as an abscess or inflammatory lesions, which may be difficult to differentiate on imaging.

Management

Initial management is of the complications arising from the physical presence of the tumour: corticosteroids for cerebral oedema and anticonvulsants for seizures.

Further treatment depends on the type and grade of the tumour. Surgical resection is preferred if possible. External beam radiotherapy can be curative and can be the treatment of choice for secondary tumours. Whole-brain radiotherapy or involved-field radiotherapy (normal brain tissue exposed to smaller amounts of radiation) is used for some types of tumours, including medulloblastomas, oligodendrogliomas and glioblastomas. In stereotactic radiosurgery, high-intensity radiation is delivered to a small target area reducing exposure of healthy tissue. In patients not suitable for surgery or radiosurgery, whole-brain radiotherapy is the only treatment option. Chemotherapy is used for CNS lymphomas. The benefits are limited for other types of tumours but it is used as an adjunct to surgery and radiotherapy and in palliative care.

A watch-and-wait policy is sometimes adopted for small, indolent tumours such as low-grade meningiomas.

CLINICAL NOTES

COMPLICATIONS OF INTRACRANIAL TUMOURS

- Hydrocephalus as a result of CSF flow obstruction. If left untreated it creates a mass effect on brain tissue eventually leading to brain herniation (where the brain is squeezed down through the openings in the skull) and compression of brainstem centres causing respiratory and cardiovascular instability (Fig. 34.8).
- Haemorrhage into the tumour.
- Complications of chemotherapy, radiotherapy (subacute encephalopathy, impaired cognitive function) and surgery.

MOVEMENT DISORDERS

Parkinson's disease

Parkinsonism is a syndrome of tremor at rest, rigidity, bradykinesia and later, postural instability; it has several causes. The differential diagnosis is detailed in Table 34.6. This section will focus on Parkinson's disease (PD), which is the idiopathic syndrome of parkinsonism.

First described by James Parkinson's in 1817, PD is due to degeneration primarily affecting dopaminergic neurones of the zona compacta of the substantia nigra. Eosinophilic inclusion bodies (Lewy bodies) are characteristic pathological features of this chronic, progressive neurodegenerative disorder. PD is thought to arise as a result of genetic and environmental factors; however, the exact cause is unknown.

The incidence increases with age and is estimated at 33.4 per 100,000 person-years. It is more common in males. PD is associated with reduced life expectancy and increased risk of dementia.

COMMUNICATION

It is essential to have a holistic approach to the care of patients and their carers in chronic conditions such as Parkinson's disease. As such, a multidisciplinary approach, involving geriatricians, Parkinson's disease specialists, GPs, hospital and community nursing staff, pharmacists, physiotherapists, occupational therapists and speech and language therapists should be instituted. This hopefully culminates in the formation of a supportive therapeutic alliance.

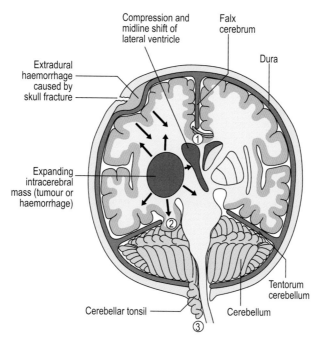

Compression and midline shift of lateral ventricle

Falx cerebrum

Dura

Extradural haemorrhage caused by skull fracture

Expanding intracerebral mass (tumour or haemorrhage)

Tentorum cerebellum

Cerebellar tonsil

Cerebellum

1. Subfalcine herniation.   3. Tonsillar herniation.
2. Uncal herniation.

Fig. 34.8 Schematic showing the neuroanatomical basis for brain herniation syndromes. An increase in the volume of the contents in the skull, such as a brain tumour or intracranial bleed, can cause brain tissue to be displaced at one of the three sites shown. (From Michael-Titus AT, Shortland PJ. *The Nervous System: Basic Science and Clinical Conditions*, 3rd ed. Elsevier; 2023.)

Table 34.6 Differential diagnosis of parkinsonism

Differential diagnosis		Suggestive features
Idiopathic Parkinson's disease		Asymmetry of onset, not ascribable to other cause
Parkinson's plus syndromes	Progressive supranuclear palsy	Supranuclear ophthalmoplegia, pseudobulbar palsy, postural instability, cognitive impairment. Rigidity and bradykinesia are symmetrical in onset
	Multisystem atrophy	Autonomic dysfunction, parkinsonism, cerebellar or pyramidal involvement. Symmetrical in onset
	Dementia with Lewy bodies	Dementia preceding or simultaneous to movement disorder
	Corticobasal degeneration	Disorder of movement and higher-order functions (apraxia, cognitive impairment). Difficult to diagnose without neuropathological examination
Drug-induced parkinsonism	Neuroleptics, antiemetics, antipsychotics, antidepressants, MPTP, lithium, calcium channel blockers, cholinesterase inhibitors, amiodarone, cinnarizine, sodium valproate, methyldopa, pethidine	Relieved by removal of causative agent
Vascular parkinsonism		History of vascular disease, evidence on CT scan
Metabolic disorders	Wilson disease, neuroacanthocytosis	Young age at onset, features on laboratory investigation
Post infectious	Encephalitis lethargica	Preceding episode of illness
Toxic	Heavy metals, carbon monoxide	Known history of exposure, often occupational

MPTP, *1-Methyl-4-phenyl-1,2,3,6-tetrahydropyridine.*

Table 34.7 Nonmotor complications of Parkinson's disease

Mental health	• Depression, anxiety, apathy • Dementia with visual hallucinations and delusions and frequent fluctuations with lucidity • Cognitive impairment
Autonomic dysfunction	• Postural hypotension • Constipation • Urinary dysfunction • Sexual dysfunction • Excessive salivation • Dysphagia
Other	• Weight loss • Reduced or absent sense of smell (anosmia) • Pain • Sensory disturbance • Sleep disorders • Fatigue

Clinical features

Early in the progression of PD, the patient may report fatigue, muscular discomfort or restlessness. Fine movements may be difficult. Onset is unilateral, becoming bilateral after months or years, although severity may remain asymmetric for the duration of the disease. Muscle power and tendon reflexes are usually normal. See Table 34.7 for nonmotor complications of PD.

HINTS AND TIPS

Bradykinesia or hypokinesia (poverty of movements) with one of: rigidity, tremor or postural instability (not resultant from another condition) are required for the diagnosis of PD.

Tremor

Initially, this is intermittent and may appear only when the patient is tired. The frequency of the tremor is 4 to 6 Hz and the tremor is most marked at rest (whereas a cerebellar tremor is more marked on intention). It often improves with movement and with mental concentration. There is a 'pill rolling' movement of the thumb over the index finger. Lips, chin and jaw can also be affected.

Rigidity

There is resistance to passive movement, which may be smooth throughout its range ('lead pipe' rigidity). When combined with tremor and increased tone, resistance to passive movement is jerky and intermittent and is termed 'cogwheel' rigidity. Rigidity likely contributes to the features of stooped posture and reduced arm swing that are commonly seen in PD (Fig. 34.9).

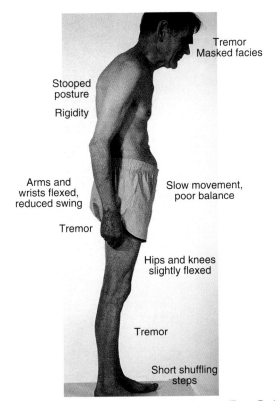

Fig. 34.9 Stooped posture of Parkinson's disease. (From Perkin DG, et al. *Mosby's color atlas and text of neurology.* 2nd ed. London: Mosby; 2002.)

Bradykinesia

Bradykinesia means difficulty in initiating movements. Dexterity is often affected first, and it may be difficult for the patient to rise from a chair. Impairment of fine movement can manifest as difficulty with buttoning clothes or opening jars. Writing becomes small (micrographia), spidery and cramped. Repeated movements show slowing and reduced amplitude. The face is expressionless and mask-like, the frequency of spontaneous blinking reduces and the voice is monotonous and unmodulated. There is reduced arm swing while walking and a shuffling, festinant gait with unsteadiness on turning (gait freezing may occur).

HINTS AND TIPS

To examine a patient for bradykinesia, ask the patient to unbutton and button his or her shirt.

Postural instability

Postural instability occurs late in the disease and results in a significant risk of falls and serious injury. Bone health should be monitored.

CLINICAL NOTES

DIAGNOSING PARKINSON'S DISEASE

The diagnosis of Parkinson's disease is clinical. Investigations help exclude other causes such as metabolic disorders or structural lesions.

Management

The disease is treated symptomatically. Physiotherapy can improve gait and help build confidence. Physical aids such as high chairs and rails may help with daily activities. Patients should have access to occupational therapy and speech and language therapy. Patient and carer information, education and support are very important.

Drug therapy

Drug therapy aims to correct the neurochemical imbalance. This may greatly improve the quality of life but does not prevent the progression of the disease; 10% to 20% of patients are unresponsive to pharmacological treatment.

Treatment is started at low doses and increased in small increments. Common side effects include motor (more frequent in young patients; loss of drug effect, motor fluctuations, dyskinesia) and neuropsychiatric complications (more frequent in older patients).

First-line treatments

Levodopa—Levodopa (L-DOPA) is the first-line treatment and most effective agent in PD. It is usually offered to patients in the early stages of the disease. It acts by replenishing depleted striatal dopamine which helps reduce bradykinesia and rigidity more than tremor. It is administered with a peripheral dopa decarboxylase inhibitor (e.g., benserazide or carbidopa), which prevents the peripheral breakdown of L-DOPA to dopamine but, unlike L-DOPA, does not cross the blood–brain barrier; decreased peripheral levels of dopamine reduce peripheral side effects such as nausea, vomiting and cardiovascular effects. The most commonly used preparations include co-beneldopa and co-careldopa. Late complications of L-DOPA use include sudden unpredictable swings of the 'on–off' syndrome, dyskinesia and 'end-of-dose' deterioration (the duration of benefit after each dose becomes progressively shorter).

Dopamine agonists—These act at the endogenous neuroreceptor, and are effective in treating motor features of the disease. Dopamine agonists are less effective than L-DOPA.

The most common side effects are nausea due to stimulation of the area postrema in the medulla (which can be alleviated with domperidone) and dyskinesias. Impulsive behaviour such as gambling, overeating and hypersexuality can also occur. Drugs in this group include rotigotine, pramipexole, ropinirole and apomorphine (given subcutaneously). Ergot-derived dopamine agonists (cabergoline, bromocriptine, pergolide) can cause cardiac fibrosis and are not to be used first-line.

Monoamine oxidase-B (MAO-B) inhibitors—Selegiline, rasagiline and safinamide inhibit the breakdown of dopamine and offer modest symptom control with fewer adverse effects. They are licensed as first-line therapy but are more often used as an adjunct.

Adjuvant treatments

Catechol O-methyltransferase (COMT) inhibitors—These reduce the peripheral breakdown of L-DOPA and thus reduce the fluctuation in plasma levels and prolong the benefit from each dose. Entacapone is an example.

Anticholinergics—Examples include benzhexol and procyclidine. Tremor and rigidity are reduced more than akinesia. They are best avoided in the elderly because of their side effects.

Amantadine—Mechanism of action includes dopamine agonism and nicotinic and NMDA antagonism. It reduces bradykinesia and rigidity more than tremor. It may be helpful in the late stages of the disease as an adjunct.

Other therapy

Surgery to alter brain regions affected by PD (subthalamotomy, thalamotomy or pallidotomy) may be considered in patients with poor response to medication/intolerable side effects, or those with severe fluctuations in response to drugs (on–off syndrome). This may involve the destruction of parts of these nuclei or the implantation of electrodes to enable electrical stimulation (thalamic, pallidal or subthalamic deep brain stimulation).

RED FLAG

Patients with PD should always receive their medication. If the oral route is unavailable due to concurrent illness or other causes, alternatives should be instituted. These include subcutaneous patches/infusions or nasogastric/intragastrointestinal delivery systems. Seek help from the neurology and pharmacy teams.

Tremor

A tremor is defined as a rhythmic oscillatory movement of a body part, most commonly the hands. It results from the contraction of opposing muscle groups and may be a sign or a symptom of the underlying disease. In the evaluation of a tremor, important points to consider are the frequency and amplitude, when it is present or most pronounced (at rest, on action or in fixed posture), how disabling it is and whether the patient has symptoms or signs suggestive of a clear underlying disorder. The differential diagnoses of tremor are summarized in Table 34.8.

Essential tremor

This is the most common type of tremor. Often family history is present. Onset can be at any age. Usually, it is bilateral and symmetrical of variable amplitude and rapid frequency (4–12 Hz). The hands are most commonly affected (but the head, trunk or legs can be involved). It is a postural tremor that is maintained on movement and can be severely disabling. It does not occur during sleep. Classically it is alleviated by alcohol, but this is an inadvisable treatment. Caffeine, stress and sleep deprivation exacerbate symptoms. Some patients will respond to β-blockers (propranolol). Botulinum toxin injections can help treat head tremor. In severe intractable cases, thalamotomy or deep brain stimulation is sometimes used.

Cerebellar tremor

This is classically a coarse low-frequency (<5 Hz) intention tremor. The amplitude increases as the movement approaches its endpoint. The tremor is usually perpendicular to the direction of movement. It is caused by dysfunction of the cerebellum or its outflow. Other features of cerebellar disease may be present (see Chapter 21).

Huntington disease

This is an autosomal dominant inherited disorder caused by an abnormal expansion (>35 repeats) of a normal repetitive cytosine–guanine–thymine (CAG) sequence at the start of the gene on chromosome band 4p16.3 which encodes the protein huntingtin. The mutation causes a progressive neurodegenerative disease characterized by chorea (irregular, involuntary, 'dance-like' movement), dystonia, behavioural problems and cognitive decline. It usually starts in middle age, although earlier onset and more severe disease may be seen with successive generations: this is termed 'anticipation'. Generally, patients survive for about 20 years after the onset of symptoms. Neuroleptics, benzodiazepines or tetrabenazine (dopamine-depleting drug) may help control chorea, but there is no disease-modifying or curative treatment.

Sydenham chorea

This is a neurological manifestation that occurs weeks to months after group A beta-haemolytic streptococcus infection and is one of the features of acute rheumatic fever. Clinical features include involuntary movements, hypotonia and weakness. It is usually self-limiting.

Other movement disorders

For a description of dystonias, tics, myoclonus and akathisia, see *Crash Course: Neurology*.

MULTIPLE SCLEROSIS

General overview

MS is an autoimmune, inflammatory, demyelinating disorder. It is the most common nontraumatic cause of neurological disability in people ≤40 years old in the UK. The prevalence of MS differs worldwide. Females are much more commonly affected. The cause of the disease is unclear. It is thought that environmental factors trigger the condition in genetically predisposed

Table 34.8 Causes of tremor

Type	Features	Causes
Resting	Seen when patient is relaxed with hands at rest	Parkinsonism
Postural	Seen when the muscles are working against gravity when, e.g., hands are held outstretched	Essential tremor
		Anxiety
		Thyrotoxicosis
		Physiological tremor – often enhanced by beta-2-agonists
Intention (also known as 'cerebellar tremor')	Seen during voluntary active movement, when, e.g., patients try to touch the examiner's finger with their finger	Cerebellar disease Midbrain lesions

individuals. Abnormal immune response to viral infections (e.g., Epstein–Barr virus) has been suggested as one of the possible causes. MS is typically diagnosed between the ages of 20 and 50 with the relapsing/remitting pattern of the disease more common in the younger group. There is no cure for the disease and the prognosis is variable.

Pathogenesis

The hallmark of MS is the presence of multiple lesions in the CNS disseminated in location and time. Inflammation, demyelination, gliosis (scarring) and axonal loss all play a role (Fig. 34.10). It is thought that the disease is started by self-reactive lymphocytes which invade the CNS, causing blood–brain barrier disruption and areas of inflammation and demyelination. Over time, repeated insults lead to sustained activation of microglia (resident macrophages of the CNS), which results in axonal loss. Sites of predilection include the optic nerve, spinal cord, periventricular areas and brainstem.

Clinical features

There is a wide spectrum of disease activity, and the course of the condition is extremely variable. It is divided into the following subtypes:

- Relapsing–remitting MS is present in 85% of patients. Here, symptom-free periods are followed by relapse. A small number of patients experience progression between relapses ('relapsing progressive' MS).
- Secondary progressive MS: Two-thirds of all relapsing–remitting patients will enter a 'secondary progressive' phase with a gradual accumulation of symptoms unrelated to relapses.
- Primary progressive MS: progressive disease from the outset. This occurs in about 10%–15% of patients.

Common presentations include optic neuritis, transverse myelitis, symptoms referable to the brainstem (diplopia) and cerebellum (ataxia, and progressive difficulties with balance) or ascending sensory disturbance and/or weakness (see Table 34.9 for other complications of MS).

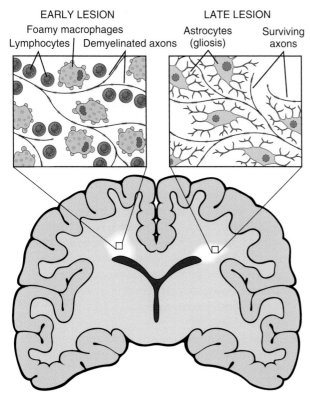

Fig. 34.10 Multiple sclerosis. Early lesions contain demyelinated axons surrounded by lymphocytes and foamy macrophages. Late lesions – that is, fully formed demyelinated plaques – consist of demyelinated axons and astrocytes. (From Damjanov I, Perry AM, Perry KD. *Pathology for the Health Professions*, 6th ed. Elsevier; 2022.)

Table 34.9 Complications of MS

Complication	Features
Eye symptoms	• Optic neuritis (see text) • Diplopia (caused by brainstem lesions of cranial nerves III, IV and/or VI) • Oscillopsia
Sensory symptoms	*See text*
Motor symptoms	• Fatigue • Spasticity • Ataxia • Tremor • Reduced mobility • Upper motor neurone signs
Cerebellar signs	• Nystagmus, incoordination, tremor, dysdiadochokinesia, titubation (continuous rhythmical tremor of the head and trunk), dysarthria
Cognitive impairment	• Impaired memory, sustained concentration and abstract conceptual reasoning
Psychiatric abnormalities	• Depression and anxiety, emotional liability
Pain	• Neuropathic or musculoskeletal pain • Trigeminal neuralgia is 300× more common in MS
Autonomic symptoms	• Urinary frequency, urgency, incontinence • Constipation or faecal incontinence • Sexual dysfunction • Thermoregulatory dysfunction

MS, *Multiple sclerosis.*

The progression of MS is very variable and depends on the pattern of the disease. The relapsing–remitting type has a better prognosis. One-quarter of patients have a nondisabling form of the disease.

Optic neuritis

This is a common initial presentation in MS. Optic neuritis presents as unilateral eye pain (often exacerbated by eye movement) and/or loss or reduction of vision. Central vision is usually more severely affected, with scotomata developing, but complete uniocular blindness may occur. The optic nerve head appears normal unless the lesion is very anterior, when the disc may be swollen. In 90% of patients, vision improves over a few months, but colour vision may be permanently affected. Transient blurring of vision lasting minutes, associated with exercise or raised body temperature, may occur (an example of Uhthoff phenomenon – worsening of symptoms with increased temperature). Following an episode of optic neuritis, optic atrophy may ensue with pallor of the disc on funduscopic examination. The risk of MS following optic neuritis depends on whether lesions are present on MRI.

Transverse myelitis

Bilateral inflammation of a section of the spinal cord. Can present with a variety of neurological signs and symptoms depending on the level of the lesion. Typically develops over hours or days.

Sensory symptoms

Ascending sensory symptoms are very common. Paraesthesia and dysaesthesia (altered sensation), diminished proprioception and vibration sense, and reduced pain and light touch sensation may all be present. The distribution differs; it can be limited to the extremities, patchy over the limbs and trunk or present in an 'evolving sensory level' pattern. Flexion of the neck may lead to an electric shock sensation in the back and limbs (Lhermitte sign), which is associated with a lesion in the cervical cord.

> **HINTS AND TIPS**
>
> Cerebellar lesions can be remembered with the mnemonic DASHING: *d*ysdiadochokinesia, *a*taxia, *s*peech abnormalities (fluctuating, slurring), *h*ypotonic reflexes, *i*ntention tremor, *n*ystagmus and *g*ait abnormalities.

Investigations

The diagnosis of MS is made by a consultant neurologist based on established criteria, such as the revised 2017 McDonald criteria (see Further Reading). There must be evidence of lesions disseminated in space and time. MRI is used to support the diagnosis. Alternative diagnoses should be excluded (see clinical notes: differential diagnosis of multiple sclerosis).

> **CLINICAL NOTES**
>
> **DIFFERENTIAL DIAGNOSIS OF MULTIPLE SCLEROSIS**
>
> - Inflammatory conditions: primary angiitis of the central nervous system, systemic lupus erythematosus (SLE), primary Sjögren syndrome, Behçet disease and polyarteritis nodosa (PAN), and in children acute disseminated encephalomyelitis.
> - Infectious diseases: Lyme disease, brucellosis, tuberculosis, human T-lymphotropic virus type 1-associated myelopathy, HIV infection, tertiary syphilis, tropical spastic paraparesis.
> - Granulomatous disorders: sarcoidosis and granulomatosis with polyangiitis.
> - Metabolic diseases: vitamin B_{12} deficiency (classically dorsal column abnormalities), diabetic peripheral neuropathy, hypocalcaemia, copper deficiency, zinc toxicity, adult-onset leucodystrophies.
> - Other: neuromyelitis optica (previously known as 'Devic disease') involves extensive demyelination of the spinal cord and optic nerve and is more common in African and Asian populations. Familial conditions include adrenoleucodystrophy and cerebral autosomal dominant arteriopathy with subcortical infarcts and leucoencephalopathy (CADASIL).
>
> The following investigations are important in a patient with MS:
> - MRI head and spinal cord shows lesions in the vast majority of patients with clinically definite disease.
> - The CSF shows lymphocytosis and moderately raised protein levels. Oligoclonal bands of immunoglobulin G (IgG) isolated to the CSF are seen in 90% of patients with clinically definite MS but are not specific for MS.
> - Delay in the visually evoked potentials can signify early demyelination in otherwise asymptomatic patients. Delays may also occur in auditory or somatosensory evoked potentials depending on the site of the lesions.
> - Antibodies to myelin proteins may be present but are of no diagnostic use. Antibodies to aquaporin 4 are 98% specific for neuromyelitis optica.

Management

Treatment of MS has two aims: symptom management and disease modification. A short course of high-dose steroids effectively reduces the duration of acute relapses but does not alter the course of the disease and should be used sparingly to limit side effects.

Symptomatic treatment is of great importance. Physiotherapy and occupational therapy maintain maximum function. Fatigue can be reduced with amantadine, modafinil or selective serotonin reuptake inhibitors. Spasticity may respond to baclofen and/or gabapentin. Amitriptyline can be used to manage emotional lability. Bladder symptoms can be managed with convene drains, pads or intermittent self-catheterization. Anticholinergic agents (e.g., oxybutynin) may reduce urinary frequency. In men with erectile dysfunction, sildenafil may be helpful.

Several disease-modifying agents have shown promise in reducing the frequency of relapses and lesions on MRI. However, whether this translates into a reduction in the accumulation of disability and a delay in disease progression is unclear. Beta interferons, peginterferon beta-1a and glatiramer acetate remain the most commonly used disease-modifying therapy for relapsing-remitting disease. Interferon beta-1b and siponimod (antiinflammatory and neuroprotective actions) are recommended for secondary progressive disease. Fingolimod (immunomodulator) is recommended for treatment if no improvement is observed despite beta interferon therapy. Alemtuzumab (monoclonal antibody that mediates the death of B and T cells) is recommended for the treatment of highly active relapsing-remitting disease. Teriflunomide and daclizumab are alternatives. Antiinflammatory dimethyl fumarate and immunosuppressant ofatumumab and ponesimod can be used in active relapsing–remitting disease. Ocrelizumab for primary progressive disease. Natalizumab (monoclonal antibody against α_4 integrin) is reserved for patients with rapidly evolving relapsing–remitting disease because of the severe side-effect profile, including progressive multifocal leucoencephalopathy. Several other agents are being assessed in clinical trials.

CLINICAL NOTES

Pregnancy reduces the frequency of relapses, however, 25% of postpartum patients have a relapse within 3 months of delivery.

HINTS AND TIPS

Live vaccinations may be contraindicated in patients treated with disease-modifying drugs.

CENTRAL NERVOUS SYSTEM INFECTION

Meningitis

General overview
Meningitis is inflammation of the meninges. It may be caused by:

- Infection: bacteria, viruses, fungi, parasites.
- Malignant cells.
- Blood (e.g., following SAH).
- Inflammatory conditions: sarcoidosis, SLE, vasculitis.
- Air, drugs or contrast media during encephalography.

The term meningitis is usually reserved for infection of the meninges by organisms. Viral meningitis is the most common cause; however, the disease is usually mild and self-limiting. Bacterial meningitis is a life-threatening condition that is associated with high morbidity and mortality. This section will focus on bacterial meningitis.

Causative organisms
The causative organism is likely to differ with the patient's age:

- In neonates (children younger than 28 days): *Streptococcus agalactiae* (group B streptococcus), *Escherichia coli*, *Streptococcus pneumoniae* and *Listeria monocytogenes*.
- In children: meningococcus (*Neisseria meningitidis*), *S. pneumonia*, *Haemophilus influenzae* type b.
- In young adults: *S. pneumoniae*, *H influenzae* type b, meningococcus, streptococci, staphylococci, gram-negative bacilli.
- In older adults: as for young adults but prone to *S. pneumoniae*.
- In immunocompromised patients and the elderly: prone to pneumococcus, *Listeria*, gram-negative organisms, *Cryptococcus*, *Mycobacterium tuberculosis*.

Vaccination against *H. influenzae* type b, serogroup B and C meningococcus and some types of pneumococcus have reduced the incidence of infections significantly.

Clinical features

Meningism
The features of meningism include headache, neck stiffness, back rigidity, photophobia and headache. Kernig sign (Fig. 34.11) (i.e., pain and resistance on passively extending the knee with the hips fully flexed) or Brudzinski sign (head flexion elicits hip flexion) may be positive.

Infection
High temperature is typical. The patient may describe malaise and arthralgia. Any rash may occur, although a petechial/purpuric rash is strongly suggestive of meningococcal disease. Rigors, tachycardia and hypotension may occur.

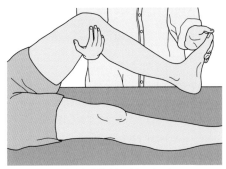

Fig. 34.11 Eliciting Kernig sign.

In tuberculous meningitis, symptoms may initially be non-specific with malaise, anorexia, headache and mild pyrexia. Symptoms may persist for days. There may be personality changes and intermittent dulling of consciousness.

Raised intracranial pressure

Headache, vomiting, altered mental state and seizures may all occur. Bradycardia with hypertension (Cushing reflex) can occur.

INVESTIGATIONS

HINTS AND TIPS

Do not delay therapy in favour of completing investigations in suspected meningitis.

- Blood: full blood count, urea and electrolytes, C-reactive protein, glucose, coagulation screen, blood cultures, whole-blood polymerase chain reaction (PCR) for *Neisseria meningitides*, arterial blood gas.
- Lumbar puncture: performed urgently once raised intracranial pressure has been excluded. Cerebrospinal fluid (CSF) is sent for Gram stain, Ziehl–Neelsen stain (for tuberculosis), culture, microbiology, sensitivity testing, cytology, virology, glucose measurement, protein measurement, rapid antigen screen for PCR and occasionally India ink stain for cryptococci. CSF changes in meningitis are summarized in Table 34.10 (see also Chapter 21).

Management

When meningitis is suspected, antimicrobials should be administered immediately. If a lumbar puncture can be performed

quickly, it may be possible to obtain a sample of CSF first, but this should not delay the administration of antibiotics.

In an out-of-hospital setting, give benzylpenicillin intra-muscularly/IV. Hospital treatment is usually empirical initially (consult local policy) (e.g., IV ceftriaxone for patients younger than 50 years and IV ceftriaxone and amoxicillin (to cover *Listeria*) in patients older than 50 years). IV acyclovir should also be given if a viral cause is suspected. Targeted therapy is started once the causative organism is known.

Supportive measures include analgesia, antiemetics, IV fluids and nutritional support. Manage any complications, including seizures, disseminated intravascular coagulation and pericardial effusion. If meningitic signs predominate, or bacterial meningitis is suspected or confirmed, give corticosteroids as soon as possible. It is also indicated in tuberculous meningitis. It should be avoided in known meningococcal disease and immunocompromised states.

COMMUNICATION

Meningitis is a notifiable disease, and cases must be reported to the Department of Health and Social Care. Prophylactic antibiotics are recommended for close contacts of the index case.

Encephalitis

This is inflammation of the brain parenchyma. There is usually some inflammation of the meninges in encephalitis and conversely some inflammation of the parenchyma in meningitis.

Viruses are the most common cause of encephalitis, with herpes simplex virus being the main pathogen. Bacteria (e.g., *Listeria*, *Mycobacterium tuberculosis*), fungi (e.g., cryptococcosis), parasites (e.g., toxoplasmosis, especially in the immunocompromised; schistosomiasis), toxins or autoimmune disorders can also lead to the condition.

The classic triad of acute encephalitis is altered mental state, headache and fever, but most patients present with features of meningitis (see earlier).

CLINICAL NOTES

The likely causative pathogen can be suggested by knowledge of local epidemics, typical radiological features (such as temporal lobe swelling in herpes

Table 34.10 Changes in the cerebrospinal fluid in meningitis

	Normal	Viral	Bacterial	Tuberculous
Appearance	Clear	Clear/turbid	Turbid	Turbid/fibrinous
Predominant cell	<5 mononuclear cells per mL	10–100 mononuclear cells per mL	200–3000 polymorphs per mL	10–300 mononuclear cells per mL 0–300 polymorphs per mL
Protein (g/L)	0.2–0.4	0.4–0.8	0.5–5	0.5–5
Glucose	More than two-thirds of the plasma level	More than two-thirds of the plasma level	Less than two-thirds of the plasma level	Less than two-thirds of the plasma level

simplex virus (HSV) encephalitis), EEG findings (periodic complexes in HSV encephalitis) CSF picture and demonstration of viruses in the CSF by serology or PCR.

HSV encephalitis is treatable and therefore, in suspected encephalitis, acyclovir is given empirically until virology results guide more specific therapy.

CLINICAL NOTES

The differential diagnosis of a ring-enhancing lesion on brain CT/MRI

- brain abscess
- toxoplasmosis
- tuberculoma
- aspergilloma
- neurocysticercosis

Subacute sclerosing panencephalitis is a late complication of measles that develops, on average, 6 to 15 years after the primary infection. The condition has very high morbidity and mortality, and there is currently no cure.

Brain abscess

This can occur via direct spread from, for example, mastoiditis or sinusitis, or from a remote region of infection such as endocarditis or chronic suppurative lung disease. Haematogenous spread often leads to multiple abscesses. There is a wide range of possible causative organisms, particularly in the immunocompromised patient, including aerobic and anaerobic bacteria, fungi, protozoa and helminths. Abscesses are often polymicrobial.

Presentation is most commonly with headache, fever, altered mental status and focal neurological signs. Features of meningitis or encephalitis may be present depending on the extent of the inflammation. MRI or CT scan with contrast enhancement will show a ring-enhancing lesion (Fig. 34.12). Treatment will require an extended course of IV antibiotics, the choice of which depends on the suspected source and identity of the organism. Surgical aspiration may be required.

SPINAL CORD DISORDERS

Spinal cord compression

Spinal cord compression is a medical emergency. The causes are summarized in Table 34.11. Symptoms include local or radicular pain, often precipitated by movement or straining, spastic paraparesis with upper motor neurone (UMN) signs (hyperreflexia, clonus, Babinski sign) below the level of the lesion and lower motor neurone (LMN) signs (hyporeflexia, muscle atrophy) at the level of the lesion, sensory loss with a characteristic 'sensory level', autonomic dysfunction (paralytic ileus, priapism) and sphincter disturbances. Injuries above C3, C4 and C5 lead to phrenic nerve paralysis and diaphragmatic dysfunction with respiratory compromise.

It is important to note that there is a discrepancy between the level of the root lesion and that of the sensory level and spastic paraparesis. This arises because the spinal cord is shorter than the spinal column (it ends at the level of L1–L2 vertebrae in the adult) and, below the cervical spine the nerve roots travel inferiorly before exiting through the vertebral foramina. For instance, a lesion at the level of the T10 cord segment may be at the T9 vertebra level and hence cause T9 root symptoms but a T10 sensory level. Compression of the cauda equina (the descending lumbar and sacral nerve

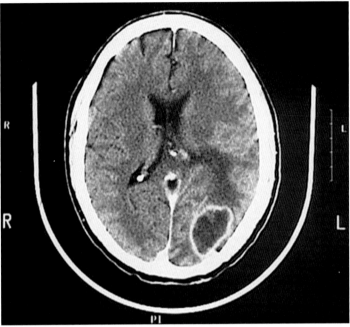

Fig. 34.12 Cerebral abscess, CT image This abscess of the left occipital lobe displays prominent 'ring enhancement' with a bright border owing to the surrounding highly vascular granulation tissue that contains many small vessels at the periphery of the abscess. Most of these cases result from staphylococcal or streptococcal infections. In addition to being destructive of brain tissue, an abscess is a mass lesion, often with surrounding oedema, that can increase ICP and cause herniation. (From Klatt EC. *Robbins and Cotran Atlas of Pathology*, 2nd ed. Elsevier; 2010.)

Table 34.11 Causes of spinal cord compression

Cause	Example
Vertebral (extradural)	Collapsed vertebrae, e.g., metastatic cancer (bronchus, breast, thyroid, kidney, prostate), osteoporosis, myeloma
	Trauma
	Spondylosis with disc prolapse
	Pott disease (tuberculosis)
	Paget disease
	Abscess
	Reticuloses
Intradural, extramedullary	Meningioma, haematoma (subdural, epidural)
	Neurofibroma
Intramedullary	Glioma, infection

roots below the level of the L2 vertebra) causes root pain and LMN pattern weakness in the legs, with saddle anaesthesia (numbness of buttocks and perineum) and sphincter disturbances. If suspected, MRI is required to visualize the spinal cord. This must be done urgently as early intervention may prevent irreversible damage. Neurosurgical opinion should be sought. Investigations should also include those of the underlying cause.

Treatment is by decompression. Radiotherapy may be useful in malignant disease. If the patient has a known or suspected malignancy, corticosteroids to reduce tissue oedema should be given.

> **RED FLAG**
>
> In a patient presenting with inability to weight bear and new bladder or bowel incontinence or saddle anaesthesia spinal cord compression should be suspected and managed urgently to minimalize potential damage.

Subacute combined degeneration of the cord

Subacute combined degeneration of the cord is also known as 'Lichtheim disease'. This is most commonly due to vitamin B_{12} deficiency and refers to patchy demyelination of the posterior and lateral columns. Vitamin E and copper deficiencies can result in similar conditions. It is associated with pernicious anaemia. The onset is usually insidious and associated with sensory peripheral neuropathy.

Clinical features include:

- Posterior columns: loss of vibration and joint position sense, and positive Romberg sign.
- Lateral corticospinal tract: weakness, hypertonia and extensor plantars.
- Peripheral neuropathy: absent knee jerks and reduced touch sensation.

Treatment is with intramuscular vitamin B_{12} injections.

Syringomyelia and syringobulbia

Syringomyelia is due to a longitudinal cyst (syrinx) usually in the central cervical spinal cord. As it enlarges it may extend into the dorsal horns and white matter, compressing the dorsal horn neurones and corticospinal and spinothalamic tracts, respectively.

Clinical features are insidious and include:

- Dissociated loss of pain and temperature sensation over the upper limbs, shoulders and trunk in a 'cape-like' distribution (Fig. 34.13). If the lesion is lower down legs are affected over the upper body. With the progressive enlargement of the cyst and involvement of other sensory tracts, light touch, vibration and proprioception can be affected.
- Loss of tendon reflexes, muscle weakness and wasting occur. Hands are affected first. The deficit spreads proximally as the syrinx extends. This reflects the involvement of the LMNs of the dorsal horn.

As the syrinx expands, it may lead to spastic paraplegia with UMN signs. Insidious loss of normal sensation may lead to joint destruction (Charcot joints) or injury. Treatment is by surgical decompression or aspiration.

If the syrinx extends into the medulla of the brainstem, this is called syringobulbia, and may affect cranial nerves, causing the following symptoms:

- Cranial nerve V: facial pain or sensory loss.
- Cranial nerve VIII: vertigo and nystagmus.
- Cranial nerves VII, IX, X and XI: facial, palatal and laryngeal palsy.
- Cranial nerve XII: wasting of the tongue.
- Sympathetic tract: Horner syndrome.

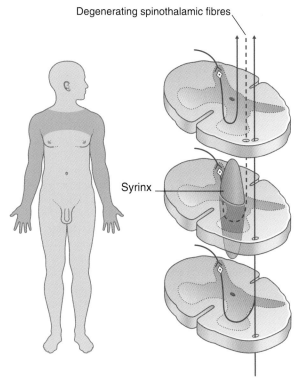

Degenerating spinothalamic fibres

Syrinx

Fig. 34.13 Syringomyelia. Shading shows distribution of pain and temperature sensation loss. (From Gruener G, Mtui E, Dockery P. *Fitzgerald's Clinical Neuroanatomy and Neuroscience*, 7th ed. Elsevier; 2016.)

PERIPHERAL NERVOUS SYSTEM DISORDERS

Peripheral neuropathy

Peripheral neuropathy is a general term referring to disorders of peripheral nerves; it can be divided into mononeuropathy, mononeuritis multiplex and polyneuropathy. The causes of these are summarized in Chapter 21. The four most common causes are diabetes mellitus, malignancy, vitamin B_{12} deficiency and drugs (notably alcohol). Treatment is aimed at the underlying disorder. Some specific peripheral nerve syndromes are considered here.

Guillain–Barré syndrome

This is an acute immune-mediated polyneuropathy with several subtypes, the most common of which is acute inflammatory demyelinating polyneuropathy. Guillain–Barré syndrome (GBS) affects motor nerves more than sensory nerves. Seventy-five percent of patients have a history of infective illness days or weeks before the condition develops. Linked pathogens include *Campylobacter* spp., cytomegalovirus, Epstein–Barr virus and HIV.

Clinical features

Clinically, there is ascending progressive, relatively symmetrical weakness accompanied by paraesthesia, hyporeflexia and numbness. Symptoms most commonly start in the lower limbs and progressively worsen to involve the upper limbs, trunk and respiratory and cranial nerves. In 10% of patients, arms or facial muscles are the first to be affected, and in the Miller Fisher subtype, there is ophthalmoplegia and ataxia.

Complications of GBS include respiratory failure, cardiac arrhythmias due to autonomic dysfunction and aspiration due to bulbar palsy. Because of immobility, patients are at high risk of deep vein thrombosis and pulmonary embolism.

Most patients with GBS start to improve within 1 month. A small proportion of patients will continue to progress or experience relapses; if this continues for more than 8 weeks, the illness is termed chronic inflammatory demyelinating polyneuropathy.

Investigations

The CSF shows a high protein concentration (up to 10 g/L) and a normal cell count. Nerve conduction studies are abnormal in most patients. Forced vital capacity helps predict respiratory outcomes. In addition, the patient's swallowing should be monitored closely as should the postural drop in blood pressure (as an indicator of autonomic function). ECG can reveal conduction abnormalities.

Management

Supportive measures include nutritional support, analgesia, skin care and thromboprophylaxis. Chest physiotherapy lowers the risk of pneumonia. Mechanical ventilation may be necessary. No definitive curative treatment exists. IV administration of immunoglobulin and plasma exchange plasmapheresis have been shown to improve outcomes, and are recommended for patients presenting up to 4 weeks after the onset of symptoms. Steroids alone are of no benefit.

Around 5% of severely affected patients will die in intensive care. Around 90% of patients have a good recovery.

Entrapment/compression neuropathies

Compression neuropathies are extremely common syndromes causing mononeuropathy with neurological symptoms and signs in the distribution of a single peripheral nerve.

Radiculopathies refer to the compression of a spinal nerve root. The injury to the nerve may be transient, changing with position, but with chronicity, demyelination and axonal degeneration may occur.

The following are some of the most frequently encountered conditions:

- Carpal tunnel syndrome: compression of the median nerve as it passes through the carpal tunnel at the wrist, causing numbness, paraesthesiae and weakness of the hand.
- Radial nerve palsy: compression of the radial nerve, frequently at the spiral groove in the upper arm, causing weakness of the wrist and finger extensors, with numbness of the dorsum of the hand and forearm ('Saturday night palsy').
- Meralgia paraesthetica: entrapment of the lateral cutaneous nerve of the thigh as it passes under the inguinal ligament, causing numbness over the lateral aspect of the thigh.

NEUROMUSCULAR DISORDERS

Muscle disorders

For more on muscle disorders, see Polymyositis and Dermatomyositis in Chapter 35.

Myotonic dystrophy (myotonia dystrophica)

This is an autosomal dominant condition characterized by myotonia: the inability of the muscles to relax normally after contraction. The peak onset is between the ages of 20 and 30 years. There is muscle wasting and weakness. Myotonia of the facial muscles results in ptosis, a wry smile or 'sneer' and a 'hang-dog' expression due to the thin face and lax jaw muscles (Fig. 34.14).

Other associated features include frontal baldness, cataracts, testicular or ovarian atrophy, cardiomyopathy with conduction disturbances, mental impairment and endocrine dysfunction, including diabetes. Reflexes are lost. The myotonia is often revealed by shaking the patient's hand (slow-to-release grip) or by asking patients to repetitively open and close their eyes or fists. It may be elicited by percussion of the thenar eminence – the induced depression is slow to fill (percussion myotonia). It increases with fatigue, cold and stress. Diagnosis is by genetic testing. There is no curative treatment. Myotonia may be relieved with procainamide or phenytoin.

Muscular dystrophies

Muscular dystrophies (MD) is a group of genetically determined diseases characterized by progressive degeneration and weakness of certain muscle groups.

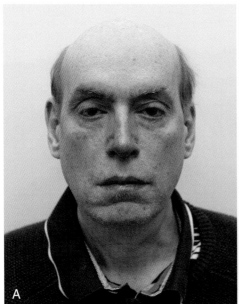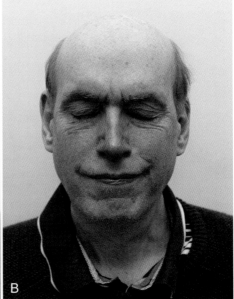

Fig. 34.14 Myotonic dystrophy. Facial features such as frontal balding, ptosis and temporal muscle atrophy. (From Goldman L, Schafer AI. *Goldman-Cecil Medicine*, 2-Volume Set, 26th ed. Elsevier; 2020.)

Duchenne and Becker muscular dystrophy (pseudohypertrophic)

These are the commonest types of MD and are X-linked recessive progressive disorders. Both involve mutations of the dystrophin gene. Duchenne MD presents in early childhood with clumsiness in walking and difficulty climbing stairs. Examination reveals a lordotic posture and 'waddling' gait due to proximal muscle weakness. The calves are hypertrophied. When rising from the floor, patients may need to use their hands to bring themselves into an upright position (Gower sign) (Fig. 34.15). Investigations show a markedly raised creatine kinase concentration. Electromyography and muscle biopsy show characteristic changes. Cardiomyopathy is common. Death usually occurs before the age of 20 years from intercurrent illnesses (e.g., chest infection). There is no specific treatment. Becker MD is less severe, with onset usually in the teenage years and survival beyond the third decade.

Facioscapulohumeral dystrophy (Landouzy–Dejerine syndrome)

This is autosomal dominant. The onset is around puberty with wasting and weakness of the upper limb-girdle and face. Life expectancy is usually normal.

Limb-girdle dystrophy

This describes a group of disorders affecting predominantly proximal muscles. Most are autosomal recessive, and onset in the most common types is in childhood. The condition is progressive, with death in middle age. There may be cardiac involvement.

Neuromuscular junction disorders

Myasthenia gravis

This is an autoimmune disease where skeletal muscle weakness is caused by a reduction in the number of functional postsynaptic acetylcholine receptors and their eventual destruction. Autoantibodies detectable in most patients include antibody to acetylcholine receptor and antibody to muscle-specific receptor tyrosine kinase (MuSK). Myasthenia gravis is associated with thymoma and thymus hyperplasia, hyperthyroidism, rheumatoid arthritis and SLE. The UK incidence is around 15 per 100,000.

Clinical features

It is more common in females and associated with other autoimmune conditions. There is painless muscle weakness, which worsens with repetitive contraction and fluctuates over the day. Most patients present with extraocular muscle weakness causing ptosis and diplopia. The facial and bulbar muscles are commonly affected, causing the 'myasthenic snarl' on smiling, dysarthria with a nasal-sounding voice and dysphagia. Proximal muscles and upper limbs are more often affected than distal muscles and lower limbs. Reflexes are usually normal. In 15% of patients, the disease remains limited to the eyes. Myasthenic crisis is a rare complication with rapidly worsening weakness often precipitated by infection or medication. Respiratory weakness is the concern in this case, and the patient may require mechanical ventilation.

Investigations

Diagnosis is mostly clinical. Anti-acetylcholine receptor antibody can be measured and, if this is negative, MuSK antibody

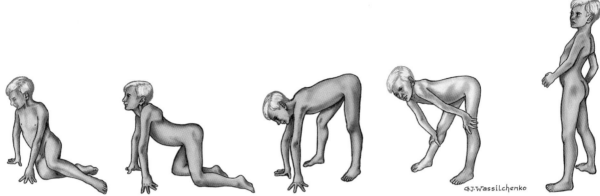

Fig. 34.15 Child with Duchenne muscular dystrophy attains standing posture by kneeling, then gradually pushing his torso upright (with knees straight) by 'walking' his hands up his legs (Gower sign). Note marked lordosis in upright position. (From Hockenberry MJ, Rodgers CC, Wilson D. *Wong's Essentials of Pediatric Nursing*, 11th ed. Elsevier; 2022.)

is checked. All patients should have thyroid function tests and a thymus scan. Neurophysiological tests can be conducted to demonstrate poor muscle responsiveness.

Management

Symptomatic control is with a long-acting anticholinesterase (e.g., pyridostigmine or neostigmine). The dose is slowly titrated against muscle power. Side effects include nausea, vomiting, increased salivation, diarrhoea and abdominal cramps. A cholinergic crisis can occur and is similar in presentation to a myasthenic crisis.

Acetylcholinesterase inhibitors are usually combined with immunosuppression. Corticosteroids on alternate days may achieve remission. If there is no remission and weakness is severe, azathioprine, methotrexate, ciclosporin or mycophenolate mofetil may be helpful. IV immunoglobulin or plasmapheresis can be used in severe relapses. The condition is usually relapsing or slowly progressive, and respiratory muscle involvement can lead to death. Thymectomy should be considered even in patients without a thymoma.

Lambert–Eaton myasthenic syndrome

This is an autoimmune condition but may be paraneoplastic; around 50% of cases are associated with small-cell lung cancer. Antibodies to the presynaptic P/Q-subtype voltage-gated calcium channels are present. This leads to impaired presynaptic release of acetylcholine.

Here, as opposed to in myasthenia gravis, weakness diminishes with exertion. Slowly progressive weakness is typical, particularly affecting the lower limbs. Autonomic involvement and hyporeflexia are characteristic. Symptomatic therapy with acetylcholinesterase inhibitors (pyridostigmine) or guanidine is possible. Acetylcholine-release enhancer amifampridine can be used. A significant increase in muscle strength can be achieved with 3,4-diaminopyridine. IV immunoglobulin or plasma

exchange can also be used. Immunosuppressants are used in severe cases. Regular chest X-rays are important to investigate patients for signs of malignancy; the neurological symptoms may predate cancer detection by months or even years.

MISCELLANEOUS DISORDERS

Motor neurone disease

This is a disease involving progressive degeneration of the motor cortex, pyramidal and corticospinal tracts, lower cranial nerve nuclei (hence the external ocular movements are normal) and anterior horn cells of the spinal cord. Both upper and lower motor neurones can be affected. Sensation is preserved. Presentation differs. Patients can report stiffness, cramps, muscle weakness and wasting. Muscle fasciculations are commonly seen on examination. As the condition progresses, muscular weakness becomes more pronounced, with swallowing and communication difficulties. Respiratory compromise may occur. Frontotemporal dementia occurs in around 10% to 15% of patients.

Motor neurone disease (MND) is slightly more common in men. Peak incidence is between the ages of 55 and 79 years, but people of any age can be affected. The cause is unknown. Familial forms account for 5% to 10% of cases and are usually due to mutations in the superoxide dismutase 1 gene (*SOD1*), although mutations of many other genes have been implicated in the pathogenesis of both the familial and sporadic forms.

Clinically there are four main patterns of disease:

- Amyotrophic lateral sclerosis (ALS): the most common type of MND. Combined LMN wasting and UMN spasticity and hyperreflexia. Weakness usually starts in the legs and spreads to the arms.

- Progressive muscular atrophy: anterior horn cell involvement, leading to LMN weakness and wasting and fasciculation of distal muscles, which spreads proximally.
- Progressive bulbar palsy: LMN weakness and wasting of the tongue and pharynx, leading to dysarthria and dysphagia. UMN features such as a stiff tongue, spastic speech and brisk jaw jerk are also usually present. Involvement of descending motor neurone pathways which arise in the cerebral cortex and brainstem (long tracts) is common.
- Primary lateral sclerosis: form limited to UMN; LMN signs may develop later in the disease. Progression is slower than for ALS.

Combinations of the aforementioned conditions may occur.

Management

Treatment is symptomatic. The aim is to help the patient with activities of daily living and to adequately manage symptoms. Quinine can be used for muscle cramps. Baclofen is an alternative and it can also help with muscle stiffness, spasticity and increased tone. Antimuscarinic drugs can be trialled for excessive drooling of saliva. Opiates should be considered for joint pains and distress. Nutrition, physiotherapy, occupational therapy and speech and language therapy teams should be involved. Difficult decisions regarding nasogastric or percutaneous endoscopic gastrostomy feeding and artificial ventilation may arise. These interventions may prolong life but also the process of dying. Riluzole, an antiglutamate drug, is licensed in MND and offers a small increase in the length of life. Other agents are used in trials. Death usually occurs 2 to 3 years after diagnosis; 25% survive to 5 years and 5% to 10% survive to 10 years.

Horner syndrome

This describes the combination of miosis (pupillary constriction), partial ptosis and ipsilateral loss of sweating (anhidrosis) caused by interruption of the sympathetic nerve supply to the face. The sympathetic nerves may be disrupted anywhere along their course:

- Brainstem: demyelination, vascular disease.
- Cervical cord: syringomyelia.
- Thoracic outlet: Pancoast tumour.
- Neck (postganglionic): carotid artery aneurysm or dissection, tumours.

Bulbar and pseudobulbar palsy

These two conditions result from disruption of lower cranial nerve motor function, affecting the tongue, muscles of chewing/swallowing (therefore causing an increased risk of aspiration) and facial muscles.

Bulbar palsy (bulbar refers to the medulla) is a LMN syndrome affecting cranial nerves VII–XII. Clinical features include flaccid, fasciculating tongue, normal or absent jaw jerk and quiet nasal speech. It is caused by diphtheria, motor neurone disease,

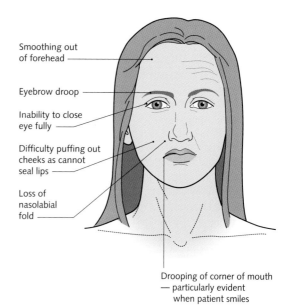

Smoothing out of forehead

Eyebrow droop

Inability to close eye fully

Difficulty puffing out cheeks as cannot seal lips

Loss of nasolabial fold

Drooping of corner of mouth — particularly evident when patient smiles

Fig. 34.16 Bell palsy.

Guillain–Barré syndrome, poliomyelitis, cerebrovascular event of the brainstem, syringobulbia and brainstem tumours.

Pseudobulbar palsy refers to bilateral UMN lesions affecting the brainstem motor nuclei (corticobulbar tracts). The tongue is spastic or paralysed, jaw jerk is increased, speech sounds like 'Donald Duck' and there is emotional lability. Pseudobulbar palsy is more common and is usually due to cerebrovascular events (e.g., bilateral internal capsule strokes). Other causes include MS, MND high brainstem tumours and neurosyphilis.

Bell palsy

This is an idiopathic unilateral LMN palsy of cranial nerve VII. Other causes must be excluded (see Chapter 2). It is thought that viral infections account for most cases.

Rapid onset of facial weakness occurs and may be accompanied by pain below the ear. There may be loss of taste in the anterior two-thirds of the tongue. The characteristic physical signs are described in Chapter 2 and shown in Fig. 34.16. Bell palsy specifically due to varicella zoster infection is termed Ramsay Hunt syndrome.

Most patients recover fully within a few weeks. Some have axonal degeneration and recovery is delayed and may be incomplete. Occasionally, aberrant reconnections are formed (e.g., eating may stimulate unilateral lacrimation – 'crocodile tears').

Steroids are effective in treating the condition if given within 72 hours. The role of antiviral drugs remains controversial. The eye must be protected when closure is incomplete: patches and artificial tears are useful.

● Chapter Summary

- Subarachnoid haemorrhage classically presents with sudden onset severe headache.
- Patients with an extradural haematoma will usually have a reduced level of consciousness, followed by a lucid interval.
- Migraine can present with features similar to a stroke.
- Carbamazepine is used as the first-line treatment for trigeminal neuralgia.
- Status epilepticus is a medical emergency and should be treated immediately. Lorazepam or other benzodiazepines are used as first line treatment.
- Multiple sclerosis is an autoimmune, inflammatory, demyelinating condition.
- *Pneumococcus*, *H. influenzae* and type b meningococcus are the most common causes of meningitis in adults in the UK.
- Listeria is a cause of meningitis in immunocompromised and elderly patients.
- Myasthenia gravis is an autoimmune condition where acetylcholine receptors are affected.

UKMLA Conditions

Bell palsy
Brain abscess
Brain metastases
Cerebral palsy and hypoxic-ischaemic encephalopathy
Encephalitis
Epilepsy
Essential tremor
Extradural haemorrhage
Meningitis
Metastatic disease
Motor neurone disease
Multiple sclerosis
Muscular dystrophies
Myasthenia gravis
Parkinson's disease
Peripheral nerve injuries/palsies
Radiculopathies
Spinal cord compression
Spinal cord injury
Stroke
Subarachnoid haemorrhage
Subdural haemorrhage
Trigeminal neuralgia

UKMLA Presentations

Altered sensation, numbness and tingling
Anosmia
Driving advice
Facial pain
Facial weakness
Fits/seizures
Headache
Limb weakness
Neck pain/stiffness
Neuromuscular weakness
Ptosis
Speech and language problems
Swallowing problems
Trauma

OSTEOARTHRITIS

Osteoarthritis (OA) is one of the most common joint conditions and is characterized by a syndrome of joint pain with various degrees of physical limitation. It is a degenerative disorder affecting mainly the weight-bearing joints and the hand (the overall prevalence of hip arthritis is 12% and that of knee arthritis is 18%). Risk factors include increasing age, family history, obesity, trauma, occupational and recreational stress on joints and female sex.

Pathology

OA is a degenerative disease of cartilage, which becomes eroded and progressively thinned as the condition proceeds. At the onset of the disease the collagen matrix of the cartilage becomes disorganized and there is marked decrease in proteoglycan content. This results in loss of water and makes cartilage susceptible to degeneration. Joint inflammation even though usually mild can also contribute to decay.

OA can affect other structures within the joint, including menisci. These can wear away and tear, ligaments become fibrotic and subchondral bone becomes hypomineralized. New bone can form and produce osteophytes usually scattered around the joint edge. Radiologically this presents as loss of joint space, subchondral sclerosis, subchondral cysts and marginal osteophytes (Fig. 35.1).

Clinical features

The clinical signs and symptoms of OA are described in Chapter 23. Diagnosis of the condition can be made clinically if all of the following are present:

- The patient is 45 years or older.
- There is activity-related joint pain.
- Lack of morning joint stiffness or stiffness lasts less than 30 minutes.

The joints commonly affected include the hips, knees, distal interphalangeal (DIP) joints, the first metacarpophalangeal (MCP) and metatarsophalangeal (MTP) joints and the lumbar and cervical spine. Pain in joints is exacerbated by movement and relieved by rest. In knees, it is often bilateral. If OA affects the hip, it can present as pain in the groin, the anterior and lateral parts of the thigh or the testicles in males. It can also be referred to the ipsilateral knee. Signs include pain and reduced range of movement in all directions, stiffness, joint swelling and synovitis. The joint deformity is often seen, and in the hands can be described as Heberden (at DIP joint) and Bouchard (at proximal interphalangeal (PIP) joint) nodes (Fig. 35.1).

The pattern of joint involvement tends to be asymmetrical. The most commonly affected joints in the hands are the DIP joints, the PIP joints and first carpometacarpal joint, giving an appearance of 'square hands'. Unlike rheumatoid arthritis (RA), there are no extraarticular manifestations of the disease.

Management

A holistic approach should be used when you are considering OA management. The impact on daily life, the support network available and appropriate pain assessment should be determined.

Lifestyle measures to prevent progression include weight loss, exercises and healthy diet. Nonsurgical and surgical treatments can be considered. The former concentrate on combinations of drugs paired with physical treatments (e.g., weight reduction and heat application), electrotherapy (transcutaneous electrical nerve stimulation), supporting exercises and mobility aids (e.g., walking sticks, special footwear, joint supports). Initially, simple analgesia (e.g., paracetamol) and topical nonsteroidal antiinflammatory (NSAIDs) should be trialled. Oral NSAIDs, cyclooxygenase 2 (COX-2) inhibitors and opioids are the next line. Intraarticular corticosteroids can be used and decrease joint inflammation. Surgical review can be considered if nonsurgical treatments have not shown desired benefits. Surgical options include joint lavage, debridement, osteotomy, arthroplasty and joint replacement.

RHEUMATOID ARTHRITIS

RA is an autoimmune, systemic disease producing symmetrical inflammatory deforming polyarthropathy with extraarticular involvement of many organs. In the United Kingdom it affects around 1% of the population and is two to four times more common in women than in men. The peak age of onset is between 30 and 50 years of age, although it can start at almost any time. Both environmental and genetic factors play a part in disease development. Smoking, silica exposure and excess alcohol use are risk factors for RA. There is often a family history of the condition and in particular certain HLA serotypes (HLA-DR4 and HLA-DR1) have been shown to be present in severe disease.

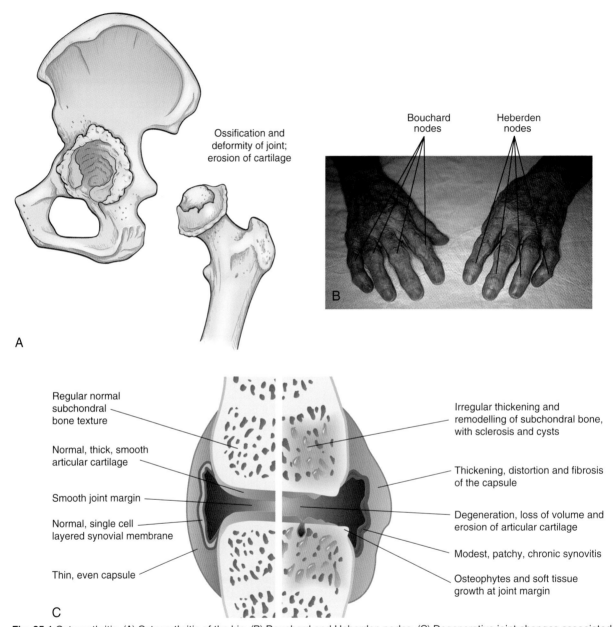

Fig. 35.1 Osteoarthritis. (A) Osteoarthritis of the hip. (B) Bouchard and Heberden nodes. (C) Degenerative joint changes associated with osteoarthritis (normal (*left*) versus osteoarthritic joint (*right*)). (A and C, from McCance K, Huether S. *Pathophysiology: The Biologic Basis for Disease in Adults and Children*. 7th ed. St Louis: Mosby; 2014; B, from Swartz MH. *Textbook of Physical Diagnosis: History and Examination*. 7th ed. St Louis: Mosby; 2014.)

Pathology

RA starts with persistent cellular activation that results in autoimmunity and inflammation. This primarily occurs within the synovial membrane, where swelling and congestion lead to infiltration of immune cells and cartilage, bone and tendon erosion.

Three distinct disease stages can be identified:

- Infiltration phase (nonspecific inflammatory features)
- Amplification in the synovium (T cell-mediated disease progression)
- Chronic inflammation (tissue injury due to cytokines interleukins (IL)-1, IL-6 and tumour necrosis factor alpha (TNF-α))

Once immune response has been established, B cell-mediated production of autoantibodies, including rheumatoid factor and antibodies to citrullinated peptides, contributes to an integral part of the condition. This includes disease progression where soft tissue inflammation surrounding the joint gives rise to granulation tissue with extensive angiogenesis and enzyme formation that damages the joint. Rheumatoid nodules (present in about 20% of cases) appear in consequence. These are usually subcutaneous nodules most commonly affecting extensor surfaces but that can also occur in other tissues (e.g., lungs, heart and sclera).

Clinical features

RA usually presents with an insidious onset of pain and stiffness (especially in the morning and after inactivity) in the small joints of the hands and feet that may progress to involve larger joints. This is symmetrical and usually associated with nonspecific systemic symptoms. Joint inflammation produces swelling, heat and redness. Persistent inflammation leads to joint and tendon destruction, muscle wasting and therefore deformity and loss of function.

In the hands the MCP joints, PIP joints and wrists are most commonly affected (Fig. 35.2). Large joints like shoulders, hips and elbows are less affected by the disease. Extraarticular manifestations are summarized in Table 35.1.

The diagnosis of RA is made on a combination of clinical and laboratory findings. Investigations should include:

- Full blood count (FBC) (may show anaemia of chronic disease (Table 35.2), thrombocytosis or thrombocytopenia and leucopoenia).
- Erythrocyte sedimentation rate (ESR).
- Rheumatoid factor, antinuclear antibodies (ANAs) and antibodies (anticyclic citrullinated peptide).
- Joint X-rays, especially of hands, wrists and feet: to aid in diagnosis and to monitor the baseline at presentation.
- Aspiration of synovial fluid.

Management

Once RA is suspect the patient should be referred to a rheumatologist. The aim is for disease remission to be achieved as soon as possible to avoid mechanical joint damage.

Paracetamol, oral nonselective NSAIDs and COX-2 selective drugs can reduce RA signs and symptoms, and low-dose oral corticosteroids and intraarticular injections can be used for short-term symptom control.

However, achieving remission will likely require use of disease-modifying antirheumatic drugs (DMARDs). Methotrexate, leflunomide and sulphasalazine are the first-line DMARDs. Others include ciclosporin, hydroxychloroquine, TNF inhibitors (infliximab, certolizumab, etanercept), monoclonal

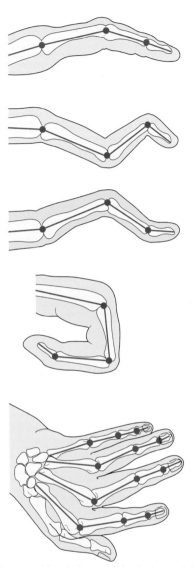

Fig. 35.2 Finger and hand abnormalities in rheumatoid arthritis. *DIP*, Distal interphalangeal; *MCP*, metacarpophalangeal; *PIP*, proximal interphalangeal.

antibodies (tocilizumab and rituximab) and T-cell modulators (abatacept).

In a new RA diagnosis, treatment with a first-line DMARDs plus short-term glucocorticoid therapy should be started within 3 months of the onset of persistent symptoms. The aim is to fully suppress the disease, and therefore close control is needed especially because of potential serious toxic side effects of DMARDs (Table 35.3).

In conventional DMARD-resistant disease, biological DMARD therapies can be useful. Their use is recommended if at least two DMARDs, including methotrexate failed to control

Table 35.1 Extraarticular features of rheumatoid arthritis

Organ system	Effects
Eyes	• Sjögren syndrome occurs in 15% of patients • Scleritis causes a painful red eye and may lead to uveitis and glaucoma • Scleromalacia perforans is an uncommon complication where a rheumatoid nodule in the sclera perforates
Nervous system	• Carpal tunnel syndrome (most common) • Peripheral neuropathy causing glove and stocking sensory loss and occasionally motor weakness • Mononeuritis multiplex due to vasculitis of vessels supplying nerves • Atlantoaxial subluxation resulting in spinal cord compression
Lymphoreticular system	• Generalized lymphadenopathy and splenomegaly may be present • Felty syndrome (seropositive arthritis, neutropenia and splenomegaly)
Blood	• Normochromic normocytic anaemia or iron-deficiency anaemia • Raised ESR; CRP level may be modestly raised or normal • Reactive thrombocytosis
Respiratory system	• Pleural effusions (more common in men) • Rheumatoid nodules • Diffuse fibrosing alveolitis • Caplan syndrome (the presence of large rheumatoid nodules and fibrosis in patients with RA exposed to various industrial dust)
Cardiac	• Pericarditis and pericardial effusions may occur
Skin	• Vasculitis may produce nail-fold infarcts, ulcers and digital gangrene • Peripheral oedema may be present and is due to increased vascular permeability
Kidneys	• Secondary amyloidosis may affect the kidneys, leading to proteinuria, nephrotic syndrome and renal failure

CRP, C-reactive protein; ESR, erythrocyte sedimentation rate; RA, rheumatoid arthritis.

Table 35.2 Causes of anaemia in rheumatoid arthritis

Anaemia of chronic disease
Hypersplenism due to splenomegaly (Felty syndrome if also neutropenic)
Chronic blood loss from peptic ulceration due to steroid and nonsteroidal antiinflammatory administration
Bone marrow suppression by disease-modifying drugs such as gold and penicillamine
Folate deficiency (increased utilization of folate)

HINTS AND TIPS

Remember to always prescribe a proton pump inhibitor when NSAIDs are used regularly, so as to prevent gastrointestinal side effects.

SPONDYLOARTHROPATHIES

This is a heterogeneous group of inflammatory rheumatoid conditions also known as 'seronegative arthropathies'. The joints predominantly affected involve the axial skeleton, peripheral joints and entheses. Other associated features include anterior uveitis and bowel disease. There is usually a strong family history, and investigations show high incidence of the presence of HLA-B27 but absence of rheumatoid factor. The following diseases are included: ankylosing spondylitis, reactive arthritis, enteropathic arthritis, psoriatic arthritis, juvenile chronic arthritis and undifferentiated spondyloarthropathy.

Ankylosing spondylitis

This is the most prevalent seronegative arthropathy that most commonly affects young men. The peak onset of age is 20 to 30 years and the male-to-female ratio is 3:1. HLA-B27 is present in more than 85% of patients.

Pathology

There is strong genetic association of the disease, and nearly half of disease susceptibility is determined by the major histocompatibility complex, a cell surface molecule manipulating leucocyte function. Bone remodelling and deposition cause the disease picture. TNF-α, interleukins, antineutrophil cytoplasmic antibodies (ANCAs) and chromosome 5 polymorphism have all been found to contribute to disease pathogenesis but the exact processes are not yet understood.

the disease after 3 months. Last resort options include surgical interventions. Furthermore, urgent surgical review is necessary if septic arthritis or any signs or symptoms suggesting cervical myelopathy are present.

The multidisciplinary team forms a very important aspect of managing a patient with RA, including occupational therapy, podiatry and psychological interventions.

Table 35.3 Recommendations regarding side effects and monitoring of disease-modifying antirheumatic drugs

Drug	Cautions and contraindications	Monitoring
Methotrexate	Ascites, active infections, immunodeficiency syndromes, bone marrow suppression, photosensitivity	FBC, LFTs and U&Es 2 weekly for 6 weeks after dose increase or disease stable. Every 2–3 months thereafter
Sulphasalazine	Salicylate hypersensitivity, acute porphyria	FBC and LFTs monthly for first 3 months
Hydroxychloroquine	Drug-induced retinopathy, acute porphyria, diabetes	Annual review by optometrist if taken for >5 years
Ciclosporin	Renal impairment, uncontrolled hypertension, active infection, malignancy	Creatinine at least twice before treatment then 2 weekly for first 3 months, then monthly for further 3
Infliximab	Severe infection, moderate heart failure	Six months pre and post treatment. Monitor for nonmelanoma skin cancer and latent TB
Etanercept	Active infection	Monitor for skin cancer and latent TB

FBC, *Full blood count;* LFTs, *liver function tests;* TB, *tuberculosis;* U&Es, *urea and electrolytes.*

Clinical features

The onset is insidious over several months or years, causing prolonged back pain. Bilateral sacroiliitis causes buttock and thigh pain that may radiate down to the legs. Most patients present with intermittent flares and periods of remission. Morning stiffness is characteristic, and improvement is seen on exercise. Systemic features are common and are summarized in Table 35.4.

With progression of the disease, spinal fusion and loss of movement occur; eventually the patient develops exacerbated thoracic kyphosis and stooped neck ('question mark' posture). Large asymmetrical joints are usually affected (hips, shoulder, chest wall). Hand joint involvement may cause dactylitis ('sausage digits'). Enthesitis occurs in about one-third of patients and affects the Achilles tendon, heel pad (plantar fasciitis) and tibial tuberosity. The diagnosis is made by the combination of a clinical and radiological presence of sacroiliitis.

CLINICAL NOTES

The extraarticular features complicating ankylosing spondylitis are (five *A*s):

- Apical fibrosis
- Aortitis and aortic regurgitation
- Anterior uveitis
- Achilles tendonitis and other enthesitides
- Amyloidosis

Management

As it is a chronic condition with a range of severity, for which currently there is no cure, all patients need to be referred to rheumatology specialists. Treatment is symptomatic with

Table 35.4 Extraarticular features of ankylosing spondylitis

System involved	Characteristics
Eyes	Anterior uveitis in 30% of people (painful, red eye with severe photophobia)
Cardiovascular system	Aortitis, aortic valve insufficiency Fibrosis of heart conducting system causing atrioventricular block
Respiratory system	Restrictive lung disease due to chest wall involvement limiting chest expansion Pulmonary fibrosis of upper lobe
Renal	Amyloidosis Immunoglobulin A nephropathy
Neurological system	Atlantoaxial subluxation Cauda equina Nerve compression due to pathological spine fractures
Metabolic bone disease	Osteopenia and osteoporosis

analgesia and lifestyle changes. NSAIDs and COX-2 inhibitors have been found to be effective.

DMARD biological agents including TNF-α inhibitors (etanercept, infliximab) have shown good effectiveness. Physiotherapy and rehabilitation play an important role and help to maintain function. Surgery is occasionally useful when deformities are to be repaired and when joint replacement is required.

Reactive arthritis

Reactive arthritis is an acute seronegative arthritis associated with inflammatory back pain and additive or migratory oligoarthritis that typically follows enteritis or urethritis. It usually affects young adults, and when composed of large joint oligoarthritis, urinary tract infection and uveitis is termed 'Reiter syndrome'.

Pathology

There appears to be strong association of reactive arthritis with HLA-B27. The syndrome is associated with precipitating infective genitourinary or gastrointestinal disease, and the most common pathogens include *Salmonella*, *Campylobacter*, *Shigella*, *Chlamydia trachomatis* and *Neisseria gonorrhoeae*. It may be associated with tuberculosis (Poncet disease) but the actual interaction between the host and the pathogen and disease manifestation is unknown.

Clinical features

Reactive arthritis usually develops 1 to 3 weeks after an infection. In about 10% of cases there are no precipitating symptoms. Asymmetrical predominantly lower limb oligoarthritis (usually not more than six joints) develops with general malaise and fatigue. There is often heel pain due to plantar fasciitis and Achilles tendinitis. Other clinical features include:

- Urethritis and balanitis
- Conjunctivitis, iritis and anterior uveitis
- Skin changes, including erythema nodosum, nail dystrophy and mouth ulcers
- Abdominal pain and diarrhoea with pathological appearances similar to inflammatory bowel disease

Management

Main goal is to eliminate underlying infective cause if still present. Otherwise treatment is symptomatic with analgesia (e.g., NSAIDs) and rest of the affected joints. Joint aspiration can help exclude septic arthritis and aid with pain management. Intraarticular or systemic steroids can be used in the acute phase. Immunosuppressants, steroids or DMARDs may be needed in patients with severe nonresponsive cases. The disease is usually self-limiting and settles within 3 to 12 months.

Psoriatic arthritis

This is a condition affecting joints and connective tissue associated with psoriasis. About 30% of patients with psoriasis will be affected. It may present with enthesitis and dactylitis, and between 40% and 60% of those affected will develop erosive and deforming joint complications. It is an autoimmune disease with strong HLA-B27 association positive in 40% to 50% of patients.

Arthritis presents as pain, swelling and stiffness, and often affects the nails. Tendosynovitis tends to affect flexor rather than extensor tendons, and enthesopathy more commonly Achilles tendonitis and plantar fasciitis. It is often relapsing and limiting, and can take five clinical forms:

- Polyarticular symmetrical arthritis: RA-like arthritis affecting small joints of the hands and feet but with DIP rather than MCP involvement to help distinguish it from RA; seen in 25% of patients
- Oligoarticular asymmetrical arthritis usually affecting less than three joints; affects 70% of patients
- Spondylitic axial arthritis: ankylosing spondylitis-like arthritis but affecting vertebrae asymmetrically
- DIP arthritis associated with nail changes
- Arthritis mutilans: variation of DIP disease producing characteristic flexion deformity of DIP joints and radiological appearance of 'pencil in cup'.

For skin as well as joint disease, management is best with monotherapy treating both. Simple analgesia, NSAIDs and corticosteroids help relieve arthritis symptoms, and in severe cases, DMARDs and anti-TNF drugs can be used.

CRYSTAL ARTHROPATHY

Gout

Gout is a result of deposition of urate crystals in joints and soft tissues and affects approximately 1 in 100 people in the United Kingdom. It can present in acute and chronic phases, and most commonly affects joints in the feet.

Pathology

Gout is a disorder of purine metabolism resulting in uric acid crystal deposition in the form of monosodium urate tophi. These can be surrounded by a ring of proteins blocking stimulation of inflammation. Once crystals become dislodged from tophi (e.g., due to physical damage), they activate an inflammatory cascade and therefore cause joint pain, stiffness and inflammation.

Triggers for uric acid precipitation include cold, rapid changes in uric acid levels brought on by trauma, medication, acidosis, proteins such as proteoglycans and collagen and stopping or starting allopurinol therapy.

CLINICAL NOTES

Risk factors for Gout development include: diet (red meat, shellfish and alcohol), obesity, family history and medication (thiazide diuretics).

Clinical features

Acute gout typically presents in the first MTP joint with a red, hot, swollen, extremely painful big toe that develops over 6 to 12 hours (Fig. 35.3). Other joints affected include knees, midtarsal joints, ankles and hands. The inflammation usually reaches its

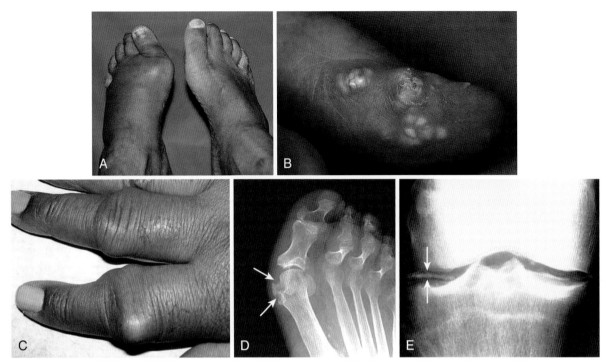

Fig. 35.3 Gout first MTP joint. *MTP,* Metatarsophalangeal. (A from Swartz MH. *Textbook of Physical Diagnosis*. 5th ed. Philadelphia, Saunders Elsevier; 2006; B from Bouloux, P. *Self-Assessment Picture Tests Medicine, Vol. 3*. London, Mosby-Wolfe; 1997; C from Goldman L, Schafer AI. *Cecil's Medicine*. 24th ed. Philadelphia, Saunders Elsevier; 2012; D from Herring W. *Learning Radiology Recognizing the Basics*. 2nd ed. Philadelphia, Elsevier Saunders; 2012; E from Marx J. *Rosen's Emergency Medicine Concepts and Clinical Practice*. 7th ed. Philadelphia, Mosby Elsevier; 2010.)

peak at 24 hours, and can be associated with fever and malaise. Left untreated, an attack should resolve within 5 to 15 days.

In the chronic stage of the disease, tophi can be seen within connective tissues, particularly the helix of the ear or around joints (commonly hands and elbows). They are hard, chalky nodules that can cause joint erosion, leading to chronic arthritis and disability.

> **COMMUNICATION**
>
> Patients with acute gout will often graphically describe the severity of their discomfort. It is a very painful condition.

For patients with typical gout presentations (MTP inflammation and high urate blood levels) diagnosis can be accurately assumed but only the presence of monosodium urate within synovial fluid confirms the diagnosis (needle-shaped, negatively birefringent crystals).

Management

An ice pack and rest may be useful in acute attacks. Pharmacological therapies in the first instance include NSAIDs and colchicine followed by corticosteroids. Last resorts in refractory disease use interleukin-1 inhibitors (canakinumab). Long-term

preventative measures need to be implemented in patient's daily life, and include weight and alcohol reduction, good hydration, avoidance of precipitating foods (red meat) and medication.

For long-term gout management, uric acid-lowering drug therapy is indicated. Allopurinol is first choice. Their use should never be started during an acute attack and treatment with them is usually lifelong. Regular monitoring is required.

> **CLINICAL NOTES**
>
> Allopurinol should not be prescribed unless there are exceptional circumstances in patients taking azathioprine because of risk of life-threatening bone marrow suppression.

Pseudogout

This is an inflammatory condition caused by deposition of calcium pyrophosphate dihydrate crystals within joints. Risk factors for development include old age, hyperparathyroidism, haemochromatosis, hypothyroidism, long-term steroid use and low phosphate or magnesium levels.

Acute attacks present with a monoarthritis or oligoarthritis, usually affecting the knees, hips or wrists. Chronic disease causes joint changes similar to OA (but more severe) and may progress to destructive arthropathy producing a neuropathic joint.

Investigation useful in diagnosis include radiographs often showing chondrocalcinosis and joint aspiration demonstrating weakly positively birefringent crystals in polarized light. Management is symptomatic with NSAIDs or colchicine and therapeutic joint aspiration. Intraarticular steroid injections can also be helpful.

CONNECTIVE TISSUE DISORDERS

Systemic lupus erythematosus

Systemic lupus erythematosus (SLE) is a multisystem, autoimmune connective tissue disorder. It is around five times more common in women and also in people of Asian and Afro-Caribbean origin. Peak incidence is at 50 to 54 years for females and 70 to 74 years for males. The cause is multifactorial, involving genetic predisposition and environmental triggers (e.g., drugs such as hydralazine and isoniazid, ultraviolet light and vitamin D deficiency).

Pathology

Lupus results from abnormal activation of the immune system and autoimmunity, mainly to proteins within the cell nucleus, producing ANAs. Other autoantibodies involved are summarized in Table 35.5. Furthermore it is thought to be type III hypersensitivity reaction where an abnormal immune system also activates and releases interleukins, interferons and complement molecules that contribute to symptoms. This in combination with abnormal programmed cell death (apoptosis) leads to cellular damage and inflammation.

Clinical features

SLE is a remitting and relapsing illness that can present in a variety of ways. The signs and symptoms are often general and nonspecific. Common early features include fever, arthralgia, malaise, tiredness, weight loss, lymphadenopathy, rashes, paraesthesia, mouth ulcers and headaches. The range of severity is broad and can include mild to life-threatening disease. Any major organ can become affected by the disease within 5 years of onset. The most common symptoms include:

- Arthralgia (nonerosive peripheral symmetrical polyarthritis with swelling and morning stiffness).
- Fibromyalgia.
- Raynaud phenomenon.
- Rashes (skin symptoms seen in 60% of patients):

Table 35.5 Autoantibodies in systemic lupus erythematous

Autoantibody	Characteristics
ANA	95% sensitivity to SLE but not diagnostic without clinical features. Present in other autoimmune conditions, including systemic sclerosis, polymyositis and Sjögren syndrome
Anti-dsDNA	High specificity but only 70% sensitivity to SLE. Levels reflect disease activity
Anti-Sm	Specific for SLE
Anti-SSA or Anti-SSB	Present in 15% of patients with connective tissue disease
Anti-RNP	Mixed connective tissue disorder
Antiphospholipid	If SLE-associated with concurrent antiphospholipid syndrome

ANA, Antinuclear antibody; dsDNA, double-stranded DNA; SLE, systemic lupus erythematous.

- Photosensitive rash (classic malar, butterfly rash on nasolabial folds that may be pruritic)
- Discoid lupus erythematous (erythematous, scaly rash on sun-exposed areas associated with scarring)
- Other rashes, including livedo reticularis rash, nonscarring alopecia and vasculitic rash.
- Respiratory fibrosis and pleurisy.
- Pericarditis, hypertension, Libman–Sacks endocarditis (nonbacterial, thrombotic endocarditis related to inflammation).
- Glomerulonephritis.
- Neuropsychiatric symptoms (almost any neurological manifestation can be seen in lupus but most commonly anxiety, depression, psychosis, seizures and neuropathy are seen).

Investigations to be considered in SLE include:

- FBC and ESR (cytopaenias are common and ESR may be raised)
- SLE autoantibodies (see Table 35.5)
- Complement investigations (C3/C4; low in active SLE)
- Urine dipstick (blood and protein suggests likely renal involvement)

Diagnosis is based on American College of Rheumatology criteria and is suggested if four or more characteristics are present.

Management

Management is multidisciplinary and often involves preventing flairs and reducing their severity. General lifestyle changes should concentrate around smoking cessation, weight management, exercising to reduce cardiovascular risks and sunlight avoidance. Initial treatment is with NSAIDs for arthritic pain and hydroxychloroquine, and corticosteroids.

In severe disease immunosuppressive drugs are used and include DMARDs (methotrexate, mycophenolate mofetil, cyclophosphamide). Biological agents such as belimumab are used in resistant disease. In cases of severe disease with organ involvement or vasculitis intravenous immunoglobulins are used. These unlike immunosuppressants do not suppress immune system therefore produce less risk of severe infection.

HINTS AND TIPS

SLE often affects young women of childbearing age. Make sure to tailor their treatment to minimize the risks to pregnancy. Family therapy and prepregnancy counselling are often helpful.

Systemic sclerosis

Systemic sclerosis (SSc) is a multisystem autoimmune rheumatic disease that results in overproduction of connective tissue. It is more common in women than men, and peak incidence is at 30 to 50 years of age. The condition is classified into two types depending on the degree of skin involvement. The more severe disease is termed 'diffuse cutaneous systemic sclerosis' (dcSSc). Limited cutaneous systemic sclerosis (LcSSc) is less severe and widespread and affects only the skin on the face, forearms and legs up to the knees. Very rarely it may occur without skin involvement when it is termed 'systemic sclerosis sine scleroderma'.

Pathology

Disease pathogenesis is driven by fibroblast overactivity leading to excessive collagen production and deposition causing fibrosis in skin, organs and small vessels. This is thought to be mediated by autoimmune response, and in most patients, autoantibodies are present:

- ANA is found most frequently but is nonspecific.
- Anti-Scl70 is SSc-specific.
- Anticentromere antibody.
- Anti-RNA polymerase III antibody is found in dcSSc.

Autoantibodies stimulate release of inflammatory molecules that together with significant vascular damage result in SSc presentation.

The cause is thought to be associated with genetic as well as environmental factors. A family history increases the risk.

Chemotherapy (bleomycin and taxane) and exposure to chemical solvents can cause SSc.

Clinical features

There is general malaise, lassitude, fever and weight loss. Raynaud phenomenon is commonly present and may precipitate all other symptoms (seen in 90% of cases). The disease can affect different systems, and its signs and symptoms are heterogeneous. The classic appearance of an affected patient shows a characteristic beaked nose, facial telangiectasia and tight skin around the mouth (Fig. 35.4). Systemic features are summarized in Table 35.6.

The course of the disease is variable but is usually slowly progressive. Prognosis depends on the extent of complications, but death occurs mostly from lung, renal or cardiac complications. The overall mean 10-year survival rate is approximately 90%.

CLINICAL NOTES

CREST syndrome (calcinosis, Raunaud's, oesophageal dysfunction, scleroderma, telangiectasia) is a feature of LcSSc).

Management

Treatment is symptomatic as currently there is no cure for the disease. It is a complex, multisystem disease with significant risk of major complications, and therefore specialist management is essential. Symptomatic control is 'organ based' and may include nifedipine to help with Raynaud phenomenon, antacids and proton pump inhibitors for reflux disease or emollients, analgesia and physiotherapy for joint disease.

Broad-spectrum immunosuppressive therapy can be used in severe cases and includes methotrexate, cyclophosphamide and mycophenolate mofetil.

Polymyositis and dermatomyositis

These are autoimmune, inflammatory disorders of mainly proximal muscle. The two conditions share many features, but dermatomyositis also affects the skin. They can occur at any age and affect women twice as frequently as men.

Pathology

These are autoimmune conditions associated with the presence of autoantibodies. Anti-Mi-2 antibodies are specific for dermatomyositis, and anti-Jo antibodies are specific for polymyositis. Other autoantibodies that are commonly present are ANAs (positive in 80% of patients) and myositis-specific and myositis-associated antibodies (MSA and MAA respectively).

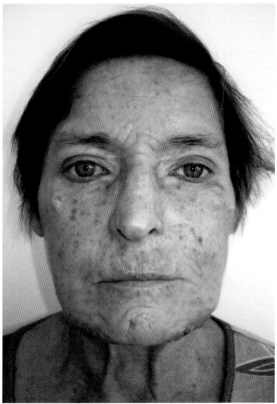

Fig. 35.4 Facial systemic sclerosis. (Reprinted with permission Nestal-Zibo et al., 2009 Calcinosis and systemic sclerosis. *Journal of Oral and Maxillofacial Surgery*. 2009.)

Polymyositis is a myopathy mediated by T cells, whereas dermatomyositis is an angiopathy that results in myopathy. Both conditions can be paraneoplastic syndromes, and dermatomyositis can sometimes be preceded by viral infections.

Clinical features

The clinical features of polymyositis and dermatomyositis show:

- Progressive, diffuse proximal muscle weakness, gradual in onset.
- Distal muscles are spared and fine movements retained.
- Flexion of the neck and torso.
- Pharyngeal weakness causes dysphagia.
- There may be muscle pain.
- In dermatomyositis there is purple 'heliotrope' coloured rash with a characteristic pattern around the eyes, face and upper trunk. There is periorbital oedema; a scaly, erythematous rash over extensor surfaces (Gottron papules if on knuckles); telangiectasia; ulcerative vasculitis and calcinosis (Fig. 35.5).

Table 35.6 Systemic manifestations of systemic sclerosis

System	Symptom
Skin	Thickening and hardening that limits function (sclerodactyly) Nonpitting oedema Digital ulcers Calcinous nodules (may protrude through skin) Thick facial skin and microstomia: Telangiectasia; skin is dry and itchy and may be hypo/hyperpigmented
Musculoskeletal	Arthritis and myositis
Gastrointestinal	Reflux disease, strictures, dysphagia Antral vascular ectasia ('watermelon stomach') may cause gastrointestinal bleed Reduced bowel motility and constipation
Respiratory	Pulmonary fibrosis causing restrictive lung disease Pulmonary arterial hypertension
Renal	Glomerulonephritis and reduced renal function Scleroderma renal crisis (malignant hypertension, hyperreninaemia, azotaemia, haemolytic anaemia) Kidney involvement is poor prognostic factor and often causes death

In both conditions association with other autoimmune diseases is high. Myasthenia gravis, Hashimoto thyroiditis and systemic sclerosis are commonly found with polymyositis and dermatomyositis. It is very important to remember that cancers can cause the conditions, and therefore patients should be investigated for underlying malignancy.

Diagnosis is confirmed by muscle biopsy, but initial clues can be found in severely elevated levels of creatine kinase.

CLINICAL NOTES

The most common cancers associated with polymyositis and dermatomyositis are breast, ovarian, gastric and lung cancer.

Management

General advice on sun avoidance and sunblock is helpful when you considering rash management. Physical activity and physiotherapy will maintain muscle strength. Topical steroids in mild disease escalated to high-dose systemic steroids are the first-line treatment. In cases of failed response, immunosuppressive

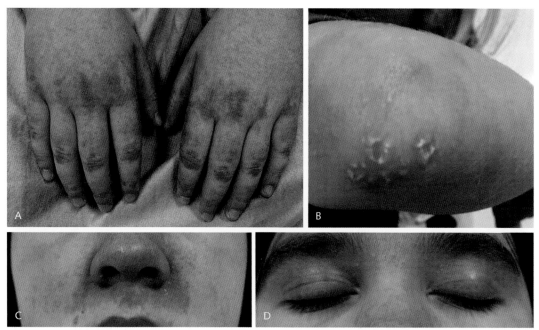

Fig. 35.5 Dermatomyositis rash. (A) Gottron papules on extensor surfaces of phalangeal joints. (B) Gottron papules on extensor surfaces of elbow. (C) Malar rash crossing the nasolabial folds. (D) Heliotrope rash. (From Tenney-Soeiro R, Devon EP. *Netter's Pediatrics*, 2nd ed. Elsevier; 2023.)

drugs (e.g., azathioprine, cyclophosphamide, rituximab) may be used.

Sjögren syndrome

This is a chronic autoimmune disease leading to destruction of exocrine glands resulting in xerophthalmia (dry eyes), xerostomia (dry mouth) and enlargement of parotid glands. It can be primary or secondary if associated with a connective tissue disorder (commonly RA and SLE). Its peak incidence is at around 30 to 40 years of age and 9 out of 10 patients with the disease are women.

The most frequent symptoms of affected patients are dry eyes and mouth causing cough, reflux disease and blepharitis and skin and vaginal dryness. Systemic features of the disorder include:

- arthralgia, polyarthritis, myalgia
- Raynaud phenomenon, vasculitis and rashes
- pancreatitis and primary biliary cirrhosis
- sleep disturbance, anxiety and depression
- mild fibrotic lung disease
- tubulointerstitial nephritis

Diagnosis is made by a combination of clinical features and investigations (e.g., presence of rheumatoid factor, ANAs).

Management concentrates on symptomatic control and includes artificial tears and saliva. Biological immunosuppressants and DMARDs are used for systemic symptoms.

VASCULITIS

General overview

Vasculitis is a group of conditions that destroy blood vessels through inflammatory change. It affects both arteries and veins, and it can be a primary condition or can result in the context of another disease (e.g., RA, SLE or infection). Primary vasculitis can be classified according to the size of the vessels affected (Table 35.7).

The common pathological feature of the vasculitides is the presence of leucocytes in the vessel wall causing inflammation and ultimately necrosis. This may lead to obstruction of the vessel and ischaemia, or the vessel may rupture, causing bleeding.

Eosinophilic granulomatosis with polyangiitis

Eosinophilic granulomatosis with polyangiitis (EGPA) is a diffuse vasculitis affecting coronary, pulmonary, abdominal, cerebral and skin small and medium-sized vessels and was previously known as 'Churg–Strauss syndrome'. Its cause is

Table 35.7 Classification of vasculitis

Vessel size	Types
Large arteries	Takayasu arteritis (affects branches of aorta) Giant cell arteritis Polymyalgia rheumatica
Medium-sized arteries	Polyarteritis nodosa Kawasaki disease (children, often affects coronary arteries) Primary CNS vasculitis
Small arteries	Behçet syndrome Eosinophilic granulomatosis with polyangiitis Microscopic polyangiitis Granulomatosis with polyangiitis Henoch–Schönlein purpura

CNS, Central nervous system.

unknown, but in 30% to 40% of cases, peripheral ANCAs are present. It is often associated with asthma and an eosinophilia.

EGPA is a rare condition and can affect various age groups. Its clinical presentation depends on the system affected, but generally may include fever, diffuse muscle and joint pains and weight loss. The most prominent systemic signs and symptoms are:

- Upper respiratory tract: rhinitis, sinusitis, nasal polyposis.
- Pulmonary: asthma, haemoptysis and pneumonitis.
- Cardiac: myocardial infarction, heart failure, myocarditis (heart disease causes 50% of deaths in EGPA).
- Gastrointestinal: bowel ischaemia, pancreatitis.
- Skin: vasculitis rash, purpura, nodules, livedo reticularis and digital ischaemia.
- Renal: glomerulonephritis and chronic kidney disease
- neurological: stroke and peripheral neuropathy (mononeuritis multiplex).

Management is with high-dose glucocorticoids or immunosuppressive medication. Recently monoclonal antibody mepolizumab has been trailed as specific first-line treatment for EGPA.

Granulomatosis with polyangiitis

This type of small-vessel vasculitis was previously known as 'Wegener granulomatosis'. It is a rare disease that involved formation of granulomas and inflammation of blood vessels as a result of ANCAs (cytoplasmic ANCAs are more specific).

It is a multisystem disease that most commonly affects the upper respiratory tract, causing rhinorrhoea (erosive sinusitis) and cough with ulcers and sores around the mouth and nose. Scleritis, episcleritis and conjunctivitis are seen. Lung involvement can result in pulmonary haemorrhage manifesting as haemoptysis and respiratory failure. There is often renal

involvement and the condition can cause a rapidly progressive glomerulonephritis. Other features include arthritis, weakness and rashes.

Management should be prompt and aim to prevent organ damage. Rituximab and cyclophosphamide in conjunction with high-dose corticosteroids is a treatment of choice. Plasma exchange is recommended if the patient presents with severe renal involvement.

CLINICAL NOTES

Granulomatosis with polyangiitis can be categorized by the ELK classification:

- E: upper respiratory tract (ear, nose sinusitis) present in almost all patients.
- L: lungs (most patients).
- K: kidneys (>75% of patients).

Henoch–Schönlein purpura

Henoch–Schönlein purpura (HSP) is an IgA-induced hypersensitivity reaction resulting in vasculitis. It is the most common in children (90% of cases), with peak prevalence at 2 to 6 years of age. It is associated with conditions precipitating its onset, including infections (group A streptococcus, herpes simplex, mycoplasma), vaccinations and environmental exposure to foods, drugs or allergens.

Its occurrence is highest in the winter months, and it usually presents with mild flu-like illness and low-grade fever. Purpura, arthritis and abdominal pain are characteristic. Purpuric rash is symmetrical and macular usually on the back of the legs, buttocks and ulnar sides of the arms. In about 40% of cases the renal system is involved. This is usually a delayed reaction and may present a few months later. In most severe cases it can result in end-stage kidney disease.

Treatment is primarily supportive, and HSP is usually self-limiting. In cases of kidney disease (with evidence of vasculitis and crescents on renal biopsy) immunosuppressive drugs are used including methylprednisolone and cyclophosphamide.

Kawasaki disease

This is a self-limiting, idiopathic vasculitis of young children. It most frequently affects children under the age of 5 years and is most common in boys and Asian countries.

It usually presents with fever that lasts more than 5 days and irritability and is not affected by usual medication. There is a marked vasculitic rash resulting in erythema, swelling and desquamation of the skin on extremities. Cervical lymphadenopathy, mouth and tongue ulcers and conjunctivitis are common

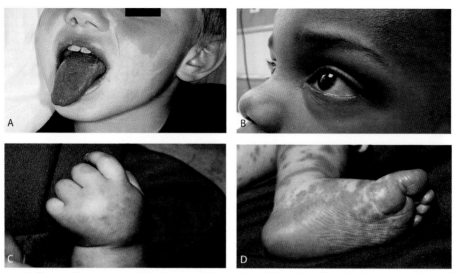

Fig. 35.6 (A) Kawasaki disease. Hyperaemia of the tongue with prominent lingual papillae ('red strawberry tongue'). (B) Conjunctivitis. (C) Nonpitting oedema of the hand. (D) Confluent, erythematous patches and plaques of the sole of foot. (From Paller AS, Mancini AJ. *Hurwitz Clinical Pediatric Dermatology*. 5th ed. Philadelphia, PA: Elsevier; 2016.)

(Fig. 35.6). The disease progresses in distinct phases, starting with the acute phase (1–2 weeks), followed by the subacute phase with marked relief of symptoms (up to 8 weeks), and then the convalescent phase. When considering diagnosis other similar conditions need to be excluded like scarlet fever and COVID-19-associated 'Kawasaki-like' disease.

It is linked to a range of potentially serious complications, the most sinister being coronary artery aneurysm. Management is with high dose of aspirin and intravenous immunoglobulins. Follow-up echocardiogram is needed to ensure normal function. Prognosis is usually good but depends on the degree of cardiac involvement.

Polyarteritis nodosa

Polyarteritis nodosa (PAN) is a necrotizing medium-sized vessel and small-vessel vasculitis. Typically it does not involve the lung and is not associated with ANCAs. 'Rosary sign' is an important diagnostic feature and results from small aneurysms strung like beads of rosary. It may be triggered by viral infection (hepatitis B virus is present in 30% of cases) but in most cases is idiopathic.

PAN often presents in a vague manner with nonspecific symptoms including fever, weight loss and myalgia. It can affect single or multiple organs and can cause peripheral neuropathies, rash and ulcers, hypertension and bowel ischaemia.

Treatment is with high-dose corticosteroids and cyclophosphamide in relapsing disease. The most severe complication is hypertension-induced kidney injury, from which 50% of patients will die if left untreated.

POLYMYALGIA RHEUMATICA AND GIANT CELL ARTERITIS

These inflammatory conditions frequently occur together; around half of patients with giant cell arteritis (GCA) have polymyalgia rheumatica (PMR). The underlying pathogenic mechanisms are incompletely understood and may be common to both conditions.

Polymyalgia rheumatica

PMR is about three times more common than GCA. It is a clinical syndrome characterized by proximal muscle pain and stiffness. The incidence increases with age, with those younger than 50 years rarely affected, and it is more common in women than men.

Its presenting symptoms may be nonspecific, but the condition should be suspected if there is acute or subacute, bilateral, severe and sustained pain in the neck, shoulders and pelvis. Severe morning stiffness that persists for more than 45 minutes and makes it difficult to brush hair or teeth is characteristic. There may be systemic features of weight loss and malaise. True muscle weakness does not occur, although power and range of movement may be limited by pain.

If there is clinical suspicion of PMR, assessment for GCA should be undertaken immediately.

Investigations may show raised levels of acute phase proteins (C-reactive protein) and raised ESR. Treatment is with high-dose glucocorticosteroids tapered down to appropriate response and is continued for longer than a year. Many patients respond well.

Giant cell arteritis

This is a systemic immune-mediated vasculitis with peak incidence between 70 and 79 years of age affecting medium-sized and large arteries. It can cause acute and bilateral vision loss in the elderly, and therefore is considered a medical emergency.

Its presentation is characterized by recent onset temporal headache with tender, reddened nonpulsatile arteries, malaise and fever. The headache may be severe and is often worse at night (see Chapter 16). Involvement of cranial arteries may cause tender scalp and pain in the jaw (jaw claudication). Involvement of the vertebral arteries may lead to TIA or stroke. Disease of the ophthalmic arteries may lead to retinal ischaemia or infarction and amaurosis fugax, blurred vision or irreversible blindness. About 25% of patients have features of PMR.

Investigations may show raised ESR (>60 mm/h), but temporal artery biopsy is diagnostic.

Urgent referral for specialized assessment is required if GCA is suspected. Treatment is with high-dose corticosteroids tapered down accordingly to symptom relief for around 12 and 18 months. Many patients recover and can stop therapy within 2 years, but spontaneous relapses are common and unpredictable. Tocilizumab (humanized monoclonal antibody) has been found to minimize GCA recurrence and flares.

HINTS AND TIPS

Use of steroids should never be delayed if giant cell arteritis is suspected. Temporal artery biopsy findings may remain positive for several weeks after the start of steroid treatment.

ANTIPHOSPHOLIPID SYNDROME

This condition is an autoimmune hypercoagulable state caused by antibodies against phospholipid (particularly anticardiolipin antibody and lupus anticoagulant). It manifests itself as an increased risk of arterial and venous thrombosis and adverse pregnancy outcomes (both for the mother and the foetus).

It may be present secondary to other autoimmune conditions such as SLE. Diagnosis is based on the presence of at least one clinical and at least one laboratory criterion from the following list.

Clinical criteria:

- Vascular thrombosis
- Pregnancy morbidity
  - Unexplained death of otherwise normal foetus at more than 10 weeks of gestation
  - Preterm birth of otherwise normal foetus at more than 34 weeks' gestation because of eclampsia, preeclampsia or placental insufficiency
  - Three or more consecutive miscarriages at less than 10 weeks' gestation in an otherwise normal pregnancy

Laboratory criteria:

- Lupus anticoagulant in plasma on two occasions at least 12 weeks apart
- Anticardiolipin antibody in medium or high titre on at least two occasions 12 weeks apart
- Anti-β_2-glycoprotein I antibody on two or more occasions 12 weeks apart

The presentation is variable as virtually any system can be affected. Management concentrates on effective anticoagulation that is usually lifelong following a thrombotic complication, but asymptomatic individuals do not need treatment.

Fibromyalgia

This is a multisystem chronic pain condition (pain lasting for 3 months or more) associated with widespread pain, fatigue, cognitive, sleep disturbances and mental health issues (anxiety and depression).

Women are 10 times more likely to be affected than men. Other risk factors include low income and socioeconomic status, depressive mental health disorders and rheumatic disease.

Although the cause is unknown it has been suggested that an interplay between genetic predisposition, hormonal imbalances, abnormal stress response and triggering events (e.g., trauma) are involved. Pathophysiological processes include altered pain perception, somatization and peripheral and central neuronal hyperexcitability and sensitization.

Pain generally occurs at multiple sites including muscles, tendons and ligaments, but patients also often complain of unrefreshing sleep, morning stiffness, a sensation of joint swelling, headaches and paraesthesia. Stress, cold and humidity generally exacerbate symptoms.

Management focuses on symptom reduction and improvement of quality of life. A multidisciplinary approach should be instituted. Each component of the condition should be managed with an appropriate strategy. The nonpharmacological approach is encouraged: aerobic and strengthening exercises, mindfulness, psychotherapy, physiotherapy, acupuncture and hydrotherapy. Pain management is described in Chapter 27.

● Chapter Summary

- A vast range of conditions affect muscles, bone and joints. These can be one phenotype or a combination of several phenotypes, including inflammatory (rheumatoid arthritis), degenerative (osteoarthritis), vasculitic (polyarteritis nodosa) or connective tissue (systemic lupus erythematous) diseases.
- These diseases can be extremely debilitating. They can affect most simple daily living activities, which can then have a negative effect on a person's psychological state.
- Musculocutaneous disease is often progressively degenerative and challenging to manage. Pain associated with the condition is chronic and severe, and it is very important to address its management when considering treatment. New therapies, including biological agents, are continuously being trialled to best manage these conditions.

UKMLA Conditions

Aneurysms, ischaemic limb and occlusions
Ankylosing spondylitis
Compartment syndrome
Crystal arthropathy
Idiopathic arthritis
Fever
Fibromyalgia
Kawasaki disease
Limp
Lower limb soft tissue injury
Lower limb fractures
Nonaccidental injury
Osteoarthritis
Osteomyelitis
Osteoporosis
Pathological fractures
Polymyalgia rheumatica
Reactive arthritis
Rheumatoid arthritis
Septic arthritis
Spinal cord compression
Spinal cord injury
Spinal fracture
Systemic lupus erythematosus
Trauma
Upper limb fractures
Upper limb soft tissue injury

UKMLA Presentations

Cold, painful, pale, pulseless leg/foot
Chronic joint pain/stiffness
Lacerations
Muscle pain/myalgia
Soft tissue injury
Trauma

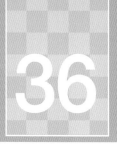

SKIN MANIFESTATIONS OF SYSTEMIC DISEASE

Systemic disease often involves the skin, ranging from the life-threatening purpuric rash of meningococcal septicaemia to rare lesions providing clues to a diagnosis. The following describes most common presentations not described in previous chapters.

Diabetes mellitus

Skin manifestations include recurrent infections (flexural candidiasis, folliculitis), ulcers, necrobiosis lipoidica diabeticorum (shiny reddish plaques on shins that can become atrophic and yellow), acanthosis nigricans (symmetrical tan, brown pigmentation over neck, axilla and groin) and granuloma annulare (red or red-brown ring-like lesions).

Inflammatory bowel disease

Both ulcerative colitis and Crohn disease are causes of erythema nodosum (Fig. 36.1; ill-defined, tender and at times necrotic subcutaneous nodules often on shins lasting 6–8 weeks) and pyoderma gangrenosum (Fig. 36.2; recurring nodulopustular ulcers with a tender necrotic edge usually healing with a pitting scar also seen in myeloma and granulomatosis with polyangiitis).

Crohn disease is associated with aphthous ulceration, perianal skin tags, fistulas and abscesses.

Coeliac disease

Dermatitis herpetiformis is a chronic manifestation of gluten-sensitive enteropathy. It manifests as itchy symmetrical blistering on elbows, the scalp, shoulders and ankles that quickly respond to treatment with dapsone.

Hyperthyroidism

Pretibial myxoedema is seen in Graves disease. It presents as skin thickening over the shins due to glycosaminoglycan deposition.

Hyperlipidaemia

This can manifest itself by deposition of lipids anywhere on the body, and includes:

- Tendon xanthomata: associated with familial hypercholesterolaemia.
- Eruptive xanthomata: yellow-orange small papules appearing all over the body.
- Xanthelasmata: yellow plaques commonly found on the eyelids.

Sarcoidosis

Erythema nodosum may occur. It is a hypersensitivity reaction resulting in granulomatous inflammation of the skin. It presents as papules, nodules, plaques most commonly on shins or lupus pernio (diffuse bluish plaque with papules over the nose).

Rheumatic fever

This may cause erythema marginatum. Round erythematous lesions with a central clearing that mostly affect the torso and extensor surfaces, and may come and go over hours.

Neurofibromatosis

A condition that results in nerve tissue tumours with distinct skin features:

- café au lait spots (light brown macules)
- axillary freckling
- violaceous dermal neurofibromata
- subcutaneous nodules

Lyme disease (borreliosis)

Caused by *Borrelia burgdorferi*, a spirochaete spread by ticks, presents with a classical rash, erythema chronicum migrans (Fig. 36.3). It starts off as a red papule before enlarging to form a ring with a raised border. It can last from days to months. Treatment is with doxycycline, amoxicillin or a third-generation cephalosporin (e.g., cefuroxime).

Malignant disease

There are many skin manifestations of internal malignancy, including:

- Acanthosis nigricans (gastric cancer and lymphoma) also seen in diabetes mellitus (Fig. 36.4).
- Dermatomyositis (ovarian, breast and lung cancer): can present as heliotrope rash and swelling, often around eyes

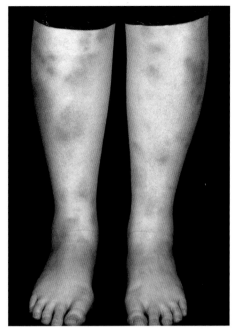

Fig. 36.1 Erythema nodosum. (Courtesy Scott Norton, MD.)

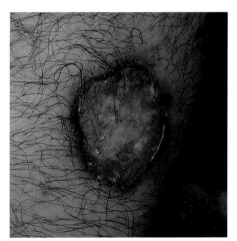

Fig. 36.2 Pyoderma gangrenosum. (From Paller AS, et al. *Hurwitz clinical pediatric dermatology: a textbook of skin disorders of childhood and adolescence*. 5th ed. Philadelphia, Elsevier; 2016.)

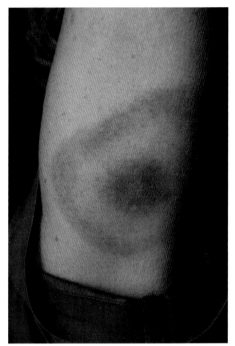

Fig. 36.3 Erythema chronicum migrans. (Courtesy James Gathany; Content Providers CDC/James Gathany—this media comes from the Centers for Disease Control and Prevention's Public Health Image Library [PHIL], with identification number #9875. From Borchers AT, Keen CL, Huntley AC, et al. Lyme disease: a rigorous review of diagnostic criteria and treatment. J Autoimmun. 2015;57:82–115.)

- Sweet syndrome: also called acute febrile neutrophilic dermatoses is well-demarcated red papules on head, neck and dorsum of the hands seen in haematological cancers (Fig. 36.7).
- Paraneoplastic pemphigus: severe oral and conjunctival ulceration (Fig. 36.8) associated with leukaemia, bronchogenic cancers and skin cancers (melanoma, basal cell carcinoma).
- Secondary skin metastases, which are most often from breast, kidney and lung cancers and non-Hodgkin lymphoma and leukaemia.

SKIN DISEASE

Psoriasis

Psoriasis is a chronic, relapsing, autoimmune inflammatory skin disease that occurs in roughly 2% of the UK population. It affects men and women equally, and even though it may occur at any age, it usually manifests itself before the age of 35 years. It presents

and the neck (V sign) or with Gottron sign (red, scaly papules at finger joints) (Fig. 36.5).
- Acquired ichthyosis: dry, scaly skin, associated with lymphoma.
- Thrombophlebitis migrans (Trousseau sign): seen with pancreatic and lung cancer and involves thrombophlebitis often recurring in a different location over time (Fig. 36.6).

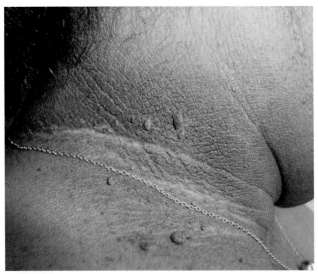

Fig. 36.4 Erythema chronicum migrans. (Source: © E. Baubion.)

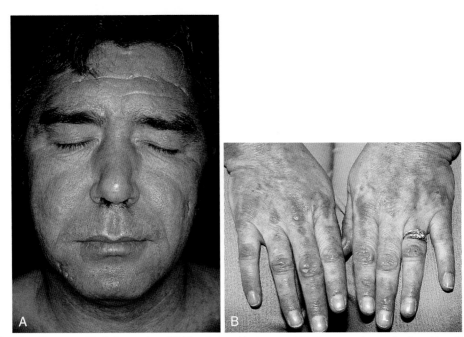

Fig. 36.5 (A) Facial erythema and heliotrope sign. (B) Classic hand lesions and Gottron papules on the knuckles. (From High WA, Prok LD. *Dermatology Secrets,* 6th ed. Elsevier; 2021.)

with a multifactorial pattern of inheritance, where 30% of cases are thought to have a familial correlation. The remaining cases may be triggered by multiple environmental factors, including sunlight and infection (streptococcal and HIV infection), stress, trauma or drugs (e.g., lithium, chloroquine and β-blockers).

The most common type is chronic plaque psoriasis. Other types include guttate (widespread raindrop lesions usually after streptococcal infection) (Fig. 36.9), seborrhoeic (nasolabial and retroauricular areas), pustular (palmar–plantar), flexural (body flexures) and erythrodermic (widespread body redness).

It is a T cell-mediated disease characterized by hyperproliferation of keratinocytes and blood vessels within the skin producing epidermal thickening.

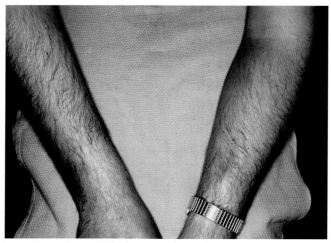

Fig. 36.6 Thrombophlebitis migrans. (From James WD, Elston DM, Treat JR, Rosenbach MA. *Andrews' Diseases of the Skin: Clinical Dermatology,* 13th ed. Elsevier; 2020.)

Clinical features

The lesions in psoriasis are typically clearly defined, salmon-pink plaques topped by a silvery scale, most frequently found on the extensor surfaces of the limbs (e.g., elbows and knees) and over the scalp. They may be severely itchy. Plaques may differ in size and shape, and can be discoid, serpiginous or circinate (ring-like). Scale scraping can accentuate the plaque or cause pinpoint bleeding (Auspitz sign) (Fig. 36.10). New lesions often occur at the site of injury to skin typically within 1–2 weeks (Köbner reaction). Most patients will have nail changes at some point in time. These include pitting, onycholysis and subungual hyperkeratosis. Thirty percent will have associated psoriatic arthropathy – symmetrical polyarthritis, asymmetrical oligomonoarthritis, psoriatic spondylosis and arthritis mutilans (distal interphalangeal joints flexion deformity) (Fig. 36.11).

The prognosis of the condition can be difficult to establish, with frequent treatment failure and recurrent relapses; however, in 75% of patients skin involvement responds to treatment with creams alone. Complications of disease are often associated with significant physiological stress and lowered quality of life.

Management

Education and avoidance of precipitating factors is very important in management of psoriasis. For mild conditions, emollient therapy and reassurance are sufficient. In more troublesome cases, topical therapy can be highly effective. Corticosteroids are most effective treatment when used consecutively for 8 weeks. Other agents include vitamin D analogues. Coal tar preparations and vitamin A analogues are of limited benefit. Phototherapy and photochemotherapy can be used in extensive disease. Systemic agents are reserved for severe or refractory disease and require regular blood testing to check for medication toxicity (Table 36.1).

Eczema/dermatitis

This is a nonspecific inflammation of the skin characterized by papules and vesicles on an erythematous base. It is a chronic and relapsing condition, and in most cases presents in childhood. It has strong environmental and genetic correlates, which are summarized in Table 36.2. Different types can be recognized, but by far the most common is atopic dermatitis (Table 36.3).

Clinical features

It affects around 1 in 5 children and 1 in 10 adults. The characteristics of the condition change with age. In infants there are exudative, crusted, itchy areas over extensor surfaces and cheeks. By childhood and adulthood, the lesions are more localized and are seen on the flexor areas of antecubital and popliteal fossae, wrists and ankles and the face and neck. There is pruritus of the inflamed skin, and long-term scratching often leads to thickened hard areas (Fig. 36.12). Skin can often become inflamed, and it is important to look for signs of underlying infection.

Investigations to characterize atopic eczema include prick tests for common allergens and raised serum immunoglobulin E level (condition association with asthma and hay fever). Common complications include infections with bacteria (*Staphylococcus aureus*), viruses (herpes simplex virus (HSV), eczema herpeticum) or fungi. Eczema is often a relapsing condition that gradually abates with adult life. By the early teenage years, atopic eczema will have cleared in 60% to 70% of individuals, bearing in mind predictors of worsening prognosis, which include early onset and co-occurrence of asthma.

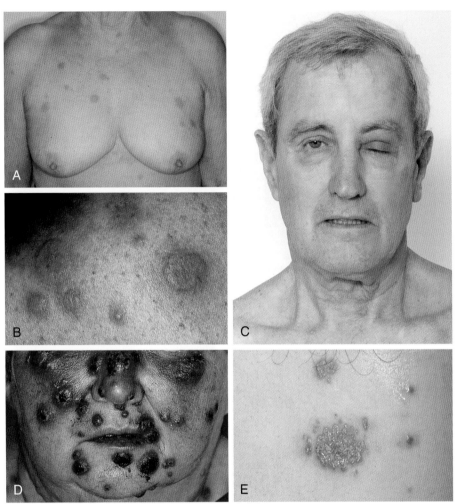

Fig. 36.7 Sweet syndrome. (A) Scattered edematous pink papules and plaques on the chest. (B) Markedly edematous plaques on the upper back, some of which are pseudovesicular while others are becoming bullous. (C) The periocular lesion demonstrates how some lesions can mimic cellulitis (pseudocellulitis). This patient also had neutrophilic esophageal ulcerations and subsequently developed colon cancer. (D) Central hemorrhagic crusts within facial plaques. (E) Plaques can also have a pseudomammillated appearance due to the associated edema. (A, C, Courtesy, Mark Davis, MD; B, D, Courtesy, Kalman Watsky, MD; E, Courtesy, Mark Davis, MD.)

Management

Education and reassurance with regard to effective treatments are paramount. Advice regarding lifestyle, environmental adaptations, recognition of irritants and flare-ups will decrease physical and psychological stress associated with the condition. Medical treatment is often long-term but successful and concentrates on the use of emollients, steroids and immunomodulators, which protect skin from breaking and concurrent infections:

- Bathing once daily in warm water with addition of bath oils for 5 to 10 minutes is recommended. Soap should not be used.

- Emollients: best applied on moist skin, liberally and frequently (every 4 hours). The general rule of thumb states 500 g of moisturizer should be used each week for an adult and 250 g for a child.
- Topical steroids should not be used long-term (2 weeks at a time), and in cases of atopic eczema not more than twice a day. A mild steroid is used for mild exacerbation and on more sensitive skin areas such as the face. More potent steroids are required for severe flare-ups and lichenified areas.
- Antibiotics are used if there is underlying infection.

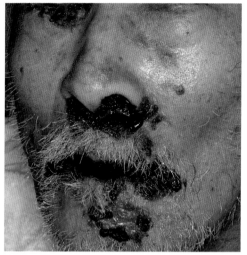

Fig. 36.8 Paraneoplastic pemphigus. (Courtesy Department of Dermatology, Keio University School of Medicine, Tokyo, Japan.)

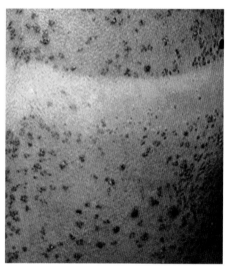

Fig. 36.9 Guttate psoriasis. (Reprinted with permission from Bolognia JL, et al. *Dermatology*, 3rd ed.)

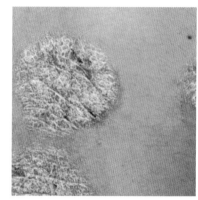

Fig. 36.10 Plaque psoriasis with Auspitz sign. (Reprinted with permission from Bolognia JL, et al. *Dermatology*, 3rd ed.)

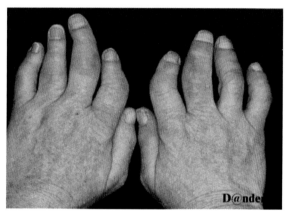

Fig. 36.11 Arthritis mutilans with psoriatic nail changes. (Reprinted with permission from Niels K. Veien.)

CLINICAL NOTES

Referral to a specialist is recommended when diagnosis has become uncertain, the disease is not controlled and flare-ups are frequent, or if the patient has marked psychological stress.

- Bandages containing ichthammol paste and zinc oxide can reduce pruritus.
- Phototherapy, azathioprine, ciclosporin, alitretinoin or oral steroids should only be used for severe refractory eczema and under specialist care.
- Immunomodulators such as tacrolimus and pimecrolimus are used when eczema does not respond to strong corticosteroids or they are contraindicated.

Acne vulgaris

Acne vulgaris a disorder of pilosebaceous follicles stimulated during puberty by androgens to produce increased amounts of sebum. This can consequently lead to blockage of ducts, which can be infected by commensal *Propionibacterium acnes*. Distended by sebum and desquamated keratinocytes, follicles become comedones that can be described as open (blackheads) or closed (whiteheads) (Fig. 36.13). Acne is most

Table 36.1 Available management options of psoriasis

	Agent	Description
Topical	Emollients	Apply three or four times per day May need as much as 500 g per week Can include creams, shampoos and bath preparations
	Corticosteroids	Avoid long-term use
	Vitamin D analogues	More effective when used in combination with corticosteroids. Be aware of hypercalcaemia if overused (e.g., Dovonex)
Phototherapy	Narrowband ultraviolet B	Used two or three times per week Advise not to use sunbeds as self-treatment
	Photochemotherapy	Photosensitive drug (e.g., PUVA) used two or three times per week with 2–4 weekly maintenance therapy
Systemic	Methotrexate	First-line treatment but with several side effects and so needs close monitoring
	Ciclosporin	Not to be used as 'flare-up' treatment
	Other agents	Retinoids (acitretin) Fumaric acid esters Hydroxycarbamide
	Biological modulators	Third-line treatment in unresponsive disease/patient is intolerant Examples include infliximab, etanercept and efalizumab

PUVA, *Psoralen and ultraviolet A.*

Table 36.2 Most common triggers of eczema

	Triggers	Description
Environmental factors	Allergens	Dietary and inhaled allergens, including nuts or dust mites (most commonly associated with eczema in children)
	Irritants	Both contact irritants (rough fabric such as wool) and chemical irritants (soaps, creams etc.)
	Infections	*Staphylococcus aureus*
	Temperature	Extremes of temperature and humidity with most patients improving in summer
	Diet	Food allergens as well as irritant foods such as chillies and chocolate
Endogenous factors	Genetic	Genetic mutation affecting production of filaggrin (protein required for maturation of stratum corneum keratinocytes)
	Hormones	Mainly in women (deterioration in pregnancy, premenstrual flare-ups)
	Stress	Exacerbated and prolonged flare-ups, poor healing

prominent on the face and upper trunk and usually abates after adolescence.

Acne is usually mild and self-limiting, but if it persists both topical and systemic treatments can be considered (Table 36.4). First-line treatment includes a trial of antimicrobial and comedolytic agents, salicylic or azelaic acids and benzoyl peroxide. Topical antibiotics and retinoids can be used alone or in combination with benzoyl peroxide. Systemic treatments often take long to show improvement and should be continued for 3 to 4 months. Options include oral antibiotics, antiandrogens and retinoids. Alternatively, blue light and 140-nm laser therapy have been found to show results. Severe acne is a serious, disfiguring condition, and its management should be coordinated by dermatology specialists.

COMMUNICATION

Even mild acne can be a distressing condition for young people and requires a sympathetic systemic approach. It is important to reassure patients there are effective treatments, and that the options are vast.

Table 36.3 Different presentations of eczema

Type of dermatitis	Characteristics
Contact dermatitis	Erythema, vesicles, fissuring due to contact with irritant/allergen
Seborrhoeic dermatitis	Erythematous, scaly, itchy, yellow eruption mostly on oily areas of skin (scalp, flexures, face)
Discoid eczema	Round, itchy, vesicular lesions around body
Dyshidrotic eczema	Itchy, erythematous, vesicular eruptions mostly on palms, soles and fingers

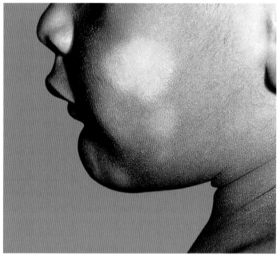

Fig. 36.12 Atopic dermatitis in a child. (Reprinted with permission from Bolognia JL, et al. *Dermatology*, 3rd ed.)

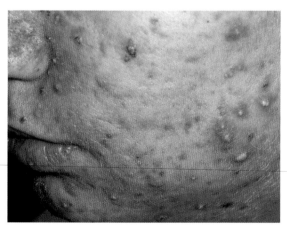

Fig. 36.13 Acne vulgaris. (Reprinted with permission from Bolognia JL, et al. *Dermatology*, 3rd ed.)

Actinic keratosis

This is a thickened scaly growth induced by ultraviolet light. It often begins as a small rough lesion that then extends and progresses to erythematous plaque that can sometimes differentiate to a hyperpigmented area or hyperkeratotic growth (cutaneous horn). It has a malignant potential and if left untreated can progress to squamous cell carcinoma (SCC) or carcinoma in situ (Bowen disease). It is seen more commonly in light-skinned individuals on areas most exposed to the sun. It is characterized by ultraviolet-induced gene mutations within keratinocytes that share common histological features with SCC. It can resolve spontaneously, stay chronic and stable or progress to skin cancer (5%–10%).

Treatment is by limitation of sun exposure, 5-fluorouracil cream (cytotoxic agent), imiquimod cream (immune enhancing agent), cryotherapy, photodynamic therapy and curettage or excision.

Seborrhoeic keratosis

This a common condition characterized by benign warty hyperpigmented raised lesions associated with ageing. The lesions have 'stuck-on' appearance with a usually well-defined border. Their surface often shows granules of visible keratin and can be covered by greasy scale. Most lesions are seen on the trunk and face, and they are usually asymptomatic; often, however, they can become irritated and consequently infected due to their size.

The condition is benign and management concentrates around reassurance and cosmetic removal by cryotherapy, curettage or shave excision.

Herpes simplex

Two types of HSV have been identified. HSV-1 usually causes cold sores, but in the United Kingdom is also the leading cause of genital herpes. HSV-2 is associated with recurrent anogenital infection (Fig. 36.14). Primary infection is usually asymptomatic, following which the virus survives latent in cell bodies of nerve ganglia. Reactivation, which may occur in times of stress or immunosuppression, causes a burning, stinging neuralgia, which precedes or accompanies the development of erythematous vesicular lesions. Diagnosis is clinical, but vesicular fluid or scrapings can show HSV. HSV antibodies can also be detected by serology in asymptomatic individuals.

Transmission is through contact with infected secretions on a mucosal surface or lesion on another anatomical site. Treatment is supportive, with pain relief and skin soothing. Topical antivirals have been found to have little effect and therefore are not recommended. Oral therapies should be started within 5 days of the onset of symptoms and include

Table 36.4 Different types of acne treatment

Treatment	Type	Action
Topical	Salicylic acid Azelaic acid	Keratolytic preparations, effective initial treatments. May cause irritation and depigmentation
	Benzoyl peroxide	A concentration of 5% to be used initially then increased to 10%. Very effective with antiseptic properties, may cause irritation
	Antibiotics	Usually erythromycin and tetracyclines used in combination with, e.g., benzoyl peroxide
	Retinoids	Isotretinoin and tretinoin are antiinflammatory and reduce comedones. Patient need to avoid exposure to strong sunlight and pregnancy
Systemic	Antibiotics	There is no strong evidence to prefer one antibiotic to another, but generally doxycycline and clindamycin are first choices
	Antiandrogens	The combined oral contraceptive pill is an effective treatment for acne. Dianette is licensed solely for use in acne as it has an associated much higher risk of thrombosis
	Retinoids	Isotretinoin is very effective in decreasing sebum production. Its toxicity and side effects, however, allow its use only under specialist care (teratogenic, dry mouth, myalgia)

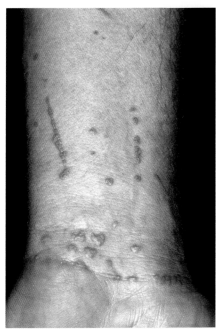

Fig. 36.14 Lichen planus. (From Micheletti RG, James WD, Elston DM, McMahon PJ. *Andrews' Diseases of the Skin Clinical Atlas*, 2nd ed. Elsevier; 2023.)

aciclovir and valaciclovir. Prophylactic oral antivirals are used for patients with recurrent infections. Intravenous aciclovir treatment can be used in severe or immunocompromised patients at high risk of developing HSV complications such as encephalitis.

Herpes (varicella) zoster

Primary infection with varicella zoster virus causes chickenpox (varicella), usually in childhood, that presents as fever and widespread vesiculopapular rash. Following recovery, the virus lies dormant in the dorsal root ganglia until immunosuppression or illness causes reactivation, termed 'shingles'. Typically, dermatomal pain and paraesthesia (preeruptive phase) precede the appearance of maculopapular vesicular lesions restricted to that dermatome (eruptive phase). The chronic phase is characterized by persistent or recurring eruptions at the site of healed infection.

It is most commonly seen in the thoracic region or in the ophthalmic division of the trigeminal nerve (trigeminal neuralgia). Treatment is with appropriate analgesia and oral antivirals (aciclovir, valaciclovir, famciclovir), and should be started within 72 hours of the onset of rash. Intravenously administered aciclovir should be considered in immunocompromised patients and those with ophthalmic involvement.

Ramsay Hunt syndrome is when varicella zoster virus affects the geniculate ganglion of the facial nerve and includes the classical triad of ipsilateral facial paralysis, otalgia and vesicles in the auditory canal or on the auricle.

> **HINTS AND TIPS**
>
> Shingles is confined to one dermatome only, which is why any rash crossing the midline is not shingles!

Lichen planus

This mainly affects middle-aged adults. The cause is unknown but may be related to disturbances of immune function. Lichen

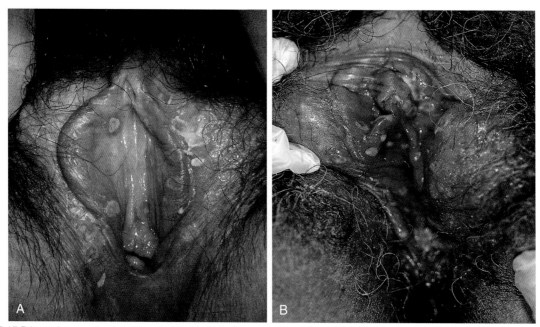

Fig. 36.15 Primary herpes simplex. (From Habif TP. *Clinical dermatology*, 4th ed. Philadelphia, Mosby; 2004)

planus-like reactions occur with certain drugs, such as sulphonamides, sulphonylureas, methyldopa, thiazides, β-blockers and drugs that alter immune function (e.g., antimalarials, gold salts, penicillamine).

The lesions are pruritic, purple, polygonal and planar or flat-topped papules, with a largely peripheral and symmetrical distribution most commonly seen on extensor surfaces, genitalia or mucosal membranes (Fig. 36.15). Wickham striae (fine white lacy lines coursing over the papule) are characteristic of the disease, and it can be precipitated by trauma (Köbner phenomenon). Postinflammatory hyperpigmentation and scarring can occur with chronic disease. Lesions usually last for 9 to 18 months if untreated. Treatment can be with steroids, phototherapy and retinoids but is often at best only partially effective.

Erythema multiforme

This is a hypersensitivity of the skin to infection or drugs. It presents as a reaction characterized by target lesion (circular with central intensity or blistering). Mucosal membranes can be involved (if >1 erythema multiforme major). It usually starts on the extremities and symmetrically spreads centrally. It may be itchy but is nontender. Management concentrates on withdrawal or treatment of the precipitant and skin conditioning with steroids. The most common infectious agents causing the condition include viruses (HSV), mycoplasma pneumonia and fungi. Precipitating drugs include barbiturates, penicillins, sulphonamides, phenothiazines, NSAIDs and anticonvulsants.

Stevens–Johnson syndrome and toxic epidermal necrolysis

These conditions are severe dermatological reactions to medication (e.g., allopurinol, antibiotics, antiepileptics) or infection. They range from mild to severe mucosal membrane involvement and form a spectrum of conditions described as 'severe cutaneous adverse reactions' that constitute dermatological emergencies. They usually start with a prodrome period of mild upper respiratory tract infection, fever and malaise but mucocutaneous lesions quickly develop. Lesions can present as macules or papules that then become vesicles with extensive erythema. Characteristically, target lesions are present and Nikolsky sign is positive (blistering of skin within minutes of applied pressure).

Skin involvement differentiates between Stevens–Johnson syndrome (<10% of skin involvement) and toxic epidermal necrolysis (TEN) (>30% of skin involvement). The only approved treatment is supportive with optimal nutrition, fluid balance and prevention of infection. The offending medication should be stopped, and any causative infection should be treated. Use of corticosteroids is controversial but recent trials suggest intravenously administered immunoglobulin may have a role. Mortality in TEN is 30% to 40%.

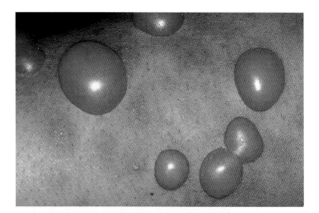

DRESS syndrome (drug reaction with eosinophilia and systemic symptoms) is a severe drug reaction with extensive rash, internal organ involvement, lymphadenopathy, eosinophilia and atypical lymphocytosis. Despite cessation of the offensive drug, flairs may continue to occur. It is a part of drug hypersensitivity syndrome that can result in multiorgan failure. Treatment is with corticosteroids and ciclosporin.

Pemphigus vulgaris and bullous pemphigoid

These are autoimmune, bullous conditions affecting mainly people aged over 60 years. In pemphigus, antibodies are directed against an epidermal cell adhesion molecule, causing flaccid, fragile blisters to develop within the epidermis. It affects the mucosa and skin, with denuded areas remaining after the blisters rupture (Fig. 36.16). Treatment is with topical steroids found to be as effective as oral steroids in this condition.

In pemphigoid, the antibodies affect the basement membrane, leading to blisters between the dermis and epidermis. It may occur spontaneously or in response to medication. The blisters are tense and widespread, occurring particularly in flexures (Fig. 36.17). First-line treatment is with monoclonal antibodies (rituximab) (Fig. 36.18).

Vitiligo

Vitiligo is characteristically well-demarcated, roughly symmetrical areas of depigmentation. There is loss of melanocytes, thought to be due to an autoimmune process. Around 30% of cases are associated with organ-specific autoimmune disease (e.g., Addison disease, pernicious anaemia, alopecia, Hashimoto thyroiditis).

NEOPLASTIC DISEASE

Basal cell carcinoma

This is the most common, locally invasive, slow-growing, malignant lesion arising from skin follicles. The lesions mainly occur in areas of long-term sun exposure such as the face, especially at the side of the nose or in the periorbital skin, head and neck. Risk factors include sun exposure, increasing age, male sex and fair skin. Early lesions are often small and pearly with a raised area of telangiectasia that then progresses to classic rodent ulcer with an indurated border (Fig. 36.19).

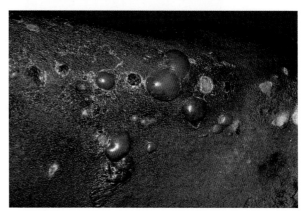

Fig. 36.16 Pemphigus vulgaris. (From Reeves JT, Maibach H. *Clinical dermatology illustrated: a regional approach*, 2nd ed. Sydney: MacLennan & Petty Pty Ltd, ©1991.)

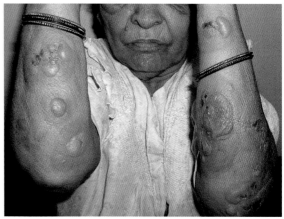

Fig. 36.17 Bullous pemphigoid. (Courtesy Shyam Verma, MBBS, DVD.)

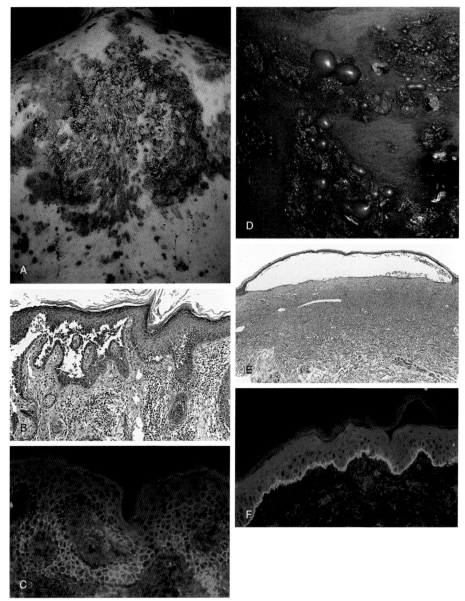

Fig. 36.18 Pemphigus vulgaris (PV) versus bullous pemphigoid (BP). (A, B, E, Courtesy, Lorenzo Cerroni, MD; C, F, Courtesy, Christine Ko, MD; D, Courtesy, Julie V. Schaffer, MD.)

There are several subtypes of basal cell carcinoma, presenting with different characteristics (Table 36.5). Treatment is by surgical excision, cryotherapy, topical therapy (5-fluorouracil, imiquimod) or photodynamic therapy can be used.

Squamous cell carcinoma

This tumour arises from keratinizing cells of the epidermis or its appendages and is most commonly seen on damaged or chronically irritated skin, especially areas of sun exposure. It is invasive and can metastasize to other organs. Risk factors include long-term sun exposure, chemical carcinogens (arsenic, chromium), human papillomavirus (HPV) infection, immunodeficiency and chronic inflammatory conditions (Marjolin ulcer).

It presents as hyperkeratotic, crusted and indurated tumour that often ulcerate, although the clinical appearance is very variable (Fig. 36.20). Bowen disease and keratoacanthoma can resemble the disease and may progress to SCC. Investigations include

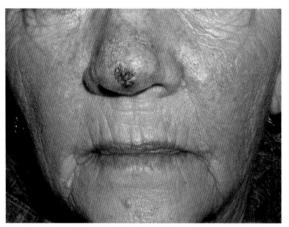

Fig. 36.19 Classic appearance of basal cell carcinoma. (Reprinted with permission from Bolognia JL, et al. *Dermatology*, 3rd ed.)

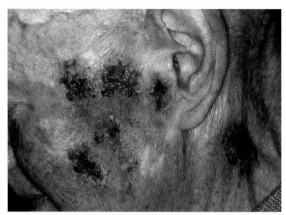

Fig. 36.20 Squamous cell carcinoma. (Reprinted with permission from Bolognia JL, et al. *Dermatology*, 3rd ed.)

Table 36.5 Types of basal cell carcinoma

Type	Characteristics
Nodular	Large, pearly, solitary, erythematous nodule with telangiectatic vessels often on the face. May ulcerate
Superficial	Usually multiple on upper trunk and limbs but also on face (more often in women). Presents as erythematous scaly plaques with central healing and well-demarcated, thread-like border. Rarely invasive
Morphoeic (sclerosing or infiltrative)	Most common on mid-facial sites with aggressive poorly defined borders. Characterized by yellow plaques. Often presents late and can recur after treatment
Pigmented	Blue, brown or grey nodular or superficial lesion, seen more often with darker skin
Basosquamous	Mixed with SCC. Potentially more aggressive than other BCC types

BCC, *Basal cell carcinoma;* SCC, *squamous cell carcinoma.*

skin biopsy and imaging to determine the extent of the disease in large tumours. Treatment is surgical excision and radiotherapy. Electrochemotherapy is useful in widespread disease.

Malignant melanoma

This tumour is increasing in incidence, and occurs particularly in fair-skinned people who are exposed to sunlight. It results from the cancerous growth of melanocytes most commonly on the skin, but melanomas affecting almost all organs in the body have been described. If melanoma is confined to the epidermis it is known as 'melanoma in situ' and does not spread to surrounding tissues. If it has infiltrated through the dermis it can metastasize and becomes invasive melanoma.

There are four types of skin melanoma: superficial spreading (most common), nodular, lentigo maligna and acral lentiginous (Fig. 36.21). Risk factors include previous invasive melanoma, naevi, family history and sun exposure. The properties that help identify malignant disease are:

- rapid enlargement
- diameter greater than 7 mm
- bleeding or crusting
- increasing variegated pigmentation, particularly blue-black or grey
- an indistinct border or irregular border
- sensory change
- small 'satellite' lesions around the principal lesion

Prognosis is related to the depth of a tumour assessed histologically (Breslow thickness), and worsens with increased depth. Metastasis are common, and in patients with in-transit metastasis, the 5-year survival rate is only 30%.

Prevention when considering melanoma management is paramount, with avoidance of exposure to direct sunlight and use of effective sunscreen lotions. Self-examination should be practised, and people should be aware of the warning signs and symptoms. Treatment is by excision (definite), radiotherapy and chemotherapy/immunotherapy.

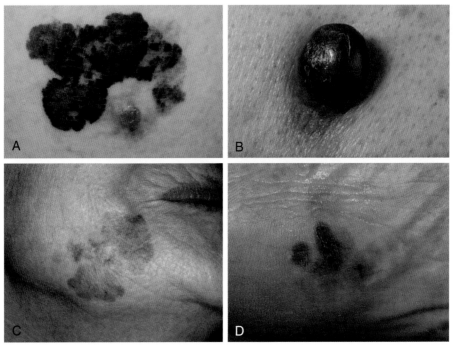

Fig. 36.21 Types of malignant melanoma: (A) superficial spreading, (B) nodular, (C) lentigo maligna and (D) acral lentiginous. (Reprinted with permission from Bolognia JL, et al. *Dermatology*, 3rd ed.)

HINTS AND TIPS

Breslow thickness (thickness of a tumour) assesses risk of spread of melanoma: less than 0.75 m, very low; 0.76–1 mm, low; 1–4 mm, high; more than 4 mm, very high.

INFECTIONS

Impetigo

This is a superficial skin infection with *Staphylococcus aureus* or β-haemolytic streptococcus, usually seen in children. Lesions begin as papules before progressing to vesicles (Fig. 36.22). These may form bullae or may break down to form a thick golden crust. Treatment is with topical and oral antibiotics, most often flucloxacillin. Recently treatment with hydrogen peroxide 1% topical ointment is recommended in favour of antibiotics for localized non bullous infection.

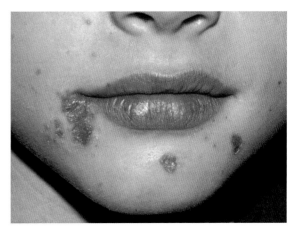

Fig. 36.22 Impetigo in a child. (Reprinted with permission from Bolognia JL, et al. *Dermatology*, 3rd ed.)

Cellulitis

This is an acute painful and potentially dangerous infection affecting skin and subcutaneous tissue. When only the dermis and superficial subcutaneous tissues are involved, cellulitis

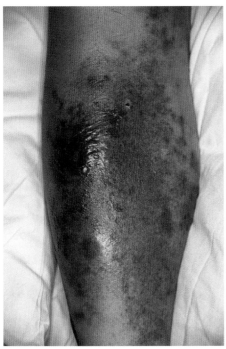

Fig. 36.23 Cellulitis of lower limb. (Reprinted with permission from Bolognia JL, et al. *Dermatology*, 3rd ed.)

takes the form of erysipelas (superficial cellulitis). Cellulitis manifests itself as erythematous, warm, oedematous rash (Fig. 36.23). *Staphylococcus* and *Streptococcus* are the most common causative organisms, but a range of aerobic and anaerobic bacteria can also be involved. Risk factors include breaks in the skin (e.g., due to trauma, ulcers or drug use), previous skin infection, elderly age, oedema, diabetes, obesity and immunosuppression. Treatment is with antibiotics (flucloxacillin/clarithromycin), and in severe cases is given intravenously.

CLINICAL NOTES

Be aware that cellulitis can very quickly spread and cause sepsis. It is useful to mark the area of infection and look for signs of spreading and tracking, which may be suggestive of ineffective treatment.

Necrotizing fasciitis

This is a potentially limb/life-threatening surgical emergency that is characterized by infection affecting one or more of the deep soft tissue compartments (dermis, subcutaneous tissue, fascia, muscle). It is often caused by group A streptococci but between 55% and 80% of cases involve more than one pathogen. Risk factors include skin injury, an underlying condition such as alcohol abuse, obesity, renal disease, diabetes and immunosuppression.

The skin is often affected but may be spared. It presents as local pain that is disproportionate to the clinical picture, rapidly advancing swelling, skin discolouration, crepitus and neurovascular compromise with raised lactate levels. Progression is rapid and unremitting; mortality is 30%. Treatment is with intravenous antibiotics and immediate surgical debridement.

BURNS

Burn is an injury caused by thermal, chemical, electrical or radiation energy. Each year estimated 0.5% to 1% of the UK population suffer from burns. Commonest causes include carelessness (35%), alcohol, and recreational accidents, most often burns occur at home. Flame burns are the most common burns in adults, scalds in children. Common complications of burns include hypothermia, infection, chronic scarring and psychological impact. The prognosis and healing are dependent on the characteristics, extent of the burn and patient comorbidities.

Clinical features

Depending on the depth of tissue damage burns can be classified as superficial or deep (Fig. 36.24). They present with characteristic presentations (Table 36.6).

Superficial burns have the ability to heal themselves by epithelization and may either be epidermal or dermal. Epidermal burns include only the epidermis and are most commonly caused by sun (sunburn). Dermal superficial burns are only to the epithelium and superficial layers of dermis (papillary dermis) and its hallmark is a blister. They heal within 7 and 14 days, respectively.

Mid-dermal burns heal much slower and present with different degrees of tissue necrosis that result in scarring. This is due to variable damage of dermal vascular plexus.

Deep burns are more severe and affect deep dermis or are full thickness. They will either not heal spontaneously or only heal after a prolonged period with significant scarring. Deep dermal burns are characterized by 'capillary blush phenomenon' that demonstrates the capillary plexus has been destroyed. Full thickness burns extend beyond the skin to subcutaneous tissue and is characterized by waxy, white, charred appearance with eschar (coagulated, dead skin).

Management

Immediate management is first aid that focuses on stopping the burning process and cooling the wound ideally with running water between 8°C and 25°C for 20 minutes. This is effective within 3 hours of the time of burn. Advanced Life Support ABCDE approach should be used for patients with focus on assessment of total body surface area (TBSA) of burn, appropriate warming, analgesia and fluid resuscitation. The greater the TBSA of the burn, the greater the mortality. It is calculated by 'rule of nines' (Fig. 36.25). Long-term management concentrates around wound management with specialist dressings and surgical debridement and reconstruction with skin grafts, xenografts or biological skin substitutes.

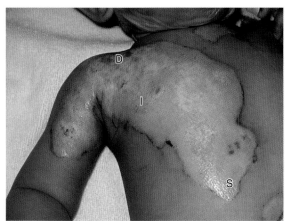

Fig. 36.24 Scald over the chest and shoulder of a child showing heterogeneity of burn depth. D, Deep (leathery, white appearance); I, mid-dermal (dark pink); S, superficial (bright red). (From Enoch S, Roshan A, Shah M. *Emergency and early management of burns and scalds*. BMJ 338:937–941, 2009.)

HINTS AND TIPS

TBSA is essential when estimating volume of fluid resuscitation needed for a burns patient. Modified Parklands formula (3–4 mL of Hartmann's solution × weight kg × % TBSA) determines fluid to be given to compensate for fluid lost as a result of burn. Half of calculated fluid should be given in the first 8 hours; the rest over the next 16 hours from the time of injury.

CLINICAL NOTES

Inhalation injury needs to be considered with burns as this is a potentially fatal injury. Some signs and symptoms include burns to mouth, nose, eyes; singed nasal hair; nasal flare; mucosal oedema; respiratory difficulty. Treatment is with high-flow oxygen and intubation.

Table 36.6 Characteristics of burn depth

Depth	Colour	Capillary refill	Blisters	Sensation
Epidermal	Red	Yes	No	Painful
Superficial dermal	Pale pink	Yes	Yes	Painful
Mid-dermal	Dark pink	Sluggish	Yes	+/–
Deep dermal	Blotchy red	No	+/–	No
Full thickness	White	No	No	No

Rule of Nines

Ignore simple erythema

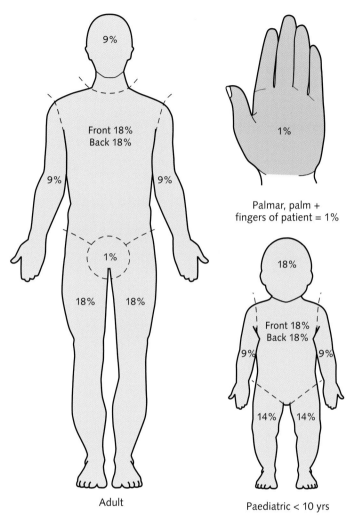

Palmar, palm +
fingers of patient = 1%

Adult

Paediatric < 10 yrs

Fig. 36.25 Rule of Nines: determining the total body surface area. (From Fulde S, Fulde G. *Emergency Medicine: The Principles of Practice*, 7th ed. Elsevier; 2020.)

Chapter Summary

- Skin disease and skin manifestations of systemic disease are vast and commonly diverse. As a clinician, it is important to familiarize yourself with common presentations and know how to assess skin for a sinister cause.
- Skin is our biggest organ and very often manifests pathological changes, and treatment of the underlying cause is vital for the best outcome. It is also important to consider the impact skin condition has on an individual in both physical and psychological manners as these are often intertwined.

UKMLA Conditions
Acne vulgaris
Atopic dermatitis and eczema
Basal cell carcinoma
Cellulitis
Contact dermatitis
Impetigo
Herpes simplex virus
Malignant melanoma
Necrotising fasciitis
Psoriasis
Squamous cell carcinoma

UKMLA Presentations
Burns
Chronic rash
Nail changes

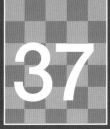
ANAEMIA

Diagnosis

Anaemia is not a diagnosis but a consequence of an underlying problem. Detailed history and examination are essential when considering the cause. Anaemia is defined as:

- Haemoglobin (Hb) <130 g/L in men over the age of 15 years
- Hb <120 g/L in nonpregnant women over the age of 15 years
- Hb <120 g/L in children aged 12 to 14 years
- Hb <110 g/L in pregnancy and <100 g/L postpartum

Following initial Hb estimation, further investigations are needed to establish the most likely cause. Remember that there may be more than one cause of anaemia. For example, folate deficiency and iron deficiency may be present together (e.g., in coeliac disease). In other diseases, such as rheumatoid arthritis, there are several potential causes of anaemia.

> **RED FLAG**
>
> Remember that the rate of drop in haemoglobin level is as important as the level itself; if blood loss is slow and chronic, very low levels can be tolerated with only mild symptoms. If the blood loss is acute, a fall of just 20 g/L can cause significant symptoms.

Management

The anaemia will recur if the underlying problem persists; therefore the cause should be sought and appropriately managed. How the anaemia is treated will depend on the type of anaemia and the presence of complications.

Iron deficiency anaemia

This is the most common cause of anaemia worldwide and is a result of long-term negative iron balance. The anaemia is microcytic (small) hypochromic (pale) and investigations show reduced mean cell volume (MCV) and mean cell haemoglobin (MCH). Serum ferritin below 30 µg/L is diagnostic for iron deficiency. Table 37.1 outlines the causes of iron deficiency anaemia.

Iron replacement

Addressing the underlying cause in the first instance is important. If a dietary deficiency is considered, commence a balanced diet with iron-rich foods (dark, green-leaf vegetables, prunes, red meat). Oral iron replacement therapy (e.g., ferrous sulphate) is the mainstay treatment. Hb levels should be rechecked within 4 weeks after initiation of treatment with the aim of an Hb rise of 20 g/L every 3 to 4 weeks. Once Hb concentration returns to normal, treatment should continue for 3 months to allow total body iron stores to be replenished.

Side effects of iron supplements include nausea, diarrhoea or constipation and abdominal pain. The stools usually become very dark or black. If side effects occur, the dose can be reduced or the preparation changed. Intravenous iron therapy can be given if oral therapy is not tolerated or if iron replacement and correction of the anaemia is time sensitive (e.g., cancer patients before major operation).

> **COMMUNICATION**
>
> Ensure patients are clear that over-the-counter preparations do not contain sufficient iron for an adequate replacement. Notably, the replacement must continue for at least 3 months to sufficiently replenish iron stores.

Vitamin B$_{12}$ and folate deficiency anaemia

This results in megaloblastic anaemia. Large immature and dysfunctional RBCs result from defects in erythropoiesis in the bone marrow and inhibition of DNA synthesis in turn halting progress through the cell cycle. Although it can be challenging to determine vitamin levels diagnostic of deficiency, it is generally accepted that folate <3 µg/L and serum cobalamin (surrogate of vitamin B$_{12}$) <200 ng/L are highly suggestive. See Table 37.2 for causes of vitamin B$_{12}$ and folate deficiency.

Table 37.1 Causes of iron deficiency anaemia

Cause	Features
Dietary deficiency	• Rarely a cause on its own.
Malabsorption	• Dietary iron is absorbed primarily in the duodenum • Coeliac disease, gastrectomy, *Helicobacter pylori*, oesophagitis, schistosomiasis, hookworm, IBD
Increased losses	• Chronic blood loss • GI tract (angiodysplasia, ulceration, cancer, NSAIDs, antiplatelets, anticoagulants) • Uterus (menstruation) • Acute haemorrhage
Increased requirement	• Pregnancy, menstruation
Other	• Epistaxis, medication

GI, *Gastrointestinal;* IBD, *inflammatory bowel disease;* NSAIDs, *nonsteroidal antiinflammatory drugs.*

Table 37.2 Causes of vitamin B_{12} and folate deficiency

Vitamin B_{12}	Folate

• Dietary deficiency
• Malabsorption (absorbed in the ileum)
  • Achlorhydria
  • Deficient intrinsic factor (produced by the parietal cells in the stomach)
  • Coeliac disease
  • Nitrous oxide exposure
• Increased needs
  • AIDS
  • Haemolysis
	• Dietary deficiency
	• Malabsorption (mainly absorbed in the jejunum)
	  • Coeliac disease
	  • Fructose malabsorption
	• Increased needs
	  • Pregnancy
	  • Lactation
	• Drugs and toxins
	  • Methotrexate, anticonvulsants, metformin, 5-fluorouracil, hydroxyurea, trimethoprim, sulphasalazine, alcohol

Vitamin B_{12} and folate replacement

Most causes of vitamin B_{12} deficiency are due to malabsorption (e.g., pernicious anaemia). Replacement is with intramuscularly administered hydroxocobalamin. Depending on whether there are any neurological symptoms, initial treatment doses differ. Maintenance is with lifelong 2- to 3-monthly injections unless the deficiency is thought to be diet related. Foods rich in vitamin B_{12} include eggs, meat, milk and dairy products.

Folate deficiency is treated with daily 5 mg oral replacement. In most people, 4 months of treatment is sufficient to correct anaemia and replace stores. A balanced diet with foods rich in folate (e.g., broccoli, brown rice, peas, chickpeas) is recommended to support treatment.

Blood transfusion

Transfusion may be necessary in cases of both acute and chronic blood loss and in patients with cardiovascular instability (e.g., due to haemorrhage). Blood is given as packed RBCs and, where possible, should be appropriately cross-matched. In cases of emergency, type O RhD-negative blood can be given. A regular blood transfusion may be necessary

for chronic anaemia which is not corrected by supplements. Table 37.3 summarizes the complications of transfusion (transfusion reactions).

Splenectomy

Splenectomy is useful in cases of anaemia related to sickle cell disease, thalassaemia and essential thrombocytopenia. Anaemias related to lymphoproliferative disease (myelofibrosis, lymphoma and leukaemia) also respond well to the procedure. Complications of splenectomy include thrombocytosis and increased susceptibility to infection with encapsulated bacteria (mainly pneumococcus, meningococcus and *Haemophilus influenzae* type b). Patients should be immunized with vaccines against these organisms 4 to 6 weeks before elective splenectomy if possible. Lifelong daily treatment with penicillin or macrolides for prophylaxis is indicated.

Erythropoietin

Erythropoietin (EPO)-stimulating agents can be used in the management of anaemia associated with chronic kidney disease

Table 37.3 Transfusion reactions

Complication	Cause
Haemolytic reaction	ABO or other antibodies (anti-rhesus, Kell) incompatibility (acute or severe), non-ABO (Kidd, Duff antigens) incompatibility (severe and intravascular), extravascular haemolysis (normally delayed by 3 days to 3 weeks; mild/clinically silent)
Anaphylaxis	Hypersensitivity to plasma proteins
Febrile reaction	Antibodies to white cells
Infective shock	Bacterial contamination of blood product
Volume overload	Particularly the elderly, and those with heart failure or chronic anaemia
Coagulopathies	Platelets and clotting factors are reduced by a dilutional effect in massive transfusion
Infection	Virus (HIV, hepatitis B virus, hepatitis C virus, EBV, CMV), gram-negative bacteria
Haemosiderosis	With repeated transfusions
Alloimmunization	Antibodies may develop into red cells, leucocytes, platelets and plasma proteins despite compatible blood being received; this may cause problems the next time the patient receives a transfusion
Graft-versus-host disease	Uncommon: preventable by use of irradiated blood (important in transplant recipients)
Transfusion-related acute lung injury (TRALI)	Due to antibodies against the patient's leukocytes. Acute respiratory distress: unpredictable, noncardiogenic pulmonary oedema, breathlessness, hypoxia

CMV, *Cytomegalovirus;* EBV, *Epstein–Barr virus;* HIV, *human immunodeficiency virus.*

(CKD). The response is dependent on the individual, the degree of anaemia, the stage of kidney disease and the presence of adverse factors (e.g., iron deficiency). Close monitoring of therapy is needed. Complications include hypertension, thromboembolic events and pure RBC aplasia.

ANAEMIA OF CHRONIC DISEASE

Clinical features

Many chronic diseases, particularly infective, inflammatory or malignant conditions, are associated with anaemia. The pathogenesis is multifactorial, with inappropriate utilization of adequate or low iron stores, dysfunctional iron transport, impaired EPO production and response and reduced survival of RBCs. In CKD, the process is related to a proportional decrease in EPO production with a decline in the glomerular filtration rate. Contributing factors include increased bleeding tendency due to uraemia-mediated platelet dysfunction, the presence of uraemic inhibitors (e.g., parathyroid hormone, cytokine inhibitors) and diminished reticulocyte response.

The presentation can be subtle in people who already have a chronic disease. Typical symptoms and signs include pallor, tiredness, breathlessness and tachycardia.

Blood tests usually show:

- Normochromic normocytic anaemia (may also be hypochromic microcytic).
- Low serum iron level but normal/high serum ferritin level.
- Increased iron stores in the bone marrow.
- Low total iron-binding capacity. Raised total iron-binding capacity helps differentiate anaemia of chronic disease from iron-deficiency anaemia.

COMMON PITFALLS

Remember that ferritin is an acute-phase protein and should not be used to diagnose anaemia in acute illness.

Management

Treatment of the underlying condition should normalize the Hb level. If anaemia is mild, no treatment is necessary. Iron supplements should be used only if iron deficiency has been established. Intravenous iron is the treatment of choice in the context of heart failure with reduced ejection fraction or CKD.

If the anaemia is severe enough to be symptomatic, or if the patient's Hb level is below a transfusion trigger for that population (generally <70 g/dL, higher in cardiovascular patients), transfusion with packed RBCs should be considered. Novel EPO-stimulating proteins or recombinant human EPO have also been recommended for use in some conditions (e.g., CKD, chemotherapy-induced anaemia, anaemia associated with rheumatoid arthritis, heart failure and cancer).

HAEMOLYTIC ANAEMIA

Clinical features

In haemolytic anaemias, the normal RBC lifespan of 120 days is reduced. RBC lysis can occur in two ways:

- Intravascular: in peripheral circulation, most commonly due to complement activation, trauma or extrinsic factors. Examples include glucose 6-phosphate dehydrogenase deficiency, prosthetic cardiac valves, thrombotic thrombocytopenic purpura and disseminated intravascular coagulation (DIC).
- Extravascular: in the monocyte–macrophage system (liver, spleen and lymph nodes). This method is most common and most likely to occur because of surface antibodies on RBCs or intrinsic RBC defects (e.g., hereditary spherocytosis).

Anaemia can be genetic (e.g., sickle cell disease, glucose 6-phosphate dehydrogenase deficiency, hereditary spherocytosis) or acquired. Acquired anaemias can be further divided into:

- Immune (e.g., haemolytic disease of the newborn, blood transfusion-related haemolysis)
- Autoimmune:
  - Warm antibody type: associated with a positive Coombs test result (lymphoma, leukaemia).
  - Cold antibody type: usually mild (paroxysmal cold haemoglobinuria, infections, e.g., *Mycoplasma pneumoniae*, or infectious mononucleosis; lymphoma).
  - Drug-related (penicillins, sulphonamides).
- Nonimmune (trauma, e.g., DIC; infection, liver disease).

The signs and symptoms are due to both anaemia and underlying disease. Jaundice can be present because of raised unconjugated bilirubin level and gallstones can occur. Blood investigations show:

- Low Hb level
- Spherocytes, fragmented and nucleated RBC on blood film
- Raised lactate dehydrogenase (LDH) level
- Raised reticulocyte count
- Reduced level of or absent haptoglobin

Management

General measures include folic acid administration (haemolysis may cause deficiency) and transfusion therapy for severe cases (as the risk of acute haemolysis of transfused blood is high). Iron replacement is needed in cases of severe intravascular haemolysis where persistent haemoglobinuria causes iron loss. Immunosuppressive therapies with steroids and biological agents and splenectomy are indicated for severe cases.

HAEMOGLOBINOPATHIES

Sickle cell disease

Sickle cell disease is an inherited group of blood disorders. The most common type is sickle cell anaemia which is an autosomal recessive condition most prevalent in the African and African-Caribbean populations. A single base mutation in the DNA on chromosome 11 causes the substitution of glutamic acid for valine at position 6 in the Hb beta chain, causing the formation of HbS which has an abnormal beta-globin chain. When the patient is heterozygous for the gene, it provides an advantage in infection with *Plasmodium falciparum* (falciparum malaria). If the patient is homozygous for the gene, it is a cause of sickle cell disease. Sickle cell disease can also be caused by other inherited disorders which result in production of the defective Hb: HbS.

Clinical features

When HbS becomes deoxygenated, it aggregates in an organized fashion, forming polymers within the RBCs that are less soluble and less deformable. As a result, the erythrocyte shape becomes distorted and changes from a biconcave disc to a sickle shape; the sickle cells cannot readily pass through the microcirculation and become trapped in small vessels (causing infarction) and clusters damage large and small blood vessels. The deformed RBCs undergo sequestration in the spleen and liver. Manifestation of this pathological process leads to anaemia of varying degrees, pain (sickle cell crisis: severe prolonged pain, often requiring hospitalization), infections, pulmonary hypertension, sickle retinopathy, impaired growth, leg ulcers, renal disease and priapism.

In the homozygous patient (HbSS), severity is variable and dependent on factors such as the level of foetal Hb (HbF) and the coinheritance of the α-thalassaemia trait. It may present from the third month of life onwards when levels of HbF start to fall. There is chronic haemolysis, with intermittent crises and complications. The most common types of sickle cell anaemia crisis are:

- Aplastic: temporary cessation of erythropoiesis causing anaemia. Commonly precipitated by parvovirus B19 infection. Profound anaemia usually requires transfusion.

- Sequestration: sudden enlargement of spleen causing a drop in Hb level, circulatory collapse and hypovolemic shock. Occurs mainly in young children and babies. If unrecognized or left untreated, the condition has a high mortality.
- Vasoocclusive: due to vascular occlusion. Can be precipitated by dehydration, hypoxia, infections or cold exposure. Almost any organ can be affected. Swollen, painful joints, lung involvement and acute abdomen are common. Large-vessel occlusion can cause serious complications, including thromboembolic stroke or acute sickle chest syndrome.
- Hyperhaemolytic: excessive haemolysis causing a fall in Hb levels.

Hb electrophoresis or chromatography demonstrates the presence of HbS and HbSS and their relative proportions.

CLINICAL NOTES

Conditions that predispose to sickling:
- dehydration
- hypoxia
- stress
- cold temperature
- infection
- pregnancy

Management

Patients should be appropriately educated regarding precipitating factors and complications. Immunization against encapsulated bacteria and prompt treatment of infection is important. During episodes of crisis, supportive care must include effective analgesia as well as optimization of hydration and oxygenation. Transfusion therapy, including exchange transfusion, is the key intervention to reduce mortality and morbidity. Other treatments include:

- Hydroxycarbamide (hydroxyurea): indicated in patients with painful crises, significant anaemia or other complications. It increases HbF levels and reduces the frequency of crises. It causes macrocytosis and myelosuppression in a dose-dependent manner, and there may be a risk of leukaemia with long-term treatment.
- Folate and zinc replacement.

Haematopoietic stem cell transplantation is the only curative treatment but is reserved for those with a severe clinical course and an HLA-matched sibling donor.

The prognosis of the condition differs because of variable clinical presentations. Median life expectancy is estimated between 40 and 60 years of age, with death most commonly due to infection.

HINTS AND TIPS

Do not deny sickle cell patients adequate analgesia during a crisis through a misplaced fear of drug dependency. Most patients nowadays will have a personalized crisis management plan that states the preferred analgesia.

Thalassaemia

Thalassaemias are a group of autosomal recessive diseases of defective Hb production. Normal Hb synthesis is summarized in Table 37.4. Thalassaemias are classified according to which

Table 37.4 Summary of normal haemoglobin synthesis

Haemoglobin feature	Characteristic
Structure	Composed of four polypeptide chains (tetramer)
	At various stages of development, different polypeptide chains are produced (ζ, ϵ, α, δ and β)
	HbF is composed of two α chains and two γ chains (α_2, γ_2) and is the major haemoglobin of intrauterine life. Its level declines rapidly around birth and it constitutes less than 1% of haemoglobin by 6 months of age. HbF is produced predominantly by the liver until 30 weeks, after which the bone marrow takes over. It has an avid affinity for oxygen
	Production of β chains increases rapidly at 36 weeks' gestation; 96% of adult haemoglobin is HbA (α_2, β_2), 3% is HbA$_2$ (α_2, δ_2), with the remainder being HbF
Genetics	The genes for the globin chains α and ζ are found clustered on chromosome 16. The genes for the remaining chains are located in a cluster on chromosome 11
	Each person has four α genes (two on each chromosome 16) and two β genes (one on each chromosome 11)

HbA, *Haemoglobin A*; HbF, *foetal haemoglobin*.

Table 37.5 Characteristics of thalassaemia

	Silent carrier	α-Thalassaemia trait	HbH disease	α-Thalassemia major (Hb Bart's hydrops fetalis)
Genetic abnormality	One α gene deleted	Two α genes deleted	Three α genes deleted	Four α genes deleted
Clinical features	Asymptomatic	Usually asymptomatic	Haemolytic anaemia Splenomegaly Bone changes May be symptomatic at birth	Hepatosplenomegaly Gross oedema Hypoalbuminaemia Extramedullary haematopoiesis
Haematological findings	Usually no abnormality	Hypochromia Microcytosis	Hypochromia Microcytosis Reticulocytosis HbH (β_4) on electrophoresis Inclusion bodies with cresyl blue	Hypochromia Microcytosis Reticulocytosis Target cells Nucleated red cells Haemoglobin Bart's on electrophoresis
Survival	Normal	Normal	Variable	Stillborn or death shortly after birth

HbH, *Haemoglobin H.*

Hb chain they affect, and the two types are α-thalassaemia and β-thalassaemia. α-Thalassaemia is commonest in Southeast Asia, Africa and India, whereas β-thalassaemia in China, the Mediterranean and the Middle East. Thalassaemia also provides an advantage in infection with *P. falciparum* (falciparum malaria).

Clinical features

The clinical presentation depends on the underlying abnormality, as described in Tables 37.5 and 37.6. Carriers with only one defective copy of the gene (or two in α-thalassaemia) are usually asymptomatic. Reduced production of one or more of the Hb chains (most importantly α or β) results in a relative excess and accumulation of the other chain (imbalanced globin chain synthesis). The unstable Hb precipitates ineffective erythropoiesis and haemolysis. Other features include:

- Skeletal change due to the expansion of erythropoietic bone marrow
- Aplastic crises with parvovirus B19 infection

Management

- Asymptomatic carriers do not generally require treatment.
- All patients should be offered disease education and psychological support.
- Transfusion to maintain an adequate Hb level, especially in periods of rapid growth, infection or pregnancy is recommended.
- In cases of hypersplenism, splenectomy should be considered.

- Iron chelation to prevent haemosiderosis using desferrioxamine.
- The only treatment for the disease is stem cell transplantation.
- Prenatal diagnosis and genetic counselling are available.

APLASTIC ANAEMIA

This refers to the failure of haemopoiesis and pancytopenia (i.e., deficiency of all three marrow cell lines) due to the hypocellular bone marrow without abnormal infiltrate or marrow fibrosis. Most cases are acquired and immune-mediated but inherited causes also exist (Table 37.7).

Clinical features

Most commonly patients present with symptoms of anaemia (pallor, fatigue, dyspnoea and palpitations) and thrombocytopenia (skin or mucosal haemorrhage, petechial rashes). Susceptibility to infection due to leucopoenia is less common.

Investigations show pancytopenia in the absence of compensatory reticulocytosis and hypocellular bone marrow on biopsy.

Management

- Treatment is based on the degree of cytopenia and not marrow cellularity (asymptomatic individuals may not need treatment).
- Supportive measures include platelet and blood transfusion, and prompt treatment of infection.

Table 37.6 Clinical features of β-thalassaemias

	β-Thalassaemia minor	β-Thalassaemia intermedia	β-Thalassaemia major
Genetic abnormality	Heterozygous abnormality in β-globin gene	Homozygous or mixed heterozygous abnormality in β-globin gene	Homozygous abnormality in β-globin gene
Clinical features	Usually asymptomatic Splenomegaly on imaging	Variable – possible features: extramedullary haematopoiesis, hepatosplenomegaly, skeletal deformity, gallstones, leg ulcers, thrombosis, pulmonary hypertension	Failure to thrive (3–6 months) Jaundice Extramedullary haematopoiesis Hepatosplenomegaly Skeletal deformity Haemosiderosis Recurrent infections Cardiac failure Gallstones Leg ulcers
Haematological findings	Mild anaemia Microcytosis with normal RDW Hypochromia Target cells Poikilocytosis HbA_2 level high HbF level may be raised	Moderate anaemia but usually not transfusion dependent Microcytosis Hypochromia Target cells Poikilocytosis	Transfusion-dependent severe anaemia Microcytosis Hypochromia Target cells Anisopoikilocytosis Reticulocytosis Nucleated RBCs Basophilic stippling Inclusion bodies on supravital staining with methyl violet HbA absent or very low level HbF level high
Survival	Normal	Variable. Usually survive to adulthood even without treatment	Death in childhood without treatment; bone marrow transplantation may be curative

HbA, *Haemoglobin A*; HbF, *foetal haemoglobin*; RBC, *red blood cell*; RDW, *red blood cell distribution width*.

Table 37.7 Causes of aplastic anaemia

Acquired	Congenital
Idiopathic Infection (5%–10% of cases are preceded by hepatitis infection) EBV, HIV, mycobacteria Toxic exposure (e.g., benzene) Drugs (chloramphenicol, gold, sulphonamides, penicillamine, chloroquine, carbamazepine) Pregnancy Sickle cell disease: aplastic crisis	Fanconi anaemia Diamond–Blackfan syndrome

EBV, *Epstein–Barr virus*; HIV, *human immunodeficiency virus*.

- Immunosuppressive therapy can be used. The most commonly used regimen combines antithymocyte globulin and cyclosporin. Other agents include biologics such as alemtuzumab.
- Bone marrow stem cell transplantation is recommended, especially for younger patients.

HAEMOCHROMATOSIS

This describes body iron overload from any cause. Hereditary haemochromatosis is an autosomal recessive genetic disorder where dysregulation in iron regulatory hormones leads to excessive intestinal iron absorption and progressive accumulation in

413

various tissues. Most commonly affected organs include the liver (leading to cirrhosis, liver fibrosis and hepatocellular carcinoma), pituitary (hypopituitarism), heart (cardiomyopathy), pancreas (diabetes), skin (discolouration) and joints (arthritis). Patients can present with nonspecific symptoms of fatigue, weakness and body pains that reveal iron deposits on investigation.

CLINICAL NOTES

INVESTIGATIONS IN SUSPECTED HAEMATOCHROMATOSIS

Serum ferritin is the most sensitive marker for iron overload but is an acute phase protein and can be falsely elevated in a range of other conditions.

Serum iron concentration and transferrin saturation should not be used in isolation to support the diagnosis as they do not adequately reflect total body iron stores. Genetic testing should be performed in all patients with otherwise unexplained elevated body iron stores markers.

The most frequently implicated gene is the *HFE* gene (chromosome 6), involved in iron uptake regulation. Other genetic mutations resulting in the condition include genes coding for the transferrin receptor, transferrin, hepcidin and caeruloplasmin.

Treatment relies on lowering iron levels. This can be achieved with phlebotomy, low iron diet and iron-chelating agents (e.g., deferoxamine). Disease resulting from organ iron deposition will also need to be treated.

LEUKAEMIA

Leukaemias are a group of conditions characterized by the malignant proliferation of leucocytes in the bone marrow. See Fig. 37.1 for stages of haematopoiesis.

In acute leukaemias, there is a proliferation of early lymphoid and myeloid precursors (blasts), which do not mature. The clinical course is very aggressive, and they are rapidly fatal without treatment. Chronic leukaemias have a more indolent course and are characterized by the proliferation of lymphoid and myeloid cells that would have reached maturity.

COMMUNICATION

Leukaemia is a frightening diagnosis for most patients. Clear communication about disease prognosis and treatment is essential.

Acute lymphoblastic leukaemia

Aetiology

Acute lymphoblastic leukaemia (ALL) is the most common malignancy in children, with about three in four cases occurring in children below the age of 6 years. It represents 12% of all leukaemias but 80% in children. Peak incidence is between 2 and 4 years of age.

Its cause is unknown but is thought to be multifactorial. Genetic, environmental and infectious predispositions have been suggested. It is more common in people with Down syndrome, Fanconi anaemia and Bloom syndrome.

Pathology

ALL results from the malignant transformation of a clone of lymphoid progenitor cells. In most cases, it is from B-cell precursors (75%). Produced lymphoblasts replace normal marrow components, resulting in a marked decrease in the production of normal blood cells, which then causes anaemia, thrombocytopenia and neutropenia.

Abnormal blasts can spill out of bone marrow and infiltrate other structures (particularly visible in the spleen, lymph nodes and the liver).

Clinical features

The history is short and usually, the initial complaint is fatigue and generalized malaise that quickly progresses to bone marrow failure (Table 37.8). The signs and symptoms can include:

- Fatigue, dizziness, palpitations
- Joint and bone pain
- Recurrent and severe infections
- Fever without obvious infection
- Haemorrhagic or thrombotic complications due to low platelets or DIC, including frequent nosebleeds, menorrhagia and petechial rash
- Lymphadenopathy and hepatosplenomegaly on examination
- Symptoms or signs due to involvement of other organs (e.g., meningism or cranial neuropathies with central nervous system (CNS) involvement)

Investigations will show:

- Normochromic normocytic anaemia with low reticulocyte count
- Normal, high or low white cell count but there is usually neutropenia
- Thrombocytopenia
- Hypercellular bone marrow dominated by lymphoblasts (>20% required for diagnosis)

Immunophenotyping (e.g., using flow cytometry) will reveal the subtype of leukaemia.

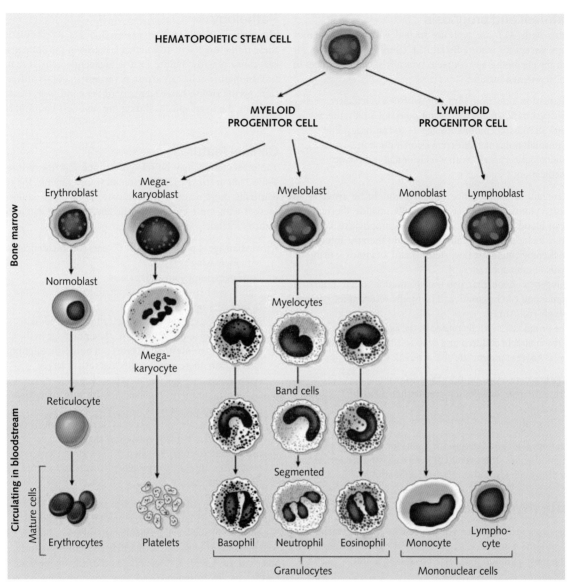

HEMATOPOIETIC STEM CELL

MYELOID PROGENITOR CELL

LYMPHOID PROGENITOR CELL

Bone marrow

Erythroblast

Mega-karyoblast

Myeloblast

Monoblast

Lymphoblast

Normoblast

Mega-karyocyte

Myelocytes

Band cells

Segmented

Circulating in bloodstream

Reticulocyte

Mature cells

Erythrocytes

Platelets

Basophil

Neutrophil

Eosinophil

Monocyte

Lympho-cyte

Granulocytes

Mononuclear cells

Fig. 37.1 Stages in blood cell development (haematopoiesis). All blood cells originate from haematopoietic stem cells. Progenitor cells are derived from haematopoietic stem cells. Myeloid progenitor cells give rise to erythroblasts, megakaryoblasts, myeloblasts and monoblasts. Lymphoid progenitor cells give rise to lymphoblasts. Notice that the suffix -blast indicates immature forms of all cells. (From Pemde H, Datta V, Harish K. *Clinical and Practical Paediatrics,* 2nd ed. Elsevier; 2020.)

Table 37.8 Symptoms of bone marrow failure

Cells affected	Result	Manifestation
Red cell precursors	Anaemia	Lethargy, dyspnoea, pallor
White cell precursors	Neutropenia	Recurrent infections, fever
Platelet precursors	Thrombocytopenia	Bleeding, bruising, purpura

Treatment and prognosis

Patients with ALL are typically treated with staged chemotherapy, except for mature B-cell ALL (Burkitt lymphoma), for which the chemotherapy course is typically short. The stages of a typical regimen include:

- Remission induction: elimination of 99% of leukaemic cells and restoration of normal haemopoiesis. Usually, therapy is with steroids, chemotherapy agents and anthracycline.
- Consolidation: intensifies remission induction.
- Maintenance: usually with weekly or daily cytotoxic medication.

Generalized maintenance measures should be available to support cytotoxic treatment and usually include the replacement of blood cells and antibiotics. CNS prophylaxis is essential and includes intrathecal methotrexate therapy, intrathecal triple therapy (methotrexate, steroids and a cytotoxic drug) or systemic combination therapy.

Allogeneic bone marrow transplantation often improves outcomes and can be curative. It is usually reserved for patients with high-risk ALL.

The prognosis is strictly related to the age of the patient. Cure rates reach 90% in children and drop to 10% in frail and elderly patients. Adverse prognostic characteristics include:

- Age less than 1 year or more than 10 years
- Presenting leucocyte count greater than 50×10^9/L
- Male sex
- CNS involvement

An important good prognostic indicator is an early response to chemotherapy. The overall 10-year survival rate for ALL is about 60% in children and 25% to 35% in adults.

Acute myeloid leukaemia

Acute myeloid leukaemia (AML) results from a malignant arrest of bone marrow cells in the early stages of development. It is the most common form of leukaemia in adults.

Aetiology

Most cases arise with no clear cause, although many risks are recognized:

- Ionizing radiation and chemical exposure (e.g., survivors of the atomic bomb dropped on Hiroshima).
- Previous chemotherapy: alkylating agents.
- Predisposing diseases: myeloproliferative disorders, aplastic anaemia and myelodysplasia can transform to acute leukaemia; congenital diseases, including Down syndrome, Fanconi's anaemia and neurofibromatosis are risk factors.

Pathology

The malignant cells in AML are myeloblasts. Accumulation of these immature haematopoietic blast cells in the bone marrow can cause marrow failure (>20% leukaemic cells is diagnostic). Immature cells can arrest at various stages of differentiation, giving rise to heterogenicity of the condition. Blasts can infiltrate the liver, spleen, skin, gums and, less commonly, the CNS.

Clinical features

The presentation may be related to bone marrow failure (see Table 37.8) or to organ infiltration. In young patients, the course is usually more acute when compared with older adults, who present with more chronic fatigue and malaise. Characteristic features include:

- Median age at presentation is 67 years (the incidence rises with increasing age).
- Bone pain, joint pain and malaise.
- Significant hepatomegaly and splenomegaly (lymphadenopathy is rare).
- Bleeding that may be caused by thrombocytopenia, coagulopathy and resulting DIC (haemorrhage in the CNS, lungs or gastrointestinal systems can be life-threatening).
- On the skin, there may be petechial rash or larger ecchymoses and leukaemia cutis.
- Gums are commonly involved, resulting in gingivitis and swollen bleeding gums.
- White blood cells (WBCs) count can be high and, even in the presence of neutropenia, cause persistent fever. If WBC counts are extremely elevated (>100×10^9/L) leukostasis (a hyperviscosity state), respiratory distress and altered mental status can occur.

Investigating the patient with suspected AML requires a blood film and bone marrow analysis for diagnosis. Cytochemistry will allow classification into subtypes. Bone marrow is hypercellular with blasts that may contain Auer rods (characteristic of AML). Cytogenetic studies can be performed to further assess prognosis and consider individually tailored treatment.

Treatment and prognosis

A good response to treatment is blast clearance in the bone marrow to less than 5%, morphologically normal haemopoiesis and normal peripheral blood count. Broad principles of management include:

- Supportive care as for all leukaemias (see ALL).
- Intensive cytotoxic chemotherapy: induction of remission and postremission (consolidation) therapy. The exact regimen is determined by patient factors and AML subtype.

- Stem cell transplantation, which has been shown to have high survival benefits in patients with intermediate-risk and high-risk AML.

The prognosis is patient and AML subtype dependent. In children, around 80% of patients achieve remission following induction chemotherapy, and overall survival rates are around 70%. In younger adults, the survival rate is about 40% at 5 years, and in those older than 60 years the survival rate can be as low as <10%.

Poor prognostic factors include very high white cell count, secondary leukaemia (e.g., previous myelodysplasia), certain cytogenetic abnormalities and the presence of DIC.

Chronic lymphocytic leukaemia

Aetiology

Chronic lymphocytic leukaemia (CLL) is the most common leukaemia in the developed world, representing about a quarter of all leukaemias. It is largely a disease of the elderly, with an incidence that increases with age. Around 40% of new cases are diagnosed in those over the age of 75 years. Incidence is higher in white ethnic groups. Genetic correlations of CLL are seen, with a sevenfold increase in the risk of CLL development in first-degree relatives of CLL patients, but the mechanisms of that are unknown.

Pathology

This leukaemia comprises malignant monoclonal expansion of B lymphocytes. Abnormal cells can accumulate in the blood, bone marrow, lymph nodes, liver and spleen. Although the morphological appearance of these cells is normal, they are nonreactive and immature, and therefore lead to immunological compromise.

Diagnosis is made when:

- Monoclonal B-cell lymphocyte count in peripheral blood is 5,000/μL or greater for at least 3 months with clonality confirmed by flow cytometry.
- Blood smear shows characteristically small, mature lymphocytes with a dense nucleus lacking nucleoli and partially aggregated chromatin.

Clinical features

The presentation can be variable, with CLL being an incidental finding for some asymptomatic patients, while others may describe malaise, weight loss, night sweats, recurrent infections, bleeding or symptoms of anaemia.

- Symmetrical lymphadenopathy is usually found.
- Hepatosplenomegaly can cause abdominal pain.

- Skin involvement is common with pallor or thrombocytopenic rash.

Investigations are with simple blood tests:

- Lymphocytosis is seen on full blood count (FBC), with peripheral blood smear showing smudge cells.
- Autoimmune haemolytic anaemia can be present and should be investigated with a direct antiglobulin test (direct Coombs test).
- A lymph node biopsy is necessary to establish the possibility of transformation to high-grade lymphoma.
- Patients should be tested for the presence of tumour protein 53 gene (*TP53*) mutation before treatment. This tumour suppressor gene deletion is associated with a lower response to treatment and a worse prognosis.

Treatment and prognosis

Except for stem cell transplantation, there is no curative treatment for CLL. Treatment is based on the disease stage. Only symptomatic patients or those with active or advanced disease require therapy. Treatment options include chemotherapy (alkylating agents, monoclonal antibodies, purine analogues, protein kinase inhibitors), steroids (may be used to treat autoimmune complications and improve marrow function) or targeted agents for those with a del (17p) or TP53 mutation (venetoclax, obinutuzumab). Relapse is managed with further chemotherapy.

CLL is usually associated with long overall survival. The median survival differs depending on the stage and extent of the disease. Patients with del (17p) or TP53 gene deletion have the worst prognosis.

Chronic myeloid leukaemia

Chronic myeloid leukaemia (CML) accounts for about 15% of adult leukaemias. It can present at any stage of life but is uncommon in the young. The median age at diagnosis is around 65 years. CLL typically progresses through three stages:

- Chronic phase (where 90% of patients present): competent immune system with patient asymptomatic for prolonged periods (4–5 years).
- Accelerated phase: 15% to 29% of blasts present in the patient's marrow, causing marrow failure and resistance to treatment. About two-thirds of chronic phase patients will transform into accelerated phase at some stage.
- Blast crisis or blastic phase: usually results from a transformation of the accelerated phase but in about 25% of patients, transformation is from the chronic phase. This is an aggressive acute leukaemia with marrow arrest that is resistant to treatment and has a high mortality.

Aetiology

The cause is unknown. There are no obvious familial, geographic, economic or ethnic associations.

Pathology

CML is a myeloproliferative disorder of pluripotent haemopoietic stem cells. It can affect one or all stem cell lines (erythroid, platelet and myeloid). Although failed apoptosis and increased production play a role, the detailed mechanisms are unknown. Over 95% of cases have been shown to result from cytogenetic abnormality known as the Philadelphia chromosome: a reciprocal translocation between chromosome 9 to 22 (9:22) which results in fusion gene *BCR–ABL*. *BCR–ABL* is a chimeric oncogene with high tyrosine kinase activity and the potential to alter cellular properties.

Clinical features

The signs and symptoms can differ and can be insidious in onset. Most commonly they include:

- Lethargy, weight loss, sweats and abdominal discomfort (enlarging spleen)
- Symptoms of anaemia or thrombocytopenia
- Splenomegaly, which may be massive
- Lymphadenopathy and hepatomegaly

    Investigations show:

- Leucocytosis with granulocytes in various stages of development on FBC and blood film
- Normocytic normochromic anaemia and thrombocytosis

    Bone marrow aspiration is crucial to determine the percentage of blasts and basophils and for cytogenetic analysis.

Treatment and prognosis

Treatment goals include haematological remission (i.e., normal FBC, no organomegaly and no cytogenic or molecular abnormalities), cytogenic remission and molecular remission. As first-line treatment, chemotherapy is considered to be superior to stem cell transplantation because of the mortality associated with transplantation. The mainstay of CML treatment is with tyrosine-kinase inhibitors (imatinib, nilotinib, dasatinib, asciminib) which have led to a dramatic increase in 10-year overall survival of 80% to 90%. Frequent monitoring of response to treatment is extremely important.

MULTIPLE MYELOMA

Aetiology

Multiple myeloma is the second most common haematological cancer. It is usually a disease of the elderly, with nearly 50% of cases diagnosed after the age of 75 years. It is more common in Afro-Caribbean patients and men.

Multiple myeloma is a progressive malignant disease that results from the accumulation of neoplastic plasma cells in the bone marrow. This process seems to be proceeded by monoclonal gammopathy of undetermined significance (MGUS) which is thought to be a premalignant stage (paraproteinaemia is <3 g/dL, plasma cells <10% in the bone marrow and no end-organ damage). In health, plasma cells produce various levels of monoclonal free light chains. They are then filtered and reabsorbed in the kidneys. If reabsorption capacity is exceeded, light chains (Bence Jones proteins) will accumulate in the kidneys as casts and cause acute kidney injury.

Multiple myeloma is thought to be due to a genetic mutation occurring before the terminal differentiation of B cells into plasma cells. As myeloma develops, further genetic mutations occur.

Pathology

The neoplastic proliferation of plasma cells leads to diffuse bone marrow infiltration and failure. The malignant cells oversecrete a monoclonal immunoglobulin (paraprotein) that is detectable in serum and urine. Osteoclast activity is increased, resulting in osteolytic bone lesions and hypercalcaemia. Renal failure and immunodeficiency are also caused by paraprotein. Myelomas are classified by the type of antibody they produce, and the most common form is immunoglobulin G myeloma.

Clinical features

A variety of signs and symptoms can be a feature of myeloma:

- Bone pain due to osteolytic lesions and pathological fractures.
- Hypercalcaemia is often present (see Chapter 33).
- Renal impairment is due to light chain or amyloid deposition and dehydration.
- Recurrent infections.
- Spinal cord and nerve compression.
- Polymerization of the monoclonal antibody can result in hyperviscosity syndrome.

Investigations commonly show:
- Normochromic normocytic anaemia
- Leucopoenia
- Hypercalcaemia
- Impaired renal function
- Persistently raised plasma viscosity and erythrocyte sedimentation rate
- A monoclonal paraprotein as demonstrated by serum protein electrophoresis (used to assess response to treatment)

- Free light chains in the urine (Bence Jones protein) as detected by urine electrophoresis, or in the serum as detected with a serum-free light chain assay
- Generalized osteopenia, 'punched-out' lytic lesions and pathological fractures as revealed by a skeletal survey

Bone marrow aspirate is diagnostic when plasma cells account for more than 10% of bone marrow cells.

> ### HINTS AND TIPS
>
> Psychological care of very sick or terminally ill patients is an important part of their management, and referral to a clinical psychologist may help patients cope with their illness.

Treatment and prognosis

Myeloma is a chronic, relapsing and remitting illness that is incurable. Treatment is aimed at disease control and improvement of survival. Patients with MGUS and asymptomatic myeloma are monitored only.

Treatment is based on corticosteroids, chemotherapy agents and immunomodulatory drugs. In younger patients, where the prognosis is better, stem cell transplantation is considered first line. Bisphosphonates reduce bone disease and EPO analogues can help in anaemic patients.

The prognosis is variable. In just under 30% of patients, survival exceeds 10 years, whereas, in aggressive disease, death usually occurs within 12 months. Response to treatment and the patient's age are independent prognostic factors.

LYMPHOMA

Lymphomas are blood cell tumours that result from the neoplastic proliferation of lymphocytes. There are two main types of lymphoma, split on the basis of histological findings: Hodgkin disease (Reed–Sternberg (RS) cells present) and non-Hodgkin lymphoma (NHL; all others).

Hodgkin lymphoma

Aetiology

Although Hodgkin lymphoma accounts for only about 10% of all lymphomas, it is one of the most common malignancies in young adults. There is a bimodal age distribution with peaks at 20 to 40 years and >70 years, with a male preponderance. Its cause is unknown but there is a link with Epstein–Barr virus (EBV), which is found in about 40% of RS cells of patients with Hodgkin lymphoma. Other risk factors include immunodeficient states (e.g., HIV infection, immunosuppressant therapy), previous NHL and family history.

Pathology

This is a malignant tumour of the lymphatic system characterized by presence of RS cells in a background of inflammatory infiltrate. There are also associated abnormal mononuclear cells that are smaller and originating from B cells in germinal centres.

Hodgkin lymphoma is further classified into subgroups (Table 37.9), with classic Hodgkin lymphomas present in 95% of cases. This divide is important as accurate classification will determine management and prognosis.

Clinical features

The most common presentation is with enlarged, otherwise asymptomatic lymph nodes typically in the cervical or supraclavicular area. Mediastinal nodes are also common, and can result in shortness of breath and a dry cough. Affected lymph nodes feel rubbery and are nontender. Pruritus is common, and alcohol-induced lymph node pain can occur. Systemic symptoms include B symptoms. Hepatosplenomegaly or features of paraneoplastic syndrome can also occur.

Diagnosis requires lymph node biopsy, and excision of a whole node is performed if possible to provide adequate structural information. A computed tomography (CT) or a positron emission tomography (PET) scan of the chest, abdomen and pelvis is performed to stage the disease (Fig. 37.2).

Table 37.9 Classification of Hodgkin lymphoma

Subtype		Feature
Classic Hodgkin lymphoma	Lymphocyte rich	More common in males
	Lymphocyte depleted	Associated with EBV
	Nodular sclerosis	Most common worldwide
	Mixed cellularity	Most common in older adults
Nodular lymphocyte-predominant Hodgkin lymphoma		No or very few RS cells

EBV, *Epstein–Barr virus*; RS, *Reed–Sternberg*.

CLINICAL NOTES

B SYMPTOMS

- Fever
- Drenching night sweats
- Unintentional weight loss (more than 10% over 6 months)

This refers to some symptoms that can be associated with lymphomas that when present should prompt investigations for the possible disease. Presence or absence of B symptoms is also significant to prognostication and staging of the disease.

CLINICAL NOTES

STAGING LYMPHOMAS

When staging a lymphoma, you give a number (I–IV) and a letter (A or B). The letter *A* denotes the absence of B symptoms and the letter *B* denotes the presence of B symptoms. For example, stage IIA corresponds to stage II lymphoma without B symptoms.

Sometimes a letter 'E' is added which signifies that the lymphoma has invaded an extralymphatic organ.

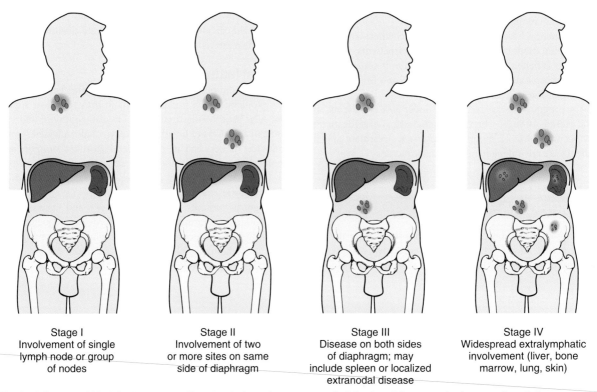

Stage I
Involvement of single lymph node or group of nodes

Stage II
Involvement of two or more sites on same side of diaphragm

Stage III
Disease on both sides of diaphragm; may include spleen or localized extranodal disease

Stage IV
Widespread extralymphatic involvement (liver, bone marrow, lung, skin)

Fig. 37.2 Staging of Hodgkin lymphoma. The classical staging system called the Ann Arbour staging has now largely been replaced by the Lugano staging classification. (From Perry AM, Damjanov I, Perry KD. *Pathology for the Health Professions,* 6th ed. Elsevier; 2022.)

Treatment and prognosis

Before treatment, staging and assessment of risk factors is essential. Radiotherapy, chemotherapy and combined therapies are used in disease management. Both radiotherapy and chemotherapy have been found to increase the risk of developing secondary solid tumours such as cancers of the breast or lung. Chemotherapy itself is effective, but carries a risk of developing leukaemia. The choice of treatment depends on the stage of disease, histological pattern and prognostic factors. Autologous stem cell transplantation is used for management of resistant disease or relapse.

The prognosis is generally good, and 5-year survival rates reach around 81%.

CLINICAL NOTES

PARANEOPLASTIC SYNDROME

Occurs as a result of an abnormal host immune response to a tumour. Symptoms are often related to the signalling molecules produced by the neoplasm such as hormones and cytokines and may be cardiovascular, neuromuscular, mucocutaneous or endocrine in nature. Fever is the most common presentation.

Non-Hodgkin lymphoma

Aetiology

NHL is a highly heterogeneous group of lymphoproliferative malignancies. Given the heterogeneity, its presentation is variable, as is response to treatment. NHL is five times more common than Hodgkin disease. The median age of presentation is >50 years. Exceptions are high-grade lymphoblastic and small noncleaved lymphomas, which are most commonly found NHLs in children and young adults.

The cause is multifactorial and includes:

- Genetic predisposition.
- Immunosuppression (particularly HIV infection, also transplant recipients).
- Pathogens: viruses (e.g., EBV, hepatitis C virus, T cell lymphoma virus 1) and bacteria (*H. pylori* causes the mucosa-associated lymphoid tissue (MALT) lymphoma).
- Autoimmune disorders (Sjögren syndrome, rheumatoid arthritis, Hashimoto thyroiditis, systemic lupus erythematosus).

Pathology

It is a heterogeneous malignancy showing diverse histological cell patterns and clinical course. It is characterized by neoplastic proliferation of B lymphocytes (usually) or T lymphocytes forming solid tumours within the lymphoid system which do not contain RS cells.

NHL can be classified by the cell origin (see Table 37.10).

Clinical features

The clinical presentation is diverse and can differ among different NHL types.

Low-grade lymphomas:

- Slowly progressing, painless lymphadenopathy, usually peripheral. Sometimes associated with spontaneous regression of enlarged lymph nodes.
- Hepatosplenomegaly and bone marrow involvement causing cytopenia can occur.
- Systemic symptoms including fatigue, fevers, weight loss and extranodal involvement are uncommon at early stages but become prominent in advanced disease.

High-grade lymphomas:

- Rapidly growing, bulky lymphadenopathy is the most frequent feature at presentation.
- Systemic symptoms and extranodal involvement (gastrointestinal and genitourinary tract, skin, CNS, bone marrow) are common.
- Hepatosplenomegaly.
- Depending on the system involved, specific features resulting from a mass effect can occur, and most commonly involve hydronephrosis due to ureter obstruction, testicular mass, mediastinal mass causing superior vena cava syndrome and abdominal mass mimicking bowel obstruction.

Diagnosis is confirmed by lymph node biopsy for histology, immunohistochemistry and cytogenetics. Fluorescence in situ hybridization (FISH) to identify *MYC*, *BCL2* and *BCL6* mutations should be considered in all patients with a new diagnosis of high-grade B-cell lymphoma. Staging should then be performed to determine the extent of disease (see Fig. 37.2). This usually comprises PET/CT imaging.

Treatment and prognosis

Treatment options differ because of high heterogeneity. Options include observation and waiting in asymptomatic disease, local or extended radiotherapy and single-agent or multiagent chemotherapy. Rituximab can be useful. Autologous stem cell transplant can be considered in some cases. MALT is initially managed with *H. pylori* eradication therapy that can be followed

Table 37.10 Simplified World Health Organization classification of non-Hodgkin lymphoma

B cell	T cell
Precursor B-cell neoplasm • Precursor B-lymphoblastic lymphoma	Precursor T-cell neoplasm • Precursor T-lymphoblastic lymphoma

Mature (peripheral) B-cell neoplasms
• High grade
  • Diffuse large B-cell lymphoma; 40% of all non-Hodgkin lymphomas in adults
  • Mediastinal large B cell
  • Primary central nervous system lymphomas
  • Primary effusion lymphoma
  • Burkitt lymphoma
  • Mantle cell lymphoma
• Low grade
  • Follicular lymphoma; 19% of all non-Hodgkin lymphomas in adults
  • Mucosa-associated lymphoid tissue lymphoma
  • Waldenström macroglobulinaemia
	Mature (peripheral) T-cell neoplasms
	• High grade
	  • Enteropathy-type T-cell lymphoma
	  • Peripheral T-cell lymphoma
	  • Subcutaneous panniculitis-like
	  • Systemic anaplastic
	  • Angioimmunoblastic
	• Low grade
	  • Mycosis fungoides and cutaneous T-cell lymphomas

by chemotherapy or radiotherapy in resistant disease. First-line treatment for Burkitt lymphoma is immunochemotherapy.

All patients should have polyvalent pneumococcal and influenza vaccinations. *Haemophilus influenzae* type b and meningococcal vaccination are also recommended. In patients with neutropenia, antibiotic prophylaxis is needed.

Low-grade NHL has a good prognosis, generally with median survival of around 10 years. Advanced disease is incurable. High-grade lymphomas are more aggressive but are also more responsive to treatment.

Poor prognostic factors include lymphoma with features of both high- and low-grade disease.

MYELODYSPLASTIC SYNDROMES

Myelodysplastic syndromes (MDSs) are a group of malignant haemopoietic diseases characterized by ineffective haemopoiesis and dysplastic changes of one or more lineages of cells. There is also a high risk of transformation into AML.

Bone marrow shows hypocellularity or hypercellularity with disordered maturation of abnormal cells. This causes blood cytopenia because of ineffective haemopoiesis. It can affect myeloid (WBCs), erythroid (RBCs) and megakaryocyte (platelet) cell lines.

About 10% of MDSs are secondary to an initial insult (secondary MDSs); for example, chemotherapy, radiotherapy or occupational exposure to radiation. Secondary MDSs have been shown to have poorer prognosis than primary cases.

MDSs are mainly diseases of the elderly, with over 80% of cases occurring in those aged 60 years or older.

Classification

MDS classification is constantly evolving because of continual improvements in our understanding of the disease. Currently, the most up-to-date classification is set by the WHO which divides the syndromes based on the cell lines affected, presence of ring sideroblasts, numbers of blasts in the peripheral blood and bone marrow and proportion of cytogenic marrow abnormality.

Clinical features

The symptoms are nonspecific and reflect the underlying cell deficiency. Patients may present with symptoms due to one or a combination of anaemia, leucopoenia and thrombocytopenia.

The examination can show signs of a thrombocytopenic rash, like petechiae or ecchymoses. Splenomegaly and lymphadenopathy are usually not seen.

Diagnosis is made by elimination of non-MDS causes of cytopenia with abnormal cell morphology and increased bone marrow blasts.

On investigation, the FBC can show various abnormalities ranging from anaemia to monocytosis, neutropenia, neutrophilia, thrombocytosis or thrombocytopenia.

Blood film classically shows RBCs with anisocytosis (unequal size) and poikilocytes (abnormally shaped RBCs), Pappenheimer bodies, basophilic stippling and irregular, large platelets.

Management

New approaches to management with novel agents are continuously being developed. In cases of indolent, low-risk MDS, supportive treatment may be all that is required. Although chemotherapy can be used with curable results in a small number of patients, the gold standard curative treatment is currently allogeneic haemopoietic stem cell transplantation.

In low-risk patients, survival is longer and transmission rates to AML are lower when compared with high-risk MDS patients. The main goals of treatment are symptomatic control of cytopenia, mainly anaemia that eventually requires transfusion.

MYELOPROLIFERATIVE DISORDERS

Myeloproliferative neoplasms are a group of rare cancers of the bone marrow caused by malignant proliferation of abnormal myeloid cells. The conditions are closely related to MDS. They can develop in any MDS and AML but usually have a much better prognosis. There are four main syndromes: CML (associated with the Philadelphia chromosome and discussed earlier), essential thrombocythaemia (ET), polycythaemia vera (PV) and primary myelofibrosis associated with *JAK2* mutation.

Polycythaemia vera

In PV there is an increased number of circulating erythrocytes (raised haematocrit). PV can also result in raised numbers of WBCs and platelets. Primary PV is associated with low levels of EPO, caused by a mutation of a tyrosine kinase gene (*JAK2*), encoding a myeloproliferation regulator, the Janus kinase, which results in overproduction of cells independently of the hormone. Over 95% of cases are associated with this mutation.

The usual age of presentation is between 60 and 70 years, and patients can be asymptomatic. The disease starts with a plethoric stage and then moves on to the spent stage. The array of signs and symptoms seen include:

- Symptoms of raised haematocrit (headache, weakness, sweating, dizziness)
- Symptoms of thrombosis (deep vein thrombosis (DVT), myocardial infarction, stroke, Budd–Chiari syndrome)
- Arthralgia and pruritus
- Plethora (red complexion) and the presence of splenomegaly

On investigation, there is raised haematocrit, thrombocytosis and leucocytosis.

Management aims to control cardiovascular risks and is with venesection (to lower the haematocrit) and low-dose aspirin. In high-risk patients, cytoreductive treatment is also recommended, and includes chemotherapy, hydroxycarbamide, interferon alfa, ruxolitinib (JAK2 inhibitor), allopurinol and radioactive phosphorus.

> **CLINICAL NOTES**
>
> #### SECONDARY POLYCYTHAEMIA
>
> This is due to overproduction of EPO which leads to increased red-cell mass. Causes include:
>
> - Physiological response to chronic hypoxia (e.g., chronic lung disease, at altitude)
> - Renal disease (e.g., renal artery stenosis, renal cell carcinoma)
> - Hepatomas
> - Anabolic steroid use

Essential thrombocythaemia

In ET the platelet count is markedly elevated and the platelets are functionally abnormal. The mean age at diagnosis is 60 years, but initial stages of the disease can be asymptomatic. 60% of patients have a mutation in the *JAK2* gene.

Clinical features are related to increased tendency of bleeding and thrombosis, and include:

- Headache, light-headedness or syncope
- Fatigue
- Burning pains, arthralgia, swollen digits
- Transient ischemic episodes and parasthesiae
- Bleeding gums, nosebleeds or gastrointestinal bleeds
- Splenomegaly and hepatomegaly

Investigations in a patient with suspected ET include FBC, which usually shows elevated platelet levels (>600 × 10^9/L). A blood film may show bizarre-looking platelets and platelet aggregates.

Treatment is with observation alone in patients with low risk of thrombosis. Low-dose aspirin can also be used. In high-risk patients cytoreductive therapy (as per treatment of PV) is necessary.

Primary myelofibrosis

In primary myelofibrosis there is proliferation of abnormal cells in all three cell lines, accompanied by release of growth factors, which cause bone marrow fibrosis. There is a characteristic leucoerythroblastic blood film appearance and elevated levels of various cytokines. The disease can present in a patient with no previous associated condition (primary myelofibrosis) or develop secondarily (e.g., from PV or ET).

The disease may be asymptomatic initially, and clinical features are variable. They may reflect progressive anaemia, leucopoenia or leucocytosis, thrombocytopenia or thrombocytosis and multiorgan extramedullary haemopoiesis (mostly hepatomegaly and/or splenomegaly). Organ enlargement can cause symptoms due to a mass effect, including spinal cord compression or seizures. Constitutional symptoms, including fatigue, weight loss and night sweats, are common.

The only curative treatment is with allogeneic stem cell transplantation. General management otherwise is palliative and concentrated around symptomatic control. Hydroxyurea has traditionally been the preferred agent, however, any cytoreductive therapy (described earlier) can be effective.

BLEEDING DISORDERS

An increased tendency for bleeding can result from abnormalities of platelets, the coagulation pathway or blood vessels. The differential diagnosis, clinical findings and investigation of these disorders are discussed in detail in Chapter 26. Specific conditions and their management are considered here.

Haemophilia A

Haemophilia A is a bleeding disorder caused by deficiency of clotting factor VIII (Fig. 37.3). It affects 1 in 4000–5000 males worldwide. The vast majority of cases result from an X-linked recessive mutation, meaning males are affected from carrier mothers. There is usually a strong family history predicting the condition however acquired forms do exist. Females born to affected fathers can have mild symptoms because of homozygosity.

The disease can have marked phenotypical variability leading to a wide spectrum of severity. Severe disease usually presents in infancy. Signs and symptoms can include excessive bleeding from minor procedures or trauma, spontaneous haemarthroses, intramuscular or intracranial haemorrhage and haematuria. Moderate disease often becomes apparent with excessive bleeding at venepuncture or during surgery. In mild forms, only major trauma or a surgical procedure will cause excessive bleeding.

On investigation, activated partial thromboplastin time (APTT) is usually prolonged and factor VIII level is low. Percentage activity represents severity of the disease.

Management is divided into prophylaxis and treatment. Prophylaxis includes factor VIII infusion. In episodes of acute bleeding, management is with monoclonal-antibody purified factor VIII, recombinant factor VIII and fresh frozen plasma, and at times with desmopressin and antifibrinolytic agents to boost factor VIII activity.

Special care is needed in haemophilia A patients when surgery or pregnancy are planned. A specialist team should be involved with planning and intensive monitoring to minimize patient risk and complications. With current therapies and specialist multidisciplinary approach life expectancy for patients is normal. Any pregnant woman with a family history of the condition should be offered genetic screening.

Haemophilia B (Christmas disease)

This is caused by a deficiency in clotting factor IX. As in haemophilia A, this is also an X-linked recessive condition but it is about five times less prevalent than haemophilia A. The clinical features of haemophilia B are similar to those of haemophilia A but less severe.

On investigation, APTT is prolonged and factor IX activity is low.

Treatment with recombinant factor IX is the first-line therapy. If this is unavailable, plasma-derived factor IX can be used. Additional treatment with antifibrinolytic therapy can be used in cases of acute bleeding. Care should be taken to monitor patients for the development of inhibitors to factor IX. The risk of an immune response to factor IX is higher than in haemophilia A and can cause a severe anaphylactic reaction.

Von Willebrand disease

Von Willebrand disease (vWD) is the most common coagulopathy worldwide (1%–2% of the general population). It is more common in females, and is more severe in people with

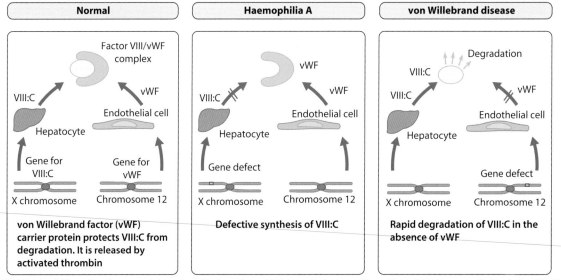

Fig. 37.3 Factor VIII synthesis: normal, haemophilia A and von Willebrand disease. (From Carroll W, Lissauer T. *Illustrated Textbook of Paediatrics*, 6th ed. Elsevier; 2022.)

blood group O. In most of those with vWD, it is an inherited, autosomal dominant condition (rarely autosomal recessive) but acquired forms also exist (pseudo-vWD, associated with myeloproliferative disease or solid tumours). It results from the abnormal function, or deficiency of von Willebrand factor (vWF).

vWF is a plasma protein that mediates platelet adherence to the subendothelium and therefore, platelet aggregation (Fig. 37.3). It also binds and stabilizes factor VIII, preventing its clearance from plasma.

Presentation differs depending on the severity of the deficiency, and in many cases remains undetected until an episode of abnormal bleeding occurs. Most patients present with bleeding characteristic for platelet disorders: bruising, bleeding into the skin, mucosal bleeding (epistaxis, bleeding gums, gastrointestinal bleeding). Spontaneous bleeding (e.g., into joints) or internal bleeding occurs only in severe cases. Menorrhagia and bleeding following surgery, dental extractions, trauma and delivery are common.

Investigations include prolonged APTT and low vWF level. Factor VIII can also be low.

Management includes patient education and avoidance of precipitating factors; minor disease does not require specific treatment. If intervention is required, antifibrinolytics (tranexamic acid) and desmopressin (releases endothelial stores of factor VIII and vWF) combined with vWF concentrates are used.

Immune thrombocytopenic purpura

Immune thrombocytopenic purpura (ITP) is an autoimmune condition that results in low platelet levels. There is antibody-mediated destruction of platelets in the spleen and liver and antibody-mediated reduced platelet production. This can happen alone (primary ITP) or can be associated with other conditions (secondary ITP). The cause is often unclear, but it may occur following viral illnesses, in the context of other autoimmune diseases (such as SLE) or lymphoproliferative disease, or following administration of certain drugs.

ITP can be acute or chronic, and it can affect both adults and children. The presentation can be relatively mild with clinical features including:

- Easy bruising, petechial or purpuric rash
- Mucosal bleeding and menorrhagia
- Haematuria and gastrointestinal bleeding (less common)
- Splenomegaly, which rarely occurs in isolated ITP and should prompt consideration of an underlying diagnosis if it is present

Treatment is considered on the basis of symptoms and factors such as platelet count, patient age and comorbidities. General measures include advice and close monitoring. If pharmacological treatment is indicated, first-line measures include steroids, intravenously administered immunoglobulin and intravenously administered anti-D. If these prove ineffective, splenectomy or biological agents (e.g., rituximab) can be indicated.

DISSEMINATED INTRAVASCULAR COAGULATION

Aetiology

The condition is characterized by a specific haematological response to a secondary disease. There are no predisposing factors in terms of sex, age and race. Risk factors include:

- Infection: septicaemia, most commonly gram-negative sepsis.
- Malignancy: mainly leukaemias.
- Some connective tissue disorders: antiphospholipid syndrome.
- Obstetric complications: amniotic fluid embolism, placental abruption, preeclampsia, HELLP syndrome, septic abortion.
- Major trauma causing tissue damage, burns.
- Immunological factors: incompatible blood transfusion, drug reaction, anaphylaxis.
- Other factors: snake bites, acute pancreatitis, heat stroke, recreational drugs.

Pathology

In DIC, normal haemostasis and processes of coagulation and fibrinolysis are dysregulated (Fig. 37.4). There is an inappropriate, diffuse activation of the clotting cascade (especially thrombin) in response to an insult. This may lead to acute or chronic thrombosis that compromises tissue oxygenation and leads to organ damage. Moreover, because of thrombosis exhausting the supply of clotting factors, severe haemorrhage can occur.

Initially, intravascular coagulation is precipitated by the release of tissue factor from injured or malignant cells. This glycoprotein is present on the surface of many cells, including endothelial cells, monocytes and macrophages, and is not normally in contact with the general circulation unless vascular damage has occurred. On exposure to blood and platelets, tissue factor binds activated factor VII, triggering the common coagulation pathway and formation of thrombin and fibrin. As a result, thrombi form throughout the microcirculation, causing ischaemia and infarction. Simultaneously, an excess of thrombin leads to activation of plasmin so as to commence fibrinolysis. Fibrin breakdown leads to formation of fibrin degradation

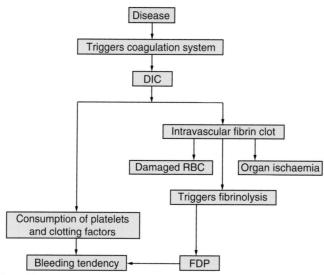

Fig. 37.4 Pathology of disseminated intravascular coagulation *(DIC)*. *FDP*, Fibrin degradation product; *RBC*, red blood cell. (From Pagana TN, Pagana TJ, Deska K. *Mosby's® Diagnostic and Laboratory Test Reference*, 16th ed. Elsevier; 2023.)

products, which have further anticoagulant properties contributing to haemorrhage.

Clinical features

DIC is a manifestation of a primary disease and therefore, usually the most immediate signs and symptoms are those of the underlying condition. Additionally, large bruises and spontaneous bleeding (e.g., from sites of venepuncture) may be apparent. In subacute and chronic cases the clinical presentation is frequently associated with thrombosis; however, in acute settings various features can be found:

- Bleeding from at least three unrelated sites (e.g., nose, ears, respiratory tract or gastrointestinal tract)
- Signs of haemorrhage
- Petechiae, purpura
- Thrombosis can cause widespread ischaemia or infarction leading to renal failure, liver failure and central nervous involvement

Investigations show:

- Low platelet count and/or dysfunctional platelets
- Prolonged prothrombin time and APTT
- Low fibrinogen levels
- High D-dimer/fibrin degradation product levels

Treatment and prognosis

Treatment of the underlying disease is the first priority and will resolve the DIC in most cases. Replacement of platelets and clotting factors (fresh frozen plasma or cryoprecipitate) may be used if there is haemorrhage or a risk of haemorrhage (e.g., in surgery). Pharmacological inhibitors of coagulation or fibrinolysis (e.g., heparin or tranexamic acid) may be beneficial in DIC with predominate thrombosis but risk of bleeding versus risk of embolism must be carefully evaluated.

DIC is associated with high mortality. It commonly results in organ failure and long-term complications. Prognosis is based on the nature of the underlying condition, comorbidities and the severity of DIC.

> **HINTS AND TIPS**
>
> Administration of blood products can be guided by laboratory tests (e.g., FBC, clotting, fibrinogen levels) or point-of-care tests such as thromboelastography (TEG) and rotational thromboelastometry (ROTEM) which can quickly provide answers as to which part of the clotting cascade is defective and therefore, what exact treatment to administer.

THROMBOTIC DISORDERS AND THROMBOEMBOLISM

General information

Venous thromboembolism (VTE) most commonly occurs in the deep veins (deep vein thrombosis, DVT) of the lower limbs and pelvis. Clots in the upper limbs, CNS, lungs, renal vessels or mesenteric vessels are less common. DVT can be classified into provoked or unprovoked. Provoked disease is associated with a transient risk factor (Table 37.11) while unprovoked DVT occurs in the absence of such (higher risk of recurrence due to inability to remove the risk factor). VTE is common and often asymptomatic. It is a serious disease that can result in death (most frequently due to PE).

Pathology

- Clotting of blood can be caused by abnormal vessel walls, venous stasis or hypercoagulable blood.
- Thrombosis may be precipitated by a specific event such as surgery or a physiological state such as pregnancy.
- Clots may break off and embolize to other organs (e.g., the lungs (pulmonary embolus)) or, very rarely, cause cerebral infarction by paradoxical embolus in patients with a patent foramen ovale or intracardiac defect.

Clinical features

- DVT causes unilateral localized pain, swelling, redness and oedema.
- Pulmonary embolus classically causes sudden onset of pleuritic chest pain, dyspnoea and haemoptysis.
- Patients with inherited hypercoagulable states may present with venous thromboses without obvious precipitants, in unusual places (e.g., Budd–Chiari syndrome), at an early age or with spontaneous abortions.

The pretest probability of DVT should be evaluated with an accepted scoring system (Table 37.12). If concerns arise,

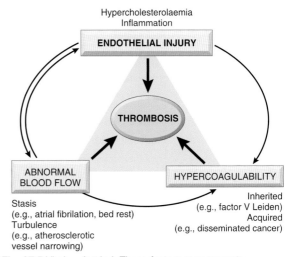

Fig. 37.5 Virchow's triad. These factors may promote thrombosis independently or in combination. (From Aster JC, Mitchell RN, Abbas AK, Kumar V. *Pocket Companion to Robbins and Cotran Pathologic Basis of Disease,* 10th ed. Elsevier; 2024.)

appropriate imaging such as ultrasound scan or CT pulmonary angiogram scan can be considered.

Treatment and prognosis

Although local protocols may differ, general management considerations for patients who have thrombotic disease should include appropriate anticoagulation and lifestyle advice. Compression stockings and avoidance of risk factors are important. Pharmacological interim anticoagulant treatment includes direct oral anticoagulants (DOACs) such as apixaban or rivaroxaban as first-line drugs and low-molecular-weight heparin

Table 37.11 Risk factors for thromboembolic events

Cause	Risk factor	Associated factors
Inherited (decreasing order of thrombotic risk)	Antithrombin III deficiency	
	Protein C deficiency	
	Protein S deficiency	
	Factor V Leiden mutation (activated protein C resistance)	
	Prothrombin 20210A mutation	
	Hyperhomocysteinaemia	
	Dysfibrinogenaemia (10% have thrombophilia, 90% have coagulopathy)	
Acquired	Physiological	Pregnancy and postpartum period
		Obesity
		Age over 60 years
		Male sex
		Smoking
	Initiating events (immobilization)	Surgery
		Trauma
		Long-distance travel (>4 hours)
		Recent hospitalization
		Significant immobility (bedbound, unable to mobilize unaided)
	Pathological	Malignancy
		Venous trauma
		Oestrogens
		Nephrotic syndrome
		Antiphospholipid syndrome
		Hyperviscosity syndromes
		Inflammatory bowel disease
		Dehydration
		Varicose veins
		Heart failure
		History of deep vein thrombosis

(LMWH), dabigatran or edoxaban if these are not suitable. Unfractionated heparin (UFH) should be considered in patients with a high risk of bleeding or those with established renal failure (UFH has a shorter half-life and can be reversed with protamine). Maintenance treatment is achieved with a DOAC or warfarin. DOACs do not need regular monitoring while warfarin therapy requires regular INR testing.

The length of treatment is variable and depends on the cause of the thrombus. Therapy is normally for at least 3 months after which it is reevaluated on the basis of comorbidities, current patient status and the cause of the initial event. In provoked disease, treatment can usually be stopped. In unprovoked DVT the preference is for continuation beyond the initial 3 months, and length of treatment is individualized with careful risk balance consideration.

HINTS AND TIPS

Warfarin alone is a *pro*coagulant when used initially because of its more rapid inhibition of *pro*tein C and *pro*tein S.

Table 37.12 Two-level Wells score algorithm

Score 1 point for each of the following. Subtract 2 points if an alternative diagnosis is as likely or more likely.
1–2 points: moderate risk of DVT
Perform high-sensitivity D-dimer: if positive a leg ultrasound is indicated.
3 points or more: likely DVT
All patients should receive a leg ultrasound and a D-dimer test.
Interim therapeutic anticoagulation is offered where appropriate.

1. Active malignancy (current, previous 6 months or palliative)
2. Paralysis, paresis or recent immobilization of legs with, e.g., plaster
3. Recently bedridden for 3 days or more, or major surgery within last 12 weeks
4. Pitting oedema in the symptomatic leg
5. Localized tenderness along deep veins
6. Swollen entire leg
7. Calf swollen by more than 3 cm when compared with the asymptomatic leg
8. Collateral superficial veins
9. Previous DVT

DVT, *Deep vein thrombosis.*

THROMBOTIC THROMBOCYTOPENIC PURPURA

Thrombotic thrombocytopenic purpura (TTP) is a rare form of thrombotic microangiopathy. It is more common in adults (peak occurrence is in the fourth decade of life), although cases in children and neonates have been reported. It is usually immune-mediated and associated with a deficiency of ADAMTS13 enzyme. Pregnancy and the postpartum period account for 10% to 25% of cases, and it has higher prevalence in those with autoimmune disease and cancer.

It is characterized by:

- Severe thrombocytopenia
- Microangiopathic haemolysis
- Neurological abnormalities such as lethargy, confusion, headache and seizures
- Acute kidney injury (AKI)
- Pyrexia that is not caused by infection

Clinical examination can show purpuric rash and splenomegaly.

Investigations include:

- Blood film: shows the fragmented RBCs (schistocytes), which are characteristic of the disease.
- Raised bilirubin, raised LDH and low haptoglobins because of haemolysis.
- Renal function tests, which may show elevated creatinine level.
- Urinalysis may show proteinuria and haematuria.

Diagnosis is a medical emergency and characteristically there is a rapid deterioration. Mortality without treatment can be as high as 90% and therefore, prompt management with intravenous plasma exchange is key. The monoclonal antibody fragment, Caplacizumab should be used alongside plasma exchange to reduce microvascular thrombosis and improve time to platelet count recovery.

Despite very low platelets, platelet transfusion should be avoided as this 'fuels the fire'.

HAEMOLYTIC URAEMIC SYNDROME

Haemolytic uraemic syndrome (HUS) consists of a triad of acute kidney injury, thrombocytopenia and microangiopathic haemolytic anaemia (negative Coombs' test). Similar to TTP there will be anaemia with evidence of haemolysis, fragments on the blood film (schistocytes), and is associated with a raised bilirubin, raised reticulocyte count and low haptoglobins. There is thrombocytopenia, although classically less severe than with TTP, and AKI is a prominent feature.

HUS is classified as typical and atypical. Typical HUS, is associated with the Shiga toxin producing *Escherichia coli* O157:H7, that damages endothelial cells. It is one of the main causes of AKI in children under the age of three. Cells particularly susceptible include those in the renal, gastrointestinal and CNS. Damage to the microvasculature causes deposition of thrombin and fibrin and narrowing of the blood vessels, preventing erythrocytes from passing and causing damage to cells and tissues.

It classically presents with profuse diarrhoea that becomes bloody at 1 to 3 days. There is often abdominal pain, vomiting and fever.

Treatment is supportive, with hydration and blood transfusion if required. Platelet transfusion, antibiotics and antimotility agents should be avoided. Dialysis is sometimes required.

Atypical HUS (aHUS) is complement mediated, and may be caused by heritable complement gene mutations or autoantibodies to complement proteins. If there is clinical suspicion for an aHUS (i.e., positive family history, absence of Shiga toxin) then anticomplement therapy, e.g., eculizumab is used.

Chapter Summary

- Haematological diseases are a group of conditions primarily affecting blood.
- They can be roughly divided into myeloid disease, including haemoglobinopathies, anaemias, myeloproliferative disorders, coagulopathies and/or disorders that reduce the number of blood cells (e.g., myelodysplastic syndrome or thrombocytopenia) and haematological malignancies.
- The malignancies include lymphomas, leukaemias and myelomas.
- Miscellaneous haematological diseases can be acquired (e.g., hyposplenism due to splenectomy), related to other underlying conditions (e.g., anaemia of chronic disease) or caused by genetic abnormalities (e.g., haemochromatosis).

UKMLA Conditions
Anaemia
Arterial thrombosis
Deep vein thrombosis
Disseminated intravascular coagulation
Epistaxis
Haemochromatosis
Haemoglobinopathies
Haemophilia
Hyposplenism/splenectomy
Leukaemia
Lymphoma
Multiple myeloma
Myeloproliferative disorders
Pancytopenia
Polycythaemia
Sickle cell disease
Transfusion reactions

UKMLA Presentations
Bruising
Epistaxis
Fatigue
Fever
Jaundice
Lymphadenopathy
Organomegaly
Pallor
Petechial rash
Purpura

Infectious diseases

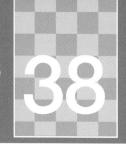

38

GENERAL OVERVIEW

Infections affecting specific systems have been discussed in the appropriate chapters. This chapter considers other important and very different infections affecting populations around the world: human immunodeficiency virus (HIV) infection, malaria, diarrhoeal disease and infection with drug-resistant bacteria. We also discuss Coronavirus disease 2019 (COVID-19), including treatment recommendations and current prevention strategies, including the global vaccination effort.

HIV AND AIDS

Epidemiology and aetiology

HIV continues to be a global health issue, with the World Health Organization (WHO) estimating 38.4 million people to live with HIV at the end of 2021, and 650,000 people to have died from HIV-related causes within that year. Approximately two-thirds of affected individuals live in sub-Saharan Africa. In the United Kingdom, Public Health England estimates that around 100,000 adults are infected with HIV.

HIV disease can be managed by treatment regimens composed of a combination of antiretroviral drugs. Current antiretroviral therapy (ART) does not cure HIV infection, but suppresses viral replication and allows an individual's immune system to recover strength and regain the capacity to fight off opportunistic infections and some cancers, which are the most common causes of death in individuals affected by HIV. Advances in ART have meant that HIV infection is now a manageable chronic disease. There has been a huge drive to increase the provision of ARTs worldwide; since 2016 WHO has recommended a 'Treat All' approach: that all people living with HIV can be provided with lifelong ART, including children, adolescents, adults and pregnant and breastfeeding women, regardless of CD4 count. By June 2022, 189 countries had already adopted this recommendation, covering 99% of all people living with HIV. Globally, 28.7 million people living with HIV were receiving ART in 2021. More efforts need to be made to upscale this treatment, particularly in children, with only 52% of children 0 to 14 years of age receiving ART at the end of 2021.

HIV can be transmitted by sexual, parenteral and vertical routes (Tables 38.1 and 38.2).

Table 38.1 Routes of HIV transmission

Route	Examples
Sexual	Vaginal intercourse, anal intercourse
Parenteral	IV drug abuse, blood transfusion, needlestick injury
Vertical (i.e., from mother to foetus)	During gestation or delivery, via breast milk

IV, Intravenous.

Table 38.2 Risk of HIV transmission

Type of exposure (source known to be HIV positive)	Risk of transmission (%)
Needlestick	0.2–0.4
Mucosal membrane exposure	0.1
Receptive oral sex	0–0.04
Insertive vaginal sex	≤0.1
Insertive anal sex	≤0.1
Receptive vaginal sex	0.01–0.15
Receptive anal sex	≤3
IDUs sharing needles	0.7
Blood transfusion	90–100

IDU, Intravenous drug user.

Table 38.3 HIV genes and the proteins they encode

Gene	Protein
pol	Reverse transcriptase (makes DNA copies of the viral RNA) and integrase (for insertion into host DNA)
gag	Core protein p24
env	Glycoprotein 41, a transmembrane protein, and glycoprotein 120, an external glycoprotein (for fusion with host cell)

Pathology

HIV is a lentivirus that belongs to a subgroup of human retroviruses, which means that its genetic information is stored in a single strand of ribonucleic acid (RNA). Three specific HIV genes produce proteins essential for virus survival (Table 38.3). Lentiviruses have a long latent phase between infection and the development of symptoms. HIV causes immunodeficiency by preferentially infecting and destroying cells of the immune system, in particular CD4 cells, which are a class of T lymphocytes. The CD4 receptor has affinity for glycoprotein 120 on the viral envelope, allowing the virus to enter the cell. Coreceptors such as CXCR4 and CCR5 are also currently being explored as potential therapeutic targets. Virus replication involves the enzyme reverse transcriptase. It makes DNA copies of the virus RNA, which then becomes integrated into the host cell's genome and results in the production of viral particles. This disrupts the normal function of the infected cells, and the host cells are eventually destroyed.

Eventually this manifests with symptoms of diseases resulting from immunodeficiency (i.e., opportunistic infections and malignancies).

Two HIV types have been identified: HIV-1 and HIV-2. HIV-1 was first identified in 1983 and is found throughout the world. It is the main cause of HIV-related disease in humans. HIV-2 has lower infectivity and relatively poor capacity for transmission compared with HIV-1 and is confined to West Africa, where it is endemic. It accounts for around 5% of HIV infections worldwide.

Diagnosis

Diagnosis is usually made by HIV antibody tests. These antibodies may be undetectable for up to 3 months after infection, which presents a window for false-negative results. Once a diagnosis has been confirmed, disease activity can be assessed by quantification of HIV RNA viral load and CD4+ cell count (Table 38.4).

> **CLINICAL NOTES**
>
> When should I offer a test for HIV?
>
> NICE guidelines suggest that in the primary care setting, an HIV test should be offered to people who:
> - request testing
> - have risk factors for HIV
> - have another sexually transmitted infection
> - have clinical features of HIV infection, or an AIDS-defining condition (see later)

> **COMMUNICATION**
>
> Do not be afraid to perform an HIV test. Remain nonjudgemental and reassure the patient of the importance of confidentiality. Stress the importance of early detection and high effectiveness of treatment.

Clinical features

The symptoms of HIV vary depending on stage of infection. NICE and The US Centers for Disease Control and Prevention (CDC) describe three stages of HIV:

'Acute' or 'primary' HIV infection

Though people living with HIV tend to be most infectious in the first few months after being infected when viral load is high, many are unaware of their status until the later stages. In the first few weeks after initial infection people may experience no symptoms, or an influenza-like illness including fever, headache, rash or sore throat. This phase is self-limiting and is known as 'primary HIV infection' or 'HIV seroconversion illness'.

Chronic HIV infection (asymptomatic phase)

Once symptoms of primary HIV infection resolve, an asymptomatic stage of infection begins. During this phase HIV is still active and continues to reproduce in the body, and people can still transmit infection. The duration of this phase varies widely between people with some progressing to advanced HIV disease (also known as acquired immunodeficiency syndrome (AIDS)) within 1 to 2 years ('rapid progressors') and others maintaining effective immune function more than 10 years later ('slow progressors'). Individuals who take ART as prescribed may never progress to stage 3 (AIDS).

Table 38.4 Investigations at different stages of HIV infection

Phase	Viral replication	p24	HIV antibodies	CD4+ count (cells/μL)
Stage 1 – Primary infection	High	Detectable until HIV antibodies appear	Detectable 3 weeks to 3 months after exposure	Transient fall because of high viral load, but returns to normal when HIV antibodies appear
Stage 2 – Chronic infection	Low	Undetectable as antibody in excess to antigen	Detectable	Normal
Stage 3 – Advanced HIV disease/AIDS	High	Detectable	Detectable	Falls; when <200, the risk of infection is very high and development of AIDS is likely

AIDS, *Acquired immunodeficiency syndrome.*

Advanced HIV infection (AIDS)

This is the most severe stage of HIV infection. A person is said to have advanced HIV disease or AIDS when the CD4 count is very low (less than 200 cells/μL). At this stage the immune system is badly damaged, and certain opportunistic infections (such as pneumocystis pneumonia) or malignancies (such as Kaposi sarcoma) develop. Some of these malignancies are associated with specific viral infections (Table 38.5). These conditions are known as 'AIDS-defining illness' (Table 38.6). Without treatment, people with AIDS typically survive around three years.

Table 38.5 Malignancies seen with increased frequency in advanced HIV, and associated viruses

Tumour	Associated virus
Kaposi sarcoma	Human herpes virus 8
Cerebral lymphoma	Epstein–Barr virus
Non-Hodgkin lymphoma	Epstein–Barr virus
Hodgkin disease	Not determined
Cervical carcinoma	Human papillomavirus
Anal carcinoma	Human papillomavirus

Suspect HIV infection in person presenting with one or more of the following:

- Flu-like symptoms that are prolonged and severe (headache, fatigue, fever, joint pain, loss of appetite, sore throat, rash, night sweats, swollen lymph nodes)
- Recurrent infections
- Glandular fever-like illness
- Conditions related to immunosuppression, such as oral candidiasis or shingles
- Lymphadenopathy of unknown origin
- Pyrexia of unknown origin
- Weight loss of more than 10 kg
- Risk factors for HIV such as living in/working in/or coming from a high prevalence area, sex between men, sex workers and IV drug use

Be aware that infants most often present with:

- Failure to thrive, and/or
- *Pneumocystis jirovecii* pneumonia
- Cytomegalovirus
- HIV encephalopathy

Features of symptomatic HIV infection per organ system are summarized in Table 38.7.

Table 38.6 AIDS-defining conditions, according to the CDC (Centre for Disease Control)

AIDS-defining conditions
Candidiasis of the oesophagus, bronchi, trachea or lungs (but NOT the mouth)
Cervical cancer, invasive
Coccidioidomycosis, disseminated or extrapulmonary
Cryptococcosis, extrapulmonary
Cryptosporidiosis, chronic intestinal (>1 month duration)
Cytomegalovirus disease (other than liver, spleen, or nodes) or cytomegalovirus retinitis
Encephalopathy, HIV-related
Herpes simplex: chronic ulcer(s) (>1 month in duration); or bronchitis, pneumonitis, or oesophagitis
Histoplasmosis, disseminated or extrapulmonary
Cystoisosporiasis, chronic intestinal (>1-month duration)
Kaposi sarcoma
Lymphoma, Burkitt, immunoblastic or primary brain
Mycobacterium avium complex, tuberculosis of any site in or out of the lungs or unidentified species
Pneumocystis jirovecii pneumonia (PJP)
Pneumonia, recurrent
Progressive multifocal leucoencephalopathy
Salmonella septicaemia, recurrent
Toxoplasmosis of brain
Wasting syndrome, HIV-related

Table 38.7 Features of symptomatic HIV infection according to body system

Organ/system	Clinical features of HIV infection
Mouth	Angular stomatitis, recurrent oral ulceration, parotid enlargement
	Oral hairy leucoplakia, oral candidiasis, necrotizing gingivitis/periodontitis
	Chronic oral herpes simplex infection
Gastrointestinal	Hepatosplenomegaly
	Persistent diarrhoea or malnutrition
	HIV wasting syndrome, HIV rectal fistula, oesophagitis (HSV, CMV, *Candida*)
	Hepatobiliary disease (*Mycobacteria*, hepatitis B virus, CMV, microsporidia), colitis (*Campylobacter*, *Salmonella*, *Shigella*, *Cryptosporidium*, *Giardia*), anal carcinoma
Cardiovascular	HIV-associated cardiomyopathy
	Pericardial effusions, conduction abnormalities, dilated cardiomyopathy, pulmonary hypertension, noninfectious endocarditis
Respiratory	Recurrent upper respiratory tract infection (e.g., tonsillitis, sinusitis)
	Pulmonary TB, severe recurrent bacterial pneumonia, lymphoid interstitial pneumonitis, chronic HIV-associated lung disease (e.g., bronchiectasis)
	Lower respiratory tract candidiasis, *Pneumocystis jirovecii* pneumonia
	Fungal pneumonia
Neurological	CNS toxoplasmosis, cryptococcal meningitis, HIV encephalopathy, progressive multifocal leucoencephalopathy, CNS lymphoma
	Myelopathy, peripheral neuropathy, inflammatory demyelinating polyneuropathy, retinitis (e.g., CMV)
Renal	HIV-associated nephropathy FSGS (collapsing variant)
Haematological	Unexplained anaemia, neutropenia or thrombocytopenia
	B-cell non-Hodgkin lymphoma
	Burkitt lymphoma, immunoblastic lymphoma
Dermatological	Herpes zoster, fungal nail infections (*Candida*, tinea), seborrheic dermatitis, itchy papular eruptions, extensive molluscum contagiosum
	Kaposi sarcoma, genital herpes simplex
	Squamous cell carcinoma, crusted scabies
Reproductive	Invasive cervical carcinoma
Other/systemic	Weight loss <10%

CMV, *Cytomegalovirus;* CNS, *central nervous system;* FSGS, *focal segmental glomerulosclerosis;* HSV, *herpes simplex virus.*

Treatment and prognosis

Currently, there is no effective cure or vaccine for HIV infection, even though in the last decade treatment of HIV infection has changed dramatically. At present, mainstay treatment is ART which slows disease progression, and has greatly improved the prognosis of HIV and AIDS.

ART is initiated with a combination of agents from at least two types of antiretroviral medication. In treatment-naïve patients, this involves a combination of two nucleoside reverse transcriptase inhibitors (NRTIs), drugs which block reverse transcriptase, an enzyme HIV needs to make copies of itself, e.g., abacavir, emtricitabine, lamivudine and tenofovir, and one of the following drugs:

- A nonnucleoside reverse transcriptase inhibitor (NNRTI): these bind to and later alter reverse transcriptase, an enzyme HIV needs to make copies of itself (e.g., efavirenz and nevirapine).
- A protease inhibitor (P): these block HIV protease, an enzyme HIV needs to make copies of itself (e.g., atazanavir, darunavir and ritonavir)
- An integrase inhibitor (INI): a drug that blocks the enzyme HIV integrase, an enzyme HIV needs to make copies of itself, e.g., dolutegravir, elvitegravir and raltegravir.

Other FDA-approved newer drug classes include fusion inhibitors – drugs that block HIV from entering the CD4

T lymphocyte, e.g., enfuvirtide; and CCR5 antagonists, drugs that block CCR5 coreceptors on the surface of certain immune cells, e.g., maraviroc (Fig. 38.1).

In the United Kingdom, treatment is recommended as soon as HIV diagnosis has been made or in the presence of AIDS-defining infection or major infection if the CD4 count is less than 200 cells/mL. It aims to deliver a long-term plasma HIV RNA concentration count of less than 50 copies per millilitre. HIV prognosis is strongly related to viral load and CD4 count. Viral load and CD4 count are also used to monitor the response to treatment.

As HIV treatment has improved, the incidence of HIV-associated infection (Table 38.8) and malignancy has changed and in many cases diminished. This means that even though long-term prognosis in people who respond well to ART (high CD4+ counts and unrecordable viral load) is not known, many are asymptomatic and living normal lives more than 15 years after diagnosis.

Prevention

No 'cure' for HIV infection means preventative measures must remain the highest priority for healthcare professionals. Such measures include education, provision of clean needles for intravenous drug abusers, use of condoms, screening of blood products and organs donated for transplantation, and postexposure prophylaxis. Research continues into new treatments and the possibility of a vaccine.

ETHICS

It is common practice to gain consent from the patient should a healthcare professional sustain a needle stick injury. Problems arise when a patient does not have the capacity to consent. The British Medical Association has established a set of ethical guidelines medical professionals can follow:

- If a patient is expected to regain capacity before testing is needed, testing should be withheld until consent can be obtained.
- If a person lacks capacity, doctors should determine whether legal arrangements have been set for the patient regarding the matter (e.g., advanced directive).
- If a patient is not expected to regain capacity before testing is required, a responsible clinician can make a decision regarding testing based on the patient's best interest.

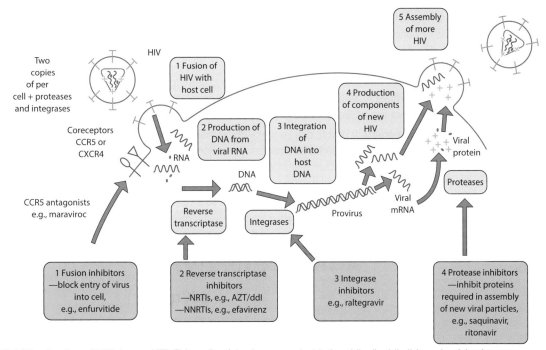

Fig. 38.1 Site of action of HIV drugs. *AZT*, Zidovudine (also known as 'azidothymidine'); *ddI*, didanosine (also known as '2′,3′-dideoxyinosine'); *mRNA*, messenger RNA; *NNRTI*, nonnucleoside reverse transcriptase inhibitor; *NRTI*, nucleoside reverse transcriptase inhibitor.

Table 38.8 Treatment and prophylaxis of opportunistic infections

Infection	Treatment	Treatment alternatives	Indication for prophy-laxis	Prophylactic drug regimes
Pneumocystis jirovecii	Orally or intravenously administered cotrimoxazole Steroids may be beneficial	Intravenously administered pentamidine, or clindamycin plus primaquine, or dapsone plus trimethoprim	Secondary prevention or CD4$^+$ count <200/μL	Orally administered cotrimoxazole, or nebulized pentamidine, or dapsone plus pyrimethamine
Toxoplasmosis	Sulphadiazine plus pyrimethamine + folate	Clindamycin replacing sulphadiazine	Secondary prevention or CD4$^+$ <200 cells/μL positive serology	Pyrimethamine plus sulphadiazine, or clindamycin, or cotrimoxazole, or dapsone
Cytomegalovirus	Ganciclovir or foscarnet		Secondary prevention	Ganciclovir or foscarnet
Herpes simplex	Aciclovir	Valaciclovir or foscarnet	Secondary prevention	Aciclovir
Herpes zoster	Aciclovir	Valaciclovir or foscarnet or famciclovir		
Cryptococcal meningitis	Amphotericin B with or without flucytosine, or fluconazole		Secondary prevention	Fluconazole
Mycobacterium avium complex	Rifampicin plus ethambutol plus clarithromycin	Rifabutin replacing rifampicin	Secondary prevention	Azithromycin or clarithromycin
Candida	Fluconazole	Ketoconazole or itraconazole	Secondary prevention	Fluconazole

MALARIA

Epidemiology and aetiology

In 2020 there was an estimated 241 million cases of malaria worldwide, with an estimated number of deaths of 627,000. It is endemic in developing countries, with the African region being disproportionately affected, home to 95% of all cases. It can easily be imported by people who have visited or come from endemic areas, and in the United Kingdom, approximately 1500 cases are notified each year. Disease is caused by infection of red blood cells with one of the species of the genus *Plasmodium* (*P. vivax, P. ovale, P. malariae* or *P. falciparum*) (Table 38.9).

Pathology

Malaria is a life-threatening illness that spreads through a bite of a female *Anopheles* mosquito. An infective, motile sporozoite travels through the bloodstream to reach the liver. There it enters a hepatocyte, where it asexually reproduces (schizogony), leading to the production of millions of merozoites. These invade new red blood cells (RBCs), in which they asexually multiply to produce 8 to 24 infective merozoites. At this point, RBCs

rupture, and the whole cycle begins again (Fig. 38.2). A burst of cells causes the release of malaria parasites, malaria antigen, cytokines (especially tumour necrosis factor) and other RBC constituents into the bloodstream, causing the typical clinical picture of periodic fevers. Depending on the *Plasmodium* species the timing of the clinical manifestations differs (see Table 38.9). *P. vivax, P. ovale* and *P. malariae* invade up to 2% of the circulating RBCs. *P. falciparum* may affect more than 10% of RBCs, producing a potentially severe illness.

Clinical features

Malaria presentation is determined by parasitaemia levels and corresponds to the parasite life cycle. Symptoms may occur from 6 days after initial infection up to several months later. It is characterized by periodic high temperature, sweating and rigors, which coincide with the release of merozoites from erythrocytes. Other nonspecific features include nausea and vomiting, abdominal pain, diarrhoea, headache, cough and arthralgia/myalgia. Splenomegaly is commonly found, but mild jaundice and hepatomegaly may also be present. Complications are almost always associated with *P. falciparum*, and are summarized in Table 38.10.

Table 38.9 *Plasmodium* species causing malaria

Organism	Clinical features
Plasmodium falciparum	Most common worldwide and responsible for most deaths. Incubation period is 7–10 days, with most travellers presenting within 8 weeks. A classic features is paroxysmal episodes of symptoms every 36–48 hours. Causes fulminating disease.
Plasmodium vivax	Incubation period is 12–17 days. Presents as 'benign tertian malaria' with temperature spikes every 48 hours. Relapse of disease is common due to persistent dormant parasite in the liver.
Plasmodium ovale	Incubation period is 15–18 days. May produce relapse similarly to infection with *P. vivax*
Plasmodium malaria	Incubation period is long at 18–40 days. Can present with quartan malaria (also known as 'quartan fever') with temperature spikes every 4 days. Can present late, 1 year after initial infection. Dormant parasites reside in the blood for up to 50 years. It is rarely fatal, but can cause glomerulonephritis.

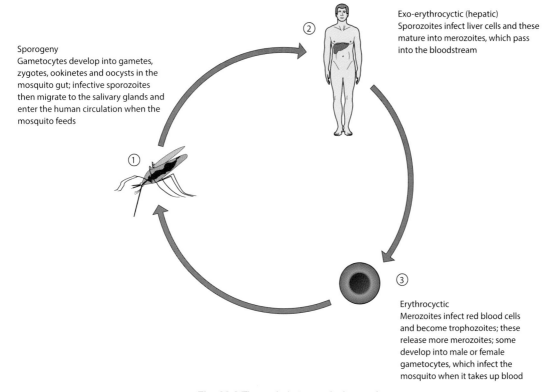

Sporogeny
Gametocytes develop into gametes, zygotes, ookinetes and oocysts in the mosquito gut; infective sporozoites then migrate to the salivary glands and enter the human circulation when the mosquito feeds

Exo-erythrocyctic (hepatic)
Sporozoites infect liver cells and these mature into merozoites, which pass into the bloodstream

Erythrocyctic
Merozoites infect red blood cells and become trophozoites; these release more merozoites; some develop into male or female gametocytes, which infect the mosquito when it takes up blood

Fig. 38.2 The malaria transmission cycle.

Early diagnosis and treatment of malaria reduce disease burden, prevent deaths and contribute to reducing transmission. Diagnosis is confirmed by using parasite-based diagnostic testing:

- Microscopy: thin and thick blood films are the gold standard tests. If there is clinical suspicion of malaria but the blood film is negative, a further two samples over the subsequent 48 hours are necessary to rule out the infection.
- Antigen detection test: rapid diagnostic tests that detect parasite antigens. These are dipstick based and can be used by staff who have not been trained in microscopy. They are more expensive, but together with microscopy

Table 38.10 Complications of infection by *Plasmodium falciparum*

Cerebral malaria (hyperpyrexia, coma, death)
Hypoglycaemia
Acute respiratory distress syndrome
Seizures
Severe intravascular haemolysis with haemoglobinuria (blackwater fever)
Acute renal failure
Hepatic necrosis
Jaundice
Haemolytic anaemia
Lactic acidosis
Coagulopathy (including disseminated intravascular coagulation)

studies are recommended as diagnostic tests for malaria by WHO.

- Polymerase chain reaction (PCR): this is more sensitive than microscopy, but takes much longer and is most useful when you are considering epidemiological testing.

Other investigations frequently used include:

- Full blood count: this may show anaemia, leucocytosis and thrombocytopenia.
- Liver function tests: enzyme levels are often deranged.
- Urea and electrolyte measurements: these may show raised creatinine level and hyponatraemia.
- Hypoglycaemia may be seen.

Treatment and prognosis

All patients suspected of having malaria should be urgently discussed with an infectious disease specialist, and all confirmed cases must be reported to Public Health England. Treatment is under constant review, and depends on a number of factors including the severity of disease, species of *Plasmodium* parasite, tolerability of specific drugs, and patterns of drug resistance. Drugs currently in use in the United Kingdom, as recommended by CDC and WHO guidance, include:

- Artesunate: recommended as first-line use to treat severe or complicated malaria. IV use can cause haemolysis, and this must be monitored.
- Quinine: may be used initially to treat severe or complicated malaria if artesunate is unavailable.
- Artemisinin combination therapy (ACT): used to treat uncomplicated malaria, and is the preferred treatment for mixed infection.

- Atovaquone–proguanil: may be used to treat uncomplicated malaria where ACT is unavailable.
- Quinine *plus* doxycycline: may also be used to treat uncomplicated malaria if ACT is unavailable. (NB. Doxycycline should not be given to children <12 years of age.)
- Chloroquine: may be used to treat uncomplicated *P. malariae, P. ovale, P. knowlesi* and most cases of *P. vivax* malaria but use depends upon patterns of resistance and tolerance.
- Primaquine: currently the only effective drug for eradication of hypnozoites (dormant parasites which persist in the liver after treatment of *P. ovale* and *P. vivax*). Screening for G6PD deficiency is essential before treatment is started as it can cause haemolysis in G6PD-deficient individuals which can be fatal. It is contraindicated in pregnancy and with breastfeeding.

If left untreated malaria can be fatal (Table 38.10). Of particular concern is cerebral malaria, with a mortality rate of 20%. Improvement of management and prevention, however, has led to a decrease in overall worldwide mortality rates by 60% in the last decade.

Prevention

Use of chemoprophylaxis together with insecticide-treated nets results in a prevention rate of 90%. Medications used include chloroquine, proguanil–atovaquone, mefloquine and doxycycline. Other protective behaviours to avoid mosquito bites, including wearing full-length/long-sleeved clothes and using insect repellent, are also important.

> ### COMMUNICATION
>
> Travellers need careful instruction about the need for malaria prophylaxis: both medication (drug, dose, adherence and cessation) and precautions against mosquito bites (e.g., insecticide/repellents). It is important to stress preventative measures are effective but are not a guarantee against the infection.

DIARRHOEAL DISEASE

Diarrhoeal disease constitutes a major global health challenge, particularly in children where it is the second leading cause of death in children younger than 5 years of age (after respiratory disease), with children under the age of five accounting for 63% of the global burden. It can last for days, and causes death by

Table 38.11 Causes of diarrhoea

Organism type	Causes of diarrhoea	Length of symptoms
Viruses	*Norovirus* (most common cause of diarrhoea worldwide) *Rotavirus* *Sapovirus*	2–3 days
Bacteria	*Salmonella* *Campylobacter jejuni* *Shigella* *Escherichia coli* (most common in the elderly)	3–5 days
Parasites	*Cryptosporidium parvum* *Giardia intestinalis* *Entamoeba histolytica* *Cyclospora cayetanensis*	Weeks to months if untreated

Table 38.12 Causes of bloody diarrhoea

Organism type	Causes of bloody diarrhoea
Bacteria	*Campylobacter jejuni* Salmonella *Escherichia coli* O157:H7 *Clostridium difficile* Shigella *Vibrio parahaemolyticus* Yersinia Aeromonas
Viruses	*Cytomegalovirus*
Parasites	*Entamoeba histolytica* Schistosomiasis

depletion of essential stores of water and electrolytes resulting in profound dehydration. Around 88% of diarrhoeal-disease-associated deaths are attributable to unsafe water, inadequate sanitation and insufficient hygiene.

The WHO defines diarrhoea as the passage of three or more loose or liquid stools per day, or more frequent than is normal for the individual. It is usually caused by infective bacteria, viruses or parasites Table 38.11. Most commonly it spreads through the enteral route, and this is through contaminated water or poor hygiene. Underlying malnutrition also increases vulnerability to diarrhoea.

Clinical features

Three distinct forms of diarrhoea can be characterized:

- Acute watery diarrhoea: caused by infection, drugs and allergies.
- Acute bloody diarrhoea (or dysentery): caused by infective organisms (Table 38.12).

- Persistent diarrhoea (>14 days): associated with chronic bowel conditions (inflammatory bowel disease, irritable bowel syndrome, diverticular disease and malignancy), infection, coeliac disease and malabsorption, constipation and drugs.

The degree of dehydration is rated on a scale of three:

1. No dehydration
2. Some dehydration (two or more of the following signs):
   - restlessness/irritability
   - sunken eyes
   - thirst
3. Severe dehydration (at least two of the following signs):
   - lethargy/altered level of consciousness
   - sunken eyes
   - decreased skin turgor
   - unable to drink

Treatment and prevention

Most dangers of diarrhoeal disease come from dehydration. Management involves initial assessment of the severity, the presence of red flag symptoms and determination of a cause. Investigations are not always necessary but may include stool sample for culture and sensitivity testing and blood tests. Treatment focuses on fluid replacement to manage dehydration. Preferred means of rehydration is with oral rehydration salts (ORS), which is a mixture of clean water, salt and sugar. In cases of severe dehydration or shock, however, intravenous fluids are required.

In most instances diarrhoea is self-limiting, however, in severe cases of infection (persistent diarrhoea or dysentery), antibiotics are required. The emergence of antibiotic-resistant strains of enteric pathogens is becoming a huge threat (see later). Prevention therefore is key. Measures to prevent diarrhoea include:

- Access to safe water
- Adequate sanitation and human waste disposal
- Promoting hand hygiene
- Promoting breastfeeding (WHO recommended exclusively for first 6 months of life)
- Vaccination for rotavirus in children

CLINICAL NOTES

Red flag symptoms include blood in stool, recent hospital treatment or antibiotic administration, persistent vomiting or high-volume diarrhoea, weight loss and nocturnal symptoms.

DRUG-RESISTANT BACTERIA

Antibiotic resistance is one of the largest global health threats today, killing at least 12.7 million people worldwide, with nearly 5 million of these deaths occurring in 2019 alone. This accounts for more deaths than was caused by HIV and malaria in the same year. It can affect anyone, of any age, in any country, and occurs when changes in bacteria cause the drugs used to treat infections to become less effective. Though antibiotic resistance occurs naturally, overuse and misuse of antibiotics are a huge contributing factor. It is an important problem, leading to increased healthcare costs, prolonged hospital stays and increased mortality. Without action, the concern is that common treatable infections will begin to cause death again. As a healthcare professional the single biggest contribution to be made to limiting spread is adherence to local infection control protocols.

Methicillin-resistant *Staphylococcus aureus*

Infection with methicillin-resistant *Staphylococcus aureus* (MRSA) results in the same range of presentations as other *S. aureus* infections, including skin, respiratory and urinary tract infections, but is highly resistant to antibiotic therapy. It is often acquired during exposure in healthcare facilities but most of the time does not cause harmful infection. MRSA is resistant to most β-lactam antibiotics, but is often sensitive to tetracyclines, glycopeptides (vancomycin and teicoplanin) rifampicin and sodium fusidate.

In hospital, patients are routinely screened (nose/axilla/groin) for MRSA. Those who test positive have eradication therapy and barrier nursed.

Other resistant bacteria

Vancomycin-resistant enterococci may have emerged because of the increased use of vancomycin for treatment of MRSA and *Clostridium difficile* infections. Enterococci are common gut flora, but in at-risk patients may cause urinary tract infection, wound infections and bacteraemia.

Carbapenem-resistant *Enterobacteriaceae* (CRE) infections are currently on the rise, and CRE are resistant to nearly all available antibiotics. It is estimated almost 50% of patients with CRE-positive blood culture die of the infection.

Resistant gram-negative bacteria such as *Pseudomonas* are a common problem in chronic suppurative respiratory conditions, such as bronchiectasis and cystic fibrosis, as well as in intensive care units, where they may cause ventilator-associated pneumonia.

WHO response

Tackling antibiotic resistance is a high priority for the WHO, and a global action plan was endorsed at the World Health Assembly in May 2015. This plan has five strategic objectives:

- To improve awareness and understanding of antimicrobial resistance.
- To strengthen surveillance and research.
- To reduce the incidence of infection.
- To optimize the use of antimicrobial medicines.
- To ensure sustainable investment in countering antimicrobial resistance.

COVID-19

Coronavirus disease 2019 (COVID-19) is an infectious acute respiratory disease caused by a novel coronavirus called SARS-Cov-2 virus. The virus gained attention after clusters of pneumonia of unknown aetiology were reported in Wuhan, the Hubei province of China, on 31 December 2019. The World Health Organization (WHO) later announced that a novel coronavirus had been detected in samples taken from these patients. The epidemic escalated and rapidly spread around the world, with the WHO first declaring a public health emergency of international concern on 30 January 2020, and then formally declaring it a pandemic on 11 March 2020. Worldwide the response to tackling the pandemic varied, though some form of 'lockdown' was implemented across almost all countries of the world. This global lockdown was initiated to stop the spread of the virus and 'flatten the curve' of the pandemic. Two years later the end of the pandemic is in sight, and globally we are beginning to adapt to the shift in behaviours, medicine and economy brought about by the pandemic.

Epidemiology

Since first reports of cases from Wuhan, China, cases of COVID-19 were reported across all continents. To date, 600 million confirmed cases and over 6.5 million deaths have been reported globally. In the United Kingdom, at the time of writing, there had been 24.4 million confirmed cases, and 212,000 deaths. Older people >70 years of age and males are at increased risk of infection and severe disease. Adolescents appear to be at similar risk to adults, while children have lower susceptibility to infection. Evidence does however suggest racial variation, with Black race and Hispanic ethnicity at higher risk than White race or non-Hispanic ethnicity. There was also an association between use of personal protective equipment (PPE) and decreased risk for infection. Risk factors are summarized in Table 38.13.

Table 38.13 Risk factors for infection with COVID-19

Older age
Male sex
Ethnic minorities
Comorbid disease (hypertension, cardiac disease, diabetes mellitus, chronic pulmonary disease, chronic kidney disease, cancer have all been linked to higher rates of hospitalization)
Obesity
Smoking
Immunosuppression (people with primary immunodeficiency disorder, solid organ or blood stem cell transplant, prolonged use of corticosteroids or other immunosuppressant medication are at increased risk of severe disease)

The 2019 emergent SARS-CoV-2 strain, usually referred to as the 'wild-type' strain, has mutated with time. These mutations have given rise to several new variants, of varying virulence. On 31 May 2021, the WHO recommended a naming system for these variants that uses the Greek alphabetic system. The Alpha variant was first identified in the United Kingdom in late 2020, and was the dominant variant until the emergence of the Delta variant. Compared with the Alpha variant, the Delta variant was identified as more transmissible, and to be related to more severe disease and higher rate of hospitalization. Currently the Omicron variants dominate in the United Kingdom. The Omicron variant was first reported in Botswana, and very soon thereafter from South Africa in November 2021. In South Africa, it was associated with an increase in regional infections, and was promptly identified in multiple other countries, where it was similarly associated with sharp increases in reported infections. Several Omicron sublineages have a replication advantage over the Delta variant and evade infection and vaccine-induced humoral immunity to a greater extent than prior variants. They also appear to be associated with less severe disease. Currently there are three Omicron variants labelled as variants of concern (VOC) within the United Kingdom.

Pathology

Coronaviruses are a large family of related viruses that cause disease in humans and animals. They are enveloped positive-stranded RNA viruses. Full genomic sequencing indicated that the coronavirus that caused COVID-19 is of the same subgenus as the severe acute respiratory syndrome (SARS) virus (as well as several bat coronaviruses), and therefore it was designated SARS-CoV-2. The host receptor for SARS-CoV-2 cell entry is the same as for SARS-CoV, the angiotensin-converting enzyme 2 (ACE2), which is highly expressed on pulmonary epithelial cells. SARS-CoV-2 binds to ACE2 through the receptor-binding domain of its spike protein. The cellular serine protease TMPRSS2 also appears important for SARS-CoV-2 cell entry,

promoting viral uptake by cleaving ACE2 and activating the SARS-CoV-2 S protein, which mediates coronavirus entry into host cells. Similar to other respiratory viral diseases, such as influenza, profound lymphopenia may occur in individuals with COVID-19 when SARS-CoV-2 infects and kills T lymphocyte cells. In addition, the viral inflammatory response impairs lymphopoiesis and increases lymphocyte apoptosis. This leads to a decreased ability to fight off the infection.

In later stages of infection, when viral replication accelerates, the epithelial–endothelial barrier integrity is compromised, triggering an influx of monocytes and neutrophils. These inflammatory infiltrates are evidenced as ground-glass opacities on CT imaging. Pulmonary oedema follows, compatible with early-phase acute respiratory distress syndrome (ARDS). This leads to dysfunctional alveolar-capillary oxygen transmission and impaired oxygen diffusion capacity.

In severe COVID-19, fulminant activation of coagulation and consumption of clotting factors occurs. This is indicated by increase in prothrombin time and international normalized ratio (INR), and is linked to microthrombi within the lungs and other organs.

Viral transmission

Route of transmission is person-to-person, mainly airborne. Infection may also occur if an individual's hands are contaminated by these secretions or by touching contaminated surfaces and then touching mucous membranes such as the eyes, nose or mouth. The incubation period is 5 to 6 days, though can be up to 14 days.

Clinical features

Patients of COVID-19 most commonly present with fever, dry cough and shortness of breath. Anosmia (loss of sense of smell) or ageusia (loss of sense of taste) is the sole presenting symptom in approximately 3% of cases. Other common features are headache, myalgia, sore throat and malaise. Gastrointestinal symptoms such as anorexia and abdominal pain are more common in children than in adults. A rash which may be erythematous, vesicular, petechial, urticaria and livedo reticularis occurs in less than 20% of individuals.

Cough, shortness of breath and fatigue may persist for weeks after infection. 'Long covid' is used to describe the effects of COVID-19 persisting for weeks or months beyond the initial illness. The National Institute for Health and Care Excellence (NICE) defines someone with 'long covid' to be:

- Experiencing the signs and symptoms of COVID-19 for 4 to 12 weeks postacute illness

  or

- Experiencing the signs and symptoms of COVID-19 for >12 weeks postacute illness, that cannot be explained by an alternate diagnosis

Research published in July 2022 by King's College London identified three distinct types of long covid based on the type of symptoms participants experienced:

- The largest group of long Covid sufferers reported symptoms such as fatigue, 'brain-fog' and headache.
- A second group experienced respiratory symptoms such as chest pain and severe shortness of breath. These symptoms were the most common in the early stages of the pandemic, before widespread vaccination.
- A third, smaller group experienced a diverse range of symptoms including heart palpitations, muscle ache and pain, and changes in skin and hair.

Long covid is more common in those who had severe acute disease, but may occur in mild disease.

Management

COVID-19 is diagnosed by positive rapid antigen test or real-time reverse transcription polymerase chain reaction (RT-PCR). Recommendations for management differ based on disease severity.

WHO definitions of disease severity:

- **Critical COVID-19:** defined by the criteria for ARDS, sepsis, septic shock, or other conditions that would normally require the provision of life-sustaining therapies such as mechanical ventilation (invasive or noninvasive) or vasopressor therapy.
- **Severe COVID-19:** defined by any of:
  - Oxygen saturation <90% on room air.
  - Signs of pneumonia.
  - Signs of severe respiratory distress in adults, accessory muscle use, inability to complete full sentences, respiratory rate >30 breaths per minute; and in children, rib recessions, grunting, central cyanosis, or presence of any other general danger signs including inability to breastfeed or drink, lethargy, convulsions or reduced level of consciousness.
- **Nonsevere COVID-19:** defined as the absence of any criteria for severe or critical COVID-19.

Nonsevere COVID-19

Treatment for nonsevere COVID-19 is with home isolation and symptom management, e.g., rehydration, antipyretics and analgesia. NICE also recommends treating with a neutralizing monoclonal antibody (nMAB) for nonhospitalized adults and children aged 12 and above who are at high risk of symptom progression. The typical characteristics of people at higher risk of symptom progression include those with older age, immunosuppression and/or chronic diseases. Lack of COVID-19 vaccination is an additional risk to consider. As of April 2022, NICE recommended treatment with the antiviral remdesivir for those at highest risk of hospitalization. This should be administered as soon as possible after onset of symptoms, ideally within 7 days. Other antiviral options include nirmatrelvir/ritonavir and molnupiravir.

Severe COVID-19

Patients with severe and critical COVID-19 should be managed in the hospital/critical care setting. Decisions about escalating treatment should be made early based on the patient's likelihood of recovery and their expectations of treatment. This should be done in the multidisciplinary (MDT) setting, with involvement of the patient's next of kin, taking into account any advanced directives issued by the patient. Supplemental oxygen therapy should be administered immediately to any patient with emergency signs (severe respiratory distress, central cyanosis, shock). Once the patient is stable, the general target is SpO_2 >90% (92%–95% in pregnant women). Oxygen flow rate should be appropriate for delivery device (nasal cannulae/venturi mask/face mask with reservoir bag). Consider awake prone positioning for people in hospital with COVID-19 who are not intubated and have higher oxygen needs.

In-hospital monitoring of stable patients

- Patients hospitalized with COVID-19 require regular monitoring of vital signs (including pulse oximetry), utilizing medical early warning scores (e.g., NEWS2, PEWS) that facilitate early recognition and escalation of treatment of the deteriorating patient.
- Haematology and biochemistry laboratory testing, and ECG and chest imaging should be performed at admission and as clinically indicated to monitor for complications, such as ARDS, acute liver injury, acute kidney injury, acute cardiac injury, disseminated intravascular coagulation (DIC) and/or shock.
- Patients should be monitored for signs or symptoms suggestive of venous or arterial thromboembolism, such as stroke, deep venous thrombosis, pulmonary embolism or acute coronary syndrome, and proceed according to hospital protocols for diagnosis (such as laboratory tests and/or imaging) and further management.
- After resuscitation and stabilization of the pregnant woman, foetal well-being should be monitored. The frequency of foetal heart rate observations should be individualized based on gestational age, maternal clinical status (e.g., hypoxia) and foetal conditions.

Critical COVID-19

In selected patients with COVID-19 and mild ARDS, a trial of noninvasive ventilation (NIV), i.e., continuous positive airway pressure (CPAP) or bi-level positive airway pressure (BiPAP) may be used. Patients with hypoxaemic respiratory failure and haemodynamic instability, multiorgan failure or abnormal mental status, however, should not receive NIV in place of other options such as invasive ventilation. Endotracheal intubation should be performed by a trained and experienced provider using airborne precautions, as patients with ARDS may desaturate quickly during intubation. In adult patients with moderate to severe ARDS prone ventilation for 12 to 16 hours per day is recommended.

Therapeutics

- Corticosteroids: NICE recommends use of a corticosteroid, e.g., dexamethasone or hydrocortisone for patients requiring supplemental oxygen to meet their prescribed oxygen saturation levels. Treatment should be for a 7- to 10-day period.
- Antivirals: NICE recommends *against* the use of remdesivir in hospitalized patients on high-flow nasal oxygen, CPAP, noninvasive mechanical ventilation, or invasive mechanical ventilation, except as part of a clinical trial. This recommendation is based on moderate-certainty evidence that suggests remdesivir may increase the risk of mortality in people who are on these interventions.
- Interleukin-6 (IL-6) inhibitors: the WHO strongly recommends an IL-6 inhibitor (tocilizumab or sarilumab) in patients with critical disease. IL-6 inhibitors may be administered in combination with corticosteroids and Janus kinase (JAK) inhibitors, and should be initiated at the same time as systemic corticosteroids. This recommendation is based on high-certainty evidence that shows IL-6 inhibitors reduce mortality and the need for mechanical ventilation, and low-certainty evidence that suggests that IL-6 inhibitors may also reduce the duration of mechanical ventilation and hospitalization.
- JAK inhibitor: NICE recommends baricitinib in hospitalized adults who need supplemental oxygen (or other respiratory support including high-flow nasal oxygen, CPAP, noninvasive ventilation or mechanical ventilation), are having or have completed a course of corticosteroids (unless contraindicated) and have no evidence of infection (other than SARS-CoV-2) that might be worsened by baricitinib.
- Low-molecular-weight heparin (LMWH): all adults should be treated with a standard prophylactic dose of LMWH.

Complications

- Septic shock: recognize septic shock in adults when infection is suspected or confirmed AND vasopressors are needed to maintain mean arterial pressure (MAP) ≥65 mmHg AND lactate is ≥2 mmol/L, in the absence of hypovolaemia. Standard care should be performed according to septic shock bundles.
- Coagulopathy: common in patients with severe COVID-19, and both venous and arterial thromboembolism have been reported. If clinically suspected, proceed immediately with appropriate diagnostic and management pathways.
- Delirium: common in patients with a prolonged critical care admission. Manage any underlying cause of delirium by monitoring oxygenation and fluid status, correcting metabolic or endocrine abnormalities, addressing coinfections, minimizing the use of medications that may cause or worsen delirium, treating withdrawal from substances and maintaining normal sleep cycles as much as possible. Antipsychotic medication for agitation should be avoided where possible.

Prevention strategies

Prevention strategies against COVID-19 include infection control measures in the healthcare setting, and personal preventative measures in the community setting. In the healthcare setting these include early identification and isolation of those with suspected disease, the use of appropriate PPE and following general measures of hand/respiratory hygiene. Local guidelines on mask-wearing in the community depend on the level of community transmission and vaccination rates.

Vaccines to prevent SARS-CoV-2 infection are considered the most promising approach for curbing the pandemic. Several COVID-19 vaccines are available globally, of which the WHO maintains an updated list. Countries around the world have taken up the opportunity to protect their populations using safe and highly effective vaccines. This protection includes booster doses, which are a critical part of sustaining protection. Vaccination strategies differ across countries, and here we focus on the UK policy for vaccination against COVID-19.

The first vaccine for COVID-19 was approved for use in the United Kingdom on 2 December 2020. To date six vaccines have been approved for use in the United Kingdom, of which three are currently available. These are: the Moderna vaccine, Pfizer/BioNTech vaccine and Nuvaxovid vaccine. COVID-19 vaccination has been shown to reduce the risk of infection, severe illness, hospitalization and death. It also protects against COVID-19 variants. However, fully vaccinated individuals can still become infected with SARS-CoV-2 and transmit the infection to other people.

Chapter Summary

- Infectious diseases including HIV-related disease and malaria are currently a growing problem in both the developed world and the developing world. The World Health Organization provides general guidelines to master disease prevention and improve patient survival. Research aims to improve management and develop a treatment.
- Unfortunately, there is no current cure for HIV infection but hopes have been raised with the use of antiretroviral treatment, which reduces HIV-associated mortality and morbidity. This is drawn from great experience gained from a successful fight with currently preventable and treatable infectious diseases such as malaria.
- Because of overuse of antibiotics and a high mutation rate, new treatment-resistant pathogens arise quickly. It is important to continue to take caution when you are considering infectious disease and ensure all appropriate precautionary measures are used.
- COVID-19 represents the biggest acute global health crisis of this century, and according to The WHO continues to be a public health emergency 3 years since it was first recognized in January 2020.
- The global vaccination effort continues to be the best strategy to curb the pandemic, with complete vaccine schedules, including booster doses as recommended by WHO, being an essential part of building immunity against virus strains circulating in communities worldwide.

UKMLA Conditions
COVID-19
Diarrhoea
Fever
Hospital-acquired infections
Human immunodeficiency virus
Influenza
Night sweats
Travel health advice
Vaccination
Weight loss

UKMLA Presentations
Diarrhoea
Fever
Night sweats
Travel health advice
Vaccination
Weight loss

Drug overdose and abuse 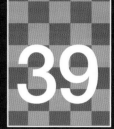 39

GENERAL OVERVIEW

Drug overdose and illicit drug use result in a significant proportion of all acute hospital admissions with death related to drug poisoning and overdose increasing by over 80% between 2012 and 2021. Over 60% of suicides involve a deliberate drug administration or overdose. Commonly used substances are described in Tables 39.1 and 39.2.

Overdose may be:

- Accidental: particularly in children or patients with impaired memory or cognition.
- Deliberate: in suicide, attempted suicide or deliberate self-harm, homicide or abuse of vulnerable adults or children.
- Iatrogenic: for example, drug interactions, reduced metabolism/excretion (renal failure, liver failure) or medical error.
- Environmental (e.g., pesticides, stings or bites).

In many patients, drug overdose results in a mild illness requiring little intervention but if sufficient amounts or mixtures of drugs are taken the result can be a life-threatening situation. In all patients, particularly the unconscious, further history from family, friends, the patient's general practitioner and the ambulance staff is likely to be helpful and should be actively sought. Establish what drugs were taken and when. It is very common for the patient to have taken more than one drug, and many patients will have consumed alcohol as well.

Try to assess the suicide risk. Features conferring higher suicide risk are detailed later. Cover the events leading to the overdose, and try to identify whether the intent was to end life i.e., a premeditated act, may include the patient collecting tablets over some time, leaving a suicide note or making attempts to minimalize the chances of being found.

- Chronic debilitating illness (psychiatric or physical)
- Drug or alcohol abuse
- Mental disorders (especially depression)
- History of violence, abuse or loss
- Vulnerable groups experiencing discrimination (e.g., refugees, migrants, LGBTI community)

 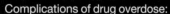
Investigations

- Collect blood and urine for a toxicology screen in addition to a full set of bloods (full blood count (FBC), urea and electrolytes (U&Es), bone profile, clotting, liver function tests, blood glucose).
- Paracetamol and salicylate levels should be measured in all patients. Paracetamol levels should be measured as close to 4 hours after ingestion as possible.

Table 39.1 Specific measures in the management of drug overdose with some of the more common drugs

Drug	Toxic side effects	Specific management
Benzodiazepines	Drowsiness, dysarthria, nystagmus, ataxia, coma, respiratory depression	Flumazenil for reversal of sedative effects: 100–400 mcg/hour, adjusted according to response. Should be used cautiously. It is contraindicated in life-threatening conditions controlled by benzodiazepines (e.g., status epilepticus)
Digoxin	Nausea, vomiting, diarrhoea, hyperkalaemia, bradyarrhythmias, tachyarrhythmias, altered colour vision, delirium	Correct electrolyte disturbances, cardiac pacing in atrioventricular block, digoxin-specific antibody fragments (Digibind) in severe overdose
β-Blockers	Bradycardia, hypotension, cardiac failure, hypoglycaemia, hyperkalaemia, convulsions, coma, asystole	Atropine intravenously for bradycardia, cardiac pacing if refractory bradycardia, Glucagon intravenously in severe overdose Inotropes, chronotropes and vasopressors are useful Intravenous calcium Haemodialysis High-dose insulin therapy
Calcium channel blockers	Cardiac toxicity with haemodynamic instability, bradycardia and hypotension, hyperglycaemia, seizures, coma, pulmonary oedema, renal failure	Treatment is as per β-blockers overdose with the addition of intravenous calcium administration
Heparin	Haemorrhage	Protamine sulphate intravenously
Warfarin	Haemorrhage	Vitamin K intravenously, 4- or 3-factor prothrombin complex concentrate (e.g., octaplex), fresh frozen plasma, prothrombin concentrate.
Selective serotonin reuptake inhibitors	Generally mild symptoms in isolated overdose such as mydriasis, diaphoresis, somnolence, gastric irritation and hyponatraemia. However, serotonin syndrome can occur in addition to seizures, CNS depression and cardiac dysrhythmias (wide complex bradycardia, AF and QTc prolongation arrhythmias)	Discontinuation of all serotonergic therapies, control of agitation and seizures with benzodiazepines. Cooling can be instituted in severe cases of hyperthermia. Antiserotonergic agents such as cyproheptadine or chlorpromazine can be used in cases refractory to supportive care
Tricyclic antidepressants	Tachycardia, dry mouth, drowsiness, nausea and vomiting, urinary retention, mydriasis, increased reflexes, seizures, confusion, coma. Prolonged QT interval may cause VT/SVT	Acidosis and hypoxia are common. Sodium bicarbonate resolves the metabolic acidosis and reduces the risk of cardiovascular complications. Seizures can be managed with lorazepam or diazepam

Activated charcoal should be considered if the presentation is within 1 hour of ingestion. Supportive measures should be instituted in all overdose cases.
AF, Atrial fibrillation; CNS, central nervous system; SVT, supraventricular tachycardia, VT, ventricular tachycardia.

Table 39.2 Features and management of common illegal drug overdose

Substance	Clinical features	Management
Cocaine/crack cocaine (coke, Charlie, snow)	Euphoria, tachycardia, agitation, hyperthermia, coronary artery spasm, seizures, acidosis	Sedation, active cooling, glyceryl trinitrate. β-Blockers are contraindicated
Ketamine (K, special K)	Dissociation, hypertension, arrhythmia, respiratory depression	Supportive measures
Mephedrone (miaow miaow, M-cat)	Agitation, tachycardia, hypertension, seizures	Supportive measures
γ-Hydroxybutyrate (GHB)	Euphoria, dizziness, hypotonia, bradycardia, respiratory depression	Supportive measures. γ-Hydroxybutyrate is rapidly metabolized and cleared
MDMA/amphetamines (ecstasy, speed, pills, molly)	Agitation, tachycardia, psychosis, hyperthermia, rhabdomyolysis, serotonin syndrome	Supportive measures, sedation, β-blockers

- Arterial blood gas to assess respiratory depression or stimulation (opiates, salicylate) and acid–base status.
- ECG: many drugs can cause arrhythmia in overdose.
- If the patient is unconscious, consider further imaging to rule out an intracranial event.

Management

The management of drug overdose can be divided into general supportive measures for all patients; specific measures according to the drug taken; and psychiatric assessment and social input when the patient recovers physically. TOXBASE run by the National Poisons Information Service should be the first point of contact for information about the management of poisoning and overdose. It contains a vast amount of detailed information, including specific antidotes, and is available 24/7.

Supportive care

- Follow the ABCDE approach. If the patient is unconscious, assess the airway and give oxygen. Intubation and assisted ventilation may be necessary.
- Treat hypotension and arrhythmias. Attach a cardiac monitor if the patient is known to have taken tricyclic antidepressants or other medications known to cause cardiac instability (e.g., β-blockers, digoxin).
- Convulsions should be treated with benzodiazepines.

Preventing absorption

Activated charcoal may be used to bind poisons in the stomach to prevent their absorption.

- It is more effective the sooner it is given, and usually needs to be given within 1 hour of ingestion.
- Repeated doses are not routinely recommended but may be indicated in cases of tricyclic and aspirin overdose.
- It is contraindicated in drowsy patients (risk of aspiration). The administration of activated charcoal is associated with aspiration and gastrointestinal obstruction.
- Activated charcoal is ineffective in the case of iron, lithium, alcohol and cyanide poisoning or overdose.

> **RED FLAG**
>
> Removal of the drug from the gastrointestinal tract is controversial. The potential benefits of reducing drug absorption may be outweighed by the hazards of the methods used (e.g., aspiration of stomach contents) or may cause a paradoxical increase in drug absorption. It should be considered only for people who present early, are fully conscious with a protected airway and are at risk of significant harm because of the poisoning. Induced emesis is not recommended.

Increase elimination of drug

Elimination of drugs can be increased by urinary alkalinization or through extracorporeal circuits, including haemodialysis, or haemoperfusion.

- Urinary alkalinization increases renal excretion of mildly acidic drugs. It is used in severe salicylate, phenobarbital and amphetamine overdose. High urinary output is required, and fluid balance, electrolyte levels and acid–base status need careful monitoring.
- Haemodialysis is especially useful for overdose of salicylate, lithium, ethanol, methanol and polyethylene glycol.

Psychiatric and social assessment

Once the acute event and medical management are completed, the patient's psychiatric state, ongoing risk of suicide and social circumstances should be assessed, however trivial the overdose may have appeared. Where appropriate, psychiatrists and social care workers should be involved.

> **CLINICAL NOTES**
>
> Serotonin syndrome, see Table 39.1, occurs in around 15% of selective serotonin reuptake inhibitor (SSRI) overdoses, a predictable consequence of excess serotonin on the central nervous system.
>
> Symptoms vary depending on the degree of serotonin toxicity but include high blood pressure, tachycardia, hyperthermia, agitation, increased reflexes, tremor, hypertonicity, diaphoresis, dilated pupils and diarrhoea. Spontaneous or ocular clonuses are classical symptoms. Complications such as seizures and rhabdomyolysis can occur. Diagnosis is clinical. Treatment is mainly supportive.

SPECIFIC DRUGS

Paracetamol

Paracetamol is the most common agent of intentional self-harm. Overdose, even in small amounts, can cause fatal liver damage. Plasma concentrations should be measured and compared against a nomogram (paracetamol treatment graph); see Fig. 39.1. Paracetamol metabolism is described in Fig. 39.2. Patients with plasma concentrations above the treatment line should be administered N-acetylcysteine (NAC) which, amongst other functions, replenishes glutathione stores and reduces the toxic effects of N-acetyl-p-benzoquinone imine (NAPQI).

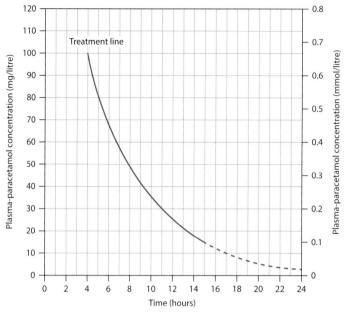

Fig. 39.1 Paracetamol nomogram. (Reprinted with permission from the Royal College of Emergency Guidance. https://www.rcem.ac.uk/docs/Paracetamol%20Overdose/Annex%201_The%20treatment%20nomogram%20and%20Annex%202_Technical_info.pdf.)

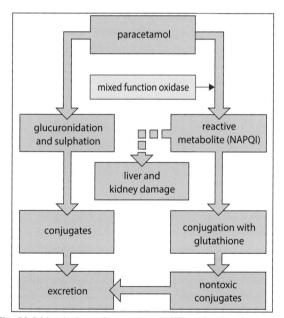

Fig. 39.2 Metabolism of paracetamol. When the drug is taken in therapeutic doses, the toxic metabolite formed, NAPQI, is detoxified by conjugation with glutathione; when taken in overdose, glutathione supplies are rapidly exhausted and NAPQI accumulates, causing cell damage. *NAPQI*, N-acetyl-p-benzoquinone imine. (From Marshall WJ, Lapsley M, Day A, Shipman K. *Clinical Chemistry*, 9th ed. Elsevier; 2021.)

If given within 8 hours of overdose NAC is virtually 100% effective; efficacy decreases significantly after that. In staggered overdose or where the time of ingestion cannot be established NAC is given regardless of drug levels. Synthetic liver function needs regular monitoring (prothrombin time, INR, albumin and platelet count). Hypoglycaemia is a late and worrying sign of fulminant liver failure. King's College Criteria for paracetamol toxicity that help determine the need for specialist referral are described later. The prognosis is good in early treatment. Poor prognostic factors include persistent metabolic acidosis (pH <7.30) 48 hours after an overdose and progressively worsening synthetic liver function despite supportive measures.

HINTS AND TIPS

Individuals at higher risk of paracetamol-induced liver disease:

- Preexisting liver disease
- Alcohol abuse
- HIV, eating disorders, cystic fibrosis, malnutrition (glutathione-depletion)
- Patients taking liver enzyme-inducing drugs (e.g., phenytoin, carbamazepine, rifampicin)

Clinical features

- Early symptoms (first 24 hours) are minimal but may include malaise, nausea and vomiting.
- After 24 hours hepatic necrosis begins giving rise to acute liver failure signs and symptoms (see Chapter 2). Acute hepatocellular damage is maximal 3 to 4 days after ingestion and can cause jaundice, encephalopathy, hypoglycaemia and abdominal pain; renal tubular necrosis may also occur. Coma and death may ensue.

CLINICAL NOTES

KING'S COLLEGE CRITERIA FOR PARACETAMOL OVERDOSE

Referral/transfer to a liver transplantation centre if one of the following is present:

- Arterial pH <7.3 *OR*
- Grade III or IV hepatic encephalopathy, *AND* coagulopathy (INR >6.5 (PT >100 s)) *AND* acute kidney injury (creatinine >300 µmol/L) *OR*
- High lactate (>3.5 mmol/L at 4 hours or >3.0 mmol/L at 12 hours) *OR*
- High phosphate (>1.2 mmol/L at 48–96 hours)

Aspirin (salicylate)

Salicylate overdose stimulates the respiratory centre, resulting in hyperventilation and respiratory alkalosis. There is a compensatory renal excretion of bicarbonate, sodium, potassium and water, resulting in a metabolic acidosis, dehydration and electrolyte imbalance. Acidosis alters the ionization of aspirin resulting in increased absorption, worsening the situation. Symptoms include nausea, vomiting, abdominal pain and tinnitus. In severe cases cerebral and pulmonary oedema, convulsions, coma and eventually death can occur.

Management includes measurement of drug levels which reach peak concentration about 2 to 4 hours after ingestion. Supportive measures should be instituted. Dehydration, hypokalaemia and hypoglycaemia should be corrected. If plasma salicylate levels are >500 mg/L (3.6 mmol/L) or there is refractory metabolic acidosis urinary alkalinization with sodium bicarbonate should be performed. In severe poisoning (>700 mg/L or 5.1 mmol/L), haemodialysis is effective and may be life saving.

ALCOHOL

Alcohol is widely used throughout the world. Over 21% of adults in the UK regularly consume amounts of alcohol that increase the risk of harm. Guidelines advise that drinking more than 14 units of alcohol per week is unsafe. This is true for both men and women. Units of alcohol can be calculated by multiplying the volume of the drink in millilitres by the % alcohol by volume (ABV). Alcohol dependence is a psychiatric disorder characterized by physiological and physical addiction features of which include tolerance, persistent desire, craving, preoccupation and continued drinking despite related harm.

Alcohol misuse is a huge problem in terms of morbidity, mortality and healthcare costs.

The CAGE questionnaire is commonly used as a screening tool for alcohol problems.

COMMUNICATION

The CAGE questionnaire:

- Have you ever felt you needed to **c**ut down on your drinking?
- Has anyone ever **a**nnoyed you by criticizing your drinking?
- Have you ever felt **g**uilty about your drinking?
- Have you ever needed a drink in the morning – an '**e**ye-opener' – to make yourself feel better?

A positive answer to any of these questions is indicative of possible alcohol dependence.

Alcohol misuse can result in acute intoxication, problems associated with alcohol withdrawal and systemic complications of alcohol use:

- Acute intoxication: alcohol causes euphoria and reduced inhibition. In greater quantities it may cause reduced consciousness level, respiratory depression, atrial fibrillation, hypoglycaemia and hypotension.
- Alcohol withdrawal: tremor, sweating, tachycardia, irritability, agitation, hallucinations, delusions, seizures. Symptoms usually start within 24 hours of the last alcohol intake.
- Systemic complications; for example:
  - Gastrointestinal: gastritis, oesophagitis, varices, pancreatitis, alcoholic liver disease (including fatty liver, hepatitis, cirrhosis).
  - Cardiovascular: arrhythmia, cardiomyopathy, hypertension.
  - Neurological: cortical atrophy, cerebellar degeneration, peripheral neuropathy, Wernicke encephalopathy/Korsakoff syndrome.
  - Endocrine: gynaecomastia, testicular atrophy, osteoporosis.
  - Increased risk of cancer, particularly oesophageal, stomach, liver, breast and head and neck cancers.

Alcohol withdrawal

Patients experiencing alcohol withdrawal are difficult to treat and, despite initial willingness, often self-discharge. The standard treatment is a course of benzodiazepines, usually chlordiazepoxide, which is slowly reduced over several days; most hospitals have a dosing protocol. In patients with severe liver disease oxazepam is preferred to chlordiazepoxide as it is not metabolized by the liver. The Clinical Institute Withdrawal Assessment for Alcohol (CIWA) scale is used to quantify the severity of the alcohol withdrawal syndrome and to guide the patient's chlordiazepoxide requirement.

Delirium tremens, or delirium-associated alcohol withdrawal, is a severe form of withdrawal which occurs in approximately 5% of patients. It is associated with a high risk of morbidity and death. The onset is usually between 2 and 5 days following cessation of alcohol intake. Features include severe tremor, clouding of consciousness, delusions, tachycardia, agitation, fever and severe hallucinations (mainly visual but can be tactile or auditory and often cause extreme fear). Treatment includes calming and reorientation, and the use of oral benzodiazepines.

Wernicke encephalopathy/Korsakoff psychosis

Wernicke encephalopathy is an acute life-threatening neurological syndrome consisting of confusion, ophthalmoplegia and ataxia. The most common cause is thiamine deficiency associated with alcoholism but it can also occur in severe starvation or prolonged vomiting. If not treated, it can lead to irreversible damage resulting in amnesia, cognitive impairment and confabulations (Korsakoff syndrome).

Heavy alcohol consumption can affect the absorption of thiamine (vitamin B_1), and people with alcoholism can be at risk of this condition despite having a normal balanced diet. Treatment is with thiamine in the form of Pabrinex (IV vitamin B with ascorbic acid). At-risk patients should be given prophylactic thiamine replacement.

RED FLAG

If thiamine deficiency is suspected, thiamine should be replaced before glucose is replaced as glucose may exacerbate the acute loss of thiamine. Prolonged carbohydrate administration without thiamine supplementation has been reported to precipitate Wernicke encephalopathy.

Long-term treatment

Regular psychosocial input is essential. This may include counselling, cognitive behavioural therapy and self-help groups (e.g., Alcoholics Anonymous). Once withdrawal has been completed pharmacological aids can be considered along with individual psychological intervention. These include naltrexone (a partial agonist at opioid receptors which reduces the pleasurable effects from alcohol) and acamprosate (reduces cravings).

OPIOIDS

Opioids are substances with affinity and efficacy at the opioid receptors. They can be classified into natural derivatives of opium (e.g., heroin, morphine, codeine) or synthetically produced compounds (e.g., buprenorphine, methadone, fentanyl). Opioids are drugs commonly prescribed for pain but are also used as cough suppressants, to manage persistent diarrhoea or shortness of breath in advanced chronic lung disease. They are highly addictive and tolerance requiring repeated dose escalation is a major problem. Due to their euphoric effects and low cost they have become one of the most commonly misused and abused drugs in the world, despite being classed as controlled substances. Opioid dependence has a relapse rate of over 90% if untreated.

Opioids act by binding to opioid receptors (Table 39.3), primarily located in the nervous and gastrointestinal systems. Overdose results in respiratory depression, drowsiness, coma, pinpoint pupils, hypotension, hypothermia or pulmonary oedema. Management includes supportive measures and naloxone which is an opioid antagonist. Administer 400 mcg intravenously followed by 800 mcg for up to two doses at 1-minute

Table 39.3 Opioid receptors are G protein-coupled receptors

Receptor	Location	Function
Delta	Brain, PNS	• Analgesia • Dependence • Respiratory depression • Antidepressant effect
Kappa	Brain, spinal cord, PNS	• Analgesia • Depression • Hallucinogenic • Dysphoria • Sedation
Mu	Brain, spinal cord, PNS, GIT	• Analgesia • Dependence • Respiratory depression • Euphoria • Reduced GI motility
Nociceptin receptor	Brain and spinal cord	• Anxiety, depression, appetite stimulation • Associated with the development of tolerance
Zeta	Multiple sites	• Involved in tissue growth

GIT, *Gastrointestinal tract;* PNS, *peripheral nervous system.*

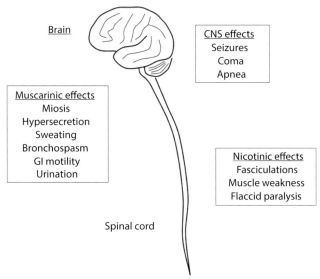

Brain

CNS effects
Seizures
Coma
Apnea

Muscarinic effects
Miosis
Hypersecretion
Sweating
Bronchospasm
GI motility
Urination

Nicotinic effects
Fasciculations
Muscle weakness
Flaccid paralysis

Spinal cord

Fig. 39.3 Clinical effects of organophosphorus poisoning. (From Das S, Thomas S, Das PP. *Sensing of Deadly Toxic Chemical Warfare Agents, Nerve Agent Simulants, and their Toxicological Aspects.* Elsevier; 2023.)

intervals (increased to 2 mg for one dose then 4 mg for one dose if no response). Naloxone has a very short half-life and therefore repeated doses or intravenous infusion may be needed.

ILLEGAL DRUGS

Table 39.2 details some of the features seen with commonly used illegal drugs.

CARBON MONOXIDE

Carbon monoxide is produced by the incomplete combustion of fuels and usually occurs as a result of inhalation of smoke, faulty heating appliances or car exhaust fumes. The affinity of carbon monoxide for haemoglobin is about 240 times higher than that of oxygen leading to its preferential binding and formation of carboxyhaemoglobin (COHb). Normal COHb levels are <3% in nonsmokers and <10% in smokers. Anything higher leads to hypoxia.

Symptoms are nonspecific including headache, nausea, flushing, confusion and, if severe, seizures, coma and death. Lips and skin appear 'cherry red' despite hypoxia. A pulse oximeter will read falsely high normal oxygen saturation levels due to similar absorption spectra of oxyhaemoglobin and COHb.

Treatment is with 100% oxygen. Hyperbaric oxygen therapy speeds up the elimination of COHb and is helpful in severe cases.

ORGANOPHOSPHATES

These are deadly unless prompt treatment is instituted. Organophosphates are used as medications, insecticides and nerve agents. Clinical presentation is the effect of inhibition of acetylcholinesterase and the resultant buildup of acetylcholine in the body (Fig. 39.3).

Management includes atropine with its anticholinergic effects and specific antidotes such as pralidoxime (bind to acetylcholinesterases inactivated by organophosphates thereby rendering it functional again). Benzodiazepines are used to treat seizures.

Chapter Summary

- In a patient with an overdose it is important to establish the risk of the overdose. What drugs were taken? Was it a mixed overdose? How many tablets were taken and at what time? Was it staggered?
- Establish whether the intent was suicide or a call for help. Planned suicide attempts with no intention to be found represent the highest risk. All patients should be seen by a psychiatrist following an overdose.
- Always consider whether an overdose has been taken in an unconscious patient. Assess the patient with a systematic ABCDE approach. Assess the consciousness level and consider if the patient can protect their airway.
- Specific drug overdoses have specific treatments. TOXBASE is a very useful guide.
- Alcohol misuse is common. Screen all patients for alcohol dependence and consider the need for oral benzodiazepines to prevent alcohol withdrawal in hospitalized patients. Have a low threshold to give thiamine replacement to reduce the risk of the patient developing a Wernicke–Korsakoff syndrome.

UKMLA Conditions
Adverse drug effects
Drug overdose
Wernicke encephalopathy

UKMLA Presentations
Overdose
Poisoning
Substance misuse

Self-Assessment

UKMLA High Yield Association Table

Chapter 28 Cardiovascular system

Key findings	Diagnoses
Chest pain radiating to the jaw and/or left arm	MI
Atypical chest pain in a diabetic patient	MI
Retrosternal chest pain radiating to the back	Aortic dissection
Chest pain 30 minutes after a meal	Oesophageal spasm
Chest pain associated with wheeze	Asthma, COPD, Heart failure (cardiac wheeze)
Chest pain associated with haemoptysis	Pulmonary embolism
Pleuritic chest pain relieved by leaning forward or sitting up	Pericarditis
Fever and sharp chest pain in a patient with a recent MI	Dressler syndrome
Continuous machine-like heart murmur	Patent ductus arteriosus
JVP with absent a waves	Atrial fibrillation
JVP with cannon a waves	Third-degree heart block
JVP with giant a waves	Tricuspid stenosis
JVP with large v waves	Tricuspid regurgitation
Palpitations	Arrhythmia
Ejection systolic murmur ('crescendo-decrescendo'), narrow pulse pressure	Aortic stenosis
Early diastolic murmur, wide pulse pressure, collapsing pulse	Aortic regurgitation
Mid-diastolic rumbling murmur loudest heard with the bell of the stethoscope	Mitral stenosis
Pansystolic murmur best heard at the apex	Mitral regurgitation

COPD, *Chronic obstructive pulmonary disease;* JVP, *jugular venous pressure;* MI, *myocardial infarction.*

Chapter 29 Respiratory system

Key findings	Diagnoses
Shortness of breath, haemoptysis and tachycardia	Pulmonary embolism
High-pitched wheeze and shortness of breath	Asthma
Respiratory symptoms in a patient with concurrent HIV	*Pneumocystis jioveci*
Dry cough and hyponatraemia in a patient who has been in contact with airconditioned air	Legionella pneumonia
Reduced FEV_1, and reduced FEV_1/FVC ratio	Obstructive lung disease
Reduced FEV_1 and FVC but increased FEV_1/FVC ratio	Restrictive lung disease
Obesity	Hypoventilation syndrome, obstructive sleep apnoea
Hyperexpanded, hyperresonant chest and history of smoking	COPD
Decreased breath sounds on that side associated with dullness to percussion	Pleural effusion
Chest symptoms in a farmer or birdkeeper	Hypersensitivity pneumonitis
Coal industry workers	Coal workers' pneumoconiosis

Continued

Key findings	Diagnoses
Mine worker, sandblaster	Silicosis
Hypoxia with increased A–a gradient	Ventilation defect, perfusion defect or shunt
Hypoxia with normal A–a gradient	Low inspiratory oxygen or hypoventilation
Sudden onset chest pain	Pneumothorax, pulmonary embolus
Shortness of breath after prolonged immobilization	Pulmonary embolus
Transudate	Often bilateral. Cardiac failure, renal failure, liver failure, nephrotic syndrome
Exudate	Often unilateral. Malignancy, inflammation, infection, trauma
Chronic cough with haemoptysis, night sweats, prevalent area	Tuberculosis
Childhood onset, malnutrition, chronic purulent cough with excessive sputum	Cystic fibrosis
Seal barking cough	Croup
Histologically most common lung cancer	Adenocarcinoma
Lung cancer strongly associated with tobacco use	Squamous cell carcinoma
Lung cancer associated with neuroendocrine phenomena (e.g., SIADH, Cushing syndrome, Lambert–Eaton syndrome)	Small cell lung cancer

COPD, *Chronic obstructive pulmonary disease;* SIADH, *syndrome of inappropriate antidiuretic hormone secretion.*

Chapter 30 Gastroenterology and hepatobiliary systems

Key findings	Diagnoses
Coffee ground vomiting	Upper GI bleed
Black or tarry stool (maelena)	Upper GI bleed
Abdominal pain worse after eating	Gastric ulcer
Abdominal pain better after eating	Duodenal ulcer
Multiple peptic ulcers	Zollinger–Ellison syndrome
Freckled lips and gastrointestinal symptoms	Peutz–Jeghers syndrome
Dysphagia to both solids and fluids	Oesophageal achalasia
Persistent dysphagia to solids	Oesophageal cancer, fixed obstruction
High ferritin, deranged liver function tests and jaundice	Haematochromatosis
Known ulcerative colitis, itch and new jaundice	Cholangiocarcinoma
A patient with history of alcohol abuse vomiting and with surgical emphysema	Boerhaave syndrome (perforation of the oesophagus)
Dermatitis, diarrhoea, mental disturbance, painful glossitis	Pellagra (lack of vitamin B_3 – niacin)
Sudden onset generalized abdominal pain	GI perforation
Burning epigastric pain aggravated by spicy or acidic foods, and occasionally cough	GORD
Right upper quadrant pain, fever, jaundice (Charcot triad)	Ascending cholangitis
Right upper quadrant pain aggravated by fatty foods	Biliary colic, cholecystitis
Right upper quadrant pain and a positive Murphy sign	Cholecystitis
Upper abdominal pain radiating to the back	Pancreatitis
Crypt abscesses	Ulcerative colitis
Cobblestone mucosa, skip lesions, transmural inflammation	Crohn disease

Key findings	Diagnoses
Nausea and vomiting, abdominal cramping, diarrhoea	Gastroenteritis
Bloody diarrhoea	Colitis
Painless jaundice	Pancreatic cancer

GI, *Gastrointestinal;* GORD, *gastro-oesophageal reflux disease.*

Chapter 34 Nervous system

Key findings	Diagnoses
Crescent shape on head CT scan	Subdural haemorrhage
Biconvex (lentiform) shape on head CT scan. History of head trauma with a lucid interval	Extradural haemorrhage
Sudden onset severe headache	Subarachnoid haemorrhage
Dementia with fluctuating level of consciousness and cognition	Lewy body dementia
Cognitive dysfunction associated with disinhibition and social inappropriateness	Frontotemporal dementia
Optic neuritis	Multiple sclerosis
Tired with repetitive movement, proximal muscle weakness	Myasthenia gravis
Ascending bilateral weakness following infection	Guillain–Barré syndrome
Bradykinesia, stiffness, tremor	Parkinson disease
Tremor that eases with alcohol	Essential tremor
Loss of pain and temperature sensation	Syringomyelia
Sharp, stabbing unilateral pain behind the eye	Cluster headache
Squeezing headache in a band-like distribution	Tension headache
Pulsatile headache associated with aura, photophobia, phonophobia or nausea and vomiting	Migraine
Chronic memory loss, confabulations, alcohol use. Thiamine deficiency (vitamin B_1)	Korsakoff syndrome
Ataxia, confusion, ophthalmoplegia	Wernicke encephalopathy

Chapter 35 Musculoskeletal system

Key findings	Diagnoses
Anti-Ro and anti-La antibodies	Sjörgen syndrome
Antimitochondrial antibodies	Primary biliary cirrhosis
Antinuclear and antismooth muscle antibodies	Autoimmune hepatitis
c-ANCA (c-antineutrophil cytoplasmic antibodies)	Granulomatosis with polyangiitis
p-ANCA (perinuclear-ANCA)	Ulcerative colitis, primary sclerosing cholangitis, ANCA associated vasculitis including (microscopic polyangitis and eosinophilic granulomatosis with polyangitis)
Antitissue transglutaminase (anti-TTG)	Coeliac disease
Antibasement membrane antibody	Goodpasture syndrome
Anti-Jo	Dermatomyositis
Antihistones antibody	Drug-induced lupus
Antinuclear, anti-double-stranded DNA, anti-Smith antibodies. Malar rash (red patches on cheeks and the bridge of the nose, nasolabial sparing)	Systemic lupus erythematosus

Continued

Key findings	Diagnoses
Rheumatoid factor, anticyclic citrullinated peptide-2 antibody	Rheumatoid arthritis
Anticentromere antibodies	Limited cutaneous systemic sclerosis
Anticardiolipin antibody	Antiphospholipid syndrome
Painful red eye in a patient with rheumatoid arthritis	Scleritis
Painless red eye in a patient with rheumatoid arthritis	Episcleritis
Bone pain, hearing loss	Paget disease
Pain better throughout the day, symmetric joint involvement, DIP sparing. Swan neck, Boutonniere and ulnar deviation deformities	Rheumatoid arthritis
Asymmetric joint pain with hard Heberden and Bouchard nodes. PIP and DIP involvement	Osteoarthritis
Painful swollen big toe	Gout
Silver scally plaques on extensor surfaces	Psoriasis

DIP, *Distal interphalangeal joint;* PIP, *proximal interphalangeal joint.*

Chapter 36 Dermatology

Key findings	Diagnoses
Target lesions	Erythema multiforme
Tender red bumps and patches on the skin, darker than the surrounding skin. Often seen on both shins. Associated with inflammatory bowel disease	Erythema nodosum
Brown lacy rash on the shins. Associated with hypothyroidism	Erythema ab igne
Circular erythema with a clear area in the middle resembling a bull's eye pattern. Associated with Lyme disease	Erythema migrans
Dry dark velvety patches of skin usually involving armpits, neck or groins	Acanthosis nigricans
Itchy blistering rash on the extensor surfaces. Associated with coeliac disease	Dermatitis herpetiformis
Painful disfiguring lesions on the face. Cutaneous tuberculosis	Lupus vulgaris
Port-wine stain birthmark on the face (purple, flat, well demarcated). Associated with seizures	Sturge–Weber syndrome
Brown macules and rubbery skin lesions that tingle on pressing	Neurofibromatosis type 1
Crusty yellow or golden scab	Impetigo
Well demarcated, raised area of erythema often on the lower limbs or face	Erysipelas
Poxvirus. Small firm spots with a dimple in the middle	Molluscum contagiosum
Thick white patches on the tongue or inside of the mouth that are difficult to scrape off	Leucoplakia
Purple nodules or patches that are painless. Associated with immunodeficiency (e.g., transplant, AIDS)	Kaposi sarcoma
Slow-growing lump with a punctum	Sebaceous cyst
Brown or black waxy or scaly lesions with stuck on appearance	Seborrheic keratosis
A rough reddish lesion with everted edges	Squamous cell carcinoma
A lesion with a rolled pearly edge	Basal cell carcinoma
Irregular pattern mole with irregularities in colour and history of change to the lesion	Melanoma
Rubbing or pressure causes separation of epidermis from dermis. Associated with staphylococcal infection	Nikolsky sign

Key findings	Diagnoses
Large tense deep blisters. Common in the elderly. Negative Nikolsky sign	Bullous pemphigoid
Fragile easily bursting blisters on the skin and mucosal membranes	Pemphigus vulgaris
Herald patch	Pityriasis rosea
Itchy, irregular flat, purple with white lines on the surface (Wickham striae) lesions	Lichen planus
Itchy white patches usually in the genital area or around the anus	Lichen sclerosus
Itch that is worse at night, most commonly in the hands and wrists	Scabies

Chapter 37 Haematological disorders

Key findings	Diagnoses
Target cells	Thalassaemia
Schistocytes (fragmented red blood cells)	Haemolysis
Auer rods (large cytoplasmic inclusion bodies)	Acute myeloid leukaemia
Reed-Sternberg cells (large, abnormal lymphocytes), lymphadenopathy	Hodgkin lymphoma
Viral association (EBV or HIV) in a patient with jaw lesion	Burkitt lymphoma
Burr cells	Uraemia or malnutrition
Acanthocytes (spur cells, red blood cells covered in spikes)	Pyruvate kinase deficiency
Spherocytes	ABO incompatibility, hereditary spherocytosis
Howell–Jolly body (nuclear remnants in the red blood cell)	Asplenia
Young patients with repeated easy bruising or joint swelling	Haemophilia
Philadelphia chromosome, splenomegaly	Chronic myeloid leukaemia
Suspicion of leukaemia in a patient with Down syndrome	Acute myeloid leukaemia
Most common leukaemia in the old age	Chronic myeloid leukaemia
Most common leukaemia in children	Acute lymphoblastic leukaemia
Back pain, fatigue, monoclonal protein in urine	Multiple myeloma
Microcytic anaemia	Iron deficiency
Macrocytic anaemia	B_{12}/folate deficiency
Renal dysfunction, thrombocytopenia and microangiopathic haemolytic anaemia (schistocytes)	Haemolytic uraemic syndrome

Chapter 39 Drug overdose and abuse

Key findings	Diagnoses
Hypoventilation	Opiate or benzodiazepine toxicity
Normal oxygen saturations in a hypoxaemic patient involved in a house fire or living in an old building	Carbon monoxide toxicity
Complication of nitrate-based treatment or use	Methaemoglobinaemia
Flumazenil	Benzodiazepine antagonist
Naloxone	Opiate antagonist

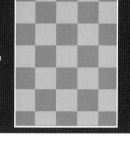

UKMLA Single Best Answer (SBA) questions

Chapter 28 Cardiovascular system

1. A 49-year-old lady is found to have a heart murmur during a routine preoperative assessment clinic. Which one statement regarding heart murmurs is correct?
   A A pansystolic murmur loudest at the apex radiating to the axilla is most likely mitral regurgitation.
   B Mitral stenosis with atrial fibrillation (AF) would give a diastolic murmur with presystolic accentuation.
   C Left-sided heart murmurs are best heard in inspiration.
   D Aortic regurgitation is best heard in the left lateral position.
   E An opening snap is heard in aortic stenosis just after the first heart sound.

2. Which one of the following findings suggests that aortic stenosis is clinically significant?
   A The apex beat is not displaced.
   B The blood pressure is 160/94 mmHg.
   C The murmur is heard all over the praecordium.
   D The murmur radiates to the carotids.
   E There is left ventricular hypertrophy on the ECG.

3. A 63-year-old man is admitted with an episode of severe, central chest pain and dyspnoea. An ECG is performed in the emergency department which shows anterior ST elevation of >2 mm. The patient receives primary percutaneous coronary intervention. He recovers well and on discharge his renal function is normal, cholesterol 4.5 mmol/L and triglycerides 3.4 mmol/L. Which of the following medications should be a part of the prescription regime on discharge?
   A Ramipril, atorvastatin, warfarin and bisoprolol.
   B Ramipril, atorvastatin, aspirin and bisoprolol.
   C Losartan, bezafibrate, aspirin and diltiazem.
   D Losartan, atorvastatin, clopidogrel and bisoprolol.
   E Ramipril, bezafibrate, aspirin and bisoprolol.

4. Which one statement regarding chronic failure with reduced ejection fraction is false?
   A Can be classified by the New York Heart Association (NYHA) scale.
   B Diuretics improve symptoms.
   C Digoxin has no role unless in atrial fibrillation.
   D May predispose to ventricular arrhythmias.
   E All patients should be on angiotensin-converting enzyme inhibitors unless contraindicated.

5. Which one of the following statements is false with regard to atrial fibrillation (AF)?
   A Can cause heart failure in previously well-controlled heart disease.
   B Results in an increased risk of stroke.
   C Is usually caused by rheumatic fever.
   D Results in absent P waves on the ECG.
   E May be a finding in acute pulmonary embolus.

6. A 23-year-old human resource manager attends the emergency department with palpitations. She described the sensation as very fast and regular. An ECG is performed and shows a regular, narrow QRS complex with a rate of 200. Shortly after admission the symptoms spontaneously resolve and a repeat ECG shows a normal PR interval with a positive delta wave in V_1. Which one of the following is the most likely diagnosis?
   A Atrial flutter.
   B Ventricular fibrillation.
   C Ventricular reentry tachycardia.
   D Atrioventricular nodal reentry tachycardia.
   E Atrioventricular reentry tachycardia.

7. Which one statement regarding the jugular venous pressure is false?
   A Is measured from the suprasternal notch with the patient sitting at 45 degrees.
   B Reflects right ventricular preload.
   C Cannon waves indicate a complete heart block.
   D An elevated noncollapsing JVP may indicate superior vena cava obstruction.
   E Tricuspid regurgitation results in large 'v' waves.

8. A 65-year-old diabetic lady with known hypertension presents to the emergency department with retrosternal chest tightness. An ECG reveals T-wave inversion in V_2–V_4. Her 12-h serum troponin level comes back as 10 times the upper limit of normal. Which single investigation will provide the most diagnostic information?
   A Cardiac catheterization.
   B Exercise tolerance test (ETT).
   C Echocardiography.
   D 24-hour ECG monitor.
   E Radionuclide cardiac perfusion scanning.

9. Which one of the following is a cause of essential hypertension?
   A Conn syndrome.
   B Phaeochromocytoma.
   C Coarctation of the aorta.
   D Renal artery stenosis.
   E Idiopathic.

10. Which statement regarding the assessment of the pulse is false?
   A The character should be assessed centrally.
   B A slow-rising pulse indicates mitral stenosis.
   C Pulsus alternans indicates poor left ventricular function.
   D Rate, rhythm, volume and character should be assessed.
   E The heart rate will increase during inspiration in sinus rhythm.

11. You are asked to see a 14-year-old boy as part of his annual health check. He is of short stature, has a short, webbed neck, small upturned nose and low-set ears. On examination you hear an ejection systolic murmur at the left upper sternal border, louder on inspiration. What is the most likely diagnosis?
   A Aortic stenosis.
   B Pulmonary stenosis.
   C Atrial septal defect.
   D Ventricular septal defect.
   E Tetralogy of Fallot.

12. A 55-year-old woman is referred to the emergency department by her GP. She complains of shortness of breath, worse on exertion and feeling tired all the time. She can no longer walk to the shops without rest. She reports the symptoms have been getting progressively worse over the past few months. On examination you find that she has bilateral pedal oedema that is pitting. What is the most useful investigation in this patient?
   A CXR.
   B CT pulmonary angiogram.
   C Coagulation screen.
   D Transthoracic echocardiogram.
   E Bloods including BNP.

13. A 59-year-old man is brought to the emergency department by the paramedics. He complains of feeling generally unwell, dizzy and not himself. On examination he is cold peripherally, with a capillary refill time of 3 seconds. His blood pressure is 68/45 mmHg. ECG shows a broad-complex tachycardia at a rate of 180 bpm. What is the best treatment option?
   A DC cardioversion.

   B IV adrenaline.
   C Amiodarone.
   D Adenosine.
   E IV metoprolol.

14. Which drug has been shown to reduce morbidity and mortality in patients with chronic heart failure due to left ventricular systolic dysfunction and NYHA functional class II?
   A Digoxin.
   B Isosorbide mononitrate.
   C Carvedilol.
   D Amlodipine.
   E Furosemide.

15. A 21-year-old male attends the emergency department with palpitations. He does not have any medical history and does not take any regular medications. His ECG shows a supraventricular tachycardia. What is the treatment of choice?
   A Nothing, but refer him for an OP cardiology appointment and an ECHO.
   B Oral bisoprolol.
   C Carotid sinus massage.
   D Intravenous fluids and electrolyte replacement.
   E Synchronized DC cardioversion.

16. What is the pharmacological treatment of choice for supraventricular tachycardia?
   A Verapamil.
   B Adenosine.
   C Amiodarone.
   D β-Blocker.
   E Digoxin.

17. A 60-year-old male is found to have elevated blood pressure through screening. He is given a home blood pressure monitor which confirms persistently elevated readings of about 145/90 mmHg. His ECG shows abnormal voltage changes and ST segment depression in the left ventricular leads. His past medical history includes type 2 diabetes.
   A Offer lifestyle advice and review in 2 months.
   B Offer lifestyle advice and discuss starting drug treatment.
   C Offer lifestyle advice and consider drug treatment.
   D Offer lifestyle advice and drug treatment.
   E Offer lifestyle advice, drug treatment and consider specialist evaluation.

18. A 17-year-old is brought to ED after he was found stabbed in the street. He is confused and shivering. His blood pressure is 92/50, his heart rate 120 and his respiratory rate 30. What stage of shock is he in?

A Stage 1.
B Stage 2.
C Stage 3.
D Stage 4.
E His signs indicate he is in between two stages.

19. Which congenital cardiac defect is most commonly associated with Down syndrome?
   A ASD.
   B VSD.
   C Atrioventricular septal defect (AVSD).
   D Tetralogy of Fallot.
   E Single ventricle defect.

20. Regarding the treatment of hypertension, which statement is correct?
   A Treatment with bendroflumethiazide can cause hypokalaemia.
   B One of the side effects of ACE inhibitors is ankle swelling.
   C Alpha-blockers are unlikely to cause postural hypotension.
   D Furosemide can result in electrolyte imbalances including hyperkalaemia.
   E All patients above the age of 50 should be on a calcium channel blocker.

21. A 56-year-old man with hypertension and known angina presents with central tight chest pain similar to his normal angina but increasing in frequency and now present at rest. ECG shows ST depression and T-wave inversion in leads V_1–V_4. What is the most likely diagnosis?
   A Dressler syndrome.
   B Posterior non-ST elevation myocardial infarction.
   C Angina pectoris.
   D Inferior non-ST elevation myocardial infarction.
   E Anteroseptal non-ST elevation myocardial infarction.

22. What is the most appropriate treatment strategy for a 65-year-old male brought to the emergency department with a 30-minute history of central crushing chest pain and an ECG showing ST elevation in V_1–V_4?
   A Immediate PCI.
   B GTN spray.
   C Oxygen and an urgent cardiology review.
   D Fibrinolysis.
   E Ensure appropriate analgesia has been given, send a full set of bloods including cardiac enzymes and repeat the ECG in 30 minutes.

23. An 82-year-old woman with a past medical history of established coronary artery disease comes to see her GP complaining of chest pain when she walks up the stairs. The pain usually settles when she sits down to rest. Her drug history includes aspirin, ramipril, bisoprolol and simvastatin. What is the next step in management?
   A Urgent referral to a cardiac centre for assessment of further myocardial ischaemia.
   B GTN spray.
   C Nonsteroidal antiinflammatory drugs.
   D Furosemide.
   E Digoxin.

24. What is the most likely diagnosis in a 60-year-old man with a pansystolic murmur loudest at the right sternal edge, a raised JVP and a pulsatile liver? He has recently returned from a two-year-long round-the-world trip.
   A Graham Steell murmur.
   B Mitral regurgitation.
   C Mitral stenosis.
   D Tricuspid regurgitation.
   E Tricuspid stenosis.

25. What would be the best treatment option in a 94-year-old patient presenting to the emergency department with dizziness and heart palpitations? Her ECG shows an irregularly irregular rhythm. She is known to have ischaemic heart disease and severe heart failure.
   A Aspirin.
   B Dual antiplatelet therapy.
   C β-Blockers.
   D Digoxin.
   E Furosemide.

Chapter 29 Respiratory system

1. A 51-year-old builder was involved in a high-speed road traffic collision. Basic first aid was provided at the scene and he was subsequently transferred to the hospital. Whilst the builder was being formally assessed, one of the FY2 doctors in the emergency department noticed the patient's oxygen saturation had dropped to 85%. He is concerned the patient may have a tension pneumothorax. Which one of the following is **not** a feature of a tension pneumothorax?
   A The trachea is deviated towards the affected side.
   B Increased percussion note over the pneumothorax.
   C Asymmetrical expansion of the chest.
   D Absent/diminished breath sounds over the pneumothorax.
   E A raised jugular venous pressure.

2. A 51-year-old Pilates instructor experienced a bimalleolar fracture of her ankle which required an open reduction and internal fixation. The operation was a success, and she was discharged with a 3-week course of low-molecular-weight heparin (LMWH). Four weeks after the operation she developed shortness of breath and a dry cough. She attended the emergency department, where a CT pulmonary angiogram reveals a pulmonary embolism (PE). Which one of the following statements is correct regarding a PE?
   A The S1Q3T3 pattern is the most common ECG abnormality.
   B An abnormal CXR is common.
   C An ABG will show T2 respiratory failure.
   D The most common finding is a sinus tachycardia.
   E An echocardiogram often shows atrial dysfunction.

3. The patient in the previous scenario is commenced on anticoagulation, which is an appropriate anticoagulation strategy for this patient?
   A Apixaban for 1 month.
   B Unfractionated heparin (UFH) for 6 months.
   C Rivaroxaban for 6 months.
   D Apixaban for 3 months.
   E Thrombolysis therapy.

4. A 19-year-old female is admitted to the hospital with a wheeze and severe dyspnoea. Which one of the following statements is true with regard to the assessment and management of an acute asthma attack?
   A The peak flow measure is unhelpful.
   B A normal Pa_{CO_2} level is reassuring.
   C Intravenous magnesium may be indicated.
   D Death is extremely rare.
   E Intravenous bronchodilator therapy is much better than nebulized therapy.

5. Following discharge, the patient in the previous scenario underwent an inhaler review. She was noted to have had multiple exacerbations in the past year. Her inhaler technique was satisfactory. Her current inhalers were salbutamol as required and a regular beclomethasone inhaler. According to BTS/SIGN guidelines, what would be the most appropriate next step in her management?
   A Increase the dose of inhaled corticosteroid inhaler.
   B Add a long-acting anticholinergic inhaler.
   C Refer to specialist care.
   D Consider the addition of theophylline.
   E Add long-acting β_2-agonist.

6. A 67-year-old gardener presents to his general practitioner with a 3-day history of productive cough, fevers and anorexia. On examination the patient has coarse crackles at the right base with bronchial breathing. The GP suspects this is pneumonia and refers the patient to be seen in the hospital for a CXR and blood cultures. Which one of the following does **not** score a point in the severity assessment for community-acquired pneumonia?
   A Blood urea level >7 mmol/L.
   B Systolic blood pressure >90 mmHg.
   C Respiratory rate >30 per minute.
   D Confusion.
   E Age more than 65 years.

7. A 72-year-old retired car mechanic presents with a 6-month history of weight loss, cough and occasional haemoptysis. A CXR reveals a mass in the right hemithorax with associated hilar shadowing. A CT scan is performed, and subsequent bronchoscopy and biopsy make the diagnosis of squamous cell carcinoma of the lung. Which one of the following statements is true regarding paraneoplastic syndromes associated with squamous cell carcinoma of the lung?
   A It is associated with the syndrome of inappropriate antidiuretic hormone secretion.
   B It is associated with hypercalcaemia.
   C It is associated with Eaton–Lambert myasthenic syndrome.
   D It is associated with Cushing syndrome.
   E It is associated with peripheral neuropathy.

8. A 60-year-old man presents with a 3-month history of worsening shortness of breath and a dry cough. He has never smoked. A CXR is requested and shows diffuse peripheral infiltrate opacifications. Which of these drugs is most likely to be associated with interstitial lung disease?
   A Amiodarone.
   B Amoxicillin.
   C Doxycycline.
   D Enalapril.
   E Sotalol.

9. A 46-year-old woman with a known diagnosis of sarcoidosis presents to the emergency department with worsening dyspnoea. A chest X-ray (CXR) is performed, and she is subsequently reported as having stage 3 pulmonary sarcoidosis. Which one of the following is the CXR most likely to show?
   A A pleural effusion.
   B Bilateral hilar lymphadenopathy.
   C Bilateral hilar lymphadenopathy with reticulonodular shadowing.
   D Fibrocystic sarcoidosis typically with upward hilar retraction, cystic and bullous change.
   E Bilateral pulmonary infiltrates.

10. A 19-year-old student is brought by ambulance to the emergency department with severe dyspnoea. His peak flow is 100 L/min (normally 650 L/min). His respiratory rate is 40 per minute, and auscultation of his chest reveals barely audible breath sounds. His mother tells you that he had been hyperventilating for approximately 30 minutes before admission. What would you expect the arterial blood gas result to be?

A pH 7.29, $Paco_2$ 6.3 kPa, Pao_2 9.2 kPa, bicarbonate 45 mmol/L.

B pH 7.51, $Paco_2$ 7.9 kPa, Pao_2 9.6 kPa, bicarbonate 37 mmol/L.

C pH 7.39, $Paco_2$ 5.3 kPa, Pao_2 7.1 kPa, bicarbonate 25 mmol/L.

D pH 7.51, $Paco_2$ 2.0 kPa, Pao_2 9.6 kPa, bicarbonate 14 mmol/L.

E pH 7.57, $Paco_2$ 3.2 kPa, Pao_2 10.2 kPa, bicarbonate 27 mmol/L.

Reference values: pH: 7.35–7.45, $Paco_2$: 4.7–6.0 kPa, Pao_2: 11–13 kPa, HCO_3-: 22–26 mmol/L.

11. A 56-year-old publican is admitted to the emergency department with dyspnoea. The nurse administers oxygen through nasal cannula at 2 L/min as his oxygen saturations were 89%. Which one of the following most accurately reflects the fraction of oxygen inspired (Fio_2)?

A 98%.

B 50%.

C 35%.

D 28%.

E 24%.

12. A 65-year-old man presents with a 1-month history of shortness of breath and pleuritic chest pain. He also reported a 6 kg weight loss in the past few months. He has a medical history of hypertension. He used to be a roofer. Based on the history, which statement is true regarding the most likely diagnosis?

A The patient has a tumour of the lung parenchyma.

B The condition usually accompanies pulmonary asbestosis.

C Diagnosis is achieved by observing pleural plaques on CXR or CT.

D The condition has a good prognosis.

E Diagnosis may result in compensation for the patient and/or family.

13. A 45-year-old male presents to the emergency department with a history of progressively worsening shortness of breath. On further questioning he admits to having a cough productive of sputum with occasional haemoptysis and night sweats. Among other tests a sputum sample is sent for culture, including AFB. This comes back positive, and tuberculosis (TB) is diagnosed. What is the appropriate drug treatment?

A Six months of combination therapy: rifampicin, isoniazid, pyrazinamide and ethambutol for 4 months followed by isoniazid and pyrazinamide alone for 2 months.

B Twelve months of combination therapy: rifampicin, isoniazid, pyrazinamide and ethambutol for 4 months followed by rifampicin and pyrazinamide alone for 2 months.

C Six months of combination therapy: rifampicin, isoniazid, pyrazinamide and streptomycin for 4 months followed by rifampicin and pyrazinamide alone for 2 months.

D Six months of combination therapy: rifampicin, isoniazid, pyrazinamide and ethambutol for 4 months followed by rifampicin and pyrazinamide alone for 2 months.

E Six months of combination therapy: rifampicin, isoniazid, pyrazinamide and ethambutol for 2 months followed by rifampicin and isoniazid alone for 4 months.

14. An 86-year-old man with a history of chronic obstructive pulmonary disease (COPD) is brought into the emergency department from a nursing home with acute onset shortness of breath. On examination he is alert and maintaining his own airway, but he is visibly in respiratory distress, gasping for air and using accessory muscles of respiration with a respiratory rate of 36 per minute. His temperature is 38.5°C. His oxygen saturations are 88% on 15 L of oxygen through a non-rebreath mask. He is tachycardic with a pulse of 110. His blood pressure is 120/80 mmHg. What is the initial treatment?

A Continue with oxygen alone. Perform further investigations before commencing other treatment as management will depend on the underlying diagnosis.

B Get senior help. Raise the head of the bed. Change the oxygen delivery system to a venturi mask. Commence back-to-back nebulized bronchodilator therapy and give steroids.

C Get senior help. Raise the head of the bed. Commence back-to-back nebulized bronchodilator therapy, steroids, IV fluids and empirical antibiotics.

D Bleep ICU so the patient can be intubated.

E Try simple manoeuvres to improve the patient's oxygenation such as raising the head of the bed and suctioning of excessive secretions. Continue with oxygen and give nebulized salbutamol. If there is no improvement, consider intravenously administered magnesium and hydrocortisone. Reassess the patient after every intervention.

15. For the patient in the previous scenario, what initial tests would be most indicated?
    A Arterial blood gas (ABG), chest X-ray (CXR), CT pulmonary angiogram.
    B Arterial blood gas (ABG), CT pulmonary angiogram, blood tests (FBC, U&Es, CRP).
    C Chest X-ray (CXR), CT pulmonary angiogram, urine dip.
    D Arterial blood gas (ABG), chest X-ray (CXR), blood tests (FBC, U&Es, CRP).
    E Chest X-ray (CXR), bloods tests (FBC, U&Es, CRP), urine dip.

16. A 63-year-old comes to the emergency department with pleuritic chest pain and shortness of breath. He returned from a trip to visit his family in Australia 2 days ago. It was a long-haul flight lasting over 15 hours. The chest X-ray is normal. A pulmonary embolism (PE) is suspected, and a CT pulmonary angiogram (CTPA) is requested. What investigation should be performed before the scan can take place?
    A Kidney function tests.
    B Peak flow.
    C D-dimer.
    D Liver function tests.
    E V/Q scan.

17. A 25-year-old goes to see her GP with a dry cough and shortness of breath. She has a fever and feels generally unwell with flu-like symptoms. She returned from a summer holiday in Spain 6 days ago. She has a diagnosis of type 1 diabetes mellitus, for which she has an insulin pump. She is a smoker. Considering the history, what pathogen causing pneumonia should you be worried about?
    A *Streptococcus pneumoniae.*
    B *Mycoplasma tuberculosis.*
    C Influenza virus.
    D *Legionella pneumophila.*
    E Methicillin-resistant *Staphylococcus aureus.*

18. A 78-year-old female presents to the emergency department with slowly progressive shortness of breath. She has a known history of lung adenocarcinoma. Her chest X-ray shows a large right-sided pleural effusion. What would you expect to find on your respiratory examination?
    A Stridor and reduced breath sounds on the left.
    B Fine inspiratory crepitations on the right with normal percussion note.
    C Hyperexpanded chest with reduced breath sounds throughout.

    D Reduced breath sound on the right with a stony dull percussion note.
    E Course inspiratory crepitations on the right with normal percussion note.

19. The patient in the previous question has a chest drain inserted and is confirmed to have a malignant pleural effusion. What is the correct position for chest drain insertion?
    A Second intercostal space, midclavicular line.
    B Within the lateral border of the pectoralis major and anterior border of the latissimus dorsi, above the fifth intercostal space.
    C Within the lateral border of the pectoralis major and posterior to the midaxillary line, above the fifth intercostal space.
    D Within the medial border of the pectoralis major and posterior border of the latissimus dorsi, above the fifth intercostal space.
    E Tenth intercostal space, midaxillary line.

20. A 45-year-old woman presents with haemoptysis. On further history she has a persistent cough with sputum production for many years. She has not had any weight loss or night sweats. On auscultation of her chest, she has coarse crepitations throughout the lung fields. What is the likely underlying cause of her haemoptysis?
    A Lung malignancy.
    B Bronchiectasis.
    C PE.
    D Heart failure.
    E Pulmonary tuberculosis.

21. A 35-year-old woman presents with a history of recurrent nose bleeds. She notes some slight shortness of breath. On further questioning you note a family history of recurrent haemoptysis. What is the possible underlying diagnosis?
    A Pulmonary embolus.
    B Antiglomerular basement membrane disease (Goodpasture syndrome).
    C Pneumonia.
    D Hereditary haemorrhagic telangiectasia (Osler–Weber–Rendu disease).
    E Cystic fibrosis.

22. A 64-year-old ex-smoker comes to see his GP. He has visible nicotine staining on his fingers. He reports that he has been having increasing breathlessness and productive cough over the past few years with increased fatigue. He has a medical history of hypertension, type 2 diabetes mellitus and osteoarthritis. On chest

auscultation you note a wheeze and increased work of breathing. He is subsequently diagnosed with COPD and commenced on a salbutamol inhaler. Despite this he remains limited by symptoms. What would be the next step in management?

A Continue salbutamol inhaler, but increase the frequency of use.

B Add salmeterol inhaler.

C Add fluticasone inhaler.

D Add salmeterol, tiotropium and fluticasone inhalers.

E Add salmeterol and tiotropium inhalers.

23. The patient in the previous scenario is later admitted to the hospital with an infective exacerbation of COPD. His arterial blood gas on admission shows the following:
pH: 7.35, $Paco_2$: 8.0 kPa, Pao_2: 7.8 kPa, HCO_3–: 31 mmol/L
Reference values: pH: 7.35–7.45, $Paco_2$: 4.7–6.0 kPa, Pao_2: 11–13 kPa, HCO_3–: 22–26 mmol/L
What does the ABG indicate?

A Mixed metabolic and respiratory alkalosis.

B Acute respiratory acidosis.

C Acute metabolic acidosis.

D Compensated (chronic) respiratory acidosis.

E Compensated (chronic) metabolic acidosis.

24. A 73-year-old who used to work on a bird farm comes in with progressively worsening shortness of breath. He is normally well, takes tablets only for high blood pressure, but has recently noted that he no longer can go for long walks with his wife as he gets short of breath and needs to stop. He has not had a cough, chest pain or fever. He also reports feeling worse when it is cold outside. What is the likely underlying diagnosis?

A COPD.

B Bronchiectasis.

C Asthma.

D Interstitial lung disease.

E Pleural effusion.

25. A 28-year-old presents to the emergency department with shortness of breath and right-sided pleuritic chest pain. He has no significant past medical history of note. He has no regular medications and is a nonsmoker. A chest X-ray demonstrates a right-sided pneumothorax with a 3-cm rim of air. What is the most appropriate management?

A Pleural drain insertion.

B Consider discharge with outpatient follow-up.

C Pleural aspiration.

D Admit for monitoring and administer oxygen.

E Give salbutamol nebulizers and oral steroids.

26. A 40-year-old female is admitted with shortness of breath, cough, fever and anosmia. Her viral PCR swab is positive for COVID-19. She is commenced on oxygen and undergoes a chest X-ray (CXR). What CXR findings would be most typical in this scenario?

A Consolidation in the right upper lobe.

B Bilateral, peripheral, patchy ground glass changes.

C Pneumothorax.

D Reticulonodular shadowing and loss of lung volume.

E Hyperexpanded lung fields.

Chapter 30 Gastrointestinal and hepatobiliary systems

1. A 67-year-old man underwent an oesophagogastroduodenoscopy (OGD) for reflux symptoms. Barrett oesophagus was diagnosed. Which one of the following statements regarding this condition is true?

A Approximately 25% of cases will progress to adenocarcinoma.

B The condition predominantly affects the middle third of the oesophagus.

C The condition is asymptomatic in most cases.

D The condition is treated surgically in the first instance.

E The condition is characterized by dysplasia from squamous cell epithelium to columnar cell epithelium.

2. A 43-year-old midwife presents with constant, epigastric pain radiating to the back. She had been suffering with intermittent episodes of right upper quadrant (RUQ) pain for the previous 6 months. Serum amylase level is 1400 U/mL. A diagnosis of suspected pancreatitis is made. Which one of the following statements is true?

A A serum amylase level of more than 2500 U/mL indicates severe pancreatitis.

B The most likely cause is gallstones.

C The Rockall score is used to assess severity.

D A recognized early complication of pancreatitis is pseudocyst formation.

E Pancreatitis is the only possible diagnosis.

3. A 58-year-old person with alcoholism with known cirrhosis presents with copious haematemesis. A variceal bleed is suspected. Which one of the following statements is true for the management of a large upper gastrointestinal (GI) tract haemorrhage?

A A detailed history and examination are a priority.

B A large bleed causes an immediate decrease in haemoglobin concentration.

C A large bleed causes a decrease in urea concentration.

D The investigation of choice is a CT scan.

E Rebleeding carries higher mortality.

4. A 24-year-old primary school teacher presents with abdominal pain and bloody diarrhoea. He has a colonoscopy which shows features of ulcerative colitis (UC). Which one of the following features is associated with UC?

A Transmural inflammation.

B Pseudopolyps.

C Perianal lesions.

D Skip lesions.

E More common in smokers.

5. A 76-year-old retired accountant presents with a change in bowel habit, tenesmus and weight loss. A colonoscopy is done and shows a carcinoma of the colon. Which one of the following statements is true about colorectal cancer?

A Most occur in patients with a strong family history.

B The cancer is likely to be in the ascending colon.

C Right-sided tumours usually present earlier.

D It may present with iron-deficiency anaemia alone.

E Only a minority of tumours can be resected surgically.

6. An 87-year-old woman was admitted for severe pneumonia and treated with a broad-spectrum β-lactamase. On the 10th day after her admission she develops perfuse diarrhoea with cramping abdominal pain. A diagnosis of pseudomembranous colitis is made after further investigation. Which one of the following statements is true?

A It is caused by *Clostridium difficile* itself.

B It can be prevented by the use of alcohol hand gel after each patient contact.

C It is diagnosed by demonstration of an erythematous, ulcerated mucosa covered by a membrane on sigmoidoscopy.

D It may be complicated by toxic dilatation of the colon.

E It is treated with intravenously administered metronidazole in the first instance.

7. A 22-year-old female medical student registers with a new GP. On her health questionnaire she states that she has received a diagnosis of irritable bowel syndrome (IBS). Which one of the following statements about IBS is true?

A The condition is rare.

B The condition is more common in males.

C It may present with rectal bleeding.

D It is a diagnosis of exclusion.

E It is usually treated with 100% success.

8. A 49-year-old mother of two presents to the emergency department with right upper quadrant (RUQ) pain and fever. On examination she is tender in the RUQ but not jaundiced. The emergency department doctor suspects she has cholecystitis secondary to gallstones. Which one of the following statements about gallstone disease is true?

A Most are radio-opaque.

B They are often asymptomatic.

C Their incidence decreases with age.

D They cannot cause bowel obstruction.

E Charcot triad is diagnostic of cholecystitis.

9. Which one of the following may be said of viral hepatitis?

A Hepatitis A may cause chronic hepatitis.

B Hepatitis B is transmitted via the faecal–oral route.

C Chronic hepatitis B infection may be complicated by hepatocellular carcinoma.

D Hepatitis C causes acute hepatic failure.

E Hepatitis E is not transmitted via the faecal–oral route.

10. Which of the following is the classic appearance of the stool in intussusception?

A Fatty stool.

B Melaena.

C Putty-coloured stool.

D Redcurrant jelly stool.

E Watery stool.

11. A 53-year-old woman with a previous diagnosis of autoimmune hepatitis and cirrhosis is seen in the acute medical assessment unit after being referred by her GP for increasing abdominal distension. On examination her body weight is 110 kg and she has bilateral pitting oedema up to her knees. She is not jaundiced. Shifting dullness is elicited on examination of the abdomen. Which one of the following is the greatest contributing mechanism to fluid retention in this patient?

A Increased sodium absorption in the renal tubules.

B Inferior vena cava obstruction.

C Lymphatic obstruction.

D Portal hypertension.

E Hypoalbuminaemia.

12. A 45-year-old man presents to the emergency department with central abdominal pain radiating to the back, associated with nausea and vomiting. He has been unable to eat or drink for the past 48 hours. He looks unwell. He has a history of alcohol abuse, depression and hypertension. You suspect acute pancreatitis. What is the initial management?

A Book an MRCP to confirm your suspicion that the cause of pancreatitis is gallstones.

B Admit the patient, commence administration of intravenous fluids, replace electrolytes, offer analgesia and refer the patient to the gastroenterology team.

C Admit the patient, commence administration of intravenous fluids, replace electrolytes, offer analgesia and refer the patient to the surgical team.

D Rehydrate the patient, replace electrolytes if necessary and send the patient home with a course of oral antibiotics with an outpatient clinic follow-up.

E None of the above.

13. A 38-year-old intravenous drug user presents with jaundice. Blood tests reveal deranged liver function test values. As part of the investigations, viral serology is requested. The results are as follows: anti-HBc positive, HBsAg negative, HCV antibody positive. What is the interpretation of the results?

A The patient has acute hepatitis B infection.

B The patient has acute hepatitis C infection.

C The patient is a carrier of hepatitis B.

D The patient is a carrier of hepatitis C.

E The patient has been vaccinated against hepatitis B and hepatitis C.

14. A patient with known ascites secondary to alcoholic liver disease presents with abdominal pain, tightness and distension. On examination the patient appears well and is warm and well perfused with a blood pressure of 108/80 mmHg and a pulse rate of 78. Peripheral stigmata of chronic liver disease are visible. Her abdomen is distended with mild generalized tenderness on palpation. Shifting dullness is present. Blood tests show no acute abnormalities. You decide that pharmacological management should be commenced. What is the best drug for this patient?

A Co-amoxiclav.

B Propranolol.

C Furosemide.

D Spironolactone.

E Piperacillin and tazobactam (Tazocin).

15. A 40-year-old man presents with central abdominal pain radiating to the back. The pain is associated with nausea but no vomiting. Blood tests reveal raised levels of inflammatory markers but are otherwise within normal range. Urine dip is negative. On further questioning he admits to having had several episodes of bloody stools in the past week. Which is the **least** likely diagnosis?

A Abdominal aortic aneurysm.

B Pancreatitis.

C Diverticulitis.

D Diabetic ketoacidosis.

E Colorectal cancer.

16. A 20-year-old woman presents to the emergency department with a 4-day history of diarrhoea. She has been unable to eat and drink normally. There is no history of vomiting. Her observations are within normal limits. What is the most likely metabolic abnormality found on an arterial blood gas test?

A Metabolic alkalosis.

B Normal anion gap metabolic acidosis.

C Mixed alkalosis.

D Metabolic acidosis with respiratory compensation.

E Raised anion gap metabolic acidosis.

17. A 45-year-old female presents to her GP with the following symptoms. Which symptom would warrant urgent investigation?

A Abdominal pain relieved by defaecation.

B Change in bowel habit.

C Rectal bleeding.

D Abdominal distension.

E Passage of mucous.

18. A 25-year-old female presents to her GP with diarrhoea and bloating. On questioning, she also states that she has lost weight recently and is feeling fatigued most of the time. She has no blood in her stool. The GP arranges for coeliac antibody tests to be done. The antibody blood test comes back suggesting coeliac disease.

What is the next investigation that should be done?

A Endoscopy with ileal biopsy.

B Colonoscopy with biopsy.

C Endoscopy with duodenal biopsy.

D Trial of a gluten-free diet.

E Endoscopy with jejunal biopsy.

19. What is the gold standard investigation for diagnosing acute diverticulitis?

A CRP.

B Colonoscopy.

C Abdominal X-ray.

D Contrast CT colonography.

E Barium enema.

20. Which of these is the commonest cause of oesophageal varices in the United Kingdom?

A Right heart failure.

B Splenic vein thrombosis.

C Hepatic vein occlusion.

D Schistosomiasis.

E Liver cirrhosis.

21. A 54-year-old woman is referred to accident and emergency through her GP with a week's history of jaundice and right upper quadrant abdominal pain. Associated symptoms include dark urine and pale stools. There is no history of weight loss and the patient does not consume alcohol. Her liver function tests reveal a bilirubin of 40 µmol/L, ALT of 40 IU/L, AST 50 IU/L and ALP of 350 IU/L. The most likely diagnosis is:
    A Gallstones.
    B Viral hepatitis.
    C Alcoholic hepatitis.
    D Carcinoma of the head of the pancreas.
    E Autoimmune hepatitis.

22. A 62-year-old man presents to his GP with a 3-month history of upper abdominal pain following meals. On questioning, he describes this pain as burning and is able to point to the pain in his epigastrium. He reports having noticed his clothes have been looser recently. Which of these is the most important investigation to arrange?
    A *Helicobacter pylori* breath test.
    B Full blood count.
    C OGD endoscopy.
    D Trial of proton pump inhibitor (PPI).
    E Abdominal X-ray.

23. A 53-year-old man staggers into A&E having vomited six times in 2 hours. He is intoxicated. His friend said his vomit was initially 'normal', but after the first couple of episodes had fresh blood in it. His blood pressure is 120/90 and HR is 70 bpm. What is the most likely diagnosis?
    A Ruptured oesophageal varices.
    B Mallory–Weiss tear.
    C Ruptured peptic ulcer.
    D Boerhaave syndrome.
    E Oesophagitis.

24. A middle-aged woman has upper abdominal pain, jaundice and rigors for several days. Her liver is tender and enlarged on palpation. A full blood count shows leucocytosis. What is the likely diagnosis?
    A Viral hepatitis.
    B Acute cholecystitis.
    C Acute cholangitis.
    D Pancreatic cancer.
    E Drug-induced hepatitis.

25. What is the most likely cause for a smooth palpable mass in the right iliac fossa of the abdomen of a 34-year-old patient with Cushingoid features?
    A Transplanted kidney.
    B Aortic aneurysm.

C Ventral hernia.
D Enlarged bladder.
E Polycystic kidneys.

26. A 38-year-old patient with a long-term history of excess alcohol consumption and multiple hospitalizations presents to his GP with weight loss and loose, offensive stools. He does not have any other medical history and has not travelled anywhere abroad recently. What is the most likely diagnosis?
    A Colorectal carcinoma.
    B Crohn disease.
    C Systemic sclerosis.
    D Villous adenoma of the rectum.
    E Chronic pancreatitis.

27. A 41-year-old woman presents with painless difficulty in swallowing associated with a dry rash at the corners of her mouth. She is otherwise fit and well. What investigation will most likely help you identify the cause?
    A Gastroscopy.
    B Colonoscopy.
    C Chest X-ray.
    D Full set of bloods including haematinics.
    E Blood film.

28. A 40-year-old woman presents with a history of Addison disease presents with lethargy and pruritus. Blood tests show an elevated serum bilirubin level and an ultrasound examination shows no evidence of obstruction. What is the most likely diagnosis?
    A Sclerosing cholangitis.
    B Biliary colic.
    C Primary biliary cirrhosis.
    D Haematochromatosis.
    E Acute cholecystitis.

29. What would you find whilst investigating a 30-year-old woman with weight loss, steatorrhoea and a blood film suggesting hyposplenism?
    A Low blood caeruloplasmin level.
    B Raised alpha-fetoprotein level.
    C Raised serum amylase level.
    D Positive antimitochondrial antibody.
    E Positive antitissue transglutaminase antibodies.

30. A 40-year-old presents with a 5-day history of bloody diarrhoea of more than 10 episodes per day. This is associated with generalized abdominal pain and nausea. The patient had two episodes of vomiting and is also complaining of night-time fever. What is the most likely diagnosis?

A   Infective colitis.
B   Variceal bleed.
C   Angiodysplasia.
D   Inflammatory bowel disease.
E   Colorectal cancer.

Chapter 31 Renal, genitourinary and sexual health

1. A 62-year-old man has an AKI in relation to diarrhoea and vomiting. He has a background of hypertension and takes ramipril regularly. On admission he is hypovolaemic and anuric. Which one of the following conditions is an indication for emergency haemodialysis/haemofiltration in AKI?
    A   Anuria.
    B   Serum creatinine level greater than 500 μmol/L (reference range 80–120 μmol/L).
    C   Bicarbonate level less than 20 mmol/L (reference range 22–28 mmol/L).
    D   Potassium level greater than 6.5 mmol/L (reference range 3.5–5.0 mmol/L) despite medical therapy.
    E   Urea level greater than 30 mmol/L (reference range 2.5–5.0 mmol/L).

2. A 62-year-old diabetic man is admitted with urinary sepsis. On routine blood tests he is found to have a serum potassium level of 6.4 mmol/L (reference range 3.5–5.0 mmol/L). An ECG is performed. Which one of the following changes would you most expect to see?
    A   Tented T waves.
    B   Absent P waves.
    C   Broad QRS complexes.
    D   U waves.
    E   Sinusoidal waveform.

3. A 5-year-old boy presents with a pale puffy face and swollen legs. There is generalized oedema on clinical examination. Which of the following best defines the triad of nephrotic syndrome?
    A   Low serum albumin level, PCR greater than 300 mg/mmol and peripheral oedema.
    B   Haematuria, proteinuria (>3 g in 24 hours) and low serum albumin level.
    C   Low serum albumin level, proteinuria (>3 g in 24 hours) and high serum cholesterol level.
    D   Low serum albumin level, more than 3 g protein in a 24-hour urine collection and an increased risk of infection.
    E   Low serum albumin level, PCR greater than 300 mg/mmol and increased risk of thromboembolism.

4. In the patient from the previous question, what is the commonest underlying cause of his nephrotic syndrome?
    A   Post-streptococcal glomerulonephritis.
    B   Rapidly progressive glomerulonephritis.
    C   Membranous glomerulonephritis.
    D   Minimal change disease.
    E   Focal segmental glomerulosclerosis (FSGS).

5. A 59-year-old woman is being investigated for an AKI with blood and protein on urine analysis (urine dipstick). She mentions to you that she had an episode of haemoptysis. Which of the following is the most important blood test to perform?
    A   Antistreptolysin O titre.
    B   Complement levels.
    C   CRP.
    D   Antinuclear antibodies.
    E   ANCA.

6. A 70-year-old old man presents with a creatinine level of 300 μmol/L (reference range 80–110 μmol/L). Which one of the following would most make you think that he has CKD?
    A   His eGFR is 18 mL/min/1.73 m^2.
    B   He is anaemic.
    C   He has small scarred kidneys on ultrasound scan.
    D   His prostate is enlarged, with a large bladder and hydronephrosis.
    E   He has a monoclonal band on electrophoresis.

7. Which one of the following statements is correct with respect to CKD?
    A   Hypertension is a rare cause.
    B   Patients with proteinuria do better.
    C   Lowering the blood pressure is dangerous.
    D   Microcytic anaemia is a feature.
    E   Dietary phosphate intake should be restricted.

8. An 18-year-old female presents with rigors, lower abdominal pain and urinary frequency. Which of the following is the best first test?
    A   Dimercaptosuccinic acid (DMSA) scan.
    B   Blood cultures and urine microscopy and culture (midstream urine).
    C   Urine β-human chorionic gonadotropin (pregnancy test).
    D   Abdominal X-ray.
    E   Full blood count.

9. Which statement regarding UTIs is true?
    A   They are more common in females.
    B   They affect 5% of the female population at least once

C   They are always symptomatic.

D   They are less common in catheterized patients.

E   They rarely ascend to involve the kidneys.

10. A 32-year-old man has a rotator cuff repair under a general anaesthetic as a day case. Routine blood tests and urine dip were unremarkable during preoperative assessment. He is discharged after an uncomplicated operation with paracetamol and ibuprofen for pain. He presents 2 weeks later to his GP with significant bilateral ankle oedema. On examination his blood pressure is 125/72 mmHg. Urine dipstick reveals 3+ protein, but no haematuria. His plasma creatinine level is 65 mmol/L (normal). What is the most likely diagnosis?

A   Membranous nephropathy.

B   Acute tubular necrosis.

C   Interstitial nephritis.

D   Lupus nephritis.

E   FSGS.

11. A 70-year-old man presents with haematuria to his GP. On further questioning, he describes intermittent colicky left loin pain, weight loss and night sweats. He has noted testicular changes, which, on examination, are a varicocele. What is the likely underlying diagnosis?

A   Acute pyelonephritis.

B   Acute cystitis.

C   Prostate carcinoma.

D   Ureteric calculi.

E   Renal cell carcinoma.

12. A 36-year-old woman presents with malaise, recurrent epistaxis, haemoptysis and microscopic haematuria. Examination reveals septal perforation and nodules on the CXR. The serum creatinine level is elevated at 307 μmol/L (reference range 80–110 μmol/L). What is the likely underlying diagnosis?

A   Antiglomerular basement membrane disease (Goodpasture disease).

B   Granulomatosis with polyangiitis (Wegener granulomatosis).

C   IgA nephropathy.

D   Primary membranous glomerulonephritis.

E   Eosinophilic granulomatosis with polyangiitis (Churg–Strauss syndrome).

13. A 39-year-old man presents to the emergency department in high summer with severe colicky right loin pain radiating down into the scrotum. Examination findings are unremarkable and the dipstick shows haematuria. What is the most appropriate imaging to confirm the underlying diagnosis?

A   MRI abdomen.

B   Ultrasound KUB (kidney, ureter, bladder).

C   CT KUB.

D   CT CAP (chest, abdomen, pelvis).

E   MRI prostate.

14. A 24-year-old woman with a history of recurrent UTIs presents with loin pain and haematuria. On examination she is noted to have hypertension. Her mother is receiving dialysis. Given the suspected diagnosis, mutations of which genes may be implicated?

A   CTFR.

B   PKD1 and PKD2.

C   FGFR3.

D   DMD.

E   NF1.

15. A 72-year-old man presents to his GP with recurrent infections and bone pain. Bloods are requested, which demonstrate a haemoglobin of 96 g/L (reference range 120–160 g/L) and a creatine 180 μmol/L (reference range 80–120 μmol/L). What further investigation would be most likely to identify the underlying diagnosis?

A   CRP.

B   Bone profile.

C   Antiphospholipase A2 receptor antibody (anti-PLA2R).

D   Serum complement.

E   Protein electrophoresis, serum-free light chains and urinary Bence Jones protein.

16. A 25-year-old man presents to his GP with haematuria. He generally feels well in himself, but did have coryzal symptoms which resolved 2 days ago. He does not have any abdominal pain or oedema. What is the most likely cause of his haematuria?

A   Minimal change nephropathy.

B   Renal caliculi.

C   Post-streptococcal glomerulonephritis.

D   IgA nephropathy.

E   Focal segmental glomerulosclerosis.

17. A 19-year-old man is seen in the sexual health clinic with penile discharge and dysuria. A urine sample and penile swab are taken which demonstrate *Neisseria gonorrhoeae*. What is the most appropriate first-line treatment?

A   Doxycycline 100 mg orally, twice daily for 7 days.

B   Ceftriaxone 1 g subcutaneously, single dose.

C   Ceftriaxone 1 g intramuscularly, single dose.

D   Benzathine penicillin 2.4 g intramuscularly, single dose.

E   Co-amoxiclav 500/125 mg orally, three times daily for 7 to 10 days.

Chapter 32 Fluid balance and electrolyte
disturbances

1. A 58-year-old man presents with polyuria, dehydration and abdominal pain. Blood tests reveal corrected calcium level of 3.2 mmol/L (reference range 2.2–2.6 mmol/L). Which of the following is correct?
   A Sarcoidosis is a cause of hypercalcaemia.
   B Treatment with bisphosphonates is urgently required.
   C If the calcium level returns to normal with treatment, no further investigation is needed on this occasion.
   D Protein-bound calcium is the relevant value.
   E Malignancy is a rare cause.

2. A 30-year-old man is in hospital for an elective cholecystectomy and is nil by mouth. He is desperately trying to find water to drink and is aggressive. He has a background of schizophrenia and has been taking lithium. In the patient's notes you read that he complains of being very thirsty and has been passing high volumes of urine. His blood test results come back, and you see that his sodium level is 150 mmol/L (reference range 135–145 mmol/L). What is the most likely diagnosis?
   A Conn syndrome.
   B Addison disease.
   C Diabetes insipidus.
   D Cushing disease.
   E Ingestion of sodium chloride tablets.

3. A 70-year-old woman is admitted to the hospital with a urinary infection. She has a background of hypertension and mild cognitive impairment, and normally lives in a residential home. Her blood test results come back showing a sodium level of 123 mmol/L (reference range 135–145 mmol/L). From her routine blood test results at her GP practice, her sodium levels are normally between 130 and 132 mmol/L. The syndrome of inappropriate secretion of antidiuretic hormone (SIADH) is suspected. How would you diagnose this condition?
   A Paired serum and urine osmolality and urinary sodium tests.
   B Fluid deprivation test.
   C Trial of fluid restriction to see if this increases the sodium level.
   D Do a cortisol level, followed by a dexamethasone suppression test.
   E Do a random cortisol level, followed by a short Synacthen test.

4. A 65-year-old woman goes to her general practitioner feeling fatigued and reports feeling forgetful. She has a background of hypertension, hypothyroidism, depression and peptic ulcer disease. Her medications include bisoprolol, bendroflumethiazide, levothyroxine, omeprazole and citalopram. Her blood test results show that her sodium level is 128 mmol/L (reference range 135–145 mmol/L). Which medication would be the most likely causative agent?
   A Bisoprolol.
   B Bendroflumethiazide.
   C Levothyroxine.
   D Omeprazole.
   E Citalopram.

5. A 30-year-old woman with depression and anxiety presents to her general practitioner (GP) with fatigue and muscle weakness. The GP finds that her body mass index is extremely low at 18 kg/m^2. On further questioning, she reports that she has been making herself vomit. Her blood test results show a potassium level of 2.6 mmol/L (reference range 3.5–5 mmol/L). Which of the following symptoms could be attributed to her hypokalaemia?
   A Abdominal pain.
   B Polyuria.
   C Urinary tract infections.
   D Seizures.
   E Perioral numbness.

6. A 60-year-old woman had a parathyroidectomy for hyperparathyroidism. She is back on the ward after surgery and you have been asked to monitor her calcium level every 4 hours and replace calcium as necessary. The calcium result comes back with a corrected calcium reading of 1.6 mmol/L (reference range 2.2–2.6 mmol/L). You perform an electrocardiogram. What features of hypocalcaemia would you be looking for?
   A Peaked T waves.
   B Delta waves.
   C Sinusoidal QRS complex.
   D Prolonged QT interval.
   E J waves.

7. A 30-year-old man presents with abdominal pain and constipation. Of note, a recent chest X-ray shows bilateral hilar lymphadenopathy. His bloods are taken. Which electrolyte disturbance is the most likely cause of his symptoms?
   A Hypernatraemia.
   B Hyponatraemia.
   C Hypercalcaemia.
   D Hypocalcaemia.
   E Hyperkalaemia.

8. A 45-year-old woman who is generally well has routine bloods taken. These show an incidental finding of a raised calcium level and low phosphate level. The rest of her bloods (FBC, renal and liver function) are unremarkable. What is the most likely cause?

A Bone metastases.

B Hypoparathyroidism.

C Multiple myeloma.

D Primary hyperparathyroidism.

E Secondary hyperparathyroidism.

9. A 30-year-old woman with vitiligo and rheumatoid arthritis complains of abdominal pain and dizziness. Her blood glucose levels have been on the low side. Her blood results demonstrate potassium of 5.6 mmol/L (reference range 3.5–5 mmol/L) and sodium of 125 mmol/L (reference range 135–145 mmol/L). What is the underlying diagnosis?

A Syndrome of inappropriate secretion of antidiuretic hormone (SIADH).

B Addison disease.

C Bartter syndrome.

D Gitelman syndrome.

E Hypothyroidism.

10. A 65-year-old woman reports feeling generally cold, fatigued and low in mood. She undergoes bloods which demonstrate she is hyponatraemic. What is the likely underlying cause?

A Diuretics medications.

B Addison disease.

C Ace inhibitor.

D Nephrotic syndrome.

E Hypothyroidism.

11. While an inpatient, a 55-year-old man is found to be hyponatraemic. What initial management plan would help you determine the underlying cause?

A Review the drug chart, fluid restrict, recheck sodium levels.

B Examine the patient's fluid status, review the drug chart, blood tests including urea and electrolytes, thyroid function, glucose and lipid levels. Paired urine and serum osmolalities and urinary sodium.

C Review the drug chart, blood tests including urea and electrolytes, thyroid function, glucose and lipid levels. Paired urine and serum osmolalities and urinary sodium. Organize short Synacthen test.

D Examine the patient's fluid status, blood tests including urea and electrolytes, thyroid function, glucose and lipid levels. Paired urine and serum osmolalities and urinary sodium.

E Examine the patient's fluid status, review the drug chart, paired urine and serum osmolalities and urinary sodium. Give IV dextrose 5%.

12. A 65-year-old man with a history of poorly controlled chronic hypertension visits his general practitioner with symptoms of fatigue, metallic taste and itch. He has a potassium level of 6.2 mmol/L (reference range 3.5–5.0 mmol/L), his phosphate level is raised and he is anaemic. What is the underlying diagnosis?

A Renal artery stenosis.

B Cushing syndrome.

C Addison disease.

D Malignancy.

E Chronic kidney disease.

13. A 70-year-old man is admitted to hospital for treatment of pyelonephritis. He is receiving Hartmann solution as intravenous fluid resuscitation and has been given gentamicin for his pyelonephritis. His potassium level is 6.2 mmol/L (reference range 3.5–5.0 mmol/L) on a venous blood gas test. What is the underlying cause of his hyperkalaemia?

A Diabetic ketoacidosis.

B Tea and toast diet.

C Renal artery stenosis.

D Acute kidney injury.

E Chronic kidney disease.

14. A 65-year-old woman is admitted with severe diarrhoea and vomiting. She is clinically hypovolaemic and blood tests demonstrate an acute kidney injury and a potassium of 6.5. Her ECG shows tented T waves. What is the initial management of her hyperkalaemia?

A IV fluids.

B IV calcium gluconate (10 mL of 5%) followed by 20 units of insulin (as Actrapid) in 100 mL of 20% dextrose IV.

C IV 10 units of insulin (as Actrapid) in 100 mL of 20% dextrose (or 50 mL of 50% dextrose).

D IV calcium gluconate (10 mL of 10%) followed by 10 units of insulin (as Actrapid) in 100 mL of 20% dextrose IV.

E An oral potassium binder, e.g., sodium zirconium cyclosilicate (Lokelma) followed by 10 units of insulin (as Actrapid) in 100 mL of 20% dextrose IV.

Chapter 33 Metabolic and endocrine disorders

1. A 55-year-old man goes to his general practitioner and is tested for diabetes. Which one of the following allows a diagnosis of diabetes to be made?

A Fasting plasma glucose level of 6.0 mmol/L.

B Random glucose level of 10.9 mmol/L.

C Random glucose level of 11.2 mmol/L and polyuria.

D Fasting glucose level of 6.9 mmol/L and 2-hour glucose level of 10.4 mmol/L.

E Fasting glucose level of 6.6 mmol/L and 2-hour glucose level of 7.5 mmol/L.

2. A 17-year-old woman with diabetes is found unconscious by her mother following a chest infection. Which one of the following is correct regarding diabetic ketoacidosis (DKA)?
   A Insulin replacement should be the first treatment.
   B In young patients there is no need to worry about fluid overload.
   C Hypoventilation is typical.
   D Antibiotics are often required.
   E Raised blood glucose level and clinical signs are sufficient for the diagnosis.

3. Which one of the following is correct regarding the long-term treatment of diabetes?
   A Type 1 diabetes can often be managed with oral medication.
   B The aim should be an HbA1c fraction below 10% (85.8 mmol/mol).
   C Sulphonylureas are the first choice in overweight patients.
   D Metformin is contraindicated in advanced CKD.
   E Once-daily subcutaneous insulin administration is the treatment of choice for type 1 diabetes.

4. A 66-year-old woman who takes low-dose steroids long-term for rheumatoid arthritis sustains a Colles fracture. Which one of the following statements is correct regarding osteoporosis?
   A It is frequently painful.
   B It is less common in women.
   C Hypocalcaemia is seen on testing.
   D A T score of –2.0 is diagnostic.
   E The prevalence is around 25% in white women aged 80 years or older.

5. A 58-year-old man presents with polyuria, dehydration and abdominal pain. Blood tests reveal a calcium level of 3.2 mmol/L. Which one of the following is correct?
   A Sarcoidosis is a cause of hypercalcaemia.
   B Treatment with bisphosphonates is urgently required.
   C If the calcium level returns to normal with treatment, no further investigation is needed on this occasion.
   D Protein-bound calcium level is the relevant value.
   E Malignancy is a rare cause.

6. A 42-year-old man comes to see you because his family are concerned his appearance has changed. He has experienced headaches over the last year. Which one of the following is a feature of acromegaly?
   A Increased interdental spacing.
   B Homonymous hemianopia.

   C Retrognathism.
   D Hypergonadism.
   E Hypoglycaemia.

7. A 60-year-old British woman with a background of vitiligo and diabetes complains of constipation, weight gain and constantly feeling cold. Which is the most likely cause of her hypothyroidism?
   A An iatrogenic cause; following radioactive treatment for hyperthyroidism.
   B Iodine deficiency.
   C Hashimoto thyroiditis.
   D Graves disease.
   E Pituitary adenoma.

8. Which one of the following statements is correct regarding Addison disease?
   A Most cases in the developed world are due to infection.
   B Blood tests demonstrating hyponatraemia and hyperkalaemia would be consistent with Addison disease.
   C Diagnosis is usually made with a random cortisol measurement.
   D Aldosterone replacement with fludrocortisone is the most important treatment in Addisonian crisis.
   E Hypopigmentation is common.

9. A 37-year-old woman presents with tremor, palpitations and loose stools. Which one of the following may be seen in thyrotoxicosis of any cause?
   A Atrial fibrillation.
   B Pretibial myxoedema.
   C Finger clubbing.
   D Menorrhagia.
   E Bilateral proptosis.

10. Which one of the following hormones is secreted by the posterior pituitary?
    A Thyroid-stimulating hormone (TSH).
    B Adrenocorticotrophic hormone (ACTH).
    C Growth hormone (GH).
    D Antidiuretic hormone (ADH).
    E Prolactin.

11. Characteristic features of untreated Cushing syndrome due to adrenocortical hyperplasia include:
    A Bitemporal hemianopia.
    B Thin fragile skin that bruises easily.
    C Muscular hypertrophy.
    D Lactation.
    E Amenorrhoea.

12. In which of the following pairings is the finding or complication on the right correctly paired with the condition on the left:
    A Familial hypercholesterolaemia – tendinous xanthoma.
    B Conn syndrome – postural hypotension.
    C Type I diabetes mellitus – weight gain.
    D Paget disease – sensorineural deafness.
    E Addison disease – hirsutism.

13. A 38-year-old female presents with symptoms of polyuria, polydipsia and dehydration. You suspect diabetes insipidus. What test would you perform to differentiate between cranial or nephrogenic?
    A Oral glucose tolerance test.
    B Dexamethasone suppression test.
    C CT scan.
    D Water deprivation test.
    E Random plasma glucose.

14. A 50-year-old female presents to clinic with a 6-month history of changes to her appearance. Her facial features have become coarse, her voice has deepened and her joints ache more than usual. What is the first-line investigation for the most likely diagnosis?
    A OGTT (oral glucose tolerance test).
    B Serum IGF-1.
    C Pituitary MRI.
    D Serum GH.
    E Serum GHRH.

15. Physical signs of thyrotoxicosis include:
    A Irregular pulse.
    B Ophthalmoplegia.
    C Tremor.
    D Abdominal distension.
    E A thyroid bruit.

16. What test would you order in a 28-year-old patient with vitiligo who is complaining of lethargy? On examination you find pigmented palmar creases and oral mucosa.
    A Short Synacthen test.
    B Insulin stress test.
    C Insulin-like growth factor 1 measurement.
    D Thyrotropin-releasing hormone test.
    E Domperidone test.

17. A 48-year-old man reports muscle cramps and weakness. He is hypertensive. Urea and electrolyte test results show hypokalaemia. Which one of the below options is the most likely cause?
    A Diabetes mellitus.
    B Conn syndrome.
    C Addison disease.
    D Hypothyroidism.
    E Prolactinoma.

18. A 25-year-old man is admitted to the hospital with hyperglycaemia, ketones and acidosis following gastroenteritis. He looks unwell. His blood pressure is 95/60, heart rate 130 and respiratory rate 30. He does not remember how he got to the hospital. What is the most important treatment in this patient?
    A Antibiotics.
    B Oxygen.
    C Intravenous fluids.
    D Fixed insulin infusion.
    E Variable rate insulin infusion.

19. A 45-year-old with long-standing type 2 diabetes, who normally takes insulin, is nil by mouth for an appendicectomy. You are the FY1 covering the wards and the nurses have called asking how he should be managed.
    A Let him eat and drink.
    B Start a variable rate insulin infusion.
    C Start a fixed-rate insulin infusion.
    D Start intravenous fluids.
    E Start metformin.

20. How would you treat a 50-year-old woman with a background of hypothyroidism and vitiligo, who presents to the emergency department profoundly hypotensive? She has had unexplained nonspecific symptoms, including abdominal pain. Her blood glucose level is low, and her potassium level is raised.
    A Intravenous fluid, hydrocortisone intravenously and T_3 intravenously.
    B Intravenous fluid, hydrocortisone intravenously, insulin and dextrose intravenously and 10 mL of 10% calcium gluconate.
    C Intravenous fluid, fixed-rate intravenous insulin infusion (0.1 units per kilogram per hour), antibiotics and low-molecular-weight heparin.
    D Intravenous fluid, propranolol intravenously, hydrocortisone intravenously and iodine and propylthiouracil orally.
    E Intravenous administration of 100 mL of 20% dextrose.

Chapter 34 Nervous system

1. Which finding favours the diagnosis of motor neurone disease?
   A Sensory loss.
   B Absent tendon reflexes.
   C Muscle fasciculation.
   D Muscle hypertrophy.
   E Optic atrophy.

2. Which is most common amongst sufferers of stroke?
   A Panic disorder.
   B Social phobia.
   C Hypomania.
   D Depression.
   E Anxiety.

3. A 22-year-old male presents with a headache that has been present for the past two days, fever and widespread purpura over his back and legs. He does not have any neck stiffness or focal neurology. He looks very unwell. Which of the below is the most useful investigation?
   A Blood culture.
   B CT head.
   C Full blood count.
   D Lumbar puncture.
   E Clotting panel.

4. A 29-year-old female is brought into the emergency department by ambulance due to severe occipital pain followed by a brief period of loss of consciousness. On assessment GCS is 14, HR 110 and BP 167/101. She has a low-grade fever and is still complaining of a mild headache. There is no neck stiffness or focal neurological signs. What is the most likely diagnosis?
   A Hypertensive encephalopathy.
   B Subdural haemorrhage.
   C Subarachnoid haemorrhage.
   D Meningoencephalitis.
   E Massive intracerebral haemorrhage.

5. A 62-year-old patient with Parkinson disease and heart failure comes to see you complaining of worsening motor symptoms. He started noticing that the medication he takes is no longer enough to control his symptoms and he now suffers from fluctuations in his motor function. He takes a maximum dose of co-beneldopa. What is the best course of action?
   A Start cabergoline.
   B Start amantadine.

   C Start entacapone.
   D Start rotigotine.
   E Seek specialist advice.

6. Which is not a feature of pseudobulbar palsy?
   A Brisk jaw jerk.
   B Tongue spasticity.
   C Dysphagia.
   D Dysarthria.
   E Tongue wasting and fasciculations.

7. A 60-year-old woman presents to her GP with a 3-month history of muscle weakness and a rash affecting her hands and eyelids. Examination reveals erythematous papules over the metacarpal and interphalangeal joints, heliotrope rash over the face and proximal muscle weakness. What is the most likely diagnosis?
   A Dermatomyositis.
   B Myasthenia gravis.
   C SLE.
   D Vitamin B_{12} deficiency.
   E Guillain–Barré syndrome.

8. A 64-year-old woman presents with progressive weakness that started in her legs. Which one of the following is correct regarding motor neurone disease (MND)?
   A It is more common in women.
   B It commonly causes sensory problems as well as motor problems.
   C It may present with diplopia.
   D The 5-year survival rate is almost 75%.
   E It may cause a mixture of upper and lower motor neurone symptoms.

9. A 45-year-old man presents following a severe sudden onset headache that occurred during exercise. CT scan shows blood in the subarachnoid space. Which one of the following statements is correct regarding this condition?
   A Mortality is low.
   B Most are preceded by a sentinel headache.
   C Reduced consciousness following initial improvement may be due to hydrocephalus.
   D He should be given β-blockers.
   E Fluid intake should be restricted.

10. A 64-year-old man presents following a 'blackout'. Which one of the following statements is correct regarding the cause?
   A Seizure is probable if urinary incontinence occurred.
   B Jerking or twitching is never seen in vasovagal syncope.

C   An ECG is unlikely to be helpful in determining the cause.

D   Biting the tip of the tongue suggests a seizure.

E   Syncope on exertion suggests a cardiac cause.

11. A 26-year-old man presents with a severe, throbbing, unilateral headache preceded by odd visual symptoms. It is worsened by loud noises, bright light or moving around. He is afebrile. Which one of the following statements is correct?

A   The most likely diagnosis is meningitis.

B   Subarachnoid haemorrhage (SAH) commonly has visual warning symptoms.

C   A triptan is a suitable treatment in this case.

D   Acute migraine headache can be treated with β-blockers.

E   Patients with cluster headache typically avoid movement.

12. A 56-year-old man is brought to the emergency department after being involved in a road traffic accident. He opens his eyes to pain and attempts to withdraw when you perform a trapezius squeeze. His speech is unclear, and he makes only incomprehensible sounds. What is his Glasgow Coma Scale (GCS) score?

A   6.

B   7.

C   8.

D   9.

E   10.

13. A 44-year-old woman presents with symptoms of raised intracranial pressure. MRI scan reveals a solitary lesion. Which one of the following statements is correct regarding intracerebral tumours?

A   Primary tumours are more common than secondary tumours.

B   If primary tumour is suspected, MRI is sufficient to determine the type of tumour.

C   Meningiomas may be cured with surgical resection.

D   Glioblastomas are indolent tumours with a good prognosis.

E   Breast cancer rarely metastasizes to the brain.

14. You see a 55-year-old man in the clinic who has noticed a gradually worsening, low-frequency tremor in his right hand over the last 6 months. Which one of the following statements is true?

A   Parkinson disease (PD) is usually symmetrical in onset.

B   The tremor of PD is more noticeable at rest.

C   L-DOPA is definitely the best treatment for this patient.

D   A radioiodine scan is necessary to make the diagnosis in this case.

E   Rigidity is an uncommon feature.

15. Which one of the following statements is correct regarding raised intracranial pressure (ICP)?

A   The headache is worse at the end of the day.

B   Tachycardia is part of the Cushing reflex.

C   Papilloedema is not caused by raised ICP.

D   Sixth cranial nerve palsy is a feature.

E   Abdominal pain is a feature.

16. From the list below choose the most appropriate first-line drug for a 45-year-old man with Parkinson disease (PD). He is complaining of resting tremor and rigidity.

A   Ropinirole.

B   Selegiline.

C   Carbidopa.

D   L-DOPA.

E   Propranolol.

17. You see a 23-year-old woman in the clinic. She experienced an episode of visual blurring in her right eye, associated with pain on movement, which came on over hours but her vision has improved over the last month. Which one of the following statements is correct?

A   This is definitely multiple sclerosis (MS).

B   It is unusual to get MS at this age.

C   Night vision is likely to be the most affected.

D   If there are lesions on MRI, her risk of developing MS is higher.

E   Vision only improves in a minority of patients.

18. A 32-year-old man presents to his GP with a few months' history of involuntary movements of both upper and lower limbs and the face. He recalls that his mother told him that his father had similar problems but unfortunately he died in his early 40s when the patient was young. What should the GP advise the patient?

A   This is most likely a space-occupying lesion, and an urgent CT scan of the head is required.

B   He most likely has Sydenham chorea. Treatment with penicillin should be started. The condition rarely leads to long-standing complications.

C   The patient has an autosomal dominant disorder, likely Huntington disease. An urgent referral to the neurology clinic is necessary.

D   Blood samples should be sent to the laboratory to investigate the presence of low levels of ceruloplasmin, indicating Wilson disease.

E   The use of haloperidol, which the patient takes for schizophrenia, should be stopped.

19. A 63-year-old woman presents 2 hours after the sudden onset of right-sided weakness. She takes warfarin for atrial fibrillation. Which one of the following statements is correct?
    A Imaging of the brain should be done within the next 24 hours but is not urgent.
    B If the CT scan shows haemorrhage, the effects of warfarin should be reversed with cryoprecipitate.
    C Because she takes warfarin, the stroke is definitely haemorrhagic.
    D Haemorrhage is the most common cause of stroke.
    E Facial weakness in stroke usually spares the forehead.

20. A 19-year-old male student is admitted with confusion, fever, photophobia and a purpuric rash. His friends say he was complaining of a severe headache and has vomited. Which one of the following is correct?
    A He should be treated urgently with intravenous antibiotics.
    B *Streptococcus* is the most likely causative organism.
    C The diagnosis should be confirmed with blood cultures before treatment.
    D *Listeria* is a common cause in young adults.
    E Lumbar puncture should be performed immediately.

21. What is the most likely nerve lesion in a 65-year-old woman presenting with loss of vibration and joint position sense in the feet with a positive Babinski sign?
    A Multiple sclerosis.
    B Pancoast tumour.
    C Spinal cord infarction.
    D Subacute combined degeneration of the cord.
    E Syringomyelia.

22. A 93-year-old woman is brought in following a sudden loss of consciousness. Two days later, she remains deeply unconscious with unreactive pupils. What is she likely to have suffered?
    A Meningitis.
    B Hepatic encephalopathy.
    C Brainstem infarction.
    D Hyponatraemia.
    E Drug overdose.

23. A 15-year-old girl is brought in by her parents after several episodes where she says she has a feeling of déjà vu and then becomes unresponsive but appears awake and picks at her clothes. She cannot remember the episodes, which last around 2 minutes. What is the likely diagnosis?
    A Febrile convulsion.
    B Glioma.

C Meningitis.
D Absence seizure.
E Temporal lobe epilepsy.

24. An 89-year-old patient with a history of vascular dementia falls and loses consciousness after getting out of bed in the morning. No ECG changes are noted on assessment in the emergency department and she has no focal neurology. What is the most likely cause for her loss of consciousness?
    A Vasovagal syncope.
    B Transient ischaemic attack (TIA).
    C Stroke.
    D Orthostatic hypotension (postural hypotension).
    E Epilepsy.

25. A 49-year-old man with a hard, irregular, palpable, right-sided thyroid swelling presents with a drooping eyelid on the same side. On examination you also notice that his right pupil is constricted. What is the diagnosis?
    A Horner syndrome.
    B Argyll Robertson pupil.
    C Bell palsy.
    D Sixth nerve palsy.
    E Ramsay Hunt syndrome.

Chapter 35 Musculoskeletal system

1. A 22-year-old female develops arthralgia and fever while away on holiday. She attends the emergency department where you notice a red scaly rash on her nose and cheeks. She tells you it got worse when she went to the beach. She is also complaining of chest pain that is worse on leaning forwards. Blood tests reveal pancytopenia and proteinuria. What is the most likely diagnosis?
    A A sexually transmitted disease.
    B Systemic sclerosis.
    C Amyloidosis.
    D Acute leukaemia.
    E Systemic lupus erythematosus.

2. A middle-aged man attends your GP practice with a fever. He is complaining of a red, hot, swollen and painful knee joint. He is unable to walk on it. This has been going on for a few days. He is normally fit and well. What is the most likely diagnosis?
    A Monoarticular rheumatoid arthritis.
    B Trauma.
    C Septic arthritis.
    D Crystal arthritis.
    E Haemarthrosis.

3. A 60-year-old female attends the emergency department with purulent discharge from a wound on her left elbow. She suffers from severe rheumatoid arthritis and had to undergo an elbow joint replacement 2 months ago. You look at her hospital notes and notice that a wound swab taken a few days after the operation has grown methicillin-resistant *Staphylococcus aureus* (MRSA). What is the most appropriate antibiotic therapy?
   A Co-amoxiclav.
   B Vancomycin.
   C Gentamycin.
   D Cefuroxime.
   E Metronidazole.

4. A 65-year-old woman with known rheumatoid arthritis (RA) presents to the clinic with her daughter. She is doing well, with no inflammation, and leads an active life. She has been maintained with the same therapy for more than 20 years. Her daughter reports that over the past year, she has developed a blue-grey discolouration on her face that has become more noticeable. Otherwise, she is well, with no other side effects. She attends her GP practice for regular blood monitoring, the results of which have been satisfactory. Which of the following disease-modifying drugs could be responsible for her skin discolouration?
   A Salazopyrin.
   B Intramuscularly (IM) administered gold.
   C Methotrexate.
   D Leflunomide.
   E Azathioprine.

5. A 25-year-old teacher presents with haemoptysis. She also has a vasculitic rash on her legs, where some areas are coalescing and forming ulcers. She has a background of sinusitis for the past few years. Her ESR is 100 mm/h. She has proteinuria and haematuria on dipstick urinalysis. A chest X-ray shows multiple focal opacities in the lungs. An autoimmune screen shows a negative result for ANA, a negative result for anti-double-stranded DNA, a negative result for rheumatoid factor but a positive result for cytoplasmic antineutrophil cytoplasmic antibodies (cANCA). What is the most likely diagnosis?
   A Polymyalgia rheumatica (PMR).
   B Granulomatosis with polyangiitis.
   C Microscopic polyangiitis.
   D Kawasaki disease.
   E Eosinophilic granulomatosis with polyangiitis.

6. A 60-year-old teacher presents with widespread joint pain. Her hands are particularly painful, notably small joints in her fingers and the joint at the base of her thumb. Her wrist is also painful, and she has a scar from Colles fracture repair

20 years ago. She also describes left groin and knee pain when walking and low back pain. Which of the following joints are *not* affected by primary osteoarthritis (OA)?
   A Wrist.
   B Metatarsophalangeal (MTP) joints.
   C Distal interphalangeal (DIP) joints.
   D Carpometacarpal joints.
   E Hip.

7. A 30-year-old woman with known seropositive rheumatoid arthritis is maintained on methotrexate (20 mg weekly) and is doing well. She is keen to start a family. What is the best advice regarding her current treatment?
   A Stop the use of methotrexate and start the use of cyclosporine.
   B Reduce the dose of methotrexate.
   C Continue with the use of methotrexate and add oral steroids.
   D Stop the use of methotrexate and start the use of another drug after consultation with the rheumatology team.
   E Stop the use of methotrexate and give oral steroids if necessary for disease flares.

8. A 25-year-old woman presents with increasing joint pain. Clinical examination reveals swollen tender distal interphalangeal (DIP) joints, pitting in her nails and swollen toes. Her spinal movements are also restricted. She also describes episodes of bloody diarrhoea and weight loss over the past year. What is most likely causing her joint pains?
   A Rheumatoid arthritis.
   B Systemic lupus erythematosus.
   C Reactive arthritis.
   D Psoriatic arthritis.
   E Fibromyalgia.

9. A history of joint pains, tiredness, oral ulceration and a rash on the hands and front of the chest in a female patient recently started on treatment for tuberculosis would point towards which antibody being present in around 90% of sufferers?
   A Antihistone antibody.
   B Antimitochondrial antibody.
   C Anti-double-stranded DNA antibody.
   D Antinuclear antibody.
   E Classical antineutrophil cytoplasmic antibody.

10. You see a 60-year-old male with a painful right lower limb. On examination the tibia is warm to the touch and there is overlying erythema. The bone is abnormally curved and appears thickened. The patient tells you that he has not suffered any trauma to the limb. He is

normally fit and well and only takes occasional paracetamol for the headache. He denies any systemic signs or symptoms. There is no travel history. What is the first-line treatment?

A Analgesia with strong painkillers and orthopaedic referral.

B Immobilization and review him in 4 weeks' time.

C CT chest, abdomen and pelvis to investigate for a possible malignancy.

D Osteoclast inhibitors.

E Antibiotics.

11. Which of the conditions listed is most likely to affect joint pain as described below? A 60-year-old man who drinks half a bottle of wine a day presents with an acutely swollen, red first metatarsophalangeal (MTP) joint and raised serum creatinine level.

A Chondrocalcinosis.

B Reactive arthritis.

C Gout.

D Pseudogout.

E Myositis.

12. A 23-year-old woman presents with two swollen fingers in her right hand, a swollen ankle and a swollen wrist. She also has colitis and has had iritis in the past. What is the most likely diagnosis?

A Septic arthritis.

B Reactive arthritis.

C Osteoarthritis.

D Rheumatoid arthritis.

E Psoriatic arthritis.

Chapter 36 Dermatology

1. You see a 68-year-old female who is complaining of a few months' history of a painless irregular lump in her right breast. On examination you find skin tethering and dimpling. What is the most likely diagnosis?

A Ductal carcinoma.

B Lipoma.

C Fibroadenoma.

D Cystic changes.

E Ductal ectasia.

2. A groin lump located below the inguinal ligament and lateral to the pubic tubercle that seems continuous with the deeper structures is most likely:

A Saphenous varix.

B Enlarged lymph node.

C Femoral hernia.

D Direct inguinal hernia.

E Indirect inguinal hernia.

3. A 50-year-old man develops weakness in his legs (examination shows proximal myopathy), an erythematous rash over his knuckles and purple discolouration around his eyes. He complains of difficulty in swallowing, and initial blood tests show his creatine kinase level to be more than 3000 IU/L. What is the most likely diagnosis?

A Polymyalgia rheumatica.

B Osteomalacia.

C Multiple sclerosis.

D Dermatomyositis.

E McArdle syndrome.

4. A 14-year-old male adolescent presents to the emergency department with a purpuric rash on his buttocks and legs. Initially, he describes lesions that began as erythematous macules. He also has bloody diarrhoea, and a urine dipstick test reveals proteinuria and haematuria. He had a viral cold 1 week ago. Given the most likely diagnosis, what is the most likely outcome?

A Full recovery.

B Chronic kidney disease.

C Acute kidney failure without full recovery.

D Recurring episodes.

E Steroid treatment followed by full recovery.

5. A 24-year-old man presents to the emergency department with arthralgia and syncope. He has a complete heart block on his electrocardiogram. He returned from a camping trip a few months ago, where he developed round, indurated, erythematous lesions on his legs. What is the most likely cause of his symptoms?

A Lyme disease.

B Tuberculosis.

C Systemic lupus erythematosus.

D Adrenal tumour.

E Granuloma annulare.

6. A 40-year-old man finds it difficult to stand from a squatting position, and develops acne, headaches, truncal obesity and very thin skin with purpura. Investigations show elevated blood glucose level. What is the most likely diagnosis?

A Reiter syndrome.

B Cushing syndrome.

C Hyperthyroidism.

D Diabetes mellitus.

E Granulomatosis with polyangiitis.

7. An elderly man is admitted to the medical assessment unit with shortness of breath and left-sided pleuritic chest pain. A chest X-ray shows a fluid level in the left hemithorax. You notice multiple well-demarcated flat segmental brown

lesions on the skin of his back. They appear stuck on. The patient denies that they cause him any symptoms but admits never having them investigated. What is the most likely diagnosis?

A Basal cell carcinoma.
B Seborrhoeic keratoses.
C Campbell de Morgan spots.
D Malignant melanoma.
E Keratoacanthoma.

8. Which one of the following is most correct about a macule, a term used in dermatology?

A A flat and well-defined area of skin less than 0.5 cm in diameter.
B A raised well-defined area of skin less than 0.5 cm in diameter.
C A localized collection of pus within the epidermis.
D A discoid elevation of the skin.
E A small collection of fluid within the skin less than 0.5 cm in diameter.

9. A male painter presents to his GP complaining of an itchy rash on his hands. This started when he started using paints gifted to him for his birthday. What is the most likely diagnosis?

A Psoriasis.
B Chemical burn.
C Lichen planus.
D Dermatitis.
E Porphyria cutanea tarda.

10. A presentation with pruritus around the elbows and knees associated with malabsorption relieved by a wheat-free diet points towards the diagnosis of which condition?

A Dermatitis herpetiformis.
B Scabies.
C Atypical eczema.
D Psoriasis.
E Polycythaemia rubra vera.

11. A bald patch in a 60-year-old man with tinea infection that he developed following a period of problems at work is most likely to be due to:

A Alopecia areata.
B Sotos syndrome.
C Aplasia cutis.
D T-cell lymphoma.
E Erythema multiforme.

12. A 67-year-old man has skin nodules that a few months ago were diagnosed as mycosis fungoides. He attends your practice because he wants to learn more about the underlying condition. What is he suffering from?

A Erythema multiforme.
B Erythema nodosum.
C Gottron papules.
D Cutaneous T-cell lymphoma.
E Ehlers–Danlos syndrome.

Chapter 37 Haematological disorders

1. A 62-year-old female presents with a few months' history of back and rib pain. A bone scan reveals osteolytic lesions in various parts, including the skull. Blood results show low haemoglobin, deranged kidney function tests, hypercalcaemia and an ESR of 100 mm/h. Liver function tests including alkaline phosphatase are normal. What is the likely diagnosis?

A Paget disease.
B Multiple myeloma.
C Bony metastases.
D Primary hyperparathyroidism.
E Osteogenesis imperfecta.

2. A 20-year-old attends his GP practice with a history of night sweats, fatigue, fever, sore throat and swollen lymph nodes. On examination there is symmetrical lymphadenopathy in the neck and axillae, enlarged red tonsils, palatal petechiae and splenomegaly. Blood counts show normal haemoglobin and white cell count with 57% segmented neutrophils, 19% lymphocytes, 26% atypical lymphocytes and 4% monocytes. What is the likely diagnosis?

A Acute lymphoblastic leukaemia.
B Toxic shock syndrome.
C Herpes simplex virus infection.
D Infectious mononucleosis.
E Streptococcal tonsillitis.

3. Which infection is particularly dangerous to immunosuppressed children with leukaemia?

A Whooping cough.
B Mumps.
C Rubella.
D Streptococcal pharyngitis.
E Chickenpox.

4. A young male presents to his GP as he has been feeling tired and fatigued for the past three months. He also reports easy bruising and night sweats. On examination a cluster of firm, mobile, enlarged lymph nodes is found in his axilla. How should he be investigated?

A Lymph node biopsy.
B Whole body PET scan.

C Lymphangiogram.
D CT of the chest, abdomen and pelvis.
E Lymphangiogram.

5. A 62-year-old female with leukaemia currently treated with chemotherapy presents to the emergency department with vomiting, thirst, abdominal pain and lethargy. Blood tests reveal hyperkalaemia, hyperuricemia, hypocalcaemia and hyperphosphatemia. She is also in metabolic acidosis. What is the most likely diagnosis?
   A Acute kidney injury and renal failure.
   B Tumour lysis syndrome.
   C Steroid-induced diabetic ketoacidosis.
   D Sepsis.
   E Malignant transformation of her leukaemia.

6. A patient with sickle cell anaemia and chronic joint arthritis develops sudden onset pain in both of her hands that she describes as 10 out of 10. Which one of the following would confirm the patient is experiencing a vasoocclusive crisis rather than her usual arthritic pain and will alter the management?
   A Haemoglobin (Hb) level.
   B Reticulocyte count.
   C Hb electrophoresis.
   D Sickle cell solubility.
   E None of the above.

7. Which one of the following best describes the pattern of incidence of acute lymphoblastic leukaemia (ALL)?
   A Peak in the first year of life followed by secondary rise at the age of 10 years and then gradual decline through adulthood.
   B Peak in first 2 to 5 years of life, less common with increasing age but gradual rise after the age of 60 years.
   C Peak in the first 10 years with secondary peak at the age of 50 years.
   D Stable but high incidence in the first 18 years followed by a gradual increase in adulthood.
   E Peak incidence after the age of 50 years.

8. A 20-year-old woman undergoes minor surgery involving incision and drainage of an abscess and bleeds profusely. On her preoperative blood test results, you notice a prolonged activated partial thromboplastin time (APTT) and normal bleeding time and prothrombin time (PT). When you take her history, she mentions that as a child she used to bruise very easily. What is the likely cause of her symptoms?
   A Von Willebrand disease (vWD).
   B Disseminated intravascular coagulation.
   C Haemophilia B.

D Thrombocytopenia.
E Liver disease.

9. A 35-year-old woman with family in Greece is found to have hypochromic microcytic anaemia with target cells. On investigation, her ferritin and iron levels are at the higher end of normal and her HbA_2 level is 5%. What is the most likely diagnosis?
   A β-Thalassaemia.
   B α-Thalassaemia.
   C Sideroblastic anaemia.
   D Iron-deficiency anaemia.
   E Anaemia of chronic disease.

10. A 55-year-old man has been complaining of fatigue and right upper quadrant pain to his GP. After ordering a blood film test, the general practitioner (GP) explains to the patient that there may be a problem with his liver. Which of the following did the GP most likely notice on the blood film results?
    A Pencil cell.
    B Schistocytes.
    C Basophilic stippling.
    D Bite cells.
    E Acanthocytes.

11. Megaloblastic anaemia is most commonly associated with the following conditions:
    A Pregnancy.
    B Alcoholism.
    C A vegan diet on most days of the week.
    D Crohn disease.
    E Following a partial gastrectomy.

12. Iron deficiency anaemia:
    A Causes dementia.
    B Is associated with a low concentration of serum ferritin.
    C Causes a macrocytic anaemia.
    D Will occur in anyone of reproductive age if total iron loss exceeds 2 mg per day.
    E Causes dysphagia.

13. A 5-year-old boy presents to his general practitioner with lethargy, weakness and petechial rash. He is pale but afebrile and on examination shows widespread lymphadenopathy and hepatosplenomegaly. What is the most likely diagnosis?
    A Chronic myeloid leukaemia (CML).
    B Acute lymphoblastic leukaemia (ALL).
    C Acute myeloid leukaemia (AML).
    D Hodgkin lymphoma.
    E Myelodysplastic syndrome.

483

14. A 70-year-old woman is seen in the emergency department with a 6-month history of progressively worsening lethargy. Her FBC shows a raised white blood cell count. Otherwise, she looks well, and the only examination finding is the presence of splenomegaly. What is your concern?
    A Myelodysplastic syndrome.
    B Acute myeloid leukaemia (AML).
    C Hodgkin lymphoma.
    D Chronic myeloid leukaemia (CML).
    E Multiple myeloma.

15. A 15-year-old male with a painless enlarged lymph node in his neck. His medical history includes treatment of Epstein–Barr virus infection last year. There is no other lymphadenopathy. A biopsy is taken. What do you suspect it will show?
    A Hodgkin lymphoma.
    B Non-Hodgkin lymphoma (NHL).
    C Essential monoclonal gammopathy.
    D Acute myeloid leukaemia.
    E Myelodysplastic syndrome.

Chapter 38 Infectious diseases

1. A 65-year-old man has had a knee joint replacement. After 2 weeks, a purulent discharge occurs, which grows methicillin-resistant *Staphylococcus aureus* (MRSA). Which antibiotic therapy is advised?
    A Nafcillin.
    B Vancomycin.
    C Cefuroxime.
    D Gentamicin.
    E Tetracycline.

2. A young woman presents with a 2-day history of a headache and fever but no neck stiffness or focal neurological signs. She has widespread purpura over the trunk and limbs. She is gravely ill. What investigation is most helpful?
    A Lumbar puncture.
    B Blood culture.
    C Full blood count.
    D Fibrin degradation products.
    E Plasma cortisol levels.

3. A 45-year-old man is known to be HIV positive. He was recently found to have mediastinal and retroperitoneal masses on a CT scan. He also complains of weight loss, sweats and fevers. What is the most likely cause of his symptoms?

A T-cell lymphoma.
B Tuberculosis (TB).
C Myeloma.
D Sarcoidosis.
E Metastatic colon cancer.

4. A 23-year-old woman with a known diagnosis of psychosis visits your general practitioner practice to seek antimalarial medication for her trip to Africa. Which medication would you not consider prescribing in this case?
    A Quinine.
    B Mefloquine.
    C Doxycycline.
    D DEET.
    E Chloroquine.

5. A 35-year-old with advanced AIDS is admitted to the hospital with high temperature. Blood cultures are performed, and you receive a call from the microbiology department that they are growing mycobacteria. Which one is the most likely?
    A *Mycobacterium leprae*.
    B *Mycobacterium avium*.
    C *Mycobacterium kansasii*.
    D *Mycobacterium marinum*.
    E *Mycobacterium bovis*.

6. A 30-year-old English journalist who is working in Africa develops fever and rigors. On examination, she has hepatosplenomegaly. Examination of a blood film shows parasitized red blood cells. What is the most likely diagnosis?
    A Amoebiasis.
    B Falciparum malaria.
    C Schistosomiasis.
    D Toxoplasmosis.
    E Cryptosporidiosis.

7. Which of the following regarding rotavirus is correct?
    A Is the commonest cause of infectious diarrhoea in the UK.
    B Is diagnosed by culturing the virus from the stool.
    C Requires antibiotic therapy.
    D Can be prevented by immunization.
    E Is easily passed from person to person.

8. Which of the following viruses does not classically give flu-like symptoms in humans?
    A Coronavirus.
    B Rhinovirus.
    C Norovirus.
    D Influenza virus.
    E Adenovirus.

9. Which of the following people have a high risk of mortality in COVID-19 infection?
   A Pregnant women.
   B Morbid obesity.
   C Immunocompromised.
   D Adults aged >70 years.
   E All of the above.

10. A 21-year-old male working in a supermarket during the COVID-19 pandemic developed a fever, fatigue and body aches similar to the flu. He was suspected of COVID-19 and advised by his GP to self-isolate at home, unless symptoms worsened, such as difficulty in breathing. All of the following statements are true about diagnosing COVID-19, except?
   A Nasal swab, throat swab and saliva can be taken as samples to detect the virus.
   B Samples taken immediately after exposure to the virus may give a false negative result.
   C A blood test is the only primary diagnostic test for detection of the virus.
   D PCR technique is the most accurate way to detect COVID-19.
   E Lateral flow tests are antigen tests.

11. Which of the following statements regarding COVID-19 vaccination are false?
    A A single dose of vaccine is sufficient.
    B The vaccine is authorized for children aged >5 years.
    C Mild to moderate side effects are common.
    D The Pfizer-BioNTECH vaccine is an mRNA vaccine.
    E It is associated with a risk of pericarditis.

12. A 19-year-year-old university student presents to her general practitioner with a short history of shortness of breath, productive cough and tiredness. She has found the symptoms limit her daily living activities when she tries to attend all university events. A chest X-ray reveals a 3-cm cavitating lesion in the upper lobe of her right lung. What is the most likely diagnosis?
    A HIV.
    B *Plasmodium ovale.*
    C *Mycobacterium avium.*
    D *Streptococcus pneumoniae.*
    E TB.

13. A 67-year-old with liver cirrhosis, fever and cough presents to the emergency department. He is tachycardia and tachypnoeic with a chest X-ray showing right-sided patchy consolidation and left-sided pleural effusion. What is the most likely diagnosis?

A *Streptococcus pneumoniae.*
B *Mycobacterium avium.*
C *Giardia lamblia.*
D *Plasmodium falciparum.*
E *Staphylococcus aureus.*

14. A 35-year-old patient presents with fever, weight loss and night sweats. She has recently developed swelling in her abdomen and is now unable to pass stool or flatus. She has a history of intravenous drug use. What are you worried is the underlying condition?
    A A blood malignancy.
    B A bacterial infection.
    C A viral infection.
    D A parasitic infection.
    E A fungal infection.

Chapter 39 Drug overdose and abuse

1. A patient who takes sertraline (a serotonin reuptake inhibitor) for a depressive disorder presents to the emergency department with a severe headache, muscle rigidity, heart rate of 150 and a blood pressure of 200/120. He also has a fever. He tells you that he recently had a bout of back pain and was prescribed a new painkiller. Which drug is the most likely to have caused his symptoms?
   A Gabapentin.
   B Codeine.
   C Paracetamol.
   D Ibuprofen.
   E Tramadol.

2. A teenage girl has had a fight with her friend and swallowed her grandmothers' diazepam tablets. She has a GCS of 10, a heart rate of 60 and blood pressure of 100/60. What is the most appropriate therapy?
   A Intravenous flumazenil.
   B Supportive treatment only.
   C Activated charcoal.
   D Gastric lavage.
   E Intubate and admit to intensive care.

3. You are the medical FY1 on-call covering the wards. You are called to see a 42-year-old patient admitted 3 days ago with vomiting and dehydration who has now become confused, agitated and appears to be hallucinating. On your arrival the nurses tell you he has been unsteady on his feet. He has a history of alcohol abuse. While you assess him he suffers a seizure. What is the most likely diagnosis?
   A Delirium tremens.
   B Acute alcohol intoxication

C Alcohol withdrawal seizure.
D Wernicke encephalopathy.
E Korsakoff syndrome.

4. A 55-year-old man presents sweaty, tachycardic and tachypnoeic. He is drowsy and complaining of tinnitus. An arterial blood gas test is done and shows a metabolic acidosis with hypokalaemia. Overdose of which one of the following drugs is most likely?
   A Aspirin.
   B Tricyclic antidepressant.
   C Benzodiazepine.
   D Opiates.
   E Digoxin.

5. A 45-year-old woman known to have alcoholism is admitted to the hospital with haematemesis and is waiting for a nonurgent endoscopy. Which of the following scores can help you assess her risk of alcohol withdrawal and guide you to the amount of benzodiazepine she will require?
   A CAGE.
   B Alcohol Use Disorders Identification Test – Consumption (AUDIT-C).
   C Clinical Institute Withdrawal Assessment for Alcohol (CIWA).
   D National Early Warning Score (NEWS).
   E Mini-Mental State Examination (MMSE).

6. A 60-year-old woman with heart failure and depression is brought to the emergency department. Her husband found her with empty blister packets around her. She is drowsy, hypotensive and tachycardic. Her pupils are dilated. She complains of a dry mouth. Her electrocardiogram demonstrates a prolonged QT interval, with a widened QRS duration of 0.6 s (reference range 0.35–0.44 s) and her venous blood gas demonstrates a metabolic acidosis, pH 7.1. A test for paracetamol is negative. Which of the following should be given to treat her overdose?
   A Oxygen, intravenous (IV) fluids and naloxone infusion.
   B Oxygen, IV fluids and flumazenil.
   C Oxygen, IV fluids and N-acetylcysteine.
   D Oxygen, IV fluids, electrolyte imbalance correction and IV sodium bicarbonate.
   E Oxygen, IV fluids, electrolyte imbalance correction and Digibind (a digoxin antidote containing digoxin-specific antibody Fab fragments).

7. A 35-year-old woman has taken an unknown mixed overdose, staggered over the last 8 hours. Which of the following is the best management plan?
   A Gastric lavage, administer activated charcoal, attach the patient to a cardiac monitor and send blood samples to the biochemistry laboratory for measurement of paracetamol and salicylate levels.
   B Administer activated charcoal, attach the patient to a cardiac monitor, send blood samples for measurement of paracetamol and salicylate levels and start N-acetylcysteine infusion, before the paracetamol level is known.
   C Attach the patient to a cardiac monitor, send blood samples for measurement of paracetamol and salicylate levels and start N-acetylcysteine infusion, before the paracetamol level is known.
   D Attach the patient to a cardiac monitor, send blood samples for measurement of paracetamol and salicylate levels and start N-acetylcysteine infusion and urinary alkalinization, before the paracetamol and salicylate levels are known.
   E Attach the patient to a cardiac monitor, send blood samples for measurement of paracetamol and salicylate levels and observe the patient.

8. A 50-year-old nonsmoker is admitted unconscious after being found in his house. He is tachycardic, has ECG changes visible on the A&E monitor and his breathing is alternating between slow and fast. His blood gas shows hypoxia, acidosis and an elevated carboxyhaemoglobin (COHb) level. The doctors are unable to wake him up and he is intubated to protect his airway and transferred to the intensive care unit. During transfer he suffers a cardiac arrest but is successfully resuscitated with a return of spontaneous circulation. What is the most appropriate treatment?
   A Treat with hyperbaric oxygen therapy as it is available in your hospital and his COHb level is significantly elevated.
   B Supportive management with 100% oxygen, vasopressors and IV fluids.
   C Start haemofiltration and 100% oxygen.
   D 100% oxygen, organ supportive measures and discussion with TOXBASE about the next steps.
   E If he is stable, try and wake him up to assess his neurology.

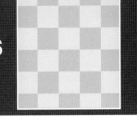

Chapter 28 Cardiovascular system

1. A. Mitral regurgitation is commonly loudest at the apex and radiates to the axilla. There is no presystolic accentuation in the context of AF due to the absence of atrial contraction. Left-sided heart murmurs are best heard in expiration, right-sided in inspiration (due to decreased venous return). Aortic regurgitation is best heard at the left sternal edge in expiration with the patient sitting up. An opening snap is a feature of mitral stenosis.

2. E. Although aortic stenosis can cause a narrow pulse pressure, the absolute value is unhelpful in assessing the degree of stenosis. The murmur may help in the initial diagnosis, neither its severity or radiation is an indicator of clinical significance (as a matter of fact in critical aortic stenosis there may be no murmur due to the severe impairment of flow). Left ventricular hypertrophy on ECG indicates functionally important aortic stenosis.

3. B. All acute coronary syndrome (ACS) patients should be on secondary prevention for atherosclerotic disease. The evidence shows an ACE inhibitor (e.g., ramipril), a β-blocker (e.g., atenolol), a statin (e.g., simvastatin) and aspirin all individually reduce mortality. Although fibrates are effective in reducing both LDL cholesterol and triglycerides, there is insufficient mortality data for these agents. An angiotensin receptor blocker (e.g., losartan) is only indicated if the patient does not tolerate an ACE inhibitor. Warfarin is not indicated in isolated ACS.

4. C. Digoxin is indicated in sinus rhythm as it improves symptoms (RADIANCE trial). The New York Heart Association classification is used to classify the degree of failure based on symptoms. Diuretics improve symptoms, but have no mortality benefit, whereas ACE inhibitors improve both morbidity and mortality. Left ventricular failure predisposes to arrhythmias, especially if the ventricle is dilated.

5. C. Although rheumatic fever may indeed result in atrial fibrillation, in the UK ischaemic heart disease and hypertension are far more common causes of AF. Atrial contraction contributes 10% to 30% of ventricular filling and AF may, therefore, cause heart failure on the background of existing heart disease. Anticoagulation should be instigated unless contraindications exist. The ECG changes associated with AF are absent P waves and irregular, narrow QRS complexes. Pulmonary embolism is a cause of AF.

6. E. The delta wave described in this clinical scenario is pathognomonic for Wolff–Parkinson–White syndrome (WPW). WPW is a form of atrioventricular reentry tachycardia since the reentry circuit is not through the AV node. The rate described is unlikely to be atrial flutter as this tends to be multiples of 75 depending on the degree of block. Ventricular fibrillation is not compatible with an awake talking patient with a cardiac output.

7. A. It is measured from the sternal angle (the angle of Louis – the angle formed between the manubrium and sternum).
    Answers B–E are all true.

8. A. This lady has suffered an NSTEMI. She will be at high risk of subsequent MI and death (GRACE score) in light of her age, comorbidities and troponin elevation. Cardiac catheterization is thus indicated as an inpatient. This investigation will be able to show the culprit lesion, but also allows for revascularization at the same time. Investigations that stress the myocardium (e.g., ETT or radionuclide perfusion scanning) in patients that have been admitted with myocardial ischaemia are contraindicated. Echocardiography may show the extent of the damage by the ischaemic event but offers no treatment potential. 24-hour ECG monitoring has no role in this scenario.

9. E. Essential hypertension is the same as primary hypertension. This idiopathic condition is responsible for 95% of cases of hypertension. Conn syndrome (hyperaldosteronism), phaeochromocytoma (catecholamine-producing tumour), coarctation of the aorta and renal artery stenosis are all causes of secondary hypertension.

10. B. A slow-rising pulse is a feature of aortic stenosis. The character of the pulse should be assessed centrally (e.g., carotid – ensure to check one side at a time!). Pulsus alternans is the physical finding of a variable pulse waveform of strong and weak beats – a feature of ventricular impairment. Venous return is decreased during inspiration which causes reduced vagal tone and results in an increased heart rate.

11. B. This patient has Noonan syndrome. The most common congenital heart defect associated with this condition is pulmonary stenosis. The murmur described is that of pulmonary stenosis.

12. D. This patient is presenting with signs and symptoms of chronic heart failure. An echocardiogram will allow confirmation of the diagnosis and assessment of cardiac function. A CXR would show cardiomegaly and evidence of pulmonary oedema but it is not diagnostic for heart failure. This is also true for BNP measurement. There is no evidence of PE.

13. A. This patient has a broad-complex tachycardia with haemodynamic instability. In situations like this, the rhythm is ventricular tachycardia until proven otherwise. DC cardioversion is the most appropriate treatment here.

14. C. Cardioselective β-blockers are of prognostic benefit in such patients. Furosemide is also of benefit but it is not specific for patients with heart failure due to left ventricular dysfunction. Amlodipine can be used in heart failure if the patient is hypertensive but otherwise it is not used. Nitrates and digoxin can be used for symptom management.

15. C. This is the initial treatment in narrow complex tachycardia if no adverse features are present (see RESUS Tachycardia algorithm).

16. B. Adenosine is the next step after vagal manoeuvres as per the RESUS guidelines.

17. B. As per most recent NICE guidelines.

18. C. The key here is confusion – young patients have high physiological reserves and can compensate very well until significant blood loss has occurred. The fact that this patient is confused indicates that cerebral perfusion is compromised and therefore compensatory mechanisms have begun to fail.

19. C. Although all of the above can occur, AVSD is the commonest.

20. A. Thiazide diuretics cause hypokalaemia. So does furosemide which can be used to treat hyperkalaemia. Calcium channel blockers cause ankle swelling and not ACE inhibitors.

21. E. The ECG changes here indicate anteroseptal ischaemia and it is the most likely diagnosis.

22. A. This patient presents with an acute STEMI. The most appropriate treatment would be immediate PCI. If this cannot be delivered within an appropriate time window he should be offered fibrinolysis. Dual antiplatelets, oxygen and analgesia are an immediate management option in STEMI; however, the question asks about the most appropriate treatment.

23. B. This is a classical presentation of stable angina. This should initially be managed with GTN. If the short-acting spray is not sufficient, long-acting preparations can be tried.

24. D. This is the murmur of tricuspid regurgitation. The travel is significant as this condition can be caused by schistosomiasis or other parasite that he was infected with on his travels. Graham Steell murmur is typically associated with pulmonary regurgitation. It is heard due to a high-velocity flow back across the pulmonary valve. Mitral murmurs are best heard at the apex.

25. D. This patient has heart failure and is in atrial fibrillation. Unless contraindicated, rhythm control should be the first treatment strategy for his AF. We do not know how long she has been in AF and therefore, immediate cardioversion would risk thromboembolic events. Digoxin is the best answer.

Chapter 29 Respiratory system

1. A. A tension pneumothorax is a medical emergency that requires immediate decompression (large-bore cannula in the second intercostal space, midclavicular line). It is a clinical diagnosis based on the presence of all or some of the following features on examination; the trachea is deviated away from the affected side; breath sounds are absent or diminished and the percussion note will be hyper-resonant. When the tension pneumothorax becomes sufficiently large to compromise cardiovascular function, venous return to the heart will be impaired, resulting in a raised jugular venous pressure.

2. D. Tachycardia is the most common finding in PE and sinus tachycardia the most common ECG abnormality. Although the $S_1Q_3T_3$ pattern is often mentioned in textbooks, it is uncommon. A CXR is commonly normal. An ABG is often normal but can show hypoxia. An ECHO may show right ventricular dysfunction, especially in significant PEs.

3. D. NICE guidelines recommend 3 months of anticoagulation in a provoked PE (in this case by immobilization post surgery). Apixaban or rivaroxaban is recommended first line with low-molecular-weight heparin (LMWH), dabigatran, edoxaban or vitamin K antagonists (warfarin) as alternatives. C would be correct in an unprovoked PE and E would be correct if the patient was haemodynamically unstable.

4. C. In severe asthma, intravenous magnesium is used alongside nebulizers (salbutamol and ipratropium) and steroids. Peak flow is a helpful tool, especially when compared with the patient's normal performance, in predicting severity. Peak flow values of <33% of normal indicate a life-threatening asthma attack. A normal P_{CO_2} level on an ABG suggests the patient is getting tired (it should be low because of hyperventilation) and is not reassuring. Death is not uncommon. There is no evidence to support the use of intravenous bronchodilators over nebulized equivalents.

5. E. According to BTS/SIGN 2019 guidelines, the patient is currently on step 1 with a regular corticosteroid inhaler (ICS) and as required short-acting β_2-agonist. The next step would be to add a long-acting β_2-agonist. If control was not achieved the subsequent step would be to increase the ICS or consider addition of a leucotriene receptor antagonist. If this then failed referral to specialist care where additional treatments (such as the addition of long-acting anticholinergic inhalers or theophylline) could be considered.

6. B. The CURB65 score is used to assess the severity of community-acquired pneumonia. Confusion, defined as an abbreviated mini-mental test score of less than 8, scores 1 point. A serum urea level of more than 7 mmol/L scores 1 point. A systolic blood pressure of *less than* 90 mmHg scores 1 point. A respiratory rate of more than 30 per minute scores 1 point. Age greater than 65 years scores 1 point. A score of 0 or 1 corresponds to mild pneumonia, a score of 2 corresponds to moderate pneumonia and a score of 3–5 corresponds to severe pneumonia. Typically, mild pneumonia is treated in the community, moderate pneumonia is potentially treated in the hospital and severe pneumonia is definitely treated in the hospital, with intravenous antibiotics.

7. B. Squamous cell carcinoma may produce parathyroid-related peptide, causing hypercalcaemia. Syndrome of inappropriate antidiuretic hormone secretion, Eaton–Lambert myasthenic syndrome, Cushing syndrome and peripheral neuropathy are all paraneoplastic syndromes which may be associated with small-cell lung cancer.

8. A. Amiodarone may cause lower-zone pulmonary fibrosis, particularly in the context of preexisting lung disease. Other causes of lower-zone fibrosis include rheumatoid arthritis, asbestosis, idiopathic causes and drugs such as bleomycin and nitrofurantoin.

9. E. There are four stages of CXR changes associated with pulmonary sarcoidosis. Answer B is stage 1, answer C is stage 2, answer E is stage 3 and answer D is stage 4. Pleural effusions are not a feature in this classification.

10. C. The scenario described above is one of a life-threatening asthma attack. The most important features here are the considerable length of the attack and the apparent lack of effective ventilation. In the acute setting, the CO_2 level would be low, with an associated respiratory alkalosis (answers D and E) due to hyperventilation. Once the patient gets tired, as indicated in the scenario by barely audible breath sounds, P_{CO_2} will be in the normal range (*this is a bad sign*) and the pH will subsequently normalize.

11. E. Although F_{IO_2} is highly dependent on respiratory rate and oxygen flow rate through the delivery system, it is useful to have a rough idea of the concentrations of oxygen given. Inspired room air has a F_{IO_2} of 21%, whereas a non-rebreather mask at 15 L/min is as close to F_{IO_2} of 100% as possible. Venturi masks have special valves that closely regulate F_{IO_2} and are commonly available at concentrations of 28%, 35%, 40% and 60%. A simple facemask delivering oxygen at 5 L/min delivers F_{IO_2} of roughly 50%.

12. E. The history points to a diagnosis of mesothelioma. The condition is usually caused by asbestos exposure and may therefore result in compensation for the patient and/or family. It is a tumour of the pleura rather than the lung parenchyma. Pleural plaques are benign and develop >20 years after asbestos exposure. Associated pulmonary asbestosis is found in only approximately 15% of cases. The prognosis is poor.

13. E. TB is an infectious disease caused by the bacterium *Mycobacterium tuberculosis*. Although the disease can involve various organs, pulmonary TB is the most common presentation. The drug regimen for pulmonary TB includes a combination therapy of four drugs: rifampicin, isoniazid, pyrazinamide and ethambutol. All four are taken for the first 2 months. After that only rifampicin and isoniazid are taken. Streptomycin is no longer recommended as first-line therapy for the treatment of pulmonary TB.

14. C. This patient is acutely unwell. His respiratory effort is inadequate, and he is at risk of suffering a respiratory arrest if not treated. Urgent management is required and senior help should be sought urgently. The patient is achieving saturations of only 88% despite 15 L oxygen and although he is at risk of carbon dioxide retention, hypoxia is more likely to kill him first. Therefore reducing his F_{IO_2} by changing to a venturi mask is incorrect at this stage. The patient is septic with a high temperature, and Sepsis Six management should be commenced. Although the help of the ICU may be indicated, lower-level interventions should be tried first before intubation. Although answer E illustrates an appropriate logical approach to management, senior help should be sought early and IV magnesium is used in an asthma exacerbation rather than COPD.

15. D. An ABG is extremely important in this case, as the results will tell you whether the patient is in respiratory failure, and if so, whether he is retaining carbon dioxide. This will help guide your treatment and in addition it will give you other useful information, such as sodium, potassium, lactate and haemoglobin levels. CXR and blood tests will also help establish the diagnosis. Raised levels of inflammatory markers will suggest an infective cause. A CXR may demonstrate consolidation, indicating an infective cause, or pulmonary oedema which will point towards a cardiac cause of shortness of breath.

Whilst a urine dip can be done simply at the bedside and should be considered in the septic screen, it is less likely to indicate the underlying diagnosis in this scenario. Although a PE could be amongst the differential diagnosis, other tests and initial management would be considered in the first instance in this scenario.

16. A. CTPA is the most sensitive noninvasive test available for the diagnosis of PE. It is a scan that requires intravenous administration of contrast, which is known to be nephrotoxic. In a previously healthy individual, with normal kidney function test results, the effect of contrast medium is usually of no clinical significance; however, in patients with preexisting renal impairment, contrast medium can lead to contrast nephropathy and worsening of kidney function. A D-dimer may be useful in a low two-level Wells score (<4); however in this scenario, the Wells score is >4 (immobilization 1.5 points, alternative diagnosis less likely 3 points). Peak flow and liver function tests are not indicated prior to a CTPA. A V/Q (ventilation/perfusion) scan may be used if a CTPA is contraindicated (e.g., contrast allergy).

17. D. Although *Streptococcus pneumonia* is the most common pathogen causing community-acquired pneumonia, in this case the history suggests that the patient may have an atypical pneumonia (travel, immunosuppression from T1DM). *Legionella pneumophila* is a bacterium that causes Legionnaires disease. The organism's natural habitat is water and human spread has been linked to contaminated water reservoirs such as air conditioning systems. Infection causes nonspecific symptoms as in the scenario.

18. D. A pleural effusion is an accumulation of fluid within the pleural space, it may be asymptomatic when it is small. The fluid causes a stony dull percussion note and reduced breath sounds/air entry on the side of the effusion. Expansion may also be reduced.

19. B. The triangle of safety for a chest drain insertion is formed anteriorly by the lateral border of the pectoralis major, inferiorly by the fifth intercostal space and laterally by the anterior border of the latissimus dorsi (midaxillary line). Chest drains are inserted under ultrasound guidance using the Seldinger technique. Answer A refers to the position used in emergency decompression of a tension pneumothorax.

20. B. Given the prolonged history of a cough with sputum production and the coarse crepitations on examination the most likely cause of the haemoptysis in this scenario is bronchiectasis. Bronchiectasis can produce bleeding from dilated blood vessels in the walls of inflamed dilated bronchi. In this scenario, a PE would not explain the duration of her history and lack of night sweats and weight loss point away from TB or malignancy. Heart failure with pulmonary oedema may cause pink frothy sputum rather than frank haemoptysis.

21. D. The key points in this scenario are recurrent epistaxis and a family history of haemoptysis. Hereditary haemorrhagic telangiectasia is dominantly inherited and associated with arteriovenous malformations in the mucosa of the mouth, nose, gastrointestinal tract, lungs and brain. The shortness of breath may be due to anaemia (secondary to epistaxis) or possibly pulmonary malformations. On examination you may find telangiectasia on the skin or in the mouth.

22. E. Following initial management with a SABA (salbutamol) or SAMA (ipratropium) inhaler, if the patient remains symptomatic or has frequent exacerbations then treatment should be up-titrated. The next step would be either to add LABA (salmeterol) + LAMA (tiotropium) inhaler or if features of asthma/steroid responsiveness then a LABA + Inhaled corticosteroid (ICS – fluticasone).
Answer D would be the next step following answer E if treatment needed further up-titrating.

23. D. The raised CO_2 indicates respiratory acidosis, but the pH is normal with a raised bicarbonate. This indicates that this is a chronic picture with metabolic compensation. The patient is also hypoxic. Oxygen delivery should be controlled, where able through a venturi mask, with target oxygen saturations of 88% to 92% to avoid precipitating type II respiratory failure.

24. D. Interstitial lung disease presents with progressively worsening shortness of breath. This patient has a history of working with birds which would predispose him to developing hypersensitivity pneumonitis (bird fancier's lung) linked to exposure to avian proteins.

25. C. Given the age and lack of underlying lung disease or smoking history, this would classify as a primary pneumothorax. Given the size is >2 cm and the patient is breathless, both of these factors would indicate pleural aspiration. In this case if the pneumothorax was <2 cm and the patient was not breathless, B could be considered. A chest drain is indicated in a >2 cm symptomatic secondary pneumothorax if no improvement after pleural aspiration in a primary pneumothorax, or small secondary pneumothorax.

26. B. Typical CXR changes in a COVID-19 pneumonitis are bilateral, peripheral, patchy ground glass changes. In the early stages of COVID-19 the CXR may be normal. D represents changes consistent with interstitial lung disease and E would be seen in COPD.

Chapter 30 Gastrointestinal and hepatobiliary systems

1. C. Barrett oesophagus is usually asymptomatic. Less than 1% of cases progress to adenocarcinoma per year. It is characterized by metaplasia from squamous to columnar epithelium in the distal part of the oesophagus. The underlying cause is GORD, which is typically managed medically with lifestyle changes and proton pump inhibitors.

2. B. Pancreatitis is an inflammatory condition of the pancreas most commonly caused by alcohol or gallstones. The history of intermittent RUQ pain is suggestive of biliary colic in a woman in her 40s. The likelihood is thus that this is gallstone pancreatitis. Severity can be assessed with the modified Glasgow or APACHE-II scoring systems. The Rockall score is used to predict mortality in gastrointestinal bleeding. Pseudocyst formation is not an early complication – it tends to occur after 2 to 6 weeks. Although a serum amylase level of 1400 U/mL is high, occasionally a perforated viscus may present in a similar manner with serum amylase concentrations higher than 1000 U/mL.

3. E. A large upper GI tract bleed is a medical emergency and should be initially managed according to advanced life support principles of airway, breathing and circulation. Fluid resuscitation is a priority. Blood results may show a raised urea level (secondary to red cell ingestion) and may initially show a normal haemoglobin concentration as there has been no chance for haemodilution in the very acute setting. The investigation of choice is an oesophagogastroduodenoscopy. Rebleeding carries immediate mortality of 40%.

4. B. Transmural inflammation, perianal lesions and skip lesions are all features of Crohn disease. Ulcerative colitis is less common in smokers, the converse of which is true for Crohn disease. Pseudopolyps are associated with ulcerative colitis.

5. D. The symptoms described here are suggestive of a left-sided tumour. The more distal the disease, the more likely it is to cause a change in bowel habit. Tenesmus is suggestive of rectal disease. Right-sided tumours typically present late and may present as iron-deficiency anaemia. More than 90% of tumours can be resected surgically.

6. D. Pseudomembranous colitis is a serious infection, commonly hospital-acquired. It is caused by the toxins produced by *C. difficile*. As is the case for all forms of colitis, toxic dilatation of the colon is a complication. Diagnosis of *C. difficile* infection is made by toxin-positive stool culture; pseudomembranous colitis is diagnosed endoscopically. Prevention is predominantly through hand washing using soap and water (to eliminate the bacterial spores) and careful use of antibiotics. Initial treatment is with orally administered metronidazole or orally administered vancomycin.

7. D. IBS is a diagnosis of exclusion that can be made only once organic causes have been excluded (such as coeliac disease, inflammatory bowel disease). The condition is more common in females between the ages of 20 and 40 years. Symptoms include central or lower abdominal pain, commonly relieved by defaecation, abdominal bloating and altered bowel habit. Rectal bleeding is not a feature. Treatment may require input from dieticians, surgeons, psychiatrists or gynaecologists, and is not always successful.

8. B. Gallstones are commonly asymptomatic. Their incidence increases with age, parity, raised BMI and they are more common in females. Occasionally, a large gallstone can erode through the gallbladder into the adjacent duodenum, causing a gallstone ileus. A minority of gallstones are radio-opaque owing to their composition: they commonly contain cholesterol and/or bile salts. Charcot triad (RUQ pain, jaundice and rigors) is suggestive of cholangitis.

9. C. Hepatitis A may relapse but does not cause chronic hepatitis. Hepatitis B transmission is parenteral, and infection may be complicated by hepatocellular carcinoma. Hepatitis C is usually asymptomatic in the acute phase. Hepatitis E is transmitted via the faecal–oral route.

10. D. Intussusception affects children more commonly than adults. In 20% of cases there may be redcurrant jelly stool, although this is a late sign. Melaena is stool containing metabolized blood (indicating an upper gastrointestinal tract bleed). Fatty stool (or steatorrhoea) or putty-coloured stool is a feature of obstructive jaundice or chronic pancreatitis. Watery stool is common in gastroenteritis.

11. A. Although portal hypertension and hypoalbuminaemia have some effect on fluid retention, renal sodium handling has the greatest effect. It is thought that aldosterone plays an important role in the mechanism, and it may be that renal sensitivity to aldosterone is enhanced in liver cirrhosis. There is no suggestion of inferior vena cava or lymphatic obstruction in this clinical scenario.

12. C. Cases of acute pancreatitis should be referred to the surgical team. Initial management is rapid fluid replacement; provided there are no contraindications, the patient should receive at least 3 L in the first 12 hours, and electrolyte replacement, analgesia and antiemetics if indicated. Chronic pancreatitis is referred to the medical team unless a surgical cause is identified.

13. D. HBV infection is present when the test for HBsAg is positive. Chronic infection is diagnosed if this persists for more than 6 months. Anti-HBc is present if the patient has immunity against the pathogen, due to previous infection. HCV infection is present if the test for HCV antibody is positive.

	Anti-HBc	HBsAg	Anti-HBs	HBV core antibody IgM
Acute infection	−	+	−	+
Chronic infection	+	+	−	−
Active immunization	−	−	+	−
Passive immunization	+	−	+	−

14. D. This patient has ascites on a background of alcoholic liver disease. The exact mechanism of why patients develop ascites is not fully understood; however, sodium and water balance are thought to play a role. Spironolactone is an aldosterone antagonist that, among other functions, promotes diuresis and hyponatraemia. Spironolactone was found to work better in reducing ascites than other types of diuretics, for instance, furosemide (a loop diuretic). It is important to remember that spironolactone can also cause hyperkalaemia, and as such, monitoring is important. Antibiotics are indicated if the patient is suspected of having spontaneous bacterial peritonitis, which can be a complication in patients with cirrhosis.
    β-Blockers, unless contraindicated, are given to patients with portal hypertension.

15. D. You would expect a positive result for ketones on a urine dip in diabetic ketoacidosis. Abdominal aortic aneurysm can present as abdominal pain or back pain. Although the patient presents with signs and symptoms suggestive of an inflammatory process, any blood passed rectally should be investigated for a possibility of cancer.

16. B. Diarrhoea would cause loss of bicarbonate with the stool and a high level of chloride in the blood and therefore lead to normal anion gap metabolic acidosis. Raised anion gap metabolic acidosis can occur because of excess acids in the body (e.g., diabetic ketoacidosis, lactic acidosis, salicylate toxicity). Metabolic acidosis with respiratory compensation is a possibility; however, the respiratory rate is then likely to be raised as the patient is breathing fast to try to blow off carbon dioxide.

17. C. Rectal bleeding is a red flag symptom that, should an obvious cause such as haemorrhoids be excluded on examination, would cause you to run further tests such as an urgent colonoscopy. Change in bowel habit is also considered to be a red flag symptom, but only in patients over the age of 50. Abdominal pain relieved by defaecation, abdominal distension (bloating) and passage

of mucous are all symptoms of IBS so would not be a cause for concern themselves.

Other red flags for GI cancer include:
A. Unexplained weight loss.
B. Anaemia.
C. Melaena (blood in faeces).
D. Rectal or abdominal mass.
E. Family history of GI cancer.

18. C. Blood tests for coeliac antibodies (IgA-tTG ± IgA-EMA) are done to give an indication of whether a biopsy is needed. However, negative serology does not necessarily rule out coeliac disease. It is the duodenal biopsies that are the gold standard investigation for diagnosis. Four biopsies are taken from the duodenum via endoscopy. The histology of the biopsies is investigated, looking for villous atrophy, crypt hyperplasia and intraepithelial lymphocytosis (proliferation and invasion of lymphocytes). The 'Marsh Scale' is used to grade the histological findings from I to IV with most coeliacs falling into the III category.
    Answers A, B and E are incorrect as it is the duodenal mucosa that is affected the most in coeliac disease and therefore exhibits the classical histological signs. Answer D is incorrect as a biopsy must be done for a definitive diagnosis to be made.

19. D. C-reactive protein (CRP) is a nonspecific marker of inflammation. A high CRP would raise the suspicion of acute diverticulitis but not diagnose it. Colonoscopy is an invasive test and is contraindicated in the acute setting due to the risk of causing perforation and bleeding. It should only be performed once symptoms have settled. An abdominal X-ray can be used to identify complications of acute diverticulitis such as perforation (looking for free air); however, again this is nonspecific. Contrast CT colonography is the gold standard investigation for acute diverticulitis – colonic wall thickening and diverticula will be seen. A barium enema can clarify the diagnosis in patients with abdominal pain and altered bowel habit but it is not the gold standard.

20. E. The most common cause of oesophageal varices in the United Kingdom is portal hypertension secondary to liver cirrhosis. This is a complication of chronic liver disease, which may be due to hepatitis infection, alcoholic liver disease, fatty liver disease or primary biliary cirrhosis. A to D are all also causes of oesophageal varices but are less common. Right heart failure is a posthepatic cause of oesophageal varices. Thrombosis in either the hepatic portal vein or the splenic vein is a prehepatic cause of varices. Obstruction of the hepatic vein is called Budd–Chiari syndrome and is a posthepatic cause of varices. Obstruction can be due to thrombosis or a tumour.

Schistosomiasis is a parasitic infection found in parts of Africa, South America, the Caribbean, the Middle East and East Asia. The parasite can damage the liver, as well as the lungs, intestine, bladder and other organs. It is the commonest cause of oesophageal varices worldwide but is rare in the United Kingdom.

21. A. The most likely diagnosis in this setting is gallstones leading to conjugated hyperbilirubinaemia. Carcinoma of the head of the pancreas would present with a more insidious cause, with a history of unintentional weight loss, and abdominal pain which radiates to the back. ALP and bilirubin are much less likely to be significantly raised in viral and autoimmune hepatitis. Both may present with constitutional symptoms such as anorexia, nausea and vomiting, malaise, fever, joint pains. C is incorrect as the history tells us that the patient does not consume alcohol.

22. C. A history of epigastric pain following meals might suggest peptic ulcer disease, in which case *H. pylori* breath test would be an appropriate answer. However, weight loss is a red flag sign of malignancy, warranting urgent investigation with OGD endoscopy. FBC and abdominal X-ray will provide us with little diagnostic information, though FBC is important to investigate for iron deficiency anaemia, and abdominal X-ray would be important if the presentation was suggestive of perforation. A trial of PPI would be beneficial if GORD was suspected.

23. B. Key to diagnosis is the history of retching and vomiting, with the initial vomitus clear of blood. Ruptured peptic ulcer and Boerhaave syndrome would both likely present with sudden onset abdominal pain and profound hypotension. Boerhaave syndrome is a complication of Mallory–Weiss tear, where there is a complete rupture of the oesophagus, leading to pneumomediastinum on erect CXR due to air entering the mediastinum. Subcutaneous emphysema in the neck is a classic finding. Oesophagitis would unlikely present with bleeding.

24. C. The features of fever/rigors, right upper quadrant pain and jaundice are cumulatively known as Charcot triad, and when present make cholangitis the most likely diagnosis. Leucocytosis with neutrophil predominance is a common finding. Viral hepatitis would more likely present with constitutional symptoms, e.g., fatigue, loss of appetite and/or muscle/joint pain, in addition to fever, abdominal pain and jaundice. Jaundice is not normally a feature of acute cholecystitis. Pancreatic cancer classically presents with abdominal pain that radiates to the back, and would not feature a tender, enlarged liver. There are no cues in the history to suggest drug-induced hepatitis.

25. A. This is a common place to put a transplanted kidney. His Cushing syndrome can be explained by steroid

therapy to prevent organ rejection. Locations of all the other options are not elsewhere on the abdomen.

26. E. In patients with alcoholism a common cause of hospitalization is acute pancreatitis – with repeated attacks and continued alcohol abuse the pancreas does not secrete sufficient enzymes, and malabsorption ensues.

27. D. This is Plummer–Vinson syndrome which is a narrowing in the upper oesophagus associated with iron-deficiency anaemia, glossitis and angular stomatitis. Gastroscopy would show the narrowing but it would not lead to the discovery of iron-deficiency anaemia which is ultimately the cause for her symptoms. The other investigations would not be helpful.

28. C. PBC is associated with autoimmune conditions such as Addison disease, Raynaud syndrome, thyroid disease and systemic sclerosis. The lack of pain and lack of evidence of obstruction on ultrasonography make other conditions less likely.

29. E. Steatorrhea occurs as a result of fat malabsorption. Hyposplenism is a known occurrence in patients with coeliac disease. In a young person antitissue transglutaminase, antibodies should be measured to further investigate this malabsorption.

30. A. Acute-onset bloody diarrhoea in a previously fit person is most likely due to infective colitis. Inflammatory bowel disease is also a possibility; however, infective colitis is the most likely diagnosis in this case.

Chapter 31   Renal, genitourinary and sexual health

1. D. Pulmonary oedema, severe acidosis, resistant hyperkalaemia and symptomatic uraemia (i.e., uraemic pericarditis) are all indications for emergency haemodialysis/haemofiltration in the context of an AKI. In this case the patient has an AKI from hypovolaemia and is at risk due to having a background of hypertension. His AKI is very likely to have been made worse by his continuing use of an angiotensin-converting enzyme inhibitor during the time of hypovolaemia and hypotension. In terms of needing to start dialysis, there is no cut-off value for creatinine, urea or bicarbonate level that would necessitate starting emergency dialysis. Hyperkalaemia resistant to medical treatment (this is the key) is an urgent indication for starting dialysis.

2. A. The first ECG feature of raised potassium level is tented T waves. At higher potassium levels the following changes occur: small or absent P waves, prolonged PR interval (progressive paralysis of atria) broadened QRS complex, atrioventricular block giving bradycardia and eventually sinusoidal waveform (this is commonly followed by ventricular fibrillation and needs *immediate* management

and escalation to seniors.). U waves are seen on an ECG in association with hypokalaemia, hypocalcaemia and hypomagnesia. This man's potassium level is 6.4 mmol/L, so the most usual features would be peaked T waves. It is important to take account of his normal potassium readings. If the patient generally has a low potassium level, then 6.4 mmol/L may result in more myocardial dysfunction and pose a greater risk to the patient.

3. A. The triad of nephrotic syndrome is hypoalbuminaemia (<30 g/L), nephrotic range proteinuria (PCR >300 mg/mmol or 24-hour protein loss of >3 g) and peripheral oedema. It is associated with increased risk of infections (from immunoglobulin loss), increased risk of thrombosis (from loss of protein C and protein S) and high cholesterol levels but this does not make up the triad.

4. D. The most common cause of nephrotic syndrome in children is minimal change disease with 80% of children in the United Kingdom who present with nephrotic syndrome having minimal change disease. It is generally very steroid responsive.

5. E. AKI, active urinary sediment and haemoptysis suggest a pulmonary–renal disease. This includes ANCA-associated vasculitis and antiglomerular basement membrane disease (Goodpasture disease). Important serological tests to help support diagnosis would be an ANCA titre and anti-GBM. In these conditions, CRP level is likely to be raised but would not help narrow down the diagnosis. Antistreptolysin O titre greater than 200 IU suggests recent streptococcal infection; complement levels are generally normal in ANCA-associated vasculitis. Complements and antinuclear antibodies should be tested, and this presentation could be compatible with a lupus nephritis, however this is less likely than ANCA associated vasculitis so would not be the single most important blood test.

6. C. Small scarred kidneys on ultrasound scan best support the likelihood that this is CKD. With any blood test measuring creatinine level, an eGFR will be estimated. However, to define CKD it requires the presence of a low eGFR measured on at least two separate occasions, 3 months apart. Anaemia is common in CKD but can occur in many other disease processes. Hydronephrosis and prostatic hypertrophy would be more in keeping with an AKI. A monoclonal paraprotein on electrophoresis is suggestive of myeloma, which can lead to AKI and if untreated CKD.

7. E. Impaired renal excretion of potassium and phosphate must be balanced by decreased oral intake. High phosphate level can lead to an increased rate of atherosclerosis, so phosphate levels are treated to bring this value down to the normal range. CKD is commonly caused by hypertension. Proteinuria is associated with a

more rapid progression of renal dysfunction. Blood pressure should be reduced to below 140/90 mmHg but with a stricter target of 130/80 mmHg in the context of proteinuria or diabetes. Decreased production of erythropoietin combined with impaired iron utilization results in a normochromic normocytic anaemia.

8. B. This is the classic presentation of pyelonephritis. Sending midstream urine for culture and blood cultures is important before antibiotic treatment is started and this should be done urgently. Any female of childbearing age presenting with abdominal pain must have a pregnancy test to rule out an ectopic pregnancy; this would be less likely to present with urinary frequency or fevers (unless the ectopic had ruptured). A full blood count would likely show a raised white cell count in keeping with infection. The preferred imaging modality would be an abdominal ultrasound. This could show evidence of pyelonephritis, renal calculus, abscess or hydronephrosis. A DSMA scan maybe useful further down the line if complications of pyelonephritis were considered, to look for scarring. If there was a strong suspicion of renal calculi, a noncontrast CT scan would be performed – an abdominal X-ray would not be indicated in this scenario.

9. A. Females are at increased risk of UTI as a result of a shorter urethra with its meatus closer to the anus. The condition will affect 25% to 35% of women at least once. UTIs are commonly asymptomatic; in pregnancy they should be treated regardless of being asymptomatic. Infection is common and hard to clear in the context of a long-term urinary catheter. A simple UTI may ascend the ureters and cause pyelonephritis.

10. C. The most likely diagnosis is NSAIDs-induced interstitial nephritis. The diagnosis would be confirmed by renal biopsy. Use of ibuprofen should be stopped, and the patient might benefit from oral steroids. Interstitial nephritis tends to present with AKI and may have an eosinophilia, occasionally with blood and protein on urine analysis. NSAID-related interstitial nephritis is an exception and can present with nephrotic syndrome and fevers. The key to treatment is recognizing the culprit drug and stopping its use. Membranous nephropathy is not associated with NSAIDs or surgical procedures. Acute tubular necrosis is often due to prolonged hypotension, and would result in a raised creatinine level, not a nephrotic presentation. There are no other features to suggest lupus nephritis. FSGS would be unlikely to give such a rapid onset of nephrotic syndrome and would tend to be associated with nonvisible haematuria.

11. E. Visible haematuria with a history of weight loss should ring alarm bells for a renal cell carcinoma. The presence of a varicocele indicates a possible tumour spread to the left

renal vein. Remember the venous drainage of the left testicle. In addition to this, renal cell carcinomas can cause fevers, and can produce erythropoietin, resulting in polycythaemia.

12. B. The presence of upper airway symptoms and signs implies this is granulomatosis with polyangiitis rather than one of the other 'pulmonary–renal' syndromes. Other 'pulmonary–renal syndromes' include SLE, antiglomerular basement membrane disease and microscopic polyangiitis. Eosinophilic granulomatosis with polyangiitis (Churg–Strauss syndrome) is a triad of raised levels of eosinophils, asthma and renal failure.

13. C. Colicky loin to groin pain suggests ureteric obstruction. The passage of a renal calculus down the ureter is the most likely cause of these symptoms. Dehydration predisposes to stone formation. The first-line imaging for renal calculi is a CT KUB.

14. B. The underlying diagnosis is adult polycystic kidney disease. The disease is characterized by the formation of cysts, which grow in number and size over time. Cyst rupture, infected cysts, loin pain and haematuria are frequent presenting features, as in this case. The patient is often hypertensive and has a family history as most cases are inherited in an autosomal dominant manner. The genes *PKD1* and *PKD2* are associated with the disease. There is an association with subarachnoid haemorrhage, mitral valve prolapse, liver cysts and malignant change. CTFR is associated with cystic fibrosis, FGFR3 with achondroplasia, DMD with Duchenne muscular dystrophy and NF1 with neurofibromatosis.

15. E. Given the history of bone pain and recurrent infections, alongside renal impairment and anaemia, the most likely underlying diagnosis is myeloma. While a CRP may be raised and a bone profile may show hypercalcaemia, the investigation which would identify the underlying diagnosis is protein electrophoresis, serum-free light chains and urinary Bence Jones protein.

16. D. IgA nephropathy can present with visible haematuria a few days following an upper respiratory tract infection. This is in contrast to a post-streptococcal glomerulonephritis, where antigens are deposited in the glomeruli and immune complexes form in situ, giving a nephritic syndrome a few weeks after the infection. Minimal change nephropathy and focal segmental glomerulosclerosis are typically present with nephrotic syndrome. His lack of abdominal pain points away from renal calculi.

17. C. *Neisseria gonorrhoeae* is a gram-negative diplococcus causing gonorrhoea. Symptoms are related to the site of infection, and may include penile/vaginal discharge, dysuria and anal bleeding/pruritus. Ceftriaxone 1 g intramuscularly as a single dose is the first-line treatment. A is a first-line treatment in chlamydia, D is a first-line treatment in primary syphilis and E may be used in pyelonephritis.

Chapter 32 Fluid balance and electrolyte disturbances

1. A. Sarcoidosis can cause hypercalcaemia. Bisphosphonates can be used to treat hypercalcaemia but such treatment should be started only after appropriate fluid resuscitation, which may be sufficient to control the calcium level. The cause of hypercalcaemia needs to be investigated. The most common causes are hyperparathyroidism and malignancy. Ionized calcium level is the relevant value, and correction for albumin should be done (although most laboratories now will give you the corrected calcium level).

2. C. He has the classic features of polydipsia and polyuria, and needs water, hence his aggression. Lithium therapy is the likely cause, and it can lead to nephrogenic diabetes insipidus. This will result in ADH not being able to act appropriately on the distal collecting duct, resulting in free water excretion (i.e., large volumes of dilute urine, with low urinary sodium level), which is inappropriate in the context of a high plasma osmolality and high serum sodium level. Conn syndrome refers to excess production of the hormone aldosterone from the adrenal gland. This abnormality can be caused by hyperplasia or by an aldosterone-producing tumour. This tends to give the clinical picture of hypertension, high sodium level (although rarely this high) and low potassium level. Polyuria and polydipsia are not a feature. Addison disease is adrenal insufficiency (i.e., low cortisol/aldosterone level), and is not a cause of hypernatraemia (biochemically associated with hyperkalaemia and low glucose level). Cushing disease and Cushing syndrome result in a high level of cortisol. Cushing disease specifically refers to when this is secondary to an adrenocorticotrophic hormone (ACTH) secreting pituitary tumour. Cushing syndrome can be caused by exogenous glucocorticoids, e.g., medications, or any tumour outside the pituitary gland that produces or results in the production of excess cortisol by the adrenal gland. This is associated with a mild hypernatraemia, hypokalaemia and hypertension, although again polydipsia and polyuria are not a clinical feature. Ingestion of salt tablets is possible, but again there is no mention of this in the vignette, and it would not cause polyuria.

3. A. SIADH is a diagnosis of exclusion. The first step in evaluating hyponatraemia is to assess the patient's fluid status. SIADH requires that the patient is euvolaemic, and that thyroid function, adrenal function, renal function and liver function are normal. To make the diagnosis, the patient must be hyponatraemic, with a serum osmolality which is low and inappropriately high urine osmolality (perform paired tests), and urinary sodium level should be inappropriately high. A fluid deprivation test is a test to confirm the presence of diabetes insipidus but is rarely performed. Fluid restriction is the treatment for SIADH, although this is not how the condition is diagnosed. A high cortisol level is a feature of Cushing syndrome/disease. A dexamethasone test is a dynamic test, looking to see whether exogenous steroid can suppress cortisol production. A short Synacthen test is a dynamic test for Addison disease; it investigates whether synthetic adrenocorticotrophic hormone can stimulate the adrenal gland to produce mineralocorticoid/glucocorticoid, the latter being measured with the cortisol level.

4. B. Bendroflumethiazide is a thiazide diuretic; it acts on the distal collecting tubule and causes sodium and potassium excretion. Through its mode of action it can lead to hyponatraemia. This would be the first agent to stop and if necessary an alternative antihypertensive should be used. Omeprazole and citalopram can both cause hyponatraemia. These would be the next medications to stop if the situation does not improve after discontinuing the thiazide. Levothyroxine and bisoprolol are not causes of hyponatraemia.

5. B. Prolonged hypokalaemia can cause nephrogenic diabetes insipidus and polyuria through distal tubular dysfunction. Abdominal pain is a feature of hypercalcaemia. There is no direct correlation between electrolyte disturbances and urinary infections. Seizures are a feature of severe hyponatraemia and hypocalcaemia. Perioral numbness is a feature of hypocalcaemia.

6. D. This is a feature of hypocalcaemia. Peaked T waves are the first abnormality seen in hyperkalaemia; at higher potassium levels this could cause a sinusoidal waveform. A delta wave is a slurring slow rise of the initial upstroke of the QRS complex which is seen with preexcitation syndromes such as Wolff–Parkinson–White syndrome. J waves can be seen with hypercalcaemia and more commonly hypothermia.

7. C. The likely underlying diagnosis is sarcoidosis, which is a multisystem disease and commonly has skin and pulmonary manifestations. Bilateral hilar lymphadenopathy is a classic feature that can be seen on chest imaging. It is a cause of hypercalcaemia.

8. D. An incidental finding of this sort is likely to be from primary hyperparathyroidism, which would lead to increased calcium loss from bone and potentiate renal phosphate excretion.

9. B. She has hyponatraemia, a low glucose level and a high potassium level which fits with Addison disease. This often presents with nonspecific symptoms (e.g., fatigue and abdominal pain) and is associated with other autoimmune conditions.

10. E. Whilst all the answers can cause hyponatraemia, hypothyroidism can cause hyponatraemia and would explain her symptoms of fatigue, cold intolerance and low mood.

11. B. Examining the patient's fluid status is extremely important in assessing for underlying causes of hyponatraemia. Ensure the drug chart is reviewed and stop any causative agents. Blood tests including potassium, thyroid function, glucose and lipid levels should be sent to assess for contributing causes. Paired urine and serum osmolalities and urinary sodium are key in diagnosing the underlying cause. Short Synacthen test is for adrenal insufficiency and should only be considered if 9 a.m. cortisol is low. Fluid restriction may be indicated if the patient is hypovolaemic, but other initial management tests and examination of the fluid status should be done prior. IV dextrose would cause a further drop in sodium.

12. E. This scenario is suggestive of CKD. He has symptoms of uraemia, with itch and metallic taste. He has a low haemoglobin level from reduced erythropoietin production by the kidney and high phosphate level from reduced phosphate excretion, in addition to the raised potassium level. He may also have a low bicarbonate level, low/normal calcium level and raised PTH level. The cause suggested is long-standing poorly controlled hypertension.

13. D. This elderly man has sepsis and is being given gentamicin, a nephrotoxic medication. Both of these may contribute to an acute kidney injury. Of note, Hartmann solution contains potassium at a level of 5 mmol/L which may also contribute.

14. D. D is the correct treatment for hyperkalaemia with ECG changes. C would treat the hyperkalaemia, but IV calcium gluconate should be given to stabilize the myocardium given the ECG changes. IV fluids would also need to be given but as her potassium is >6 this needs urgent treatment. Salbutamol nebulizers should also be given. Oral potassium binders should be considered in conjunction with acute management but will have a delayed onset so are not used in the acute management. Potassium should be repeated every 4 to 6 hours.

Chapter 33 Metabolic and endocrine disorders

1. C. Diabetes may be diagnosed based on one abnormal plasma glucose level of 11.1 mmol/L or greater or fasting glucose level of 7 mmol/L or greater in the presence of diabetic symptoms such as thirst/polyuria. If the patient is asymptomatic, two fasting glucose levels of 7 mmol/L or greater are required or a fasting glucose level of 7 mmol/L or greater followed by a positive oral glucose tolerance test result (i.e., plasma glucose concentration of 11.1 mmol/L or greater 2 hours following an oral 75-mg glucose load). An HbA1c level of 48 mmol/mol or HbA1c fraction of 6.5% can also be used to diagnose diabetes. Answer C fits this definition. A random glucose level of 10.9 mmol/L warrants further investigation. Answer D shows impaired glucose tolerance and answer E shows impaired fasting glucose.

2. D. Antibiotics are often required for underlying infection, which is a common cause of DKA. Patients are usually very dehydrated, and correction of the fluid balance is the priority. In young patients, particularly, an overzealous fluid replacement can precipitate cerebral oedema. Compensatory hyperventilation (Kussmaul respiration) to 'blow off' carbon dioxide is commonly seen. To diagnose DKA it requires an acidosis (pH 7.3; reference range pH 7.35–7.45), ketosis (serum ketone level >3 mmol/L or 2+ on urine dipstick) in a known diabetic or hyperglycaemia (glucose level greater than 11 mmol/L).

3. D. Type 1 diabetes requires treatment with subcutaneously administered insulin and is usually treated with a basal-bolus regimen of four injections per day. The aim is an HbA1c fraction between 6.5% (48 mmol/mol) and 7.5% (58 mmol/mol). Type 2 diabetes can initially be managed with oral medication. Metformin is the first-line treatment but is contraindicated in renal failure with an estimated glomerular filtration rate of less than 30 mL/min per 1.73 m^2, given the risk of developing lactic acidosis. Sulphonylureas often cause weight gain and can also cause hypoglycaemia.

4. E. Osteoporosis is not painful until a fracture is sustained. It is more common in women. Calcium, phosphate and alkaline phosphatase levels are normal. A T score of less than −2.5 is diagnostic. This is the standard deviation from the mean value for a young adult and is calculated from the bone mineral density measured on a dual-energy X-ray absorptiometry scan. A Z score is also given which is age-matched.

5. A. Sarcoidosis is one cause of hypercalcaemia. Malignancy, including myeloma, is a common cause. Even if the calcium level quickly returns to normal with treatment, it is important to find the underlying cause. Ionized calcium level is the relevant value, and correction for the albumin level should be done. Hydration alone may normalize the calcium level; bisphosphonates should be given only if there is resistant hypercalcaemia after sufficient intravenous fluids, generally more than 3 L. Allow time for the bisphosphonates to lower the calcium level.

6. A. If present, the visual field defect is bitemporal hemianopia in acromegaly, with the pituitary adenoma causing compression at the optic chiasm. Prognathism is common, along with increased size of the head, hands and feet. Hypogonadism and hyperglycaemia are common.

7. C. The most common form of hypothyroidism is primary hypothyroidism. Chronic autoimmune disease (Hashimoto thyroiditis) would be the most common cause in this middle-aged woman with coexisting autoimmune disease. There is nothing in the vignette to suggest she has been treated previously for hyperthyroidism. Iodine deficiency is now very rare in the United Kingdom. Graves disease is associated with hyperthyroidism. Secondary hypothyroidism from a pituitary disease (e.g., a pituitary adenoma) or a hypothalamic disorder is extremely rare.

8. B. Autoimmune destruction is most common in the developed world; worldwide, infection, especially TB, is more common. Diagnosis is made with the short Synacthen test. Rehydration, correction of electrolyte abnormalities and replacement of cortisol with hydrocortisone are most important in a crisis. In the long term, most patients also require fludrocortisone. Hyperpigmentation is seen in Addison disease, but there is an association with vitiligo.

9. A. Sinus tachycardia is also common. Menorrhagia occurs in hypothyroidism; thyrotoxicosis causes amenorrhoea. Pretibial myxoedema, proptosis and clubbing (thyroid acropachy) are all specific to Graves disease.

10. D. ADH (also called 'arginine vasopressin') is synthesized predominantly in the hypothalamus and is released by the posterior pituitary. Oxytocin is the other hormone secreted by the posterior pituitary. The main hormones secreted by the anterior pituitary are TSH, ACTH, GH, LH, FSH and prolactin.

11. B. Cushing syndrome describes the series of symptoms and signs caused by abnormally high serum cortisol levels. These include weight gain, fatty deposits in the midsection, face ('moon face') and between the shoulder blades ('buffalo hump'), thin skin that bruises easily, prolonged wound healing and muscular weakness.

12. A. Familial hypercholesterolaemia is a genetic disorder of abnormally high cholesterol levels, characterized by deposits of cholesterol-rich fat on various parts of the body including in tendons (tendinous xanthoma) – particularly the Achilles tendon – around the eyelids

(xanthelasma palpebrarum), and the outer margin of the iris (arcus senilis corneae). Conn syndrome is associated with high blood pressure. Weight gain is more commonly associated with type 2 DM than type 1. Conductive deafness may feature in Paget disease due to involvement of the ossicles. Hirsutism is a feature of Cushing disease.

13. D. A water deprivation test using desmopressin is used to differentiate between cranial and nephrogenic diabetes. The patient is deprived of fluids for several hours, and urine osmolality tested for both pre- and postgiving desmopressin (artificial ADH). In cranial DI, symptoms occur as the hypothalamus fails to secrete ADH. However, the kidneys can still respond to it, and therefore are able to concentrate urine when given desmopressin, leading to high urine osmolality. In nephrogenic DI on the other hand the kidneys are unable to respond to ADH, so cannot concentrate urine even when desmopressin is given, and therefore urine osmolality remains low.

14. B. This scenario describes a presentation of acromegaly, a condition caused by excessive secretion of growth hormone (GH). GH stimulated the production of insulin-like growth factor 1 (IGF-1), the main tissue mediator of the actions of GH. Serum IGF-1 level is therefore recommended as the initial screen for suspected acromegaly. OGTT is second line and confirms the diagnosis.

15. C. Clinical findings in thyrotoxicosis include tachycardia, increased sweating, and tremor. Symptoms include palpitations, heat intolerance and proximal muscle weakness.

16. A. In suspected Addison disease the test of choice is short Synacthen test. Administration of an exogenous adrenocorticotrophic hormone (Synacthen) is used to diagnose Addison disease. The Synacthen test would fail to produce an appropriate increase in serum cortisol level with Addison disease.

17. B. An aldosterone-producing adenoma, Conn syndrome, causes hypertension and is associated with hypokalaemia, mild hypernatraemia and metabolic alkalosis. It should be considered as a differential in individuals with resistant hypertension. Hypokalaemia often causes muscle symptoms.

18. C. This man has diabetic ketoacidosis and is clearly very unwell. The priority is to resuscitate with intravenous fluid, following this a fixed rate insulin infusion should be commenced to switch off further ketone production.

19. B. In an established diabetic patient using regular insulin who is going to be nil by mouth for potentially an extensive period and is clinically unwell, a variable-rate intravenous insulin infusion regimen is the treatment of choice. You may well see in practice patients being nil by mouth and not needing this variable-rate intravenous insulin infusion regimen but just being given their long-acting insulin and omitting the short-acting insulin. This is common and correct practice with elective surgery but not in the unwell patient.

20. B. This is an Addisonian crisis. The patient has other features of autoimmune disease. Hypotension, hypoglycaemia and hyperkalaemia are all features of Addison disease. Treatment involves intravenous (IV) fluids and hydrocortisone. The hypoglycaemia needs to be addressed as well as treatment of the hyperkalaemia with IV insulin and dextrose and calcium gluconate should there be evidence of myocardial irritability (i.e., an abnormal ECG).

Chapter 34 Nervous system

1. C. Muscle fasciculations are almost universally present in motor neurone disease. They often are the only symptom early in the disease. Fasciculations represent the hyperexcitability of the diseased neurons before weakness occurs.

2. D. Although any can occur, depression is by far the commonest psychiatric problem after a stroke.

3. A. This patient likely has an infection and is septic. Although most of the above investigations could be used blood cultures have the highest chance of identifying the organism responsible for his infection and therefore direct antibiotic therapy.

4. C. Severe occipital headache is a classic presenting feature of a subarachnoid haemorrhage. Subdural haemorrhage is unlikely as a presentation with a headache is uncommon, she is young and there is no history of trauma. A massive intracerebral haemorrhage would normally result in a much lower GCS and focal neurological signs. Meningoencephalitis normally presents with a slow-onset headache and progressively worsening signs and symptoms over a period of a few days; there would also be signs and symptoms of meningeal irritation.

5. E. If patients with Parkinson disease develop dyskinesia or motor fluctuations, specialist advice should be sought before modifying their antiparkinsonian drug therapy. Each sufferer should have access to a multidisciplinary team that they can contact should they require assistance, this includes a team of specialized nurses and doctors that can provide advice regarding medications.

6. E. Pseudobulbar palsy is an upper motor neurone disorder, whereas bulbar palsy is a lower motor neurone disorder. Tongue wasting and fasciculations are lower motor neurone features. All other presentations can occur in pseudobulbar palsy.

7. A. Dermatomyositis is a connective tissue disorder. Inflammation of the skin and muscle is one of the characteristics. The rash present on the dorsal aspect of the hands is known as Gottron papules. Proximal muscle weakness and heliotrope rash are also characteristic.

8. E. MND is slightly more common in men. It does not affect the sensory nerves or the extraocular muscles. Prognosis is poor; survival beyond 5 years is rare. It usually causes a mixture of upper and lower motor neurone signs.

9. C. Mortality associated with subarachnoid haemorrhage is high. Only 30% are preceded by a sentinel headache. As well as hydrocephalus, other causes of decreasing Glasgow Coma Scale score are vasospasm and rebleeding. Treatment depends on clinical presentation and the extent of the bleeding. Neurosurgery may be required. Antihypertensive medications other than nimodipine that reduces cerebral ischaemia and the incidence of vasospasm are not normally used – adequate blood pressure is needed to maintain cerebral perfusion pressure (cerebral perfusion pressure = mean arterial pressure – intracranial pressure).

10. E. Syncope on exertion should prompt investigations to look for aortic stenosis or hypertrophic cardiomyopathy. Urinary incontinence and a few jerks/twitches are commonly seen during syncope. ECG is useful and may reveal arrhythmia. Biting the side of the tongue is suggestive of a seizure.

11. C. Meningitis is not as likely as migraine – the patient is afebrile and the visual symptoms would be atypical. A minority of SAHs are preceded by a sentinel bleed but visual warning symptoms are not typical. β-Blockers are sometimes used for migraine prophylaxis. Patients with cluster headache are typically restless, as opposed to those with migraine. Triptans are effective for acute migraine.

12. C. This patient's GCS is calculated as follows: eyes – 2; voice – 2; motor – 4. See Chapter 34.

13. C. Metastases are more common than primary tumours. If a primary tumour is suspected, a stereotactic biopsy is required. Meningiomas, when small, can be simply observed. Surgery is often successful. Glioblastomas are aggressive tumours with a poor prognosis. Breast cancer, as well as lung and skin cancer, commonly metastasizes to the brain.

14. B. Symptoms are asymmetrical in onset; symmetrical onset implies an alternative diagnosis such as the Parkinson plus syndromes. He is young, and a dopamine agonist is often preferred as first-line therapy in younger patients. A radioiodine scan may be helpful if the diagnosis is in doubt, but is not required. Rigidity is one of the cardinal features of parkinsonism, the others being tremor, bradykinesia and postural instability.

15. D. Sixth cranial nerve palsy is commonly referred to as a false localizing sign. The headache is typically worse in the morning and on lying flat or coughing/straining. The Cushing reflex is a late sign consisting of hypertension and bradycardia. Fundoscopy should be performed to look for papilloedema if raised ICP is suspected. Nausea and vomiting may occur; abdominal pain is not a feature.

16. A. Dopamine agonists are usually used first in younger patients, whereas L-DOPA is the drug of choice in older patients. Selegiline is a monoamine oxidase B inhibitor and can be used in PD; however, it would not be as first-line therapy. Carbidopa is a peripherally acting L-DOPA metabolism inhibitor. Propranolol can be used for treatment of essential tremor but would not be helpful in PD.

17. D. Optic neuritis is commonly due to MS, but it can occur in isolation or can be due to other disorders such as infection or vasculitis. Colour vision is usually affected more. In 90% of patients the vision gradually improves over weeks to months following the initial event. The risk of developing MS following an episode of optic neuritis is higher if white matter lesions are present on MRI. MS typically occurs between the ages of 20 and 40 years.

18. C. Although the presentation could be due to a space-occupying lesion, a family history of a similar presentation together with an early death suggests that the condition is genetically linked. The most likely diagnosis is Huntington disease. Although Sydenham chorea and Wilson disease are possibilities, these would normally present with other signs and symptoms. Haloperidol causes tardive dyskinesia.

19. E. Facial weakness from a stroke is due to an upper motor neurone lesion which spares the forehead. A CT scan is required urgently to rule out haemorrhage and image the brain. If haemorrhage is present, the effects of warfarin should be reversed with prothrombin complex concentrate and vitamin K. Ischaemic strokes can occur in patients taking warfarin if the INR is subtherapeutic for a prolonged period, or occasionally if the INR is therapeutic. Haemorrhage accounts for around 20% of strokes.

20. A. The purpuric rash is most likely to occur in meningococcal infection. *Streptococcus pneumoniae* is a common cause but does not usually cause a purpuric rash. *Listeria* is more common in the elderly, people with alcoholism and newborns. Lumbar puncture is required but it should not delay the administration of antibiotics, and the presence of severe headache, confusion and vomiting should warn you of raised intracranial pressure. Treatment with intravenous antibiotics as per hospital

guidelines (often ceftriaxone) is urgently required along with supportive measures.

21. D. Loss of vibration sense and proprioception with upper motor neurone sign indicates involvement of neurones of the dorsal column pathway. Pancoast tumour is a cancer that is located in the apex of the lung. It can cause compression of a range of structures passing through the area, resulting in a range of symptoms. Compression of the brachial plexus can cause upper limb muscle weakness or sensory disturbances (including pain). Sympathetic ganglion compression can cause Horner syndrome. Syringomyelia presents as cape-like distribution of sensory abnormalities resulting from compression of the spinothalamic tract. This is most commonly caused by a fluid-filled cavity within the spinal cord. Classically, other sensory modalities are spared in this condition.

22. C. The sudden onset suggests a vascular cause. Loss of consciousness is uncommon in strokes unless the brainstem is affected or the stroke is massive, causing a mass or pressure effect. Unreactive pupils suggest brainstem and cranial nerve involvement. This could be either from a brainstem stroke or a pressure effect leading to brain herniation.

23. E. This is a typical history of complex partial seizures seen in temporal lobe epilepsy. There is an association with febrile convulsions in childhood.

24. D. The most likely cause here is orthostatic hypotension. The patient's blood pressure drops, causing hypoperfusion of the brain, after standing up from supine too quickly. Vasovagal syncope is induced when upright for a comparatively longer duration. There is no evidence of epilepsy or stroke. It could have been a TIA; however, an episode of postural hypotension is more likely.

25. A. The other features of Horner syndrome are enophthalmos and anhidrosis. In this case the cause is a preganglionic lesion – thyroid neoplasm. Ramsay Hunt syndrome is shingles of the geniculate ganglion.

Chapter 35 Musculoskeletal system

1. E. Systemic lupus erythematosus (SLE) is an autoimmune disorder that results in widespread inflammation and tissue damage. It is more common in females. The above signs and symptoms are classically seen in SLE. There is no evidence that she has a sexually transmitted disease although gonorrhoea can cause reactive arthritis and fever it would not normally lead to a butterfly rash that gets worse in the sunlight. Systemic sclerosis is a multisystem disorder that can have various presentations; however, skin symptoms are normally skin tightening with telangiectasia rather than a rash.

2. C. A red, hot, swollen and painful isolated joint swelling is septic arthritis until proven otherwise. All of the above could present with knee pain, but with fever septic arthritis needs to be excluded and a joint aspiration is indicated.

3. B. Vancomycin is the treatment of choice for an invasive MRSA infection. MRSA is resistant to beta-lactam antibiotics. Noninvasive MRSA can be managed with oral therapy; however, in this case the patient is at an increased risk of complications due to foreign material in the joint and concurrent systemic disease (rheumatoid arthritis). The orthopaedic team should be involved in her care, given the risk here of septic arthritis in a joint with a prosthesis.

4. B. This is a classic presentation if prolonged IM gold therapy is used. This skin discolouration is known as chrysiasis and is otherwise usually asymptomatic apart from the obvious cosmetic appearances. Often if patients are achieving good disease control with the IM gold therapy they are willing to accept the skin discolouration.

5. B. Granulomatosis with polyangiitis is a cytoplasmic ANCA-positive, small-vessel vasculitis which can affect any organ. It can be fatal if left untreated, and typically presents with respiratory signs and symptoms, including sinusitis, rhinitis, epistaxis and haemoptysis. It is characterized by the formation of necrotizing granulomata (in this case most likely in the lungs). Glomerulonephritis is also common. Treatment with severe features is with high-dose steroids and cyclophosphamide or rituximab. PMR usually affects older patients and causes pain and stiffness in the shoulder and pelvic girdles. Kawasaki disease is a systemic vasculitis presenting usually in young children.

6. A. Primary or idiopathic OA affects the DIP and carpometacarpal joints in the hands, MTP joints in the feet, the knee, hip, shoulder and spine. If other joints are affected, then this is more likely due to a secondary cause (e.g., congenital disorders, trauma, infection or metabolic, endocrine or crystal deposition diseases).

7. D. Methotrexate is teratogenic and should not be used in women planning a pregnancy. Her care should be overseen by the rheumatologists ideally with prepregnancy planning to ensure good disease control with medications which are safe in pregnancy.

8. D. Psoriatic arthritis is the most likely cause given the patient's age and pattern of involvement. DIP joint involvement and dactylitis together with nail disease are characteristic of psoriatic arthritis. She may also suffer from spondyloarthropathy (limited spinal movements) and inflammatory bowel disease (bloody diarrhoea), which are associated with psoriatic arthritis and should be further investigated.

9. A. This is drug-induced lupus due to isoniazid (one of the antituberous medications). Antihistone antibodies can be found in 90% of patients (although they are not specific to the condition). In drug-induced lupus antinuclear antibodies are positive in around half of the patients.

10. D. This is Paget disease which is a consequence of dysfunctional osteoclast and osteoblast activity. The first-line treatment is osteoclast inhibitors such as bisphosphonates. This helps prevent bone resorption and resultant uncoordinated osteoblast activity leading to unwanted bone formation.

11. C. This is the classic presentation of gout at an MTP joint. Predisposing factors include male sex, alcohol, impaired kidney function, diabetes and diuretic use.

12. E. Asymmetrical distribution, dactylitis and associated iritis and colitis are suggestive of psoriatic arthritis. Rheumatoid arthritis is normally symmetrical involvement of joints.

Chapter 36 Dermatology

1. A. A lesion like this is a ductal carcinoma until proven otherwise.

2. C. The femoral canal lies below the inguinal ligament and lateral to the pubic tubercle. An inguinal hernia will present above the inguinal ligament and medial to the pubic tubercle.

3. D. This patient has many features of this inflammatory myopathy. Cutaneous involvement with raised creatine kinase levels differentiates it from polymyositis. Muscle biopsy reveals inflammation within the muscle. Some patients will have an underlying malignancy so this must be screened for.

4. A. The most likely diagnosis is Henoch–Schönlein purpura. This is common in young males. It is vasculitis that typically follows viral upper respiratory tract infection. It is characterized by a purpuric rash on the back of the legs and buttocks. In most cases, Henoch–Schönlein purpura is self-limiting, with full recovery. It is rare in children that renal failure will develop.

5. A. Lyme disease is characterized by erythema migrans, described here to have developed on the patient's legs. Lyme disease is caused by *Borrelia burgdorferi* and can also lead to arthralgia and cardiac abnormalities. Treatment is with antibiotics.

6. B. The condition that would most likely cause the features described is excess cortisol seen in Cushing syndrome. Peripheral muscle weakness, truncal obesity and various skin manifestations are characteristic. Reiter syndrome usually follows infection, and granulomatosis with polyangiitis would present with respiratory symptoms.

7. B. This is typical for seborrhoeic keratoses. Basal cell carcinoma is the commonest malignant skin tumour that is classically described as having a pearly white appearance with areas of superficial telangiectasia and rolled edge surrounding a sunken centre. Campbell de Morgan spots are abnormal vascular regions that present as cherry-red round lesions. Malignant melanoma is aggressive cancer that if suspected needs urgent management. Keratoacanthoma often presents as a round discrete nodule with a central darker area filled with keratin.

8. A. Macules are flat and well defined. B is a description of a papule. C is a description of a pustule. D is a description of a plaque. E is a description of a vesicle.

9. D. This is a typical presentation of dermatitis which is a skin reaction to the chemicals the person has been in contact with (in this case, paints). Psoriasis presents with plaques usually in the extensor distribution. Chemical burn would be more severe than an itchy rash. Lichen planus is associated with characteristic fine white lines that lie over papules (Wickham striae). Porphyria cutanea tarda is a rare manifestation of photosensitivity.

10. A. Dermatitis herpetiformis is a skin manifestation of coeliac disease. It is characterized by itchy blisters commonly found on the scalp, elbows and knees. Scabies is most commonly found in the web spaces of the hands and feet where track marks from the mite can often be found. Polycythaemia rubra vera is a disorder affecting haemopoiesis.

11. A. This is a localized area of hair loss that can be caused by ringworm infection. Other risk factors include familial predisposition and psychological stress. In some cases hair loss can be extensive and permanent. Sotos syndrome (also called cerebral gigantism) is a rare autosomal dominant genetic condition. Birth length is often above the 90th centile, and then continues to increase rapidly. Macrocephaly, large hands and feet are features. Children also commonly have learning difficulties.

12. D. Mycosis fungoides is the most common form of cutaneous T-cell lymphoma. It presents as patchy generalized dermatitis that then develops into lesions or tumours.

Chapter 37 Haematological disorders

1. B. This is suggestive of multiple myeloma with the characteristic 'CRAB' features, hypercalcaemia, renal impairment, anaemia and bone involvement.

2. D. There are signs and symptoms of infectious mononucleosis, also known as glandular fever and caused by the Epstein–Barr virus. Toxic shock syndrome is a body reaction to bacterial toxins. Presentation includes signs and symptoms of infection, rash and skin peeling. Streptococcal tonsillitis does not normally cause splenomegaly.

3. E. In immunocompromised patients infection with varicella zoster virus can lead to dissemination and multiorgan involvement (pneumonia, encephalitis, hepatitis, coagulopathy).

4. A. The most likely diagnosis here is lymphoma. Additionally, the patient has B symptoms which is worrying. A diagnosis needs to be made as soon as possible. Lymph node biopsy is required in the first instance to establish whether this is in fact lymphoma and if so, of what type. Body scanning is used to determine disease spread and guide therapy.

5. B. Tumour lysis syndrome is a potentially fatal complication that occurs when large amounts of tumour cells die as a result of cytotoxic therapy and release their contents into the bloodstream. It most commonly complicates treatment of high cell turnover cancers such as lymphomas and leukaemias but can occur with any malignancy. It is characterized by metabolic abnormalities described above. Although this could be acute kidney injury the history points towards tumour lysis syndrome. There is no evidence of sepsis or mention of the use of steroids. Malignant transformation occurs at a cellular level.

6. E. Even though both Hb level and reticulocyte count can be useful in determining the baseline for a sickle cell anaemia patient, there is no definitive investigation that will confirm a vasoocclusive crisis. This is a clinical decision based on the history and examination findings, and even though Hb electrophoresis, sickle cell solubility and blood film can confirm the diagnosis, these should not delay prompt management.

7. B. ALL is present in both children and adults. From the answers above the most correct is B. ALL is the most common cancer of childhood. ALL is less common in adults but shows a gradual increase in incidence after the age of 60 years.

8. C. Haemophilia B is the most likely diagnosis. This is milder than haemophilia A but with a similar presentation and is due to factor IX deficiency. It is an autosomal recessive condition often picked up following exacerbated bleeding after minor surgery or trauma. Von Willebrand disease (vWD) results in prolonged APTT but also prolonged bleeding time. Liver disease is uncommon in 20-year-old healthy individuals and would also lead to prolonged PT. APTT is not prolonged in thrombocytopenia.

9. A. β-Thalassaemia is an inherited disease of defective haemoglobin (Hb) synthesis. In the case of β-thalassaemia there is malproduction of the β chain of Hb that results in abnormal haemopoiesis and microcytic hypochromic anaemia. This condition is common in people of Mediterranean origin. There is an excess of HbA_2 and more than 3.2% is diagnostic of the disease. In anaemia of chronic disease and iron-deficiency anaemia, one would expect ferritin level to be low.

10. E. This man could have chronic liver disease. Acanthocytes are spiked red blood cells (RBCs) that are commonly found in chronic liver problems. They are also present in α-thalassaemia trait. Pencil cells occur in iron-deficiency anaemia or thalassaemia traits. Schistocytes are fragmented RBCs that become damaged when passing through vessels in cases of intravascular haemolysis. Basophilic stippling is seen in disorders of erythropoiesis, and bite cells are seen in oxidative haemolysis and glucose-6-phosphate dehydrogenase deficiency.

11. B. Alcoholism causes megaloblastic anaemia. A vegan diet and associated vitamin B_{12} deficiency can cause a megaloblastic anaemia but some animal products on nonvegan days of the week should mitigate this process, furthermore alcoholism is a much more common cause. Pregnancy most commonly causes dilutional anaemia or iron deficiency anaemia (microcytic anaemia). Crohn disease causes iron deficiency anaemia. Gastrectomy can cause both microcytic and macrocytic anaemia; however, partial removal of the stomach should leave enough surface for absorption and therefore minimalize the risk of developing anaemia.

12. B. A serum ferritin level of less than 30 μg/L is diagnostic of iron deficiency anaemia.

13. B. This is the most common form of leukaemia in children, and the peak incidence occurs at 2 to 5 years. It commonly presents with constitutional features and lymphadenopathy.

14. D. CML is a myeloproliferative disorder of pluripotent haemopoietic stem cells that can affect any stem cell line. More than 90% show cytogenetic abnormality of the Philadelphia chromosome. It can present with massive splenomegaly and constitutional symptoms such as this patient.

15. B. NHL can present in various ways and is more common in adults. Exceptions are high-grade lymphoblastic and small noncleaved lymphomas, which are commonly found in children. Risk factors for disease development include viral illness, immunosuppression and autoimmune disease.

Chapter 38 Infectious diseases

1. B. By definition, MRSA is resistant to certain antibiotics. Therefore, NHS hospitals set guidelines suggesting the recommended choice of treatment. From the list above, vancomycin is the recommended treatment, showing the highest rates of success when compared with the development of resistance.

2. B. The description suggests that the patient has sepsis. National guidelines recommend following the sepsis protocol. This includes measuring lactate levels, obtaining blood cultures, measuring urine output and administering oxygen, intravenous antibiotics and intravenous fluids.

3. B. This man presents with HIV-associated disease. Weight loss and night sweats together with mediastinal and retroperitoneal masses are characteristic of late TB, which is very common in HIV-positive patients.

4. B. Antimalarial medication can cause a variety of side effects. There are guidelines in place suggesting appropriate use. From the list above, mefloquine is known to be associated with episodes of depression and psychosis, and therefore its use is not recommended in cases of past mental health problems.

5. B. *Mycobacterium avium* is a common pathogen causing infection in immunocompromised patients. It can cause respiratory symptoms, including a persistent cough, fever and malaise. It can be particularly severe in later stages of AIDS.

6. B. Falciparum malaria is diagnosed by finding ring trophozoites inside red cells on a blood smear. It is a mosquito-borne disease caused by *Plasmodium falciparum*, which presents with features of fever and flu-like illness.

7. D. Rotavirus is a virus that causes diarrhoea and other intestinal symptoms. It is very contagious and is the most common cause of diarrhoea in infants and young children worldwide. It is usually self-limiting, resolving without the need for medications, though dehydration is a concern, and could become life-threatening. The vaccine is >90% effective in preventing severe infection.

8. C. Norovirus, also known as the 'winter vomiting bug', is a highly contagious virus that causes vomiting and diarrhoea. It is the most common cause of gastroenteritis in the United Kingdom.

9. E. All of these categories of people are deemed to be higher risk of mortality if they contract COVID-19.

10. C. The simplest test for COVID-19 is through a swab from the nose and/or throat, or a saliva sample. This can be performed in the home setting or by a healthcare provider. Home lateral flow kit tests for the presence of antigens against COVID-19. It is recommended that in asymptomatic people, a swab is taken 5 days after exposure to the virus due to the risk of a false-negative result. PCR-based tests are the most reliable tests for people with or without symptoms.

11. A. At least two doses of a vaccine are required for stronger and long-lasting protection from COVID-19. Most people require booster doses to help improve protection from the first two doses of the vaccine. In the United Kingdom, everyone aged 5 years of age or older is eligible for vaccination. Mild to moderate flu-like symptoms are common. The Pfizer-BioNTECH vaccine is an mRNA vaccine. Other vaccine types include whole virus (Sinovac), nonreplicating viral vector (Oxford–Astra-Zeneca) and protein subunit (Novavax). Rare cases of myocarditis and pericarditis have been reported following vaccination with mRNA vaccines.

12. E. The most probable diagnosis is TB. This is the most common pathogen and it spreads through direct contact and air. It is likely the 19-year-old became infected in the new environment of the university. Initially, TB may be asymptomatic, but erythema nodosum, pleural effusion and a persistent cough can be troublesome. Chest X-ray characteristically shows consolidation, air space or nodular changes with loss of volume, and this is typically in upper zones.

13. A. This man has signs and symptoms of pneumonia. He is at high risk of developing the disease because of his liver cirrhosis. *Streptococcus pneumoniae* is the most common causative organism. Other common causes include *Haemophilus influenzae* and *Chlamydophila pneumoniae*. The most common signs and symptoms include fever, productive cough and shortness of breath.

14. C. This patient presents with signs and symptoms suggestive of Burkitt lymphoma. This is a rapidly growing B-cell non-Hodgkin lymphoma that is associated with Epstein–Barr virus and immunosuppression. It is common in patients with HIV-related disease. Most commonly it presents with swelling in mandibular/maxillary and abdominal areas fever and weight loss. Management is with chemotherapy.

Chapter 39 Drug overdose and abuse

1. E. These are signs and symptoms of serotonin syndrome as a result of a drug interaction. Patients on SSRIs who are prescribed another drug that affects levels of serotonin are at an increased risk of developing this syndrome. This is also true for those taking serotonin-norepinephrine reuptake inhibitors.

2. B. Flumazenil is inappropriate as she is stable and maintaining her own airway and giving the drug could lead to unnecessary side effects. Activated charcoal or gastric lavage would not be appropriate as we do not know when the overdose occurred. She does not need intubation.

3. A. Delirium tremens occurs as a result of alcohol withdrawal. It usually occurs about three days after the onset of withdrawal symptoms. Patients often experience shaking, shivering and sweating. Both visual and auditory hallucinations are common. Although it appears that he has suffered an alcohol withdrawal-induced seizure, he has all the symptoms of delirium tremens and therefore this is the most likely diagnosis.

4. A. Salicylate (aspirin) stimulates the respiratory centre resulting in hyperventilation and respiratory alkalosis. There is compensatory renal excretion of bicarbonate, sodium, potassium and water. This leads to dehydration and metabolic acidosis with electrolyte disturbance. The acidosis can increase the absorption of aspirin into the central nervous system, resulting in reduced consciousness and seizures. Tinnitus is a distinctive feature of salicylate overdose. Benzodiazepine and opiate overdoses are associated with respiratory depression. Metabolic acidosis is also a feature of tricyclic antidepressant overdose, but this is not associated with tinnitus.

5. C. The CIWA scale is a validated 10-item assessment tool that can be used to quantify the severity of the alcohol withdrawal syndrome and to monitor and medicate patients throughout withdrawal. The CAGE questionnaire and AUDIT-C are screening tools to identify individuals with alcohol dependence and alcohol misuse, respectively. NEWS is used to identify the haemodynamically deteriorating patient. MMSE is a 30-point scoring system to screen patients for cognitive impairment.

6. D. This woman has features of tricyclic overdose, with the anticholinergic effects of dilated pupils, dry mouth and tachycardia. This is in keeping with a severe overdose as there is evidence of significant QT prolongation and severe metabolic acidosis. Treatment should be directed at correcting hypoxia, correcting electrolyte imbalance and giving sodium bicarbonate to prevent arrhythmias. She needs to be attached to a cardiac monitor. Naloxone is the treatment for opiate toxicity; features would include pinpoint pupils and respiratory depression. Flumazenil is used for known benzodiazepine overdose, and lowers seizure threshold, so should not be given in the context of a tricyclic overdose. N-Acetylcysteine is the treatment for paracetamol overdose. Digibind (a digoxin antidote containing digoxin-specific antibody Fab fragments) would be used for significant digoxin overdose. Digoxin overdose classically causes altered coloured vision and is associated with a shortening of the QT interval.

7. C. This is a mixed unknown overdose. In these cases, always assume paracetamol has been taken and treat the patient for paracetamol overdose. Given it is 8 hours after ingestion, N-acetylcysteine infusion should be started. This can always be stopped when the serum paracetamol level is known. It is 8 hours after ingestion, so gastric lavage will not be effective. Paradoxically, absorption of certain drugs will increase following the administration of activated charcoal, so this should be avoided. It is essential to monitor the patient for cardiac irritability. Alkalinization of the urine is indicated for significant aspirin overdoses but should not be commenced without the salicylate level being known.

8. D. These signs and symptoms (altered level of consciousness, Cheyne Stokes respiration, arrhythmia, tachycardia) are suggestive of a COHb level of at least 50%. This patient is critically unwell and needs to be stabilized prior to transfer anywhere to prevent another cardiac arrest. Although hyperbaric oxygen therapy is successful in reducing the time it takes for the elimination of COHb risks of transferring him to a remote location need to be weighed against the benefits. Discussion with TOXBASE is always recommended in cases of overdose or poisoning.

INDEX